Implant Aesthetics

Edward Dwayne Karateew
Editor

Implant Aesthetics

Keys to Diagnosis and Treatment

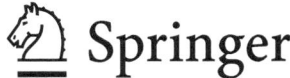

Editor
Edward Dwayne Karateew
Advanced Education in Periodontics
University of Illinois at Chicago
Chicago
IL
USA

ISBN 978-3-319-50704-0   ISBN 978-3-319-50706-4 (eBook)
DOI 10.1007/978-3-319-50706-4

Library of Congress Control Number: 2017939712

© Springer International Publishing AG 2017
This work is subject to copyright. All rights are reserved by the Publisher, whether the whole or part of the material is concerned, specifically the rights of translation, reprinting, reuse of illustrations, recitation, broadcasting, reproduction on microfilms or in any other physical way, and transmission or information storage and retrieval, electronic adaptation, computer software, or by similar or dissimilar methodology now known or hereafter developed.
The use of general descriptive names, registered names, trademarks, service marks, etc. in this publication does not imply, even in the absence of a specific statement, that such names are exempt from the relevant protective laws and regulations and therefore free for general use.
The publisher, the authors and the editors are safe to assume that the advice and information in this book are believed to be true and accurate at the date of publication. Neither the publisher nor the authors or the editors give a warranty, express or implied, with respect to the material contained herein or for any errors or omissions that may have been made. The publisher remains neutral with regard to jurisdictional claims in published maps and institutional affiliations.

Printed on acid-free paper

This Springer imprint is published by Springer Nature
The registered company is Springer International Publishing AG
The registered company address is: Gewerbestrasse 11, 6330 Cham, Switzerland

Preface

Objective: To create a comprehensive review, from diagnostics and treatment planning to reasoning and delivery of various techniques, was the raison d'être behind the development of this publication.

Often we are far too quick to look at a problem and offer a solution. For many, this can be accomplished in the 'blink of an eye' via our automated intellectual processing, a reaction to a problem which we cannot explain as to how we came to the answer. Perhaps it is the result of innate reasoning or engrained learning or a combination of both. However, with more demanding patients, anatomical difficulties of a higher and more complex order and ever-increasing technologically based tools at our disposal, collectively we need material to which we can turn and seek answers to our questions or minimally have a decision tree developed with logical reasoning.

With this publication, I have turned to friends and respected colleagues, to share their thoughts, insights and techniques in addressing the problems which we face with the 'aesthetic dental implant'. We have at our disposal incredible technology to assist us in the diagnostic processes, but of what use is it to us if we are not utilizing this correctly or optimally? If we fail to develop evidence-based algorithms for the successful and repetitive treatment of clinical situations which we face, then we as clinicians have not succeeded in learning from those who went before us.

Methodology for a multitude of procedures such as 'ridge preservation', hard tissue augmentation and soft tissue manipulation can often be difficult to find and choosing the ideal technique even more burdensome. Reviews of materials and outcomes assessments can leave clinicians, from the novice to the most experienced, at times wanting more. It was my hope that this publication can answer these and many more aspects of the treatment of the 'aesthetic dental implant'.

I have gathered a group of individuals, each of whom can be considered a leader in the field of implant dentistry, to author individual sections of this book so that it can be assembled into a greater, more comprehensive tome. From diagnostics and treatment planning, manipulation of the tissues, wound healing, prosthetics (interim and definitive), material science and trouble-shooting, when objectives do not meet treatment goals, have been covered in a logical and comprehensive manner. It is my goal that this publication is one which does not leave your desktop and remains the go-to reference of which it was intended.

I wish to thank each of the authors for their time and patience in creating this publication. It certainly has been a labour of love and an exhaustive but rewarding process which I could not foresee when I embarked upon this project.

Lastly, I wish to offer my sincere gratitude to everyone at Springer for offering this opportunity to me and for their efforts in making it become a reality. My professional 'bucket list' has now become one item shorter in length.

Chicago, IL, USA   E. Dwayne Karateew

Acknowledgements

This book is lovingly dedicated to those key individuals in my life who not only have inspired me to reach for new heights but exhibited great restraint and tolerance to many of my unique characteristics.

First and foremost, to my wife, Mitra. She is always at the ready for a new challenge and does not know how to give less than 100 % of herself to any project she signs onto.

Your unending love, encouragement and support have made this publication possible. Thank you for being the individual that you are and for both the love and guidance you have expressed over the years we have shared together.

To my departed parents, Marni and Ed. The self-sacrifice for the betterment of my education which you unselfishly bestowed upon me was perhaps never acknowledged directly, but is never forgotten. Thank you for teaching me not only how to love, smile and laugh but to also study and work hard. You may be gone, but are never out of my mind.

To my in-laws, Dr. Ali, Masoudeh and Dr. Mahtab. One could not wish for a better, more considerate and loving extended family.

To the memory of our dog Kuma. He was an integral component of our family and embodied unconditional love. His 'smile' is missed.

Special recognition is warranted for my residents and colleagues, Drs. A. Narvekar, F. Gholami, E. Kaminsky, C. Traxler, T. Newman, H. Aljewari at the University of Illinois at Chicago (UIC), Department of Periodontology, who tirelessly aided me in the proof reading of this book.

E. Dwayne Karateew

Contents

Part I Diagnostic and Treatment Considerations

1. **Recognition of Risk Factors and Patient Assessment** 3
   Lyndon F. Cooper and Homayoun H. Zadeh

2. **Determination of the Sequence of Therapy** 19
   Michael S. Block

3. **Osseointegration and the Biology of Peri-implant Hard and Soft Tissues** 31
   Clark M. Stanford

4. **Revisiting the Role of Implant Design and Surgical Instrumentation on Osseointegration** 43
   Paulo G. Coelho, Estevam A. Bonfante, and Ryo Jimbo

5. **Anatomic Considerations in Dental Implant Surgery** 57
   Mitra Sadrameli

6. **The Aesthetic Challenge: Three-Dimensional Planning Concepts for the Anterior Maxillary Aesthetic Zone** 79
   Scott D. Ganz

7. **Clinical Assessment of the Gingiva and Alveolus** 103
   Yung-Ting Hsu and Hom-Lay Wang

8. **Interdisciplinary Planning, Development, and Treatment** 117
   Keith M. Phillips

9. **Flap Design, Suturing, and Healing** 135
   Praveen Gajendrareddy, Sivaraman Prakasam, and Satheesh Elangovan

10. **Digital Photography and Digital Asset Management** 151
    Steven H. Goldstein

Part II Tissue Augmentation Considerations

11. **Preservation of Alveolar Dimensions at the Time of Tooth Extraction** 171
    Robert A. Horowitz

12	**Development of Hard Tissues with Block Grafting Techniques** 189
	John Russo

13	**Guided Bone Regeneration for Aesthetic Implant Site Development** 203
	Bach Le

14	**Development of the Soft Tissue with Gingival Grafting** 233
	David H. Wong

15	**Tissue Engineering Approach to Implant Site Development** 247
	Dan Clark, Igor Roitman, Mark C. Fagan, and Richard T. Kao

Part III Implant Placement and Restoration

16	**Optimal Implant Position in the Aesthetic Zone** 261
	Jae Seon Kim, Lance Hutchens, Brock Pumphrey, Marko Tadros, Jimmy Londono, and J. Kobi Stern

17	**Parameters of Peri-Implant Aesthetics** 287
	Henriette Lerner

18	**The Single Implant-Crown Complex in the Aesthetic Zone: Abutment Selection and the Treatment Sequencing** 301
	Stavros Pelekanos

19	**Implant Provisionalization: The Key to Definitive Aesthetic Success** 337
	Edward Dwayne Karateew

20	**Biomaterials Used with Implant Abutments and Restorations** 353
	Toru Sato, Kazuhiro Umehara, Mamoru Yotsuya, and Michael L. Schmerman

21	**Digital Implant Abutment and Crowns in the Aesthetic Zone** 369
	Nesrine Z. Mostafa, Chris Wyatt, and Jonathan A. Ng

22	**Challenging Maxillary Anterior Implant-Supported Restorations: Creating Predictable Outcomes with Zirconia** 383
	Michael Moscovitch

Part IV Complications and Their Management

23	**Peri-implantitis: Causation and Treatment** 407
	Michael L. Schmerman and Salvador Nares

Contents

24 Laser-Assisted Treatment of Peri-implantitis 417
Edward A. Marcus

**25 Prosthetic Solutions to Biological Deficiencies: Pink
and White Aesthetics** 427
Pinhas Adar

Appendix: Implant Checklist 439

Index 441

Contributors

Pinhas Adar, MDT, CDT Adar Dental Laboratory, Atlanta, GA, USA

Gustavo Avila-Ortiz, DDS, MS, PhD Department of Periodontics, University of Iowa College of Dentistry, Iowa City, IA, USA

Christopher A. Barwacz, DDS Department of Family Dentistry & Craniofacial Clinical Research Program, The University of Iowa College of Dentistry & Dental Clinics, Iowa City, IA, USA

Michael S. Block, DMD Center for Dental Reconstruction, Metairie, LA, USA

Estevam A. Bonfante, DDS, MS, PhD Department of Prosthodontics, University of São Paulo – Bauru College of Dentistry, Bauru, SP, Brazil

Daniel Clark, DDS Orofacial Sciences, Postgraduate Periodontology, UCSF School of Dentistry, San Francisco, CA, USA

Paulo G. Coelho, DDS, PhD Biomaterials and Biomimetics, Hansjorg Wyss Department of Plastic Surgery, New York University College of Dentistry, New York University College of Medicine, New York, NY, USA

Lyndon F. Cooper, DDS, PhD Department of Oral Biology, University of Illinois at Chicago College of Dentistry, Chicago, IL, USA

Satheesh Elangovan, BDS, ScD, DMSc The University of Iowa College of Dentistry and Dental Clinics, Iowa City, IA, USA

Mark C. Fagan, DDS, MS Private Practice, San Jose, CA, USA

Praveen Gajendrareddy, BDS, PhD Department of Periodontics, University of Illinois, Chicago, IL, USA

Scott D. Ganz, DMD Department of Restorative Dentistry, Rutgers School of Dental Medicine Private Practice, Fort Lee, NJ, USA

Steven H. Goldstein, DDS Private Practice Scottsdale, AZ, USA

Robert A. Horowitz, BS, DDS NYU College of Dentistry. Private Practice Scarsdale, NY, USA

Yung-Ting Hsu, DDS, MDSc, MS Department of Periodontology and Dental Hygiene, University of Detroit Mercy School of Dentistry, Detroit, MI, USA

Lance Hutchens, DDS Department of Periodontics, The Dental College of Georgia, Augusta, GA, USA

Ryo Jimbo, DDS, PhD Department of Oral and Maxillofacial Surgery and Oral Medicine, Faculty of Odontology, Malmö University, Malmö, Sweden

Georgia K. Johnson, DDS, MS Department of Periodontics, Iowa City, IA, USA

Richard T. Kao, DDS, PhD Private Practice, Cupertino, CA, USA

Department of Orofacial Sciences, University of California, San Francisco, CA, USA

Department of Orofacial Sciences, University of Pacific, Cupertino, CA, USA

E. Dwayne Karateew, DDS Advanced Education in Periodontics, University of Illinois at Chicago, Chicago, IL, USA

Jae Seon Kim, DDS Restorative Dentistry, University of Washington, Seattle, WA, USA

Bach Le, DDS, MD, FICD, FACD Oral and Maxillofacial Surgery, Los Angeles County USC Medical Center, Whittier, CA, USA

Henriette Lerner HL-Dentclinic, Baden-Baden, Germany

Jimmy Londono, DDS Department of Oral Rehabilitation, College of Dental Medicine, Augusta University, Augusta, GA, USA

Edward A. Marcus, DDS Periodontics and Periodontal Prosthesis, University of Pennsylvania School of Dental Medicine, Philadelphia, PA, USA

Michael Moscovitch, BSc, DDS, CAGS (Prosthodontics) Division of Restorative Sciences, Boston University, Boston, USA

McGill UniversityMontreal, Quebec, Canada

Nesrine Mostafa, BDS, MSc, PhD Faculty of Dentistry, University of British Columbia, Vancouver, BC, Canada

Salvador Nares, DDS, PhD Department of Periodontics, The University of Illinois at Chicago, Chicago, IL, USA

Jonathan A. Ng, DDS, MSc, Dip Pros, FRCD(C) University of British Columbia, Vancouver, British Columbia, Canada

Stavros Pelekanos, DDS, Dr med dent Department of Prosthodontics, Dental School of Athens, University of Athens, Athens, Attica, Greece

Keith M. Phillips, DMD, MSD, CDT, FACP Department of Restorative Dentistry, University of Washington School of Dentistry, Fife, WA, USA

Sivaraman Prakasam, BDS, MSD, PhD Periodontics, Oregon Health and Science University, Portland, OR, USA

Brock Pumphrey, DMD Pumphrey Periodontics, Atlanta, GA, USA

Igor Roitman, DMD, MS UCSF School of Dentistry, Department of Dentistry, San Francisco VA Hospital, Menlo Park, CA, USA

John Russo, DDS, MHSc Division of Periodontics, Medical University of South Carolina, Sarasota, FL, USA

Mitra Sadrameli, DMD, MS, Dipl. ABOMR University of British Columbia Faculty of Dentistry and Private Practice, Chicago, IL, USA

Toru Sato, DDS, PhD Department of Crown and Bridge Prosthodontics, Tokyo Dental College, Tokyo, Japan

Michael L. Schmerman, DDS Department of Periodontics, University of Illinois College of Dentistry, Chicago of Dentistry, Chicago, USA

Illinois Masonic Medical Center, Chicago, USA

Department of Dentistry, Chicago, IL, USA

Clark M. Stanford, DDS, PhD College of Dentistry, The University of Illinois at Chicago, Chicago, IL, USA

J. Kobi Stern, DMD, MSc Advanced Education in Periodontics, Department of Periodontics, Augusta University, Evans, GA, USA

Marko Tadros, DMD Oral Rehabilitation – Prosthodontics, Augusta University, Augusta, GA, USA

Kazuhiro Umehara, DDS, PhD Umehara Dental Office, Aomori, Japan

Hom-Lay Wang, DDS, MSD, PhD Department of Periodontics and Oral Medicine, School of Dentistry, University of Michigan, Ann Arbor, MI, USA

David H. Wong, DDS Private Practice Tulsa, OK, USA

Chris Wyatt, BSc, DMD, MSc, Dip Pros, FRCD(C) Division of Prosthodontics & Dental Geriatrics, Department of Oral Health Sciences, University of British Columbia, Vancouver, BC, Canada

Mamoru Yotsuya, DDS, PhD Department of Crown and Bridge Prosthodontics, Tokyo Dental College, Tokyo, Japan

Homayoun H. Zadeh, BS, DDS, PhD Advanced Education Program in Periodontology, Division of Diagnostic Sciences, Ostrow School of Dentistry of University of Southern California, Laboratory for Immunoregulation and Tissue Engineering (LITE), Los Angeles, CA, USA

List of Videos

Videos can be found in the electronic supplementary material in the online version of the book. On http://springerlink.com enter the DOI number given on the bottom of the chapter opening page. Scroll down to the Supplementary material tab and click on the respective videos link. In addition, all videos to this book can be downloaded from http://extras.springer.com. Enter the ISBN number and download all videos.

Video 18.1	Video showing the correct implant positioning according to the guide stent
Video 18.2	Video showing how to customize the impression coping according to the emergence profile
Video 18.3	Video showing the customization of the emergence profile of a single implant in the lab
Video 18.4	Video showing the digital design of a customized zirconia abutment for a cemented restoration
Video 18.5	Video showing the customization of the emergence profile, zirconia abutment and provisional crown fabrication prior to extraction and implant placement on a stereo-lithographic model
Video 18.6	Video showing tooth extraction and implant placement with the use of a stereo-lithographic stent. "One time-final abutment" and provisional crown insertion
Video 18.7	Video showing the customization of the healing abutment. The concave shape of the abutment does not exceed the dimensions of the extraction socket, thus protecting the blood clot and leaving space for the soft tissue to grow
Video 18.8	Video showing only one disconnection of the final abutment and extra-oral cementation of the final crown
Video 18.9	Video showing the correction of the screw access with the use of The LTS abutment
Video 18.10	Video showing the extraoral cementation of the veneer on the lithium disilicate implant-abutment
Video 18.11	Video showing the final cement-screw retained crown insertion

Video 18.12	Video showing a double digital impression of the implant and the achieved emergence profile
Video 18.13	Video showing the digital design of a LS_2 abutment to fit in the customized emergence profile
Video 18.14	Video showing the milling of the abutment from a pre-crystalized Lithium disilicate block (IPS e.max CAD) with a pre-manufactured connection
Video 18.15	Video showing the laboratory procedure for the cementation of LS_2 abutment on the titanium sleeve
Video 18.16	Video showing the Insertion of the final lithium disilicate abutment and cementation of the final e.max crown

Part I
Diagnostic and Treatment Considerations

Recognition of Risk Factors and Patient Assessment

Lyndon F. Cooper and Homayoun H. Zadeh

Abstract

Esthetic outcomes are of central importance to most patients. To ensure that patients' expectations are aligned with expected outcomes, a systematic risk assessment is required. Communication of the risk factors and expected outcomes is important to ensure the patient has realistic expectations. Risk reduction for implant therapy begins with collection of diagnostic information and sharing a comprehensive esthetic diagnosis with the patient. Esthetic risks for dental implants are often associated with the tissues that surround the implant, specifically the lack of interproximal tissue fill and the recession of buccal tissues following implant restoration. Diagnostic information regarding connective tissue attachment levels at adjacent teeth can clarify the risk for incomplete interproximal tissue fill, and steps to overcome buccal tissue recession include both augmentation procedures and proper dental implant placement. The establishment of ideal tooth contours for the implant crown is easily achieved when the proper volume of the supporting bone and soft tissue is provided. Integrating an ideal implant-supported restoration into a beautiful smile requires a comprehensive esthetic diagnosis, a broad approach to implant site development, and careful execution of the planned implant therapy.

1.1 Introduction

Dental implants are often preferred as a method of tooth replacement. The success of dental implants and the restorations they support are favorably reported in a large body of literature representing a broad spectrum of evidence. For example, single-tooth dental implant outcomes have been systematically reviewed to have high success at multiple levels. Full arch restorations subjected to this scrutiny in the literature have similar high

L.F. Cooper, DDS, PhD (✉)
Department of Oral Biology, College of Dentistry,
University of Illinois at Chicago,
Chicago, IL 606112, USA
e-mail: cooperlf@uic.edu

H.H. Zadeh, DDS, PhD
Herman Ostrow School of Dentistry of USC,
925 West 34th Street, Los Angeles,
CA 90089-0641, USA
e-mail: zadeh@usc.edu

reported success rates. Multiunit anterior restorations, particularly restricted to the anterior maxillary arch, where esthetics is paramount, have not received this level of direct evaluation. The survival of implants and prostheses in the anterior maxilla is reported to be high. Unfortunately, these large datasets regarding single, multiunit, and complete arch implant restorations are lacking of outcomes regarding esthetics.

Before embarking on a discussion of risk factors and patient assessment with regard to dental implant esthetics, it is worthwhile to consider what is known regarding patient-based outcomes regarding this facet of implant therapy (Yao et al. 2014). Over a decade ago, it was reported that "patient satisfaction with implant position, restoration shape, overall appearance, effect on speech, and chewing capacity were critical for patient overall acceptance of the dental implant treatment"(Levi et al. 2003). It has been reiterated that esthetic outcomes are of central importance to our patients and that their expectations may be high (even unrealistic). Yao et al. (2014) summarized the following regarding patient esthetic expectations for dental implants:

1. An inverse correlation was found between age and functional expectations, and negative correlations were found between satisfaction and age.
2. Patient expectations before treatment were higher than satisfaction after treatment, but this difference was significant only for esthetics in patients who had received implant-supported fixed partial dentures (FPDs).
3. Participants expected implants to restore their oral-related quality of life to "normal."
4. Patient expectations on implant success and predictability are high compared with their reluctance toward treatment costs.

It is vitally important to establish expectations in the context of the patients' understanding of esthetics. Patients seeking replacement of their tooth may expect esthetic improvement over their existing tooth or teeth. It is the authors' opinion that there is no better way to assure that the patient's esthetic expectations and the likely outcomes based on biological realities and clinical capabilities are aligned than to conduct a comprehensive esthetic diagnosis (one extending beyond the dental implant) prior to providing any implant-related prognosis.

1.2 Comprehensive Esthetic Diagnosis: A First Step in Dental Implant Success

A comprehensive esthetic diagnosis requires several tools, as well as a checklist to obtain sufficient information to complete this task. In addition to intraoral instruments (mirror, periodontal probe, explorer), a suitable intraoral camera and impression materials are needed. The meaningful introductory patient visit should result in obtaining a complete clinical record, high-quality clinical intraoral and extraoral photographs, screening radiographs (revealing potential pathology or aberrant anatomy), and ideal study casts. Esthetic implant therapy requires deployment of a comprehensive esthetic diagnostic toolkit (Table 1.1).

An esthetic evaluation should be performed on an objective basis to avoid untoward meaning or misunderstanding between the patient and clinical

Table 1.1 An esthetic diagnosis toolkit

Extraoral photographs
Oblique view
Facial view
At rest, speaking, smiling, and laughing
Intraoral photographs
Fully retracted facial view (molar to molar)
Oblique view
Region(s) of interest (three-tooth view)
Occlusal view
Facial view
Mounted study casts
Full representation of teeth and alveolar ridges
Careful articulation revealing interocclusal distances
Clinical chart
Tooth inventory
Caries charting
Periodontal disease
Screening radiographs (PA or panoramic)
Revealing potential pathology or aberrant anatomy
Consolidating information in HIPAA compliant, central location

team. For example, "my tooth is too big" requires understanding if it is too far facially displaced, too long incisally, too wide mesiodistally, or exposed due to gingival recession. The objective diagnosis begins with review of the extraoral photographs. The macroesthetic elements of smile design include factors influencing "the relationship between teeth, the surrounding soft tissue, and the patient's facial characteristics". Included are the facial midline, tooth display (the amount of tooth and/or gingiva displayed in various views and lip positions); the position of the intercommissure line, vestibular (negative space); the orientation of the smile line; and the orientation of the lower lip frame (Morley and Eubank 2001). These factors can be clearly discerned from carefully oriented clinical photographs made using the simplest of digital cameras and black-and-white desktop printer images (Fig. 1.1).

Any esthetic diagnosis for implant therapy involving single-tooth replacement, multiunit prosthesis, or full arch tooth replacement must be comprehensive in nature. The placement of an ideal single-tooth implant crown amidst mediocre restorations and aberrant anatomical relationships of other teeth can lead to disappointment, despite the quality of the implant therapy. Similarly, replacement of tooth/teeth, in the presence of periodontitis, may lead to increased likelihood of biologic complications. A comprehensive diagnosis is best performed objectively using a conceptual framework such as the "14 fundamental objective criteria" proposed by Mange et al. (2003) that have been repurposed specifically for the purpose of guiding single-tooth implant therapy (Cooper 2008). Several parameters overlap with the macroesthetic determinants of esthetics described above. Collectively, the objective analysis of the many esthetic determinants of the smile provides sufficient information to (a) characterize any esthetic limitations, (b) describe these objectively for presentation with the patient, and (c) provide a framework for discussion what possible features can and cannot be changed by the intervention proposed (Table 1.2).

Table 1.2 An esthetic checklist to reduce dental implant esthetic risk

Macroesthetic keys (Morley and Eubank 2001)	Fourteen objective criteria for dental esthetics (Mange et al. 2003)
Midline	Gingival/periodontal health
Occlusal plane orientation	Interdental closure
Tooth/gingival display	Tooth axis
Intercommissure line	Zenith of the gingival contour
Lower lip frame[a]	Balance of the gingival levels
	Level of the interdental contact
	Relative tooth dimensions
	Basic features of tooth form
	Tooth characterization
	Surface texture
	Color
	Incisal edge configuration
	Lower lip line[a]
	Smile symmetry

[a]Equivalent clinical parameters

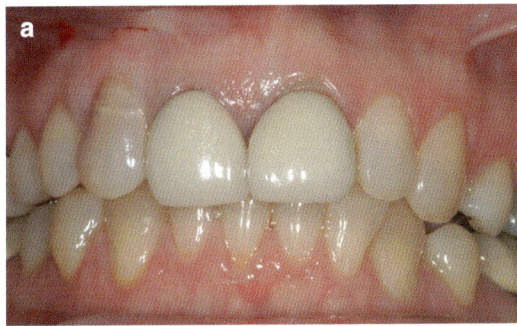 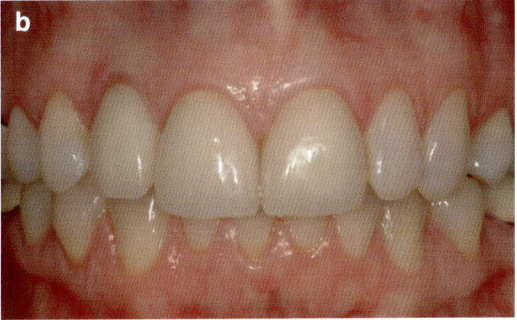

Fig. 1.1 (a) A simple color retracted photograph should be made, archived, and used for discussion with the patient. This can be printed and illustrated or shown on a simple monitor, but serves as a point of reflection in discussions. (b) The final result realized for a complex situation involving immediate implant placement (tooth #6) replacing a missing lateral incisor

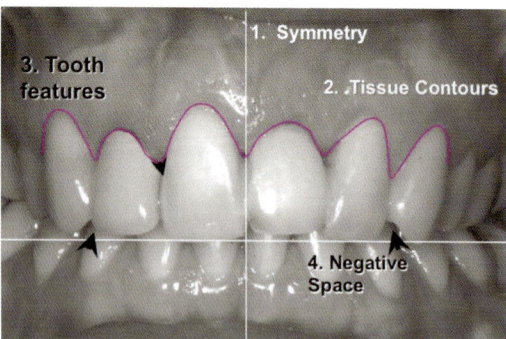

Fig. 1.2 The global aspects of esthetics include symmetry, tissue contours, tooth features, and negative space. These can be easily explored with patients by printing in a simple *black*-and-*white* format or more detailed in color presentation

The culmination of collecting information for a comprehensive esthetic diagnosis is the explanation of the esthetic determinants of each individual's smile in objective terms (Fig. 1.2). This permits rational discussion of what esthetic changes may or may not occur and what esthetic improvements may or may not be possible following the proposed dental implant therapy. The clinical photographs and mounted study casts used as data points for the diagnosis become a central part of the discussion. It is this discussion of what the preoperative realities are that initiates a mutual understanding of possible outcomes to assure favorable acceptance.

1.3 Biological Realities and Site Development

The next step in the successful management of esthetic risk involving dental implants is the careful assessment of the underlying biological realities associated with the individual scenario. There are at least four general concerns: (1) tooth display as defined by maxillary arch position, lip length, and lip mobility, (2) gingival/periodontal health and architecture, (3) general tooth health and condition of existing restorations, and (4) occlusion. The assessment of these factors involves consideration of the initial diagnostic dataset (Table 1.1).

Tooth display, or more importantly gingival display, is frequently considered a risk factor for dental implant esthetics. Unless movement of the maxilla or repositioning of the upper lip (lip switch, botox) is considered, gingival display is more a challenge than a risk to implant-based esthetic interventions. Gingival display of less than 3 mm is considered esthetically acceptable (Kokich et al. 2006) although cultural variations have been documented (Ioi et al. 2013). Irrespective, the identification of incipient or remarkable gingival display (a macroesthetic parameter) mandates that additional specific attention be paid specifically to many other criteria including gingival health, interdental closure, zenith of gingival contour, balance of gingival levels, and basic features of tooth form.

The gingival health and architecture are the principle determinants of single-tooth implant planning and outcomes. Because nearly one-half of the tooth form is defined by its framing by gingiva, the health and form of the gingiva are essential in planning (Fig. 1.2). The gingival architecture is highly dependent on the attachment of gingival fibers to the tooth root cementum, and it follows the natural tooth CEJ circumferentially. This is the cause of the often reported "risk" for single-tooth replacement, when dealing with markedly triangular teeth with highly scalloped gingival architecture (Kois 2004). Upon removal of the tooth, the architecture may be remarkably flattened and reduced.

When there exists greater than 1 mm of loss of connective tissue attachment at teeth adjacent to the planned dental implant position, the esthetic outcome of the implant intervention is negatively impacted. Loss of attachment at the adjacent tooth, a situation without regenerative solutions, invariably leads to absence of interproximal tissues and an unesthetic "black triangle" (Fig. 1.3). Clinical guidelines that direct therapy are well established; the extent of interproximal soft tissue that can be formed vertically between a tooth and an implant (with sufficient horizontal displacement from the tooth) is no more than 5 mm (Choquet et al. 2001).

The buccal soft tissue determinants at dental implants are relatively independent of adjacent

1 Recognition of Risk Factors and Patient Assessment

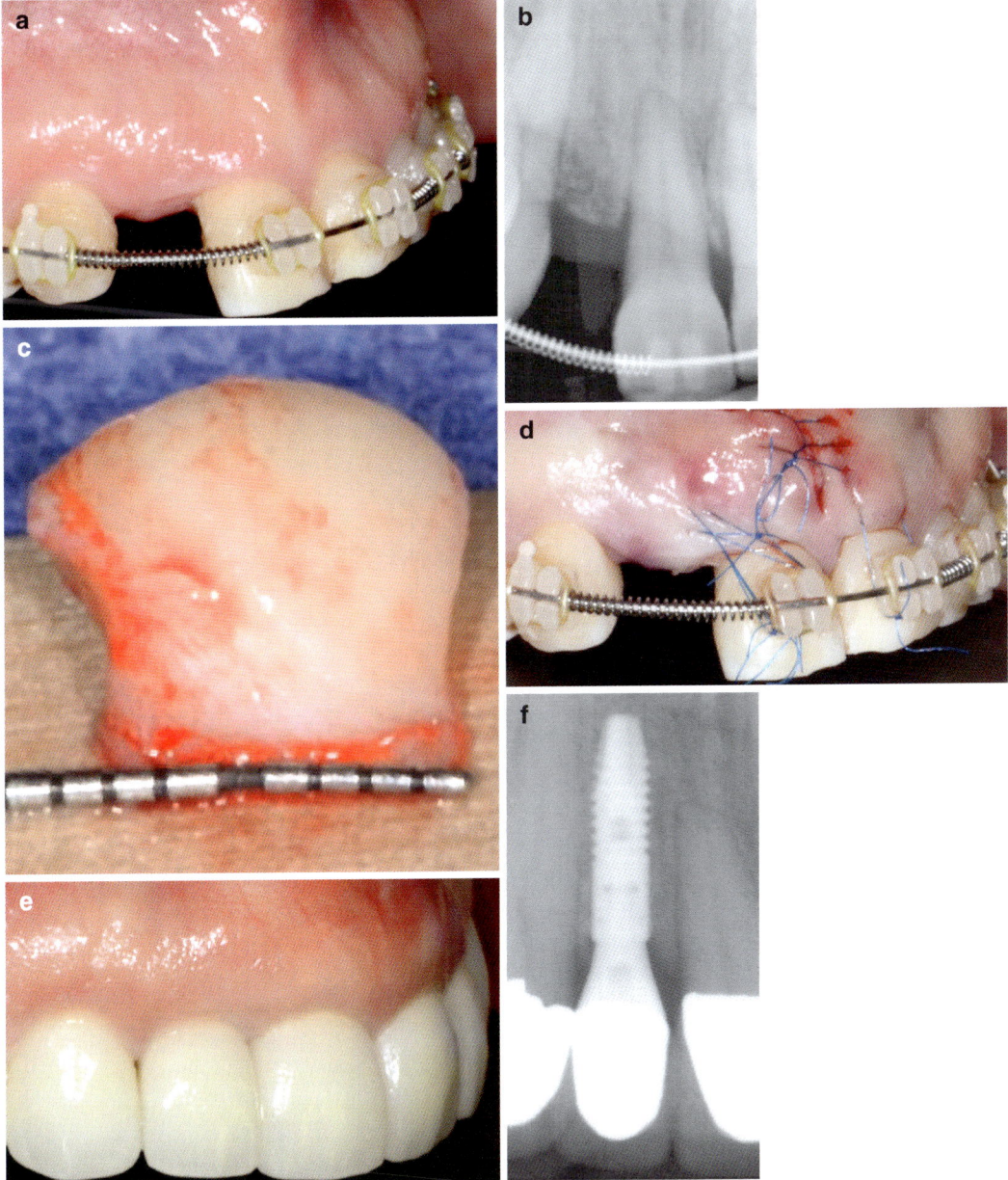

Fig. 1.3 (a) Clinical presentation revealing loss of attachment distal to central incisor. (b) Radiograph demonstrates location of the crestal bone, (c) submucosal connective tissue graft harvested for augmentation, (d) immediate postoperative photograph following insertion of the submucosal CT graft, (e) eventual implant crown with acceptable interproximal tissue levels and modest volume restoration, (f) radiograph of implant, abutment, and crown

tooth factors. Instead, the buccal soft tissue form is dependent on the location of the buccal bone, its relationship with the implant/abutment interface, the contour of the abutment, and the thickness of the facial tissue. The human periodontium consistently forms a biological width around teeth of approximately 3 mm. On the facial aspects of healthy teeth, this dimension has been reproducibly measured. For example, the distance from the tooth CEJ to the labial osseous crest was 2.79 mm on average for all anterior teeth (Vera et al. 2012). When this vertical distance is violated (e.g., by restoration), soft tissue stability is at risk of persistent inflammation and/or recession. Significant defects (dehiscence) predictably result in recession (Kan et al. 2007).

Alveolar ridge preservation procedures and ridge augmentation procedures are important steps in preparing for dental implant placement. When our diagnostic procedures identify osseous limitations to dental implant esthetics, successful ridge preservation (Mardas et al. 2015) and alveolar regeneration procedures (Sanz-Sánchez et al. 2015) should be prescribed. While these procedures are generally successful, a recent study of high-risk patients revealed that extensive alveolar process remodeling after grafting occurred more commonly at central incisors and canines and for sites where tooth abscesses existed prior to tooth extraction (Cosyn et al. 2014).

The thickness of the facial tissues overlaying the dental implant is a critical determinant of implant esthetics. Today, it is widely appreciated that when approximately 2 mm of tissue is present facial to the implant and implant abutment, longer-term stability of the peri-implant mucosa is observed (Evans and Chen 2008; Cooper et al. 2014). It may be concluded that dehiscence of extraction sockets and absence of sufficient bone volume located 3–4 mm apical to the gingival zenith are strong contraindications to implant placement and merit bone augmentation/regeneration steps preceding implant placement. The observation of thin buccal mucosa adds another relative risk to implant esthetics as related to potential recession, but also as related to discoloration.

The discoloration of peri-implant mucosa relative to the gingival tissues of adjacent teeth can limit the general esthetic outcome of an otherwise ideal implant crown. It has been concluded that mucosa thickness is a crucial factor influencing discoloration caused by titanium (as well as zirconia) abutments (Jung et al. 2007). Tissue thickness prior to tooth extraction can be assessed by visualization of the periodontal probe through the sulcus mucosa. Alternatively, tissue/bone sounding can be conducted on anesthetized patients to directly measure the thickness of the alveolar mucosa prior to definitive implant planning. Properly constructed CBCT guides may also permit assessment of peri-implant mucosal thickness. Irrespective of the situation or approach, presurgical knowledge of the peri-implant mucosal thickness is an important aspect of risk assessment.

The nature of the peri-implant mucosa is important. Although it is beyond the scope of this chapter to discuss the role of keratinized mucosa in long-term dental implant outcomes (reviewed in Brito et al. 2014), esthetic demands for mucosal color and texture harmony require that keratinized tissue be preserved and well organized when dealing with anterior maxillary implant therapy. When evidence of thin gingival or alveolar mucosal tissue is presented, augmentation with connective tissue autograft or allogenic or xenogenic materials should be considered in a discussion of obtaining an ideal esthetic result (Lorenzo et al. 2012). Regarding the mucogingival junction, if prior grafting resulted in marked advancement and disruption of the mucogingival junction, its restoration should be considered as part of the implant surgical intervention.

Although the condition of adjacent teeth and crowns may not directly influence dental implant success, the esthetic status of these restorations can markedly influence the outcome of any esthetic intervention involving even a single tooth. The periodontal attachment level of teeth adjacent to planned implant site can determine the presence or absence of interdental papillae around the implant restoration. Therefore, the condition of adjacent teeth should be carefully documented using the 14 objective criteria. Not infrequently, the esthetic enhancement sought by the patient undergoing implant therapy involves the unaffected tooth or teeth. Examples include a discolored tooth secondary to trauma and following endodontic therapy, exposed crown margins on previously restored teeth, stained restorations, and rotated teeth. These possible inadequacies may not be part of a chief complaint but, through objective exploration, may be identified as key to achieving esthetic satisfaction.

Related to the condition of the adjacent teeth, the dimensions of the bound edentulous anterior space must be carefully defined. When the space requiring restoration is not congruent with the dimension of the contralateral tooth or teeth, restorative and/or orthodontic intervention should be offered to overcome this limitation. Two central incisors of different widths are likely unacceptable to a majority of patients.

Occlusion is unfortunately infrequently discussed in the context of dental implant esthetics. However, remarkable difficulty may be encountered if the simplest of occlusal issues are not addressed in planning implant therapy. A common feature of a missing maxillary anterior tooth of longer duration is that the antagonist mandibular tooth has migrated in both the occlusal and facial directions. Small migrations that are not readily observed upon initial presentation can be observed using mounted study casts and diagnostic waxing procedures. The position of the implant may not be influenced by the antagonist tooth's malposition, but the crown may necessarily require shortening, labioversion, or rotation. In anticipation of such events, alternatives that include ameloplasty (minor), restoration (e.g., veneer), or preferably minor orthodontic tooth movement may enable more ideal crown placement.

Occlusal forces are constant and persistent. Irrespective of the individual, it is essential that anterior tooth restoration be performed in the context of function. Anterior implant restorations placed without effective posterior occlusion function or without sufficient posterior occlusal vertical dimensional determinants are at risk for remarkable failure. Under the vast majority of circumstances, anterior esthetic therapies should be reserved for individuals with intact posterior occlusion that adhere minimally to a shortened dental arch philosophy (Kanno and Carlsson 2006).

1.3.1 Diagnostic Imaging

Three-dimensional assessment of alveolar bone and its relationship to tooth/teeth planned for replacement is an important aspect of risk assessment (Fig. 1.4). If tooth/teeth are planned for extraction, careful assessment of the facial alveolar position relative to the CEJ as well as its thickness should be undertaken. Interproximal bone location can be assessed by intraoral periapical radiographs. However, the position of facial alveolar bone can assist in detecting facial bone dehiscence. Facial bone dehiscence has been correlated with increased early failure (Valentini 2006), reduced bone fill (Schropp 2003), increased bone resorption (Chen 2005, 2007), and increased incidence of mucosal recession (Kan 2007) following immediate implant placement. Conversely, the thickness of the alveolar facial plate has been

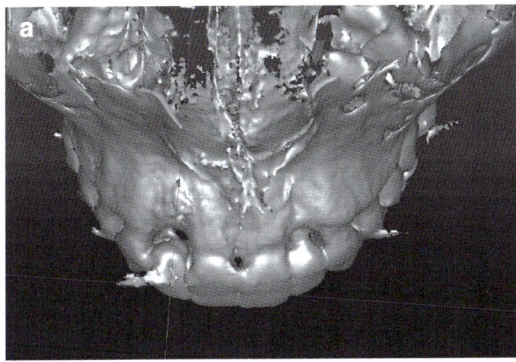

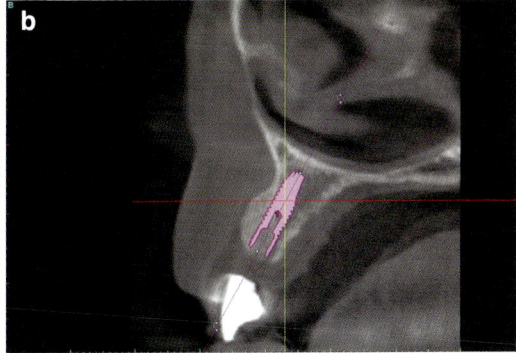

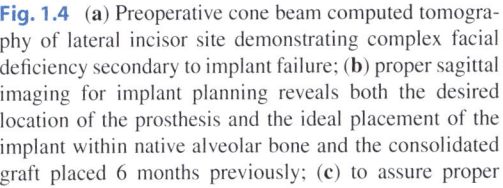

Fig. 1.4 (a) Preoperative cone beam computed tomography of lateral incisor site demonstrating complex facial deficiency secondary to implant failure; (b) proper sagittal imaging for implant planning reveals both the desired location of the prosthesis and the ideal placement of the implant within native alveolar bone and the consolidated graft placed 6 months previously; (c) to assure proper mesiodistal placement and planned orientation (both depth and buccolingual displacement), a guided surgical approach was utilized; (d) facial photograph upon attachment of the provisional abutment and crown; (e) final photograph at 1 month following placement of cement-retained lithium disilicate crown on a patient-specific abutment to complete restoration of the missing lateral incisor

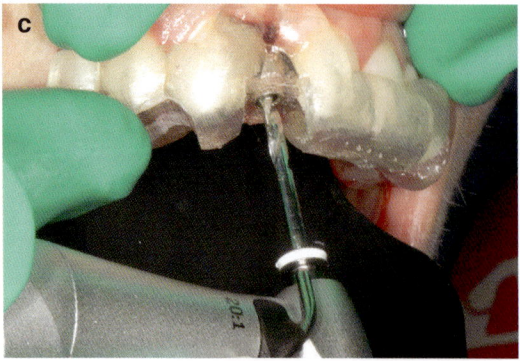
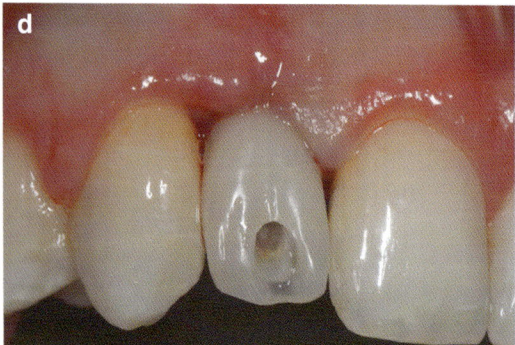
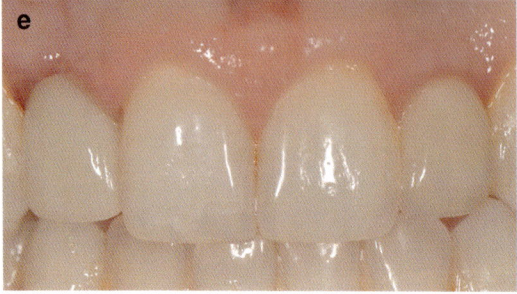

Fig. 1.4 (continued)

inversely correlated with the degree of post-extraction alveolar bone resorption (Chappuis et al. 2014; Cardaropoli et al. 2014). Interestingly, grafting extraction sockets by a ridge preservation protocol minimized the degree of post-extraction resorption so that there was no longer any correlation between initial facial bone thickness and bone resorption (Cardaropoli et al. 2014). It is important that the architecture of bone and adjacent structures be revealed prior to implant surgery.

1.3.2 Clinical Capabilities

Dental implant esthetics is often as much a result of choices as its biology. The esthetic replacement of a tooth or teeth with dental implants requires that the patient is accepting the knowledge of the existing condition, that they understand the limitations presented by these conditions, and that they understand what existing conditions can be changed or favorably addressed by the clinical team. The clinical team must possess a set of materials and techniques that can positively modify the conditions that will otherwise negatively influence the esthetic outcome of implant therapy. One major risk influencing dental implant outcomes is actually that one or another effective procedure has not been invoked in the process of developing an ideal implant restoration. Examples include the failure to select or undergo a bone augmentation procedure prior to implant therapy, the failure to identify the need for soft tissue augmentation, the failure to utilize orthodontic therapy to optimize periodontal attachment position, the inappropriate selection of abutment material or design, or ignoring occlusal factors that influenced crown placement.

The current spectrum of clinical techniques and materials that can be leveraged to the benefit of ideal dental implant esthetics is large. Most briefly, clinical photography and digital imaging methods permit submillimeter design and instrumentation of implant surgeries. The use of planning software is invaluable in communication and implementation of implant therapy. Placement of implants into sockets with dehiscence without any intervention should not be performed. When soft tissue limitations are encountered, existing data argues that autogenous connective tissue grafts or xenogenic grafts may be utilized to augment thin tissues

1 Recognition of Risk Factors and Patient Assessment   11

(Thoma et al. 2014). Thin or relatively transparent gingival tissues may require selection of zirconia versus titanium abutments to achieve improved gingival color. The ultimate restoration of the implant must be achieved in accordance with general dental esthetic principles, often requiring an integrated approach involving other teeth (Cooper 2008). Bleaching, intracoronal restoration, and veneer or crown restorations may be valuable in achieving desired esthetic outcomes. What emerges from the preceding discussion is a diagnostic protocol that leads to defining a set of "implant site development" procedures that extend beyond the conventional thoughts of bone regeneration for site development (Table 1.4). Completion of site development prior to implant placement and implant provisionalization is, second to a comprehensive diagnosis, the best guarantee against dental implant negative esthetic outcome (Fig. 1.5). Failure to recognize and prescribe these procedures is a greater risk than the success or failure of these procedures.

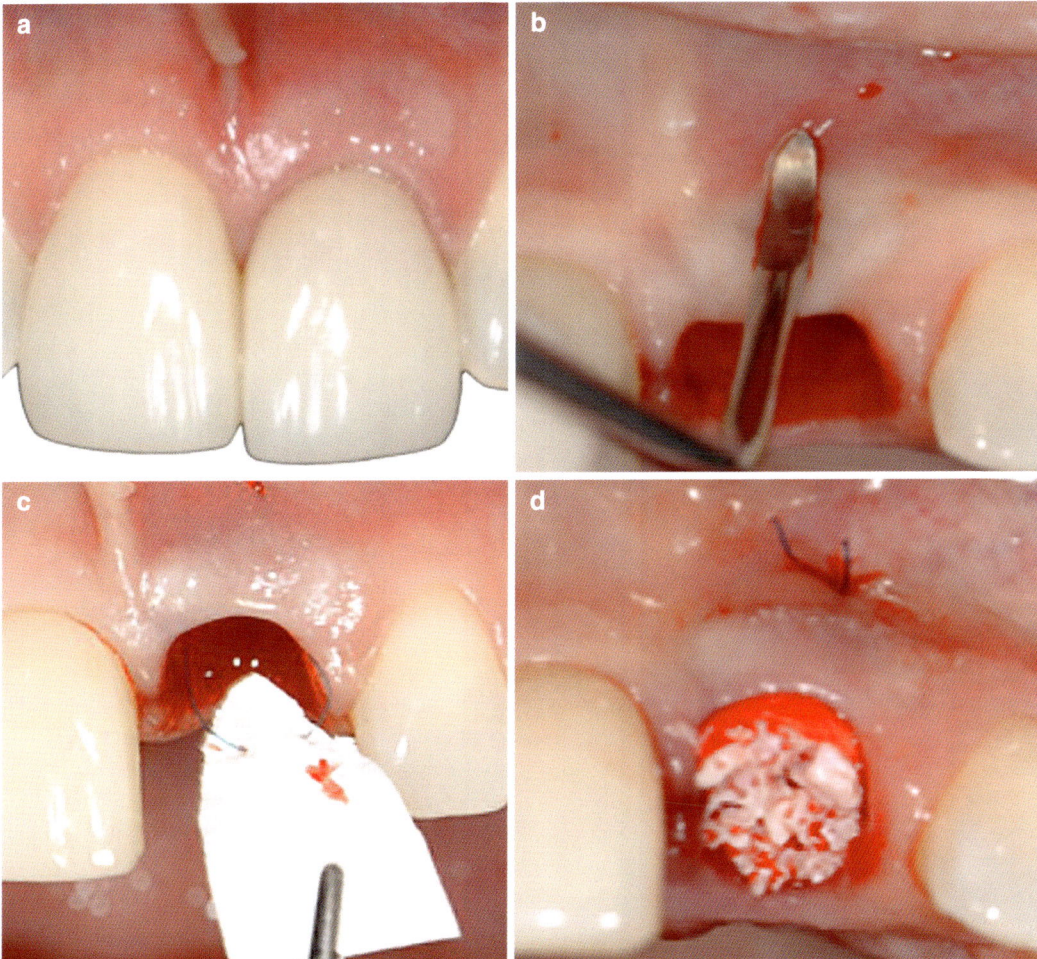

Fig. 1.5 (**a**) Initial condition of failing central incisor (tooth #9). (**b**) Extraction of the tooth reveals significant dehiscence in the buccal alveolar bone. (**c**) Placement of a resorbable collagen membrane through the mucosa and facial to the existing alveolar bone. (**d**) Placement of anorganic xenograft to achieve grafting of the deficient socket, (**e**) closure of the socket using an autogenous connective tissue graft, and (**f**) placement of a provisional restoration to aid in defining the soft tissue architecture and stabilize the graft. After 6 months, an implant was placed, and 2 months subsequently, a zirconia patient-specific abutment was placed. (**g**) Note the contour and volume of the peri-implant tissues. (**h**) A 4-year follow-up photograph reveals stability of the fully developed architecture

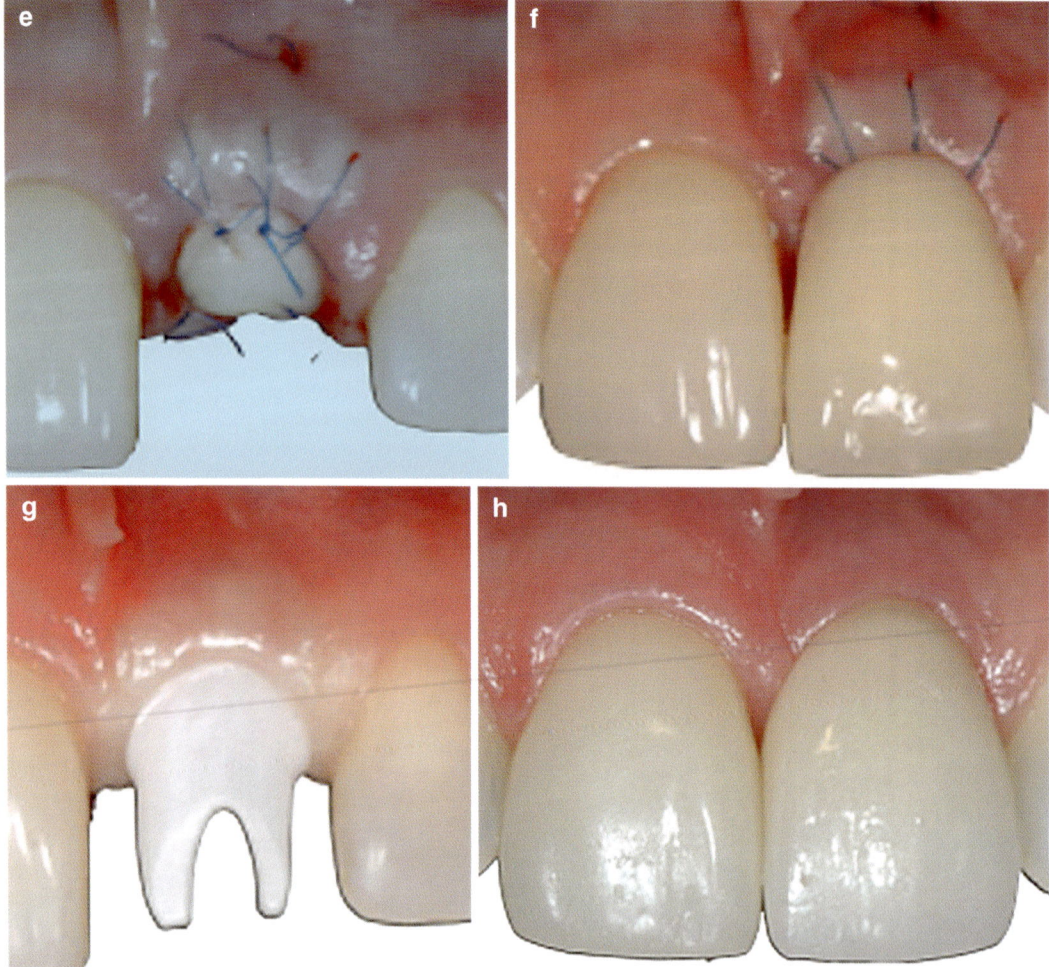

Fig. 1.5 (continued)

1.4 Providing Esthetic Implant Therapy

The preceding discussion has focused on obtaining the necessary data regarding the individual clinical scenario to inform proper decision-making. The general information regarding macroesthetic factors must be considered first. Should the agreed upon esthetic goals require more than replacement of one or more teeth, then the procedures required to address possible midline discrepancies, gingival display, gingival balance, symmetry, and occlusal concerns should be prescribed.

It may be valuable to identify the individual risk factors influencing single-tooth implant therapy in an organized and consistent manner. Regardless of an individual clinician's standardized approach to recording such risk factors, the major implant-specific observations that are required typically center on the condition of the adjacent tooth connective tissue attachments, the condition of the residual alveolar ridge, and the quality of the alveolar mucosa (Table 1.3). Although the ability to perform periodontal regenerative therapy is limited by defect morphology, orthodontic therapy may be considered as a means of changing the position of the periodontal attachment of adjacent teeth relative to the site planned for implant therapy. The key decisions are related to whether or not additional procedures are required to provide assurances that the supporting bone and soft tissues

Table 1.3 Prioritized risk factors influencing single-tooth implant esthetics

1. Existing loss of connective tissue attachment at adjacent teeth leading to lack of interproximal tissue fill
2. Combined vertical and horizontal buccal alveolar osseous defect leading to lost alveolar dimension or buccal tissue recession
3. Implant crown dimension does not equal contralateral tooth dimension mesiodistally (and occlusogingivally (see 2 above))
4. Failure to address gingival symmetry
5. Markedly thin mucosa permitting abutment discoloration
6. Failure to address discoloration of adjacent tooth
7. Defective adjacent restorations

Table 1.4 Site development procedures useful in reducing esthetic risks associated with dental implant esthetics

Management of the occlusogingival dimension of the edentulous space
    Bone augmentation procedures
    Soft tissue augmentation procedures
    Gingivectomy
    Crown lengthening
Management of the mesiodistal dimension of the edentulous space
    Orthodontic
    Restorative adhesive restorations
    Crowns and veneers
Management of the mesiodistal dimension of the alveolus
    Bone augmentation procedures
    Soft tissue augmentation procedure
Management of tooth color integration
    Bleaching
    Veneer, crowns
Management of the gingival color
    Soft tissue augmentation procedure
    Abutment material selection

will adequately provide the esthetic framework for an outstanding dental prosthesis. These issues should be reevaluated after management of the more global issues addressed above.

A standard procedural rubric can be followed as illustrated for a single-tooth implant (Fig. 1.2). Clinical photographs, clinical charting, and preliminary study casts are evaluated in terms of the 14 objective criteria for esthetics. A diagnostic waxing of the planned tooth or teeth should be performed in accordance with these criteria. The diagnostic waxing may be used to create a radiographic guide that indicates the position of the planned prosthesis in the volumetric image produced by subsequent cone beam CT imaging. After following these five diagnostic steps, sufficient information should be available to select a restorative pathway to achieve the esthetic goals.

Treatment may include one or more interventions to address site development (Table 1.4). It is not atypical that minor interventions are required to alter bone and or soft tissue dimensions. Major alterations involving bone augmentation procedures or crown lengthening/gingivectomy procedures should be discussed and encouraged in the context of ideal esthetic outcomes. Interim or provisional prosthetic management of mesiodistal dimension of the edentulous space or tooth shade can be performed in advance or coincident with implant placement and or provisionalization, but final restorative procedures are best performed at the time of final implant restoration.

While implants may be placed by different protocols (two-stage, one-stage, immediate placement, and immediate loading), efforts directed toward assuring the architectural control of implant esthetics (facial tissue thickness, depth of placement, and interproximal tissue fill related to adjacent tooth connective tissue attachment) are goals that supersede the technique. The various protocols are not the intention of this chapter; however, it must be underscored that irrespective of each of these approaches to implant placement, the data acquisition, planning, and risk management procedures do not differ. The biological principles for lasting dental implant esthetics are not dissimilar among these protocols.

The actual process and accuracy of implant placement is an essential part of achieving an ideal esthetic result. As indicated above, avoiding risks of facial soft tissue recession requires the availability of approximately 2 mm of tissue facial to the implant/abutment. Moreover, the depth of placement must permit biologic width development of 3 mm beyond the osseous crest. Advocated is the placement of dental implants with the specific orientation of 3 mm apical and 2 mm palatal to the designated mucosal zenith of the planned restoration. Surgical planning software assists in this planning, and surgical guides can be utilized to assure accuracy in placement (Fig. 1.4). When attempting to reduce the risk of advanced recession following single immediate implant treatment, a systematic review revealed four factors that reduce this risk substantially (<10%). They include (a) presence of an intact facial bone wall, (b) a thick gingival biotype, (c) use of flapless surgery, and (d) provision of an immediate implant crown (Cosyn et al. 2012a).

Consideration of risks of interproximal tissue loss is also related to placement. While diagnostic evaluation will demonstrate if connective tissue loss has occurred and will not be compensated for by implant placement, further interproximal tissue recession has been associated with (a) small implant-tooth distance, (b) multiple surgical reopening procedures, and (c) the distance from the contact position to the interproximal bone level (Cosyn et al. 2012b). Precise implant positioning using minimally invasive procedures is one aspect in esthetic risk management for dental implants.

Assuming that ideal implant placement has been provided for the patient and that the supporting architecture of the underlying bone and surrounding soft tissues has been adequately prepared in volumetric terms, the final aspects of risk reduction involve proper implant restoration using an abutment and crown to direct the peri-implant mucosal architecture and provide an esthetic integration with existing teeth. The restorative aspects of achieving esthetic integration with existing teeth are among the 14 objective criteria and include tooth axis, basic features of tooth form, tooth characterization, surface texture, and color. While the majority of these aspects of esthetic excellence are delegated to the dental laboratory technician, it is important to recognize that marked deviation in implant position and orientation can create challenges in directing tooth axis and achieving integrated tooth form. Suggested is a prioritized list of considerations for risk management in esthetic implant therapy (Table 1.4). Generally, the subsequent controlled management of the soft tissue architecture using appropriate provisional restorations and abutment design defines the soft tissue contours and strongly influence tooth shape (Fig. 1.6). Any misstep in second-stage surgery,

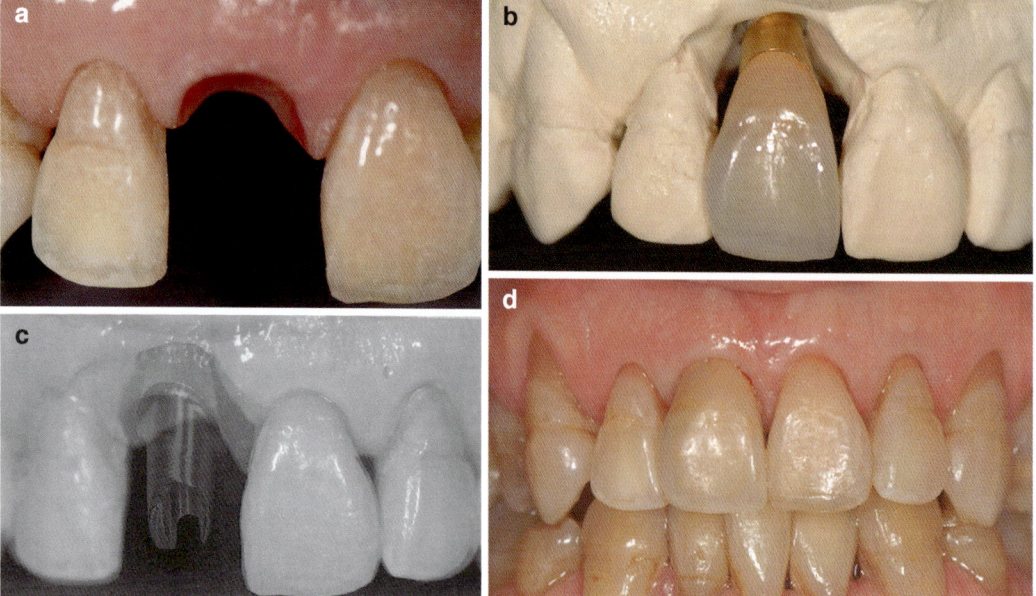

Fig. 1.6 (**a**) Facial photograph reveals the condition of the peri-implant tissues 3 months following an immediate loading and provisionalization procedure. The shape is fully dependent upon the contours of the abutment and provisional crown. (**b**) The patient-specific abutment (TiN plasma coated) and the lithium disilicate crown have been designed and manufactured to represent the contours of a central incisor tooth, (**c**) superimposed photographs reveal the precision of design for the abutment to support these peri-implant tissue, **d**) facial photograph of the implant, abutment, and crown restoring tooth #8 at the time of crown cementation

1   Recognition of Risk Factors and Patient Assessment

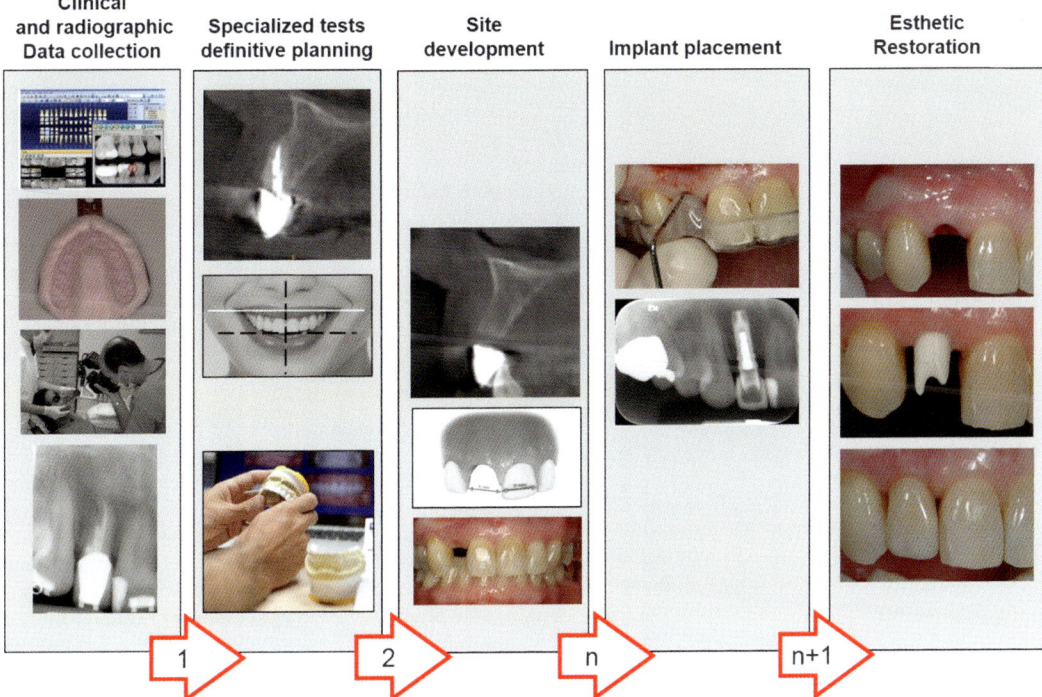

Fig. 1.7 Progressive elimination of implant esthetic risk factors; a clinical activities flow chart

provisionalization, abutment design and delivery, and crown cementation can lead to esthetic disappointment. By adopting a careful, stepwise process of eliminating risk factors for dental implant esthetics (Fig. 1.7), success can be assured.

> **Summary**
>
> For many patients and for a variety of different scenarios, ideal implant esthetics is not achieved in a single step or procedure. A comprehensive esthetic diagnosis is the first step in the reduction of esthetic risks for dental implants and requires gathering all necessary data regarding esthetics prior consideration of dental implant placement factors. The second key in reduction of esthetic risk often requires one or more steps involved in a broad approach to implant site development. When an ideal implant restoration has been planned for placement in an ideally developed site, the third key to reduction in esthetic risk is careful implant placement. When these therapeutic steps can be performed with minimal steps and with accuracy, the final steps in providing an esthetic implant restoration can be fulfilled with little drama. Providing a highly esthetic implant abutment and crown when ideal tissue volume and implant position have been provided recapitulates the value in identifying the risk factors and removing the limitations prior to implant placement. When the clinical capabilities are carefully aligned with the esthetic expectations and biological realities presented, success generally follows (Fig. 1.8).

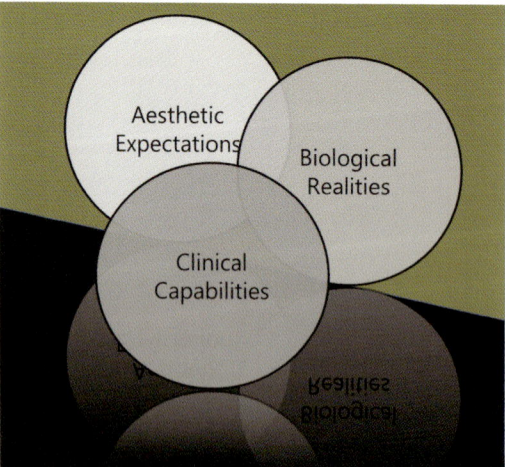

Fig. 1.8 Risk factors for dental implants are successfully addressed when the clinician understands and has communicated with the patient the ABCs of dental implant esthetic therapy; esthetic expectations of the patient, the biological realities of the clinical scenario, and the clinical capabilities are available to address the expectations and realities of the scenario

References

Brito C, Tenenbaum HC, Wong BK, Schmitt C, Nogueira-Filho GI (2014) keratinized mucosa indispensable to maintain peri-implant health? A systematic review of the literature. J Biomed Mater Res B Appl Biomater 102(3):643–650

Choquet V, Hermans M, Adriaenssens P, Daelemans P, Tarnow DP, Malevez C (2001) Clinical and radiographic evaluation of the papilla level adjacent to single-tooth dental implants. A retrospective study in the maxillary anterior region. J Periodontol 72(10):1364–1371

Cooper LF (2008) Objective criteria: guiding and evaluating dental implant esthetics. J Esthet Restor Dent 20(3):195–205

Cooper LF, Reside GJ, Raes F, Garriga JS, Tarrida LG, Wiltfang J, Kern M, De Bruyn H (2014) Immediate provisionalization of dental implants placed in healed alveolar ridges and extraction sockets: a 5-year prospective evaluation. Int J Oral Maxillofac Implants 29(3):709–717

Cosyn J, Hooghe N, De Bruyn HA (2012a) systematic review on the frequency of advanced recession following single immediate implant treatment. J Clin Periodontol 39(6):582–589

Cosyn J, Sabzevar MM, De Bruyn H (2012b) Predictors of inter-proximal and midfacial recession following single implant treatment in the anterior maxilla: a multivariate analysis. J Clin Periodontol 39(9):895–903

Cosyn J, Cleymaet R, De Bruyn H (2014) Predictors of alveolar process remodeling following ridge preservation in high-risk patients. Clin Implant Dent Relat Res. 18(2):226–233

Evans CD, Chen ST (2008) Esthetic outcomes of immediate implant placements. Clin Oral Implants Res 19(1):73–80

Ioi H, Kang S, Shimomura T, Kim SS, Park SB, Son WS, Takahashi I (2013) Effects of vertical positions of anterior teeth on smile esthetics in Japanese and Korean orthodontists and orthodontic patients. J Esthet Restor Dent 25(4):274–282

Jung RE, Sailer I, Hämmerle CH, Attin T, Schmidlin P (2007) In vitro color changes of soft tissues caused by restorative materials. Int J Periodontics Restor Dent 27(3):251–257

Kan JY, Rungcharassaeng K, Sclar A, Lozada JL (2007) Effects of the facial osseous defect morphology on gingival dynamics after immediate tooth replacement and guided bone regeneration: 1-year results. J Oral Maxillofac Surg 65(7 Suppl 1):13–19

Kanno T, Carlsson GE (2006) A review of the shortened dental arch concept focusing on the work by the Käyser/Nijmegen group. J Oral Rehabil 33(11):850–862

Kois JC (2004) Predictable single-tooth peri-implant esthetics: five diagnostic keys. Compend Contin Educ Dent 25(11):895–896 898, 900 passim; quiz 906-7

Kokich VO, Kokich VG, Kiyak HA (2006) Perceptions of dental professionals and laypersons to alter dental esthetics: asymmetric and symmetric situations. Am J Orthod Dentofacial Orthop 130:141–151

Levi A, Psoter WJ, Agar JR, Reisine ST, Taylor TD (2003) Patient self-reported satisfaction with maxillary anterior dental implant treatment. Int J Oral Maxillofac Implants 18(1):113–120

Lorenzo R, García V, Orsini M, Martin C, Sanz M (2012) Clinical efficacy of a xenogeneic collagen matrix in augmenting keratinized mucosa around implants: a randomized controlled prospective clinical trial. Clin Oral Implants Res 23(3):316–324

Mange P, Gallucci GO, Belser UC (2003) Anatomic crown width/length ratios of unworn and worn maxillary teeth in white subjects. J Prosthet Dent 89(5):453–461

Mardas N, Trullenque-Eriksson A, MacBeth N, Petrie A, Donos N (2015) Does ridge preservation following tooth extraction improve implant treatment outcomes: a systematic review: group 4: therapeutic concepts & methods. Clin Oral Implants Res 26(Suppl 11):180–201

Morley J, Eubank J (2001) Macroesthetic elements of smile design. J Am Dent Assoc 132(1):39–45

Sanz-Sánchez I, Ortiz-Vigón A, Sanz-Martín I, Figuero E, Sanz M (2015) Effectiveness of lateral bone augmentation on the alveolar crest dimension: a systematic review and meta-analysis. J Dent Res 94(9 Suppl):128S–142S

Schropp L, Kostopoulos L, Wenzel A. (2003) Bone healing following immediate versus delayed placement of titanium implants into extraction sockets: a prospective clinical study. Int J Oral Maxillofac Implants.18(2):189–99.

Thoma DS, Buranawat B, Hämmerle CH, Held U, Jung RE (2014) Efficacy of soft tissue augmentation around dental implants and in partially edentulous areas: a systematic review. J Clin Periodontol 41(Suppl 15):S77–S91

Valentini P, Abensur D, Albertini JF, Rocchesani M. (2010) Immediate provisionalization of single extraction-site implants in the esthetic zone: a clinical evaluation. Int J Periodontics Restorative Dent;30(1):41–51.

Vera C, De Kok IJ, Reinhold D, Limpiphipatanakorn P, Yap AK, Tyndall D, Cooper LF (2012) Evaluation of buccal alveolar bone dimension of maxillary anterior and premolar teeth: a cone beam computed tomography investigation. Int J Oral Maxillofac Implants 27(6):1514–1519

Yao J, Tang H, Gao XL, McGrath C, Mattheos N (2014) Patients' expectations to dental implant: a systematic review of the literature. Health Qual Life Outcomes 12:153

Determination of the Sequence of Therapy

Michael S. Block

Abstract
Patients often present with the need for replacement and reconstruction of teeth in the anterior maxilla. This chapter describes a sequence of preoperative, intraoperative, and postoperative methods to treat many of these patients in an organized and evidence-based set of methods.

2.1 The Clinical Problem

Patients present to the dental clinic with anterior teeth which are deemed non-restorable. Many of these patients have had extensive dental restorative care, which is fatiguing, and in need of replacement. The patient often wants to be reconstructed to appear and function as they did prior to compromise of their teeth. The clinician must collect information concerning the status of the tooth, soft, and hard tissues in order to fabricate a treatment plan which can predictably result in an acceptable restoration. This chapter describes a sequence that can be used for many patients who need tooth replacement in the aesthetic zone with implants.

Establishing the goals Each patient must be individually assessed to determine their expectations. If they have a tooth in the aesthetic zone which needs replacement, it is natural for them to desire the same level of aesthetics that they had prior to tooth removal. If there is gingival recession, swelling, or an obvious pathological condition, the patient may still expect an ideal result. It is the responsibility of the clinician to accurately diagnose the presenting clinical situation and predict the final result and communicate this with the patient.

If there is excessive gingival recession, it will be very difficult to obtain an ideal gingival facial margin at the conclusion of the therapy. These patients may require orthodontic eruption of the tooth prior to its removal, excessive grafting, osteotomies, and prosthesis modifications that included simulated gingiva. This chapter will focus on cases presenting with mild to moderate gingival recession within the suggested algorithms of therapy.

Data collection At the initial consultation visit, after reviewing the patient's past medical history, the physical examination must include specific details in order to formulate a treatment plan.

M.S. Block, DMD
Center for Dental Reconstruction,
110 Veterans Memorial Boulevard, Suite 112,
Metairie, LA 70005, USA
e-mail: drblock@cdrnola.com

Standardized photographs Each patient should have a uniform set of photographs that can be utilized to describe to the patient and colleagues the current situation. These photographs can also be used to compare to digital imaged plans and the final result.

The following are included in a suggested series:

Incisor show at rest with the lips slightly apart and relaxed. The patient's central incisor show at rest is documented.

Smile line – With the patient expressing an animated smile, a photograph is taken to demonstrate the incisor show. This is especially important in the patient who starts treatment with gingival recession or for those patients who have short clinical crowns and may be candidates for crown lengthening at the incisor edge at the gingival margin.

Frontal, lateral, and full occlusal photographs are taken with retractors. Another important but often forgotten photograph is a lateral view of the teeth in occlusion showing ridge relationships and lip posture.

Establishing the planned gingival margin Ideally the incisor show at rest should be 2–3 mm. The length of the central incisor should be 10.5–11 mm depending on the patient's facial length. These two data points are used to identify the ideal level of the gingival margin and set the specific location of the gingival margin. Once this specific location has been determined, the treatment plan can incorporate therapies to inferiorly or superiorly relocate the gingival margin to allow for ideal incisor show at rest and at smile with ideal tooth proportions (Block 2014).

Determination of bone height and width The cone beam CT (CBCT) scan is the most effective method to determine bone height and width. The scan is taken, data collected, and when viewed in an appropriate viewing software, a spline is drawn on the axial view through *the pulp chambers of the teeth. This is a method that can be used to standardize the comparison of one scan to another. Cross-sectional views are made perpendicular to the spline curve. The* width and height of the ridge can be seen and measured. The 3D view is used to visualize bone morphology and to identify a concavity and how it relates to the adjacent teeth. When the tooth is present, the overlying labial bone may be seen or may appear absent. It is important to note that in some scans, the labial bone may not be seen if the bone is less than 1.5 mm thick; this is related to the voxel size of the scan and in addition due to a phenomenon known as "volume averaging."

Relating the CBCT to the clinical situation Based on the abovementioned data points, the patient's existing tooth can be utilized as a reference to plan for the ideal final result.

The physical examination of the patient identifies the ideal location of the central incisor's edge and its ideal position of the gingival margin. These identifiers can then be related to the patient's current teeth. Linear markings can be drawn on the CBCT images to locate bone and to plan what is necessary to achieve these ideal tooth positions. The level of the bone is determined to be acceptable or deficient. The horizontal projection of the alveolar bone crest is also assessed to simulate the need for grafting.

Current case planning should include virtual placement of teeth to understand exactly what is surgically needed to place implants in the desired locations. By loading the data from a CBCT scan into an appropriate software, the clinician can see where the implants must be placed based on the restorative plan. This digital diagnostic methodology eliminates many of the lab procedures which add additional laboratory costs and can be inaccurate due in large part by an inherent lack of knowledge on behalf of the laboratory technician tasked with this detail. Surgical guides can then be fabricated to accurately place implants based on the ideal preoperative planning. The patient benefits from less invasive surgery and a more accurate implant placement.

The biotype of the gingiva is very important to determine as thin or thick prior to initiating treatment. Thin gingiva recedes with minimal surgical intervention. If bone loss occurs after surgery, thin gingiva will move superiorly, creating an unaesthetic situation. If the patient has thin gingiva, the treatment should include methods to convert the thin to a thickened gingiva. A thickened gingiva will recede less if bone resorbs and as well can be manipulated with provisional crown forms (Langer and Calagna 1980, 1982; Langer and Langer 1985; Bruno 1994, 1999).

Unfortunately tissue thickness is difficult to measure in a predictable objective method. The clinician can use several observations to confirm the presence of thin tissue. If the tissue is glossy and lacks stippling, it is usually thin. If the tissue is red and mobile, or when you can see the periodontal probe through the overlying gingiva, it is usually considered to be thin. Different methods to convert thin to thick tissue are used within the sequence of treatment, usually at the first surgical procedure when removing a tooth.

The lack of labial bone Usually labial bone loss is not difficult to determine by combining probing of the gingival sulcus, the presence of overlying gingival erythema and recession, and lack of bone on the CBCT scan. When there is deficiency of labial bone, grafting will be necessary and may include one to two procedures to gain thick gingiva and bone for appropriate implant placement.

Normal to thin bone When the tooth structure is present with minimal facial tooth structure fractures, the labial bone may be present but thin. In this situation, there may be options to graft bone and place the implant at the same procedure.

The decision tree is now formed:

- If there is a lack of *labial bone and thin gingiva*, the surgeon may place an allograft in the socket and, at the same session place, a subepithelial connective tissue graft under the labial mucosa (Case 1). This converts the thin to thick tissue and provides satisfactory bone for implant placement. In the presence of thick gingiva, bone resorption, if it occurs, may be masked by the thickened gingiva. The use of implants with medialized abutment-implant interfaces and a concave abutment submergence profile also increases the ability to form thickened gingiva for long-term success. The soft tissue graft combined with the allograft is often all that is required. Occasionally adding a sintered xenograft at the time of implant placement can further augment the gingival profile (Block 2014).
- *Thin bone on the labial*: If the residual ridge has adequate bone on the palatal side of the tooth socket, which it usually does, then the tooth can be removed with preservation of the labial bone. Implant placement for screw retained access if possible, and grafting the gap between the implant and intact yet thin labial bone with sintered xenograft (Case 2) can be accomplished in one procedure. The sintered xenograft is relatively non-resorbable. It will heal with some bone formation but also with dense "scar-like" response because of the relatively inert properties of the sintered xenograft. The bundle bone is expected to resorb, leaving the sintered xenograft under the facial gingiva. The xenograft will be held together by dense scar tissue, which acts as a "filler" to thicken and "plump" the gingival form (Block 2014).
- *Gingival recession with the need for 2–3 mm of coronal movement* of the gingival margin (Case 3). If the tooth is relatively intact for even a brief period of time, orthodontic forced eruption can be used to move the gingival margin coronally. In select cases, gingival movement can be enhanced by the use of removable "Essix"-type prostheses which, by overlapping the ridge, can create a negative pressure under the Essix resulting in gingival hyperplasia and coronal movement of up to 2 mm (Bachado, Personal communication 2005).

Surgical methods The following methods are suggested:

Sulcular incisions For the treatment of one or more adjacent teeth in the anterior maxilla, sulcular incisions with no vertical release incisions are very effective to prevent movement or shrinkage of the gingiva on the tooth. A 15c-type blade is used to incise within the sulcus to the bone. A thin elevator is used to gently reflect the flap to the margin of the bone and tooth. The use of full-thickness reflection over the labial cortical bone for a single- or two-tooth region in the aesthetic zone is unnecessary and further strips blood supply to the labial bone.

Choice of graft materials Graft materials include allografts, xenografts, and growth factors such as bone morphogenetic protein and recombinant platelet-derived growth factor, with or without the use of blood source products using clots and serum. For this chapter, only two materials are recommended to graft the aesthetic socket, with long-lasting membranes or foils to retain a larger graft in a severe concavity situation.

2.2 Grafting Material Characteristics

1. The graft should maintain the space of the extraction socket. When the graft material maintains the space within the socket, bone can repopulate the graft and thus recreate bone volume similar to pre-extraction size. The graft should have osteoconductive features.
2. Bone formed within the graft should allow stable placement of the implant.
3. The rate of bone formation over time should be taken into consideration to plan the sequencing of therapies such as implant placement, additional contour grafting, and pontic and site development.
4. The material should be relatively inexpensive and readily available and should not transfer pathologic conditions.

2.3 Bovine or Equine Sintered Xenograft

Bovine- or equine-derived bone is a xenograft. Sintering is removal of organic material by heating the graft under pressure. This increases the crystallinity of the graft material resulting in a very slow resorption rate. Clinically, this material is non-resorbable. Sintered xenograft is used to preserve ridge form and to augment the thin ridge (Berglundh and Lindhe 1997; Artzi et al. 2000; Wetzel 1995; Van Steenberghe et al. 2000). The relatively inert nature of this material delays revascularization and subsequent bone formation compared to more natural materials such as autogenous bone.

2.4 Mineralized Bone Allograft

Human mineralized bone in particulate form can preserve most of an extraction site's bone bulk and volume in preparation for the placement of implants. The advantages of an allograft are (Block 2014) the graft material is readily available without the need for a second surgical harvest site, and (Langer and Calagna 1980) the material is osteoconductive. Over time, the allograft resorbs and, it is hoped, replaced with bone.

Human mineralized bone is available as particulate cortical or cancellous bone. The recommended particle size ranges from 250 to 750 μm. Particles smaller than 250 μm tend to flow with blood out of the site, and larger particles can be shed through the sites. Allografts are prepared by bone banks. Sterile procedures are used to harvest the bone, which is washed with a series of delipidizing agents such as ethers and alcohol, lyophilized, and then sieved to the particle size necessary for a specific indication. The freeze-dried mineralized bone allograft usually is irradiated to sterilize it, even though the entire process for harvesting to packaging is performed under strict sterile condition.

When placed in an extraction site, mineralized bone graft material is still present at 4 months (Block et al. 2002). However, the bone forming around the mineralized bone particles usually is sufficiently mineralized to allow immediate provisionalization, with adequate primary stability after placement of the implant in the extraction site grafted with a mineralized allograft.

One goal of grafting of the extraction site is retention and preservation of the original ridge form and maintenance of the crestal bone after the implants have been restored. In one study in which no membrane was used at the time of extraction site grafting, the grafted sites felt "bone hard" at 4 months and appeared to be filled with bone (Block 2002). However, long-term studies are not confirming maintenance of ridge contour in the anterior maxilla when the thin labial-bundle bone resorbs naturally after tooth removal (Becker et al. 1996; Hurzeler et al. 2010; Perenack et al. 2002). When the labial or facial bone is not present or is minimally present, allograft may resorb resulting in a flat ridge rather than a ridge with convex form. In these situations an onlay of sintered xenograft is recommended (Block and Kaleem 2014).

The current technique for the management of premolars, canines, incisors, and maxillary palatal root sites advocates the additional use of a fast-resorbing material to retain the graft and promote epithelialization over the graft. The graft can be covered with a fast-resorbing hemostatic collagen material that resorbs in less than 7 days (Van Steenberghe et al. 2000). In mandible molar sites and for coverage of the buccal root sites for maxillary molars, coverage with advancement of the gingiva is recommended with the periosteum used to retain the graft in the extraction socket.

When to use soft tissue grafts A connective tissue (CT) graft is used to convert thin to thick tissue and is usually a subepithelial connective tissue graft placed under thin facial gingiva. In animal studies, the survival of the connective graft is marginal. There is significant scar formation when the cells within the connective graft do not survive, creating a denser tissue than prior to the graft. A sham procedure can also result in thicker tissue, but when a CT graft was placed, the sites had slightly thicker, more predictable conversion from thin to thick gingiva (Perenack et al. 2002).

A common clinical situation for the use of a CT graft is when removing an anterior tooth which has lost labial bone and has thin tissue, where gingival recession must be avoided. The patient with a high smile line and thin gingiva will have gingival recession if the tooth is removed, and the thin gingiva is left without conversion. The tooth is removed, the socket is grafted with allograft, and a CT graft is placed under the facial gingiva to convert thin to thick tissue. After the bone has formed, the implant can be placed with a flapless technique if the thickness of the tissue is adequate or with small incisions for addition of a non-resorbable graft (xenograft) as needed.

Postoperative methods to gain margin control The use of a vacuum-form can produce negative pressure on the gingiva and can result in gingival hyperplasia and 1–2 mm of gingival production. This requires a model with a spacer, followed by a vacuum-form with its margins extending beyond the soft tissue deficit, with contact on the soft tissues. The negative pressure developed under the vacuum-form can result in gingival formation to partially fill the defect (modified from 8).

Case examples:

Case 1 Thin gingiva and lack of labial bone (Fig. 2.1):

This male presents with the need for removal of his left central incisor. He suffered trauma 20 years prior and had his central incisors repositioned with orthodontics. His current problems include thin gingiva, a small draining fistula at the apex of the tooth, an apically positioned facial gingival margin, and lack of labial bone. He has exceptionally high aesthetic concerns and believes his current teeth are too long and prominent.

His treatment plan must address the superiorly positioned gingival margin as well as the lack of bone and thin gingiva. The first phase of his treatment was orthodontic extrusion of the left central incisor to reposition the gingival margin.

After this was accomplished over a period of 4 months, the orthodontic appliances were removed and the first surgical procedure was performed. A sulcular incision was used and the tooth was removed. A subperiosteal dissection was made on the facial aspect, and a subepithelial CT graft from the palate was placed under the labial gingiva to thicken the thin gingiva. Mineralized allograft was placed into the socket

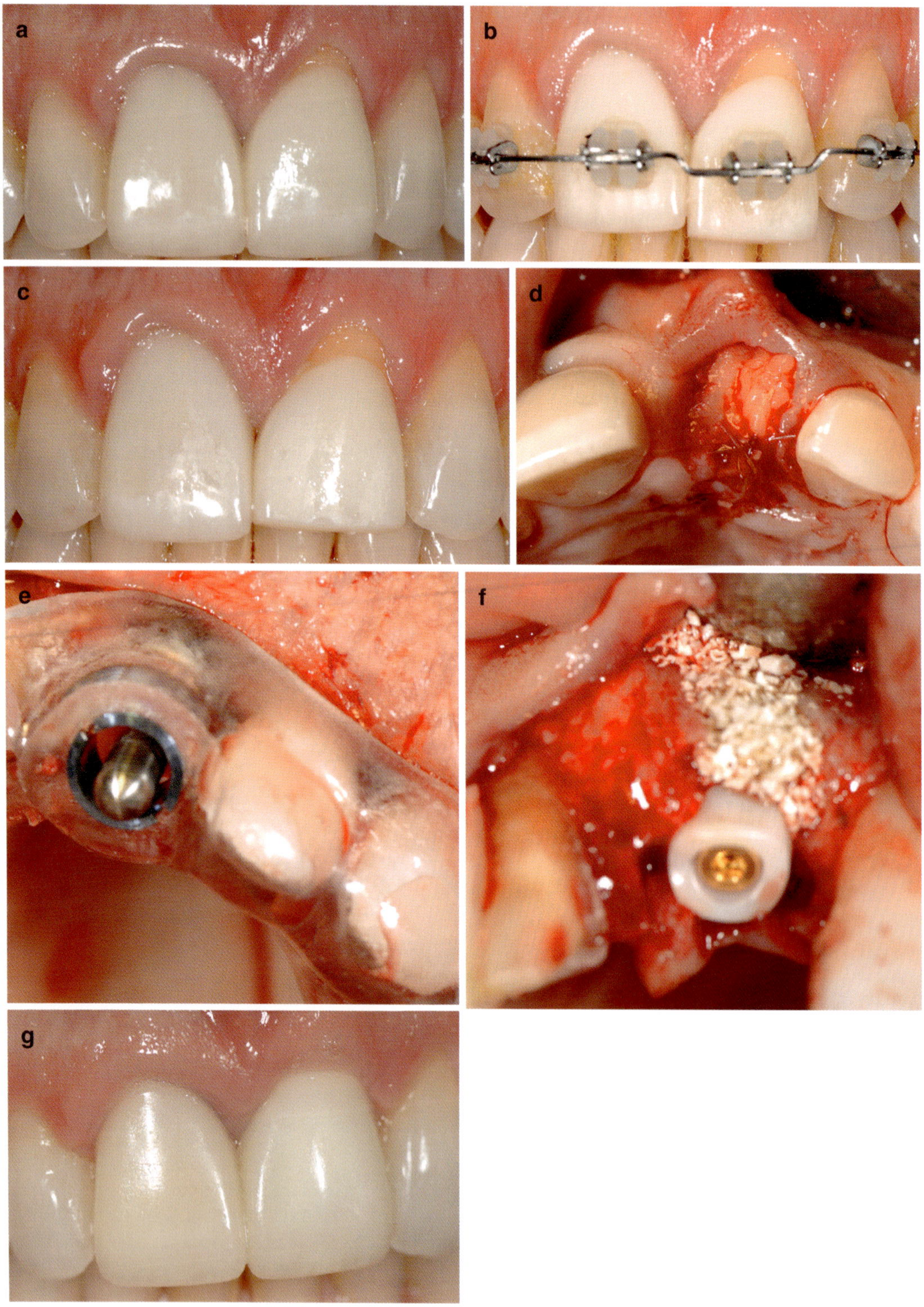
a
b
c
d
e
f
g

under the CT graft. A fixed provisional using the adjacent teeth as abutments was placed.

After 4 months CBCT guidance was used to accurately place an implant using a conservative flap. The flap was used because he needed additional graft material on the labial to finalize his gingival contour.

The final restoration was fabricated and has been stable for 5 years.

Case 2 Extraction of a central incisor and grafting the labial with xenograft, with immediate provisionalization (Fig. 2.2):

This woman presents with a fractured central incisor with minimal ferrule for restoration. Her restorative dentist discussed options with her, and she decided to have the tooth removed and an implant placed. She preferred a fixed provisional rather than a removal option.

Her gingiva tended to be thin but not translucent. She had labial bone which was less than 1 mm in thickness as seen in the cross section CBCT scan imaging. Her gingival margin was in an ideal location.

The treatment plan was to remove the tooth, place an implant engaging the palatal wall of the socket, graft the anticipated buccal gap with sintered xenograft to preserve ridge form, and place an immediate provisional to develop the subgingival contour.

The only surgery performed included a sulcular incision with elevation of the gingiva to the margin of the bone. A water cooled laser was used to separate the tooth from the labial and interdental bone. An extraction elevator subluxed the tooth which was then removed with forceps.

The labial bone was intact, but thin as expected. The implant was placed engaging the palatal slope of the extraction socket. An abutment try-in was used to determine the abutment gingival height and slope. In this patient, a 4 mm tall abutment with a 15° angle correction was chosen and screw retained to the implant. After the abutment was placed, sintered xenograft was packed firmly into the gap between the implant and the intact labial bone. A provisional crown was made over a plastic coping and cemented in place.

Four months later, an implant level impression was made, and on the second restorative visit, the final crown was placed. Two-year follow-up shows retention of the labial ridge form.

Case 3 Need to improve gingival contour with removable prosthesis (Fig. 2.3):

This patient had removal of a central incisor with socket grafting and a subepithelial graft to thicken her thin gingiva. Two weeks postoperative, she had loss of the labial aspect of the margin of the gingiva over the extraction site. In this patient, her high smile line and the current 11 mm tall central incisor required more coronal gingiva than was present 2 weeks after tooth removal.

Her Essix-type provisional was remade with its labial aspect overextended onto the gingiva, with a space maintained under the vacuum-form. Within 2 weeks, gingival healing had repopulated the defect area.

At 6 months, an implant was placed with CBCT guidance with an immediate provisional. Note at 5 weeks after the implant and provisional excellent gingival form at the correct gingival height.

Fig. 2.1 (**a**) Patient presents with left central incisor with gingival recession and a high vestibular draining fistula. He has high aesthetic demands and shows 3 mm of his gingiva on smile. (**b**) In order to move the gingival margin to an acceptable level with the adjacent central incisor, orthodontic forced extrusion was performed (Orthodontics by Dr. Bradley Gottsegen). At this level of extrusion, the soft tissue stopped moving inferiorly with the tooth; thus, the orthodontics was stopped. (**c**) The orthodontic appliances were removed, and the tooth was allowed to stabilize for 3 months. (**d**) At the time of tooth removal, a subepithelial connective tissue graft was harvested from the left palate to thicken the thin gingiva over the left central incisor. After the tooth was atraumatically removed, a subperiosteal tunnel was made, and the connective tissue graft was inserted under the facial gingiva. Allograft was placed and the connective tissue graft was used to cover the allograft. (**e**) The CBCT-generated drill guide was used to guide implant placement, with the understanding that a graft was necessary to rebuild the horizontal projection of the site. (**f**) Sintered xenograft was placed over the labial surface of the implant. (**g**) The final crown with the gingival margin within 0.5 mm level with the right central incisor tooth (Prosthetics by Dr. Joseph Collura)

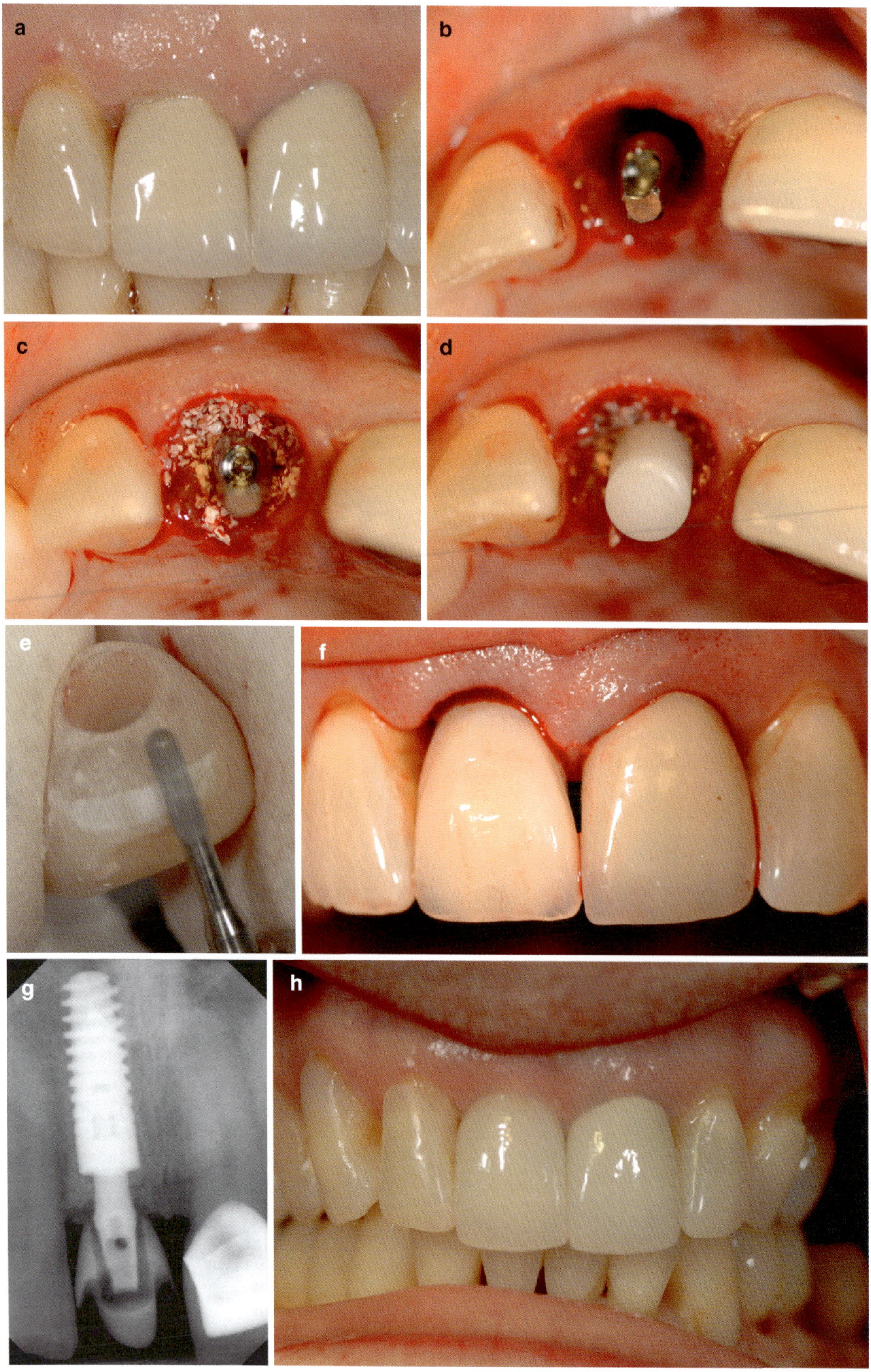
a
b
c
d
e
f
g
h

2 Determination of the Sequence of Therapy   27

Fig. 2.2 (**a**) Preoperative view of fractured right central incisor. Note that the facial gingival margin on the left central incisor is apical to the right central incisor. (**b**) Sulcular incisions were made. A water cooled laser was used to create a trough between the tooth and the labial bone. The tooth was removed. One Ankylos (A14 C/X, Dentsply Implants, Waltham, Mass) implant was placed in the resultant socket of the extraction site in contact with the palatal wall. The driving mount indicates appropriate emergence along the incisive edge of the adjacent teeth. (**c**) After a try-in abutment was used, the final abutment was chosen and screw retained to the implant. Sintered xenograft was packed firmly between the implant and intact labial bone. (**d**) A plastic cap was placed over the abutment. (**e**) The plastic cap was roughened and adhesive luted to it. A provisional crown was luted to the plastic cap using composite. Outside of the mouth, additional composite was placed and shaped to develop an ideal subgingival contour. The provisional was then cemented. (**f**) The provisional 2 weeks after surgery. (**g**) A radiograph 4 months after placement showing adequate bone implant contact for the final restoration. Note the augmentation coronal to the shoulder of the implant. (**h**) The final restoration – 1 year post-restoration, showing maintenance of the gingival margin coronal to its original position

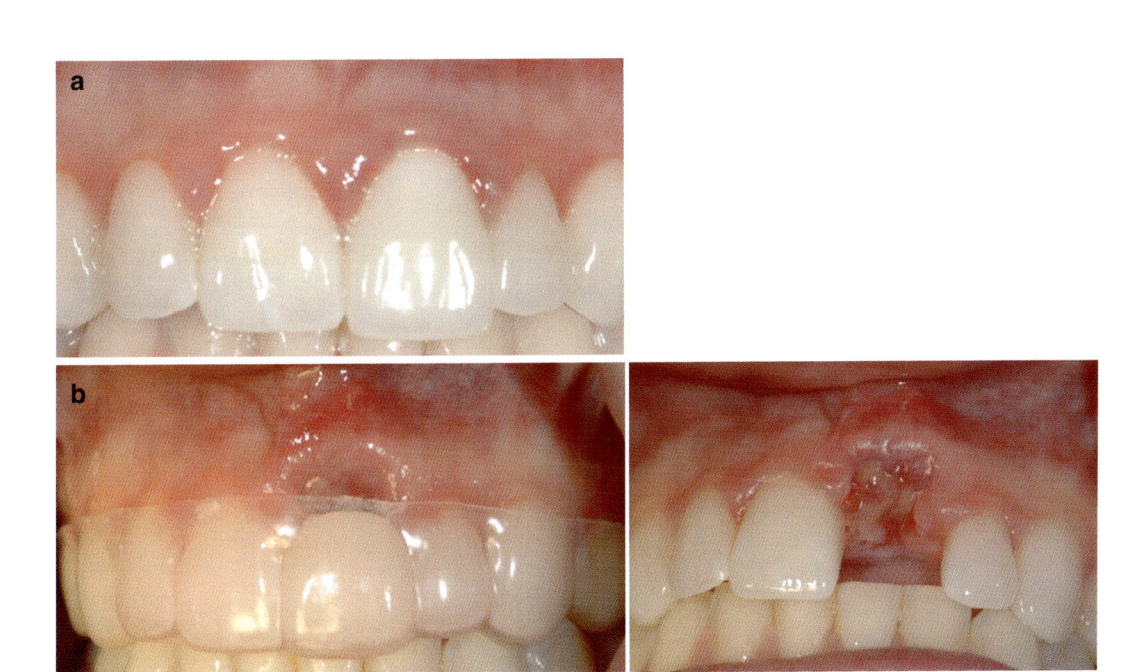

←

Fig. 2.3 (**a**) Preoperative photograph showing thin gingiva, the facial gingival margin 1 mm superior to the adjacent 11.0 mm length crown, in a high smile patient with high aesthetic concerns. (**b**) These two images show the patient 2 weeks after tooth extraction, allograft and CT graft. The socket graft was placed to allow for implant placement. The CT graft was placed to increase the thickness of the gingiva. However, there was incision breakdown from trauma and loss of 2 mm of the facial gingival margin. (**c**) The vacuum-form that held a provisional crown was remade to extend over the soft tissue defect with contact superiorly. This was made from an impression that had a negative profile designed to maintain space where gingiva was desired. (**d**) Four months later, she was ready for implant placement with immediate provisionalization. Note the excellent gingival response to the vacuum-form created gingiva. (**e**) Provisional restoration in place 5 weeks after implant placement. Note the excellent facial gingival margin restoration

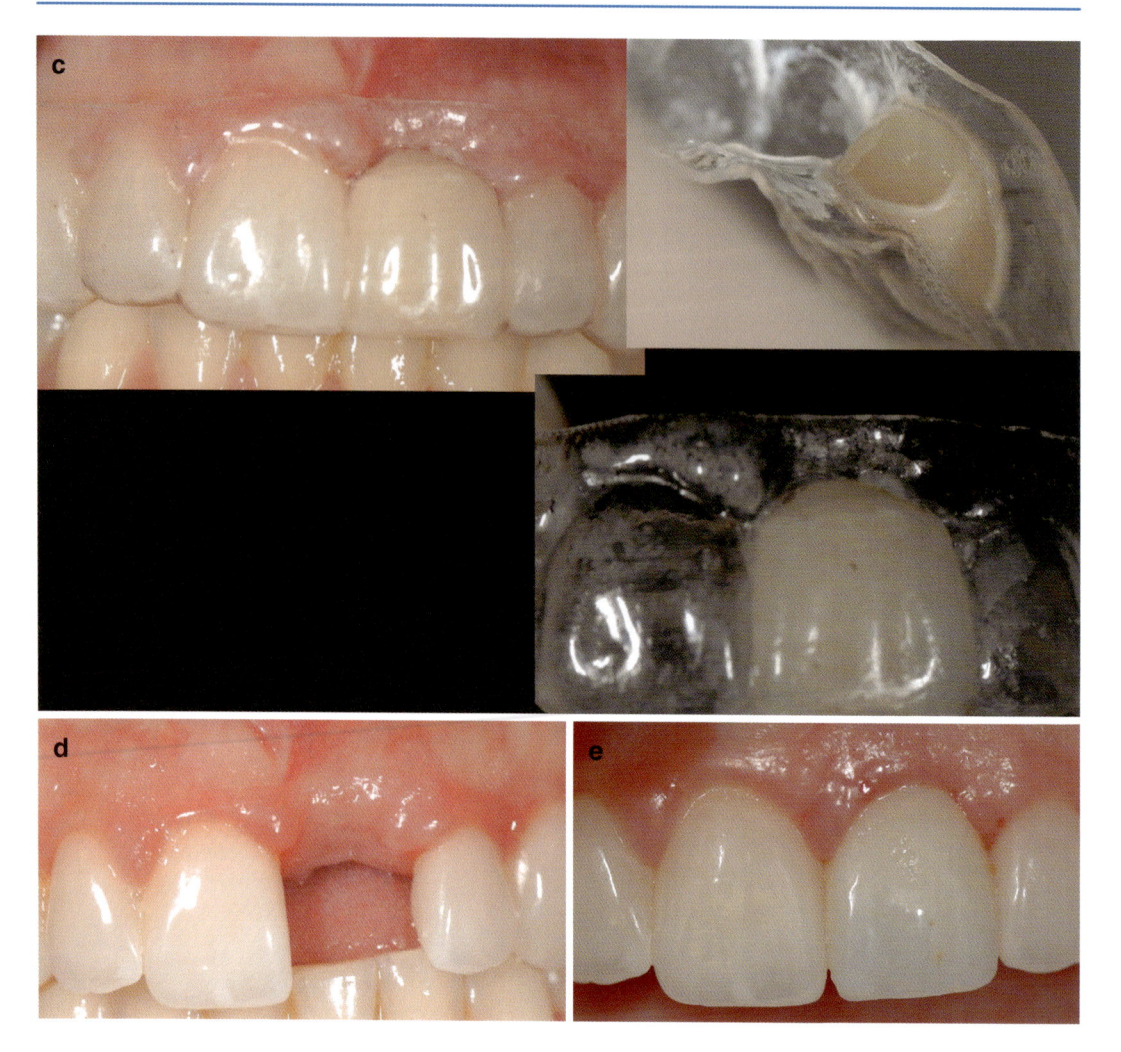

Fig. 2.3 (continued)

References

Artzi Z, Tal H, Dayan D (2000) Porous bovine bone mineral in healing of human extraction sockets. Part 1. Histomorphometric evaluations at 9 months. J Periodontol 71:1015–1023

Becker W et al (1996) Clinical and histologic observations of sites implanted with intraoral autologous bone grafts or allografts: 15 human case reports. J Periodontol 67:1025–1033

Berglundh T, Lindhe J (1997) Healing around implants placed in bone defects treated with Bio-Oss: an experimental study in the dog. Clin Oral Implants Res 8:117–124

Block MS (2014) Techniques for grafting and implant placement for the extraction site. Chapter 7. In: Color atlas of dental implant surgery. Elsevier, St. Louis

Block MS, Kaleem A (2014) Use of Sintered xenograft over allograft for ridge augmentation: technique note. J Oral Maxillofac Surg 72(3):496–502

Block MS, Finger I, Lytle R (2002) Human mineralized bone in extraction sites before implant placement: preliminary results. J Am Dent Assoc 133:1631–1638

Bruno JF (1994) Connective tissue graft technique assuring wide root coverage. Int J Periodontics Restorative Dent 14:126–137

Hurzeler MB, Zuhr O, Schupbach P, Rebele SF, Emmanouilidis N, Fickl S (2010) The socket-shield technique: a proof-of-principle report. J Clin Periodontol 37:855–862

Langer B, Calagna L (1980) Subepithelial connective tissue graft to correct ridge concavities. J Prosthet Dent 44:363–367

Langer B, Calagna L (1982) The subepithelial connective tissue graft: a new approach to the enhancement of anterior esthetics. Int J Periodontics Restorative Dent 2:22–33

Langer B, Langer L (1985) Subepithelial connective tissue graft technique for root coverage. J Periodontol 56:715–720

Perenack J, Wood RJ, Block MS, Gardiner D (2002) Determination of subepithelial connective tissue graft thickness in the dog. J Oral Maxillofac Surg 60(4):415–421

Runo JF (1999) A subepithelial connective tissue graft procedure for optimum root coverage. In: Block MS, Sclar AG (eds) Soft tissue esthetic procedures for teeth and implants, Atlas of the oral and maxillofacial surgery clinics of North America, vol 7. W.B. Saunders, Philadelphia, pp 11–28

Van Steenberghe D et al (2000) The clinical use of deproteinized bovine bone mineral on bone regeneration in conjunction with immediate implant installation. Clin Oral Implants Res 11:210–216

Wetzel AC, Stich H, Caffesse RG (1995) Bone apposition onto oral implants in the sinus area filled with different grafting materials: a histologic study in beagle dogs. Clin Oral Implants Res 6:155–163

Osseointegration and the Biology of Peri-implant Hard and Soft Tissues

Clark M. Stanford

Abstract

Restoration of missing teeth in the aesthetic zone with oral implants is a complex combination of surgical and restorative techniques along with medical device designs that optimizes the potential of biology to both rapidly heal and maintain long-term hard and soft tissue health around the implant. Rapid expansion of our knowledge regarding wound healing is allowing this knowledge to be applied to implant designs, enabling a more rapid and predicable use of oral implants in the aesthetic zone. As important as biology is for bone wound healing, the response of the mucosal soft tissue will be the most dominant aspect of the result observed by the patient. Care in planning and execution of the implant procedure is needed along with careful development of a concave transition zone from the head of the implant to the restorative margin for predicable stability of soft tissues. Through a combination of innovative biomedical device designs, clinical diagnosis, careful surgical management, and detailed understanding of the restorative aspects will allow for the provision of optimal patient care in the aesthetic zone.

3.1 Introduction

The use of oral implants has created a fundamental ground swell in the management of tooth loss for patients. The clinical success of this procedure occurs through clinical and biological steps starting with initial primary stability provided by the amount, quality, and distribution of bone within the proposed implant site (Roos et al. 1997). Following placement of an oral implant, a series of bone modeling and remodeling steps occur creating an adaptation or integration of an implant characterized by biological reactions starting with bone turnover at the interface (a process of localized necrosis) followed by repair (Stanford and Brand 1999). A common clinical end point is defined as a lack of aggressive chronic inflammation, a lack of implant mobility,

C.M. Stanford, DDS, PhD,
Dean and Professor, College of Dentistry, and
Department of Bioengineering, College of
Engineering, The University of Illinois at Chicago,
801 South Paulina Street,
DENT Room 102C (MC621),
Chicago, IL 60612, USA
e-mail: cmstan60@uic.edu

and radiographic bone adaptation to the interface (Albrektsson and Sennerby 1991; Smith and Zarb 1989). High success rates hold for certain anatomic regions of the mouth although the bony response within the thin cortical plates and diminished cancellous bone characterizing the canonical Lekholm and Zarb type IV bone can be a challenge with conventional machined-surfaced implants (e.g., 65–85%) (Widmark et al. 2001). These results relate to both the minimally rough implant surfaces used at the time and the atrophic patient population, treated. The introduction of moderately rough implant surfaces has significantly reduced these issues and has allowed the expanded use of shorter implants (<10 mm in length) and narrow diameter implants (<3 mm ⌀) for certain situations (Atieh et al. 2012; Gulje et al. 2012, 2013).

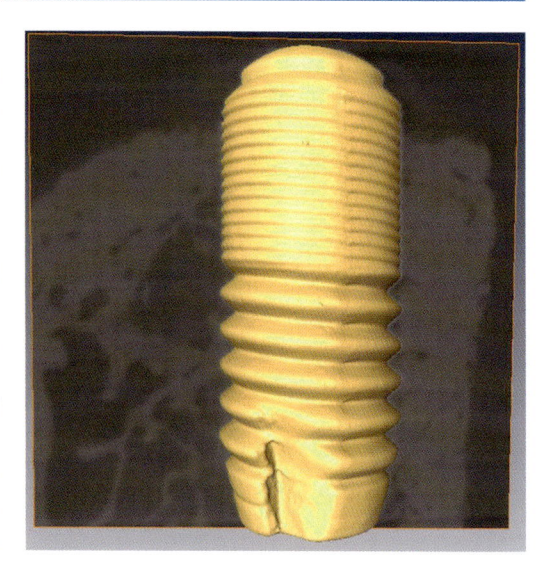

Fig. 3.1 Micro-CT imaging of cancellous and cortical bone healing around an oral implant. Image shows both the intimate contact in the transcortical region and the cancellous bone adaptation to the mid-body of the implant

3.2 Implant Macro-surface

Implants used in the oral environment have one of the three major types of macro-retentive features: screw threads (tapped or self-tapping), solid body press-fit designs, and/or sintered bead technologies. These approaches are designed to enhance initial implant stability and/or create large volumetric spaces for bone ingrowth. An important biological principle of bone is its favorable response to compressive loading (without the presence of a ligament) but not to shear forces (Stanford 1999). Therefore, screw thread implant designs have been adapted to achieve a compressive loading of the surrounding cortical or cancellous bone (Orsini et al. 2012). Other thread designs focus on reducing the surrounding shear forces by reducing the height of the thread profile (reducing the contribution of any one thread) with an increase in the number of threads per unit area of the implant surface (Hansson 1999) (Fig. 3.1). This has the additional benefit of increasing the strength of the implant body by increasing the amount of remaining wall thickness of the implant body (Binon 2000).

For the more popular threaded implant designs, implant shape, surface roughness, thread design, implant diameter, and length may

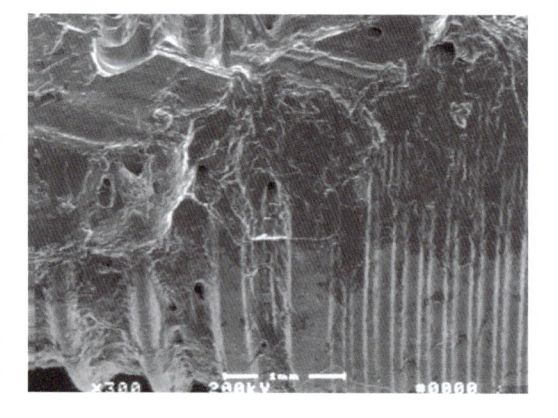

Fig. 3.2 Bone adapting to the titanium dioxide surface of a healed oral implant

impact the perception of primary stability at the time of implant placement. In general, the thread to bone contact in the transcortical region conveys the highest level of stress which may result in increased bone loss in this region (Hansson and Halldin 2009; Halldin et al. 2014) (Fig. 3.2). A moderately rough implant surface plays a role in primary stability, but its significance lies in promoting an establishment of secondary stability (Mendonca et al. 2008, 2009; Valencia et al. 2009; Stanford 2010; Thalji and Cooper 2013,

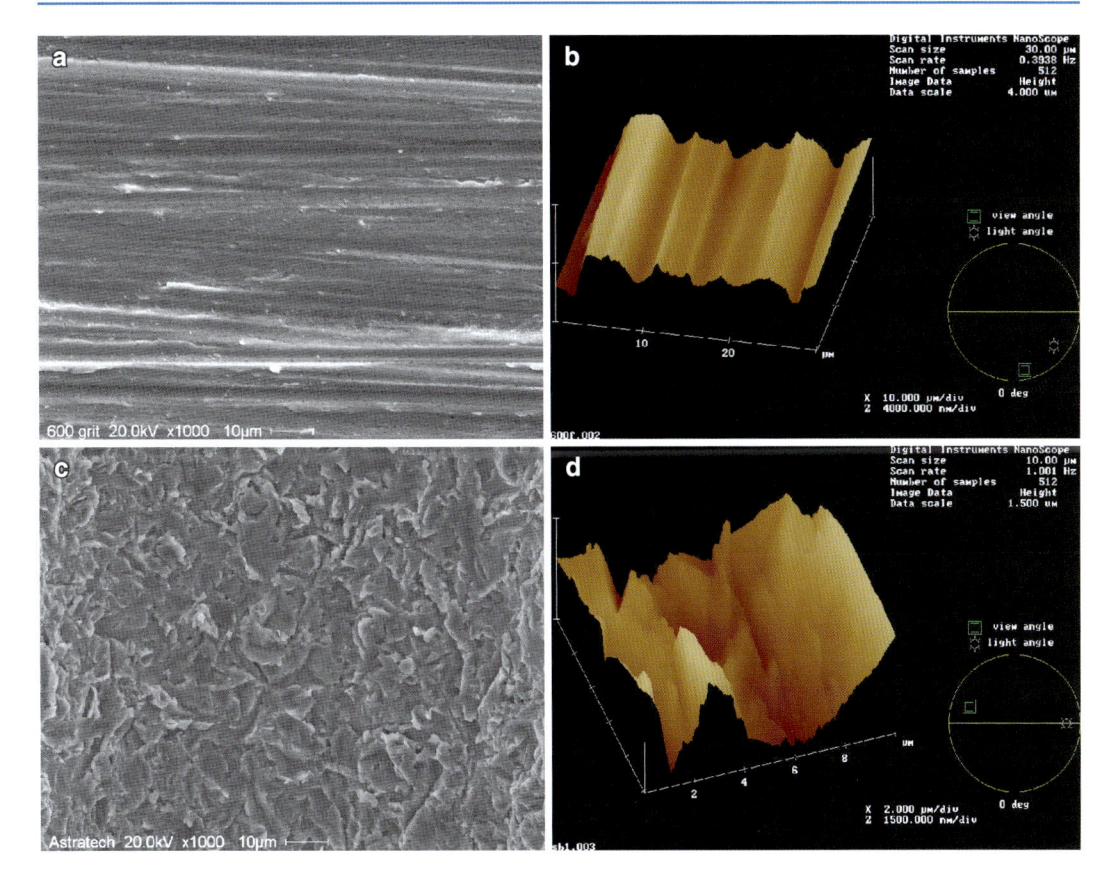

Fig. 3.3 (**a**) Scanning electron microscopy (SEM) of a turned surface implant showing a smooth surface with milling lines from the lathe process created during the turning process. (**b**) Atomic force microscopy (AFM) of the turned surface showing the grooves created but minimal complex topography. (**c**) A SEM of a complex titanium surface that was blasted with TiO to create a moderately rough surface with a subsequent mild etching. (**d**) AFM of the blasted and etched surface showing the complexity created on the titanium surface which assists in mechanical interlocking of the implant body to the healed bone tissue. This intimate process achieves a rigid fusion of the outer titanium oxide surface with the bone tissue, a process referred to as osseointegration

2014; Thalji et al. 2013) (Fig. 3.3a–d). Implant shape can enhance primary stability, especially using a tapered shaped implant body (Arnhart et al. 2012). Given that a tapered implant can put excessive transcortical strain on crestal bone, it is important to minimize the degree of compression and perform long-term clinical research on these types of designs (Norton 1998, 2013). Thread design significantly influences primary stability through features such as thread pitch, depth, width, as well as thread thickness at the tip of the thread (Ausiello et al. 2012). As discussed by Abuhussein and colleagues, thread design through reduced pitch, reduced helix angulation, and deeper threads (resulting in more surface area) are attributes that enhance primary stability (Abuhussein et al. 2010) (Fig. 3.4). More recently, Norton proposed that implant diameter may be the strongest determent factor based on the concept of maintaining a critical pressure on the transcortical bone below a level leading to excessive microfracturing (and hence, delayed healing and/or excessive bone loss) (Norton 2013; Mathieu et al. 2014). Implant length may play a role in primary stability, yet recent data indicates that with sufficient healing time, predictable secondary stability (osseointegration) can be achieved around very short implants (Atieh et al. 2012; Gulje et al. 2012; Mertens et al. 2012).

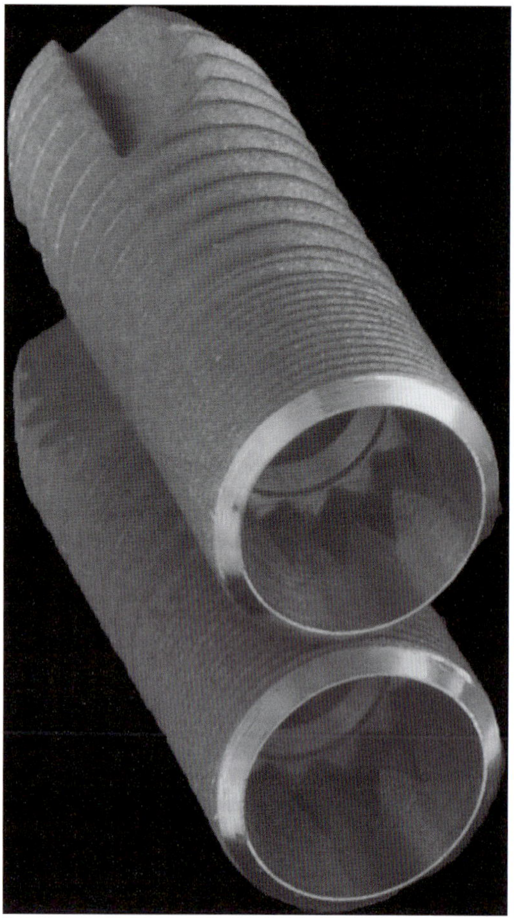

attempt to enhance the in-migration of new bone (e.g., osteoconduction) through surface topography (a.k.a., *surface roughness*), biological means to manipulate the type of cells that grow onto the surface, and strategies to utilize the implant as a vehicle for local delivery of a bioactive coating (adhesion matrix or growth factor such as BMP-2) (Davies 1998; Fink et al. 2008; Leknes et al. 2008; Wikesjo et al. 2008) (Fig. 3.2).

Many attempts have been used to enhance bone adaptation by modifying the implant surface. While increased surface roughness of implants leads to greater success, it is not clear what aspect of "roughness" is advantageous (Wennerberg and Albrektsson 2000). In dental implant design, it is usually assumed that a greater surface area (per unit of bulk metal surface) is an objective by various means to enhance the surface roughness of the implant surface (Fig. 3.3). This enhanced surface area then allows a greater area for load transfer of bone against the implant surface (Buser et al. 1991; Wennerberg et al. 1997; Hansson 1999, 2000). Micromechanical features influence the process of secondary integration (bone growth, turnover, and remodeling) (Stanford and Brand 1999). One advantage of acid etching, a technique commonly used, is to increase the roughness of the grit blasted surface with the potential for a nanometer-scale topography laid on the macroscale roughness allowing bone to adapt to the surface under elevated shear forces (Brunski 2000; Kasemo and Lausmaa 1994).

Fig. 3.4 A common oral implant showing design features of micro- and macrothread for primary anchorage, a moderately rough surface to assist with secondary stability (integration) and shape and design features to assist in placement of the device into adequate hard tissue at the site of interest

3.3 Implant Micro-surfaces

Upon the placement of an implant into a surgical site, there is a cascade of molecular and cellular processes providing new bone growth and differentiation along the biomaterial surface. Following placement, the surrounding bone undergoes an initial necrosis, bone resorption, and replacement with woven-like cell-rich bone tissue that is eventually replaced through a mechanotransduction-mediated remodeling with mature Haversian bone (Stanford and Brand 1999; Sims and Gooi 2008; Slaets et al. 2009; Thalji and Cooper 2013; Mathieu et al. 2014). Recent strategies to accelerate bone adaptation can be divided into those that

3.4 Peri-implant Mucosal Health

The long-term success of implant therapy is not just dependent on enhanced osseous stability. Recently, greater attention is being addressed to transmucosal dental implant or implant abutment interfaces (Linkevicius et al. 2014; Lops et al. 2014). Peri-implant health, especially in the premaxilla region, often necessitates a band of keratinized mucosa for improved health, reduced inflammation, and stability of the mucosa around the abutment (Bishti et al. 2014; Barwacz et al. 2015; Cooper et al. 2015; Wang et al. 2015) (Fig. 3.5). It is important that the surgical procedures follow critical rules, such as the "rule of six," to assure enough three-dimensional space for adequate volume of connective tissue, allowing the illusion of an emergent root form (Cooper and Pin-Harry 2013). Mechanical and biological stability derived from the design and abutment surfaces in this connective tissue and junctional epithelial environment are critical to a volume of connective tissue that reduces inflammatory infiltrate. Chronic inflammation in this transmucosal region is influenced by architecture (shape and contour of the transition zone) and surface roughness of the abutment surface leading to a risk for unstable and long-term tissue recession and even an elevated risk for peri-implantitis (Berglundh et al. 2002, 2005; Lang et al. 2004; Fransson et al. 2005; Roos-Jansaker et al. 2006a,

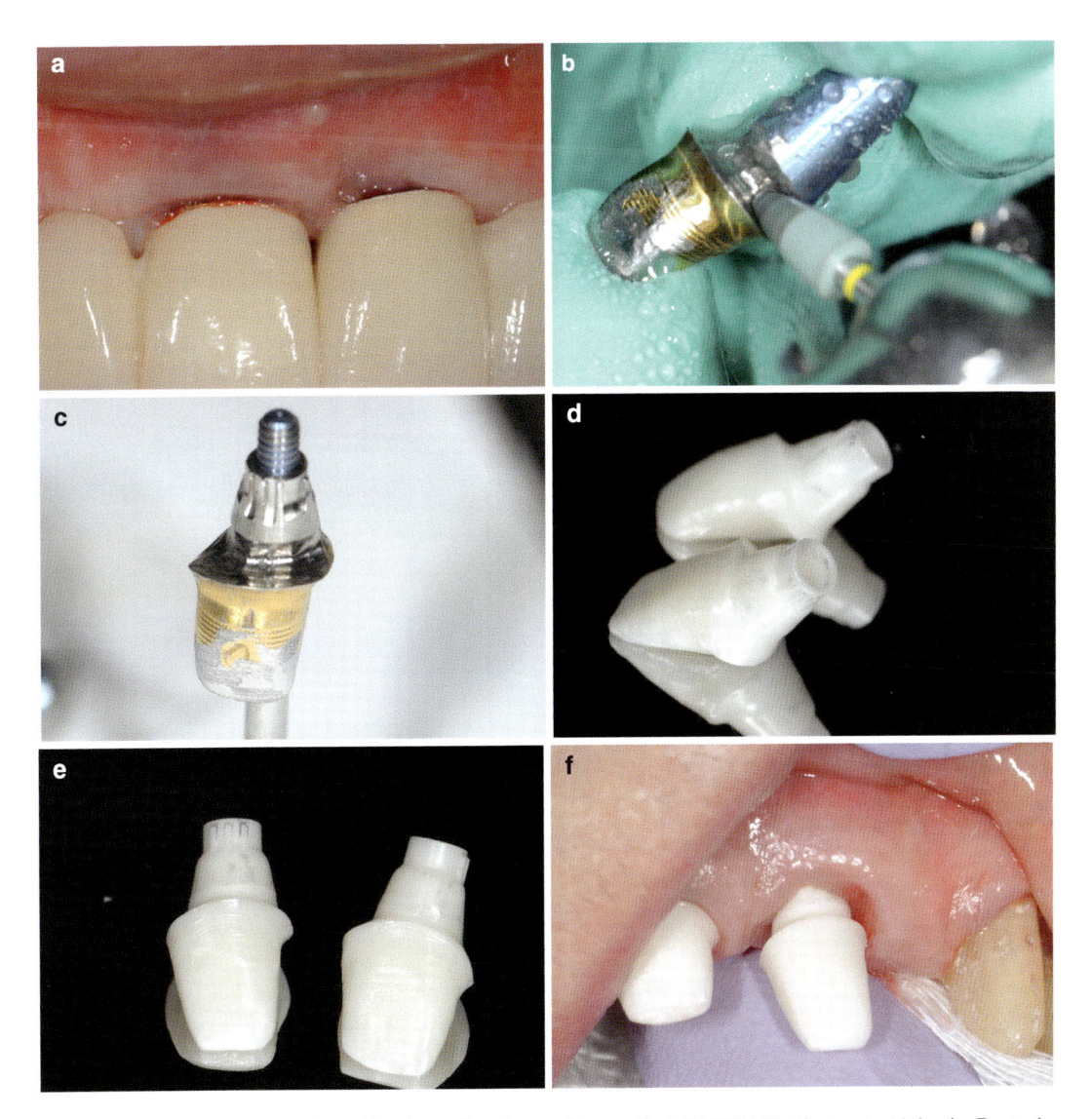

Fig. 3.5 (a) Clinical presentation of implants placed to restore the upper central incisors (11 and 21) showing recession a year following delivery. The implants had been placed with the head of the implants not adequately deep enough for development of an ideal transition zone (Cooper and Pin-Harry 2013). (b) The titanium abutments were removed and the facial transition zone diagnostically adjusted to reduce the pressure on the thin mucosa present in this region. (c) Modified abutment showing the attempt to create more of a concave facial transition zone. (d) Copy milled CAD/CAM Abutments (Atlantis, Dentsply Implants) made in Zirconia used to replace the modified abutments now designed with the concave facial profile. (e) Abutments showing the flat interproximal design for wall strength to the abutments. (f) Abutment being placed with an evaluation of tissue blanching. (g) Minimal to no tissue blanching should be present in this situation. (h) Final zirconia abutments with zirconia fixed implant prosthesis in place showing reasonable aesthetics given the shallow implant placement in the anterior aesthetic zone

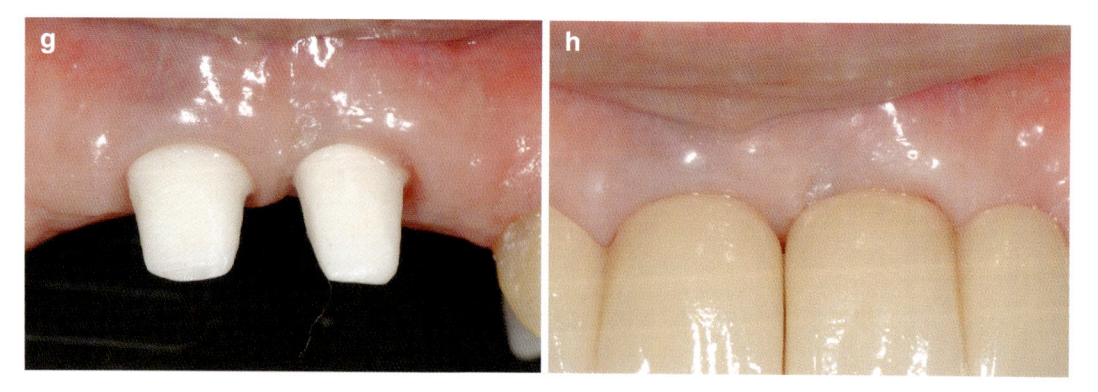

Fig. 3.5 (continued)

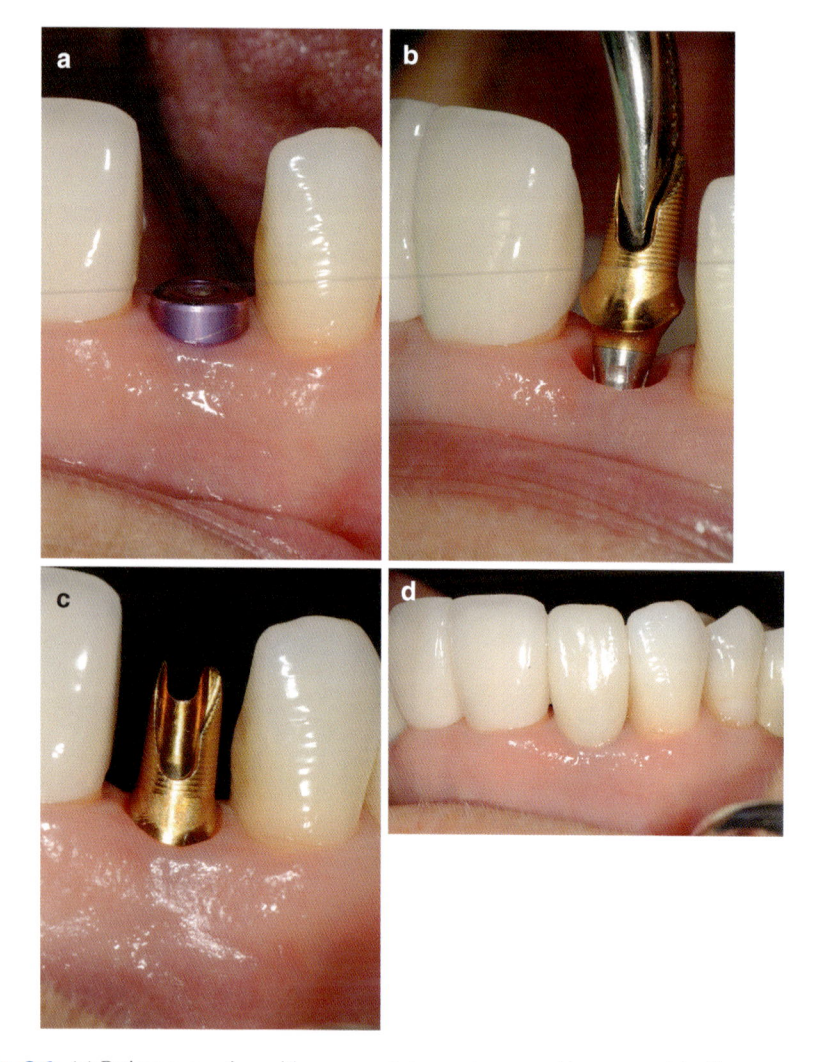

Fig. 3.6 (**a**) Patient presenting with a narrow interproximal space in which a 3.6 mm diameter implant was placed. (**b**) A gold-coated titanium abutment is placed with careful evaluation of the facial tissue contact of the transition zone. (**c**) Abutment seated with final torque, showing minimal mucosal blanching. (**d**) Final crown (EMax, Ivoclar Vivadent) in place

b, c; Renvert et al. 2007). Implant abutment often will have a thin fibroblastic layer along the lining surface with circular collagen fibers surrounding the abutment (a.k.a., scar band), but this region does not have the common collagen architecture observed around teeth including the dentogingival and alveologingival fiber network (Wennstrom and Derks 2012). Further, it has been observed that a flat or concave transition zone shape or architecture is needed to avoid placing excessive pressure on the connective tissue scar band inducing a potential for recession (Patil et al. 2013; Cecchinato et al. 2015; Ferrari et al. 2015) (Figs. 3.5 and 3.6).

3.5 Implant Wound Healing and the Potential Role of Surface Modification

Wound healing around a dental implant placed into a prepared osteotomy follows three stages of repair. Initial formation of a blood clot occurs through a biochemical activation followed by a cellular activation and finally a cellular response. These initial rapid changes during the surgical phase of implant therapy lead to activation of key biochemical pathways: clotting system, complement activation, Kinin cascade activation, and, finally, plasminogen activation of plasmin. The adhesion of platelets to the assembled fibrin scaffold as well as adhesion to the surface topography of an implant surface leads to a process of platelet activation. Platelets are a rich source of locally released growth factors (e.g., PDGF, TGF-Beta, PDEGF, IGF-1) accelerating the wound healing process through recruitment and differentiation of mesenchymal cells critical to establishing an osseous interface at the implant surface (Sanchez et al. ; Mendonca et al. 2009a, b; Bryington et al. 2012). It is the interaction with the surface and serum proteins which appear to create the primary effect of implant surface topography (Christenson et al. 2007). In fact, titanium surfaces modified through a controlled etching process have been shown to alter whole blood-derived platelet adhesion and generated thrombin-antithrombin complexes (Thor et al. 2007). Platelet activation has also been elevated on etched titanium surfaces. When platelet adhesion and activation were compared on machined versus blasted/etched titanium surfaces, in vitro, the smoother machined surfaces demonstrated higher adhesion of platelets but reduced activation, while the rougher surfaces demonstrated reduced platelet adhesion but near 100% platelet degranulation (Stanford et al. 2006).

During the initial remodeling steps, there are a number of immune cells mediating early tissue development (platelets, PMNs) followed by an in-migration of phagocyte macrophages (Mosser and Edwards 2008; Pollard 2009; Stanford 2010). The complex and pluripotent role of macrophages has recently become engaged in biomaterial research not just as mediators of debris removal but also potentially playing a key role in mediating new bone formation on the implant surface (Tan et al. 2006; Chehroudi et al. 2009; Thalji et al. 2013). There is a complex role of macrophages that range from the canonical or classically activated macrophage pathway due to bacterial derived lipopolysaccharide activated Toll-like receptors to the alternative or anabolic activated pathway (activation via IL4, IL13, and cell surface expression of CD206, arginase-1 receptor). It has been argued that there is in fact a continuum between these two cell types of macrophages and that anabolic wound healing is an important role of a subset of these cells (Mosser and Edwards 2008). Obviously, an initial role for these cells is to remove the necrotic debris created by the drilling process, but they then undergo physiological changes leading to expression of cell surface proteins (CD135) (Cao et al. 2006; Mosser and Edwards 2008). It is interesting to note that when histological studies are performed on clinically healed oral implants, there is often bone contact exceeding 50% of the implant surface area extending along the portion of the device that passes through the medullary cavity (Shalabi et al. 2006; Meirelles et al. 2007, 2008c; Veis et al. 2007). This allows rapid contact of the implant surface with marrow-derived monocytes and may be one reason for the observation of extensive adhesion of macrophages to retrieved implant surfaces (Tan et al. 2006; Thalji et al. 2013). From a biomaterial perspective, the influence on the wound healing capacity by macrophages may be strategic. These cells respond through both innate and adaptive responses which include response to basophil and mast cell release of IL-4 (Brandt et al. 2000; Loke et al. 2007). This cytokine-regulated cellular recruitment, migration, proliferation, and formation of an extracellular matrix on the implant surface can be influenced by this early population of macrophages. The end result of this complex cascade is promotion of a wound healing process that includes angiogenesis. The development of an elaborate vascular network is an important part of the implant wound healing process and may be elicited by the initial ischemia in the immediate wound site followed by the macrophage-mediated release of bFGF, TNF-α, and vascular endothelial growth factor (VEGF) (Lewis et al. 1999; Crowther et al. 2001; Okazaki et al. 2005).

The subsequent formation of a mineralized matrix during osteogenesis and bone remodeling or during osseointegration of dental implants involves the recruitment of multipotent mesenchymal stem cells and the progressive differentiation of these cells into osteoblasts (Aubin et al. 1995). Osteoblast differentiation and skeletal formation during embryonic development are mediated by an essential transcription factor protein called core-binding factor α (Cbfa1) or RUNX-2 (Ducy et al. 1997). Cbfa1 belongs to the Runt family of transcription factors (Xiao et al. 1998) and regulates osteoblast differentiation and expression of bone extracellular matrix protein genes that encode for bone sialoprotein (BSP), osteocalcin, and type I collagen (Ducy et al. 1999; Harada et al. 1999). RUNX-2/Cbfa1 plays an essential role in osteogenesis, osteoblast matrix formation, chondrocyte differentiation, and bone resorption by osteoclasts (Hoshi et al. 1999) and could therefore be a downstream target of cellular events such as extracellular matrix adhesion-mediated signaling, changes in cell shape, and responses to local paracrine environments. A second transcription factor, Osterix, has been described and has been suggested to play a key role downstream of RUNX-2 in which its expression is necessary for the ongoing differentiation within the osteogenic pathway (versus shifting to a chondrogenic pathway) (Nakashima et al. 2002). Upregulation of Ostrix and BSP was noted on alumina-coated titanium surfaces with a nanometer-level topography, relative to surfaces with just micrometer-level surface features. Human mesenchymal stem cells were grown over a 28-day period and demonstrated specific response to the etched titanium surfaces (Mendonca et al. 2009a, b; Valencia et al. 2009).

3.6 Implant Micro-retentive Features: Surface Roughness by Blasting/Etching

Currently there are two main, but interrelated, approaches being evaluated to enhance bone adaption to dental implant surfaces. Both approaches are designed to improve the adaptation of trabecular bone. The two approaches involve either the addition of biological mediators to the implant surface (e.g., cell adhesion or bioactive peptides, growth factors, etc.) or creation of reproducible nanoscale surface features.

The other direction for manipulating biological responses is to create topographical surface features at the nanoscale level on the titanium oxide surface. Relevant nanometer (10^{-9} m) scale features typically mean in the range of 1–100 nm in dimension. The interest in this area of research is that the conventional Newtonian properties of materials are very different for a nanomaterial (e.g., increased number of atoms at the surface, surface grain boundaries, enhanced surface energy and surface area, electron delocalization, etc.) (Webster and Ahn 2007; Meirelles et al. 2008a, b, c; Mendonca et al. 2008, 2009a, b; Valencia et al. 2009). At the nanoscale level molecular interactions with the surface can be targeted to create specific cell-level responses. For instance, work done with nanophase ceramics more than a decade ago demonstrated a specific increase in osteoblast cell adhesion, differentiation, and matrix expression on surfaces with a 60 nm grain size or less (Webster et al. 1999). If the grain size is 70 nm or greater, the specific biological effects are lost. Further studies suggested this effect may be related to protein orientation to the nanophase structures and specifically the mode of orientation of adhesion proteins such as vitronectin to the grain boundaries which in turn alters osteoblast adhesion and shape, both critical to formation of bone (Webster et al. 2000; Balasundaram and Webster 2007; Balasundaram et al. 2007; Christenson et al. 2007; Sato et al. 2007; Webster and Ahn 2007).

Over the past 25 years, the use of oral implants that replace missing teeth has undergone a rapid expansion. The basic biology remains the same and there are ongoing efforts to utilize our new knowledge to drive translational innovation, both the hard and soft tissue aspects of oral implant utilization. Research is helping to drive innovation both to improve the predictability of patient care and to assist the clinician in enhanced predictability, especially in challenging situations.

References

Abuhussein H, Pagni G, Rebaudi A, Wang HL (2010) The effect of thread pattern upon implant osseointegration. Clin Oral Implants Res 21(2):129–136

Albrektsson T, Sennerby L (1991) State of the art in oral implants. J Clin Periodontol 18(6):474–481

Arnhart C, Kielbassa AM, Martinez-de Fuentes R, Goldstein M, Jackowski J, Lorenzoni M, Maiorana C, Mericske-Stern R, Pozzi A, Rompen E, Sanz M, Strub JR (2012) Comparison of variable-thread tapered implant designs to a standard tapered implant design after immediate loading. A 3-year multicentre randomised controlled trial. Eur J Oral Implantol 5(2):123–136

Atieh MA, Zadeh H, Stanford CM, Cooper LF (2012) Survival of short dental implants for treatment of posterior partial edentulism: a systematic review. Int J Oral Maxillofac Implants 27(6):1323–1331

Aubin JE, Liu F, Malaval L, Gupta AK (1995) Osteoblast and chondroblast differentiation. Bone 17(2 Suppl):77S–83S

Ausiello P, Franciosa P, Martorelli M, Watts DC (2012) Effects of thread features in osseo-integrated titanium implants using a statistics-based finite element method. Dent Mater 28(8):919–927

Balasundaram G, Webster TJ (2007) An overview of nano-polymers for orthopedic applications. Macromol Biosci 7(5):635–642

Balasundaram G, Yao C, Webster TJ (2007) TiO(2) nanotubes functionalized with regions of bone morphogenetic protein-2 increases osteoblast adhesion. J Biomed Mater Res A 84(2):447–453

Barwacz CA, Stanford CM, Diehl UA, Qian F, Cooper LF, Feine J, McGuire M (2015) Electronic assessment of peri-implant mucosal esthetics around three implant-abutment configurations: a randomized clinical trial. Clin Oral Implants Res. 27(6): 707–715

Berglundh T, Abrahamsson I, Lindhe J (2005) Bone reactions to longstanding functional load at implants: an experimental study in dogs. J Clin Periodontol 32(9):925–932

Berglundh T, Persson L, Klinge B (2002) A systematic review of the incidence of biological and technical complications in implant dentistry reported in prospective longitudinal studies of at least 5 years. J Clin Periodontol 29(Suppl 3):197–212 ; discussion 232–193

Binon PP (2000) Implants and components: entering the new millennium. Int J Oral Maxillofac Implants 15(1):76–94

Bishti S, Strub JR, Att W (2014) Effect of the implant-abutment interface on peri-implant tissues: a systematic review. Acta Odontol Scand 72(1):13–25

Brandt E, Woerly G, Younes AB, Loiseau S, Capron M (2000) IL-4 production by human polymorphonuclear neutrophils. J Leukoc Biol 68(1):125–130

Brunski JB (2000) The new millennium in biomaterials and biomechanics. Int J Oral Maxillofac Implants 15(3):327–328

Bryington M, Mendonca G, Nares S, Cooper LF (2012) Osteoblastic and cytokine gene expression of implant-adherent cells in humans. Clin Oral Implants Res. 25(1):52–58

Buser D, Schenk RK, Steinemann S, Fiorellini JP, Fox CH, Stich H (1991) Influence of surface characteristics on bone integration of titanium implants. A histomorphometric study in miniature pigs [see comments]. J Biomed Mater Res 25(7):889–902

Cao S, Zhang X, Edwards JP, Mosser DM (2006) NF-kappaB1 (p50) homodimers differentially regulate pro- and anti-inflammatory cytokines in macrophages. J Biol Chem 281(36):26041–26050

Cecchinato D, Lops D, Salvi GE, Sanz M (2015) A prospective, randomized, controlled study using OsseoSpeed() implants placed in maxillary fresh extraction socket: soft tissues response. Clin Oral Implants Res 26(1):20–27

Chehroudi B, Ghrebi S, Murakami H, Waterfield JD, Owen G, Brunette DM (2009) Bone formation on rough, but not polished, subcutaneously implanted Ti surfaces is preceded by macrophage accumulation. J Biomed Mater Res A 93(2):724–737

Christenson EM, Anseth KS, van den Beucken JJ, Chan CK, Ercan B, Jansen JA, Laurencin CT, Li WJ,

Murugan R, Nair LS, Ramakrishna S, Tuan RS, Webster TJ, Mikos AG (2007) Nanobiomaterial applications in orthopedics. J Orthop Res 25(1):11–22

Cooper LF, Pin-Harry OC (2013) "Rules of Six" – diagnostic and therapeutic guidelines for single-tooth implant success. Compend Contin Educ Dent 34(2):94–98 100–101; quiz 102, 117

Cooper LF, Reside G, Stanford C, Barwacz C, Feine J, Abi Nader S, Scheyer ET, McGuire M (2015) A multicenter randomized comparative trial of implants with different abutment interfaces to replace anterior maxillary single teeth. Int J Oral Maxillofac Implants 30(3):622–632

Crowther M, Brown NJ, Bishop ET, Lewis CE (2001) Microenvironmental influence on macrophage regulation of angiogenesis in wounds and malignant tumors. J Leukoc Biol 70(4):478–490

Davies JE (1998) Mechanisms of endosseous integration. Int J Prosthodont 11(5):391–401

Ducy P, Starbuck M, Priemel M, Shen J, Pinero G, Geoffroy V, Amling M, Karsenty G (1999) A Cbfa1-dependent genetic pathway controls bone formation beyond embryonic development. Genes Dev 13(8):1025–1036

Ducy P, Zhang R, Geoffroy V, Ridall AL, Karsenty G (1997) Osf2/Cbfa1: a transcriptional activator of osteoblast differentiation. Cell 89(5):747–754

Ferrari M, Cagidiaco MC, Garcia-Godoy F, Goracci C, Cairo F (2015) Effect of different prosthetic abutments on peri-implant soft tissue. A randomized controlled clinical trial. Am J Dent 28(2):85–89

Fink J, Fuhrmann R, Scharnweber T, Franke RP (2008) Stimulation of monocytes and macrophages: possible influence of surface roughness. Clin Hemorheol Microcirc 39(1–4):205–212

Fransson C, Lekholm U, Jemt T, Berglundh T (2005) Prevalence of subjects with progressive bone loss at implants. Clin Oral Implants Res 16(4):440–446

Gulje F, Abrahamsson I, Chen S, Stanford C, Zadeh H, Palmer R (2012) Implants of 6 mm vs. 11 mm lengths in the posterior maxilla and mandible: a 1-year multicenter randomized controlled trial. Clin Oral Implants Res. 24(12):1325–1331

Gulje F, Abrahamsson I, Chen S, Stanford C, Zadeh H, Palmer R (2013) Implants of 6 mm vs. 11 mm lengths in the posterior maxilla and mandible: a 1-year multicenter randomized controlled trial. Clin Oral Implants Res 24(12):1325–1331

Halldin A, Jimbo R, Johansson CB, Wennerberg A, Jacobsson M, Albrektsson T, Hansson S (2014) Implant stability and bone remodeling after 3 and 13 days of implantation with an initial static strain. Clin Implant Dent Relat Res 16(3):383–393

Hansson S (1999) The implant neck: smooth or provided with retention elements – a biomechanical approach. Clin Oral Implants Res 10(5):394–405

Hansson S (2000) Surface roughness parameters as predictors of anchorage strength in bone: a critical analysis. J Biomech 33(10):1297–1303

Hansson S, Halldin A (2009) Re: effect of microthreads and platform switching on crestal bone stress levels: a finite element analysis. J Periodontol 80(7):1033–1035 authors response 1035–1036

Harada H, Tagashira S, Fujiwara M, Ogawa S, Katsumata T, Yamaguchi A, Komori T, Nakatsuka M (1999) Cbfa1 isoforms exert functional differences in osteoblast differentiation. J Biol Chem 274(11):6972–6978

Hoshi K, Komori T, Ozawa H (1999) Morphological characterization of skeletal cells in Cbfa1-deficient mice. Bone 25(6):639–651

Kasemo B, Lausmaa J (1994) Material-tissue interfaces: the role of surface properties and processes. Environ Health Perspect 102(Suppl 5):41–45

Lang NP, Berglundh T, Heitz-Mayfield LJ, Pjetursson BE, Salvi GE, Sanz M (2004) Consensus statements and recommended clinical procedures regarding implant survival and complications. Int J Oral Maxillofac Implants 19(Suppl):150–154

Leknes KN, Yang J, Qahash M, Polimeni G, Susin C, Wikesjo UM (2008) Alveolar ridge augmentation using implants coated with recombinant human bone morphogenetic protein-2: radiographic observations. Clin Oral Implants Res 19(10):1027–1033

Lewis JS, Lee JA, Underwood JC, Harris AL, Lewis CE (1999) Macrophage responses to hypoxia: relevance to disease mechanisms. J Leukoc Biol 66(6):889–900

Linkevicius T, Puisys A, Steigmann M, Vindasiute E, Linkeviciene L (2014) Influence of vertical soft tissue thickness on crestal bone changes around implants with platform switching: a comparative clinical study. Clin Implant Dent Relat Res. 17(6):1228–1236

Loke P, Gallagher I, Nair MG, Zang X, Brombacher F, Mohrs M, Allison JP, Allen JE (2007) Alternative activation is an innate response to injury that requires CD4+ T cells to be sustained during chronic infection. J Immunol 179(6):3926–3936

Lops D, Bressan E, Parpaiola A, Luca S, Cecchinato D, Romeo E (2014) Soft tissues stability of cad-cam and stock abutments in anterior regions: 2-year prospective multicentric cohort study. Clin Oral Implants Res. 26(12):1436–1442

Mathieu V, Vayron R, Richard G, Lambert G, Naili S, Meningaud JP, Haiat G (2014) Biomechanical determinants of the stability of dental implants: influence of the bone-implant interface properties. J Biomech 47(1):3–13

Meirelles L, Albrektsson T, Kjellin P, Arvidsson A, Franke-Stenport V, Andersson M, Currie F, Wennerberg A (2008a) Bone reaction to nano hydroxyapatite modified titanium implants placed in a gap-healing model. J Biomed Mater Res A. 87(3):624–631

Meirelles L, Arvidsson A, Albrektsson T, Wennerberg A (2007) Increased bone formation to unstable nano rough titanium implants. Clin Oral Implants Res 18(3):326–332

Meirelles L, Arvidsson A, Andersson M, Kjellin P, Albrektsson T, Wennerberg A (2008b) Nano hydroxyapatite structures influence early bone formation. J Biomed Mater Res A. 87(2):299–307

Meirelles L, Melin L, Peltola T, Kjellin P, Kangasniemi I, Currie F, Andersson M, Albrektsson T, Wennerberg A (2008c) Effect of hydroxyapatite and titania nanostructures on early in vivo bone response. Clin Implant Dent Relat Res. 10(4):245–254

Mendonca G, Mendonca DB, Aragao FJ, Cooper LF (2008) Advancing dental implant surface technology – from micron- to nanotopography. Biomaterials 29(28):3822–3835

Mendonca G, Mendonca DB, Simoes LG, Araujo AL, Leite ER, Duarte WR, Aragao FJ, Cooper LF (2009a) The effects of implant surface nanoscale features on osteoblast-specific gene expression. Biomaterials 30(25):4053–4062

Mendonca G, Mendonca DB, Simoes LG, Araujo AL, Leite ER, Duarte WR, Cooper LF, Aragao FJ (2009b) Nanostructured alumina-coated implant surface: effect on osteoblast-related gene expression and bone-to-implant contact in vivo. Int J Oral Maxillofac Implants 24(2):205–215

Mertens C, Meyer-Baumer A, Kappel H, Hoffmann J, Steveling HG (2012) Use of 8-mm and 9-mm implants in atrophic alveolar ridges: 10-year results. Int J Oral Maxillofac Implants 27(6):1501–1508

Mosser DM, Edwards JP (2008) Exploring the full spectrum of macrophage activation. Nat Rev Immunol 8(12):958–969

Nakashima K, Zhou X, Kunkel G, Zhang ZP, Deng JM, Behringer RR, de Crombrugghe B (2002) The novel zinc finger-containing transcription factor Osterix is required for osteoblast differentiation and bone formation. Cell 108(1):17–29

Norton M (2013) Primary stability versus viable constraint – a need to redefine. Int J Oral Maxillofac Implants 28(1):19–21

Norton MR (1998) Marginal bone levels at single tooth implants with a conical fixture design. The influence of surface macro- and microstructure. Clin Oral Implants Res 9(2):91–99

Okazaki T, Ebihara S, Takahashi H, Asada M, Kanda A, Sasaki H (2005) Macrophage colony-stimulating factor induces vascular endothelial growth factor production in skeletal muscle and promotes tumor angiogenesis. J Immunol 174(12):7531–7538

Orsini E, Giavaresi G, Trire A, Ottani V, Salgarello S (2012) Dental implant thread pitch and its influence on the osseointegration process: an in vivo comparison study. Int J Oral Maxillofac Implants 27(2):383–392

Patil R, van Brakel R, Iyer K, Huddleston Slater J, de Putter C, Cune M (2013) A comparative study to evaluate the effect of two different abutment designs on soft tissue healing and stability of mucosal margins. Clin Oral Implants Res 24(3):336–341

Pollard JW (2009) Trophic macrophages in development and disease. Nat Rev Immunol 9(4):259–270

Renvert S, Roos-Jansaker AM, Lindahl C, Renvert H, Rutger Persson G (2007) Infection at titanium implants with or without a clinical diagnosis of inflammation. Clin Oral Implants Res. 18(4):509–516

Roos-Jansaker AM, Lindahl C, Renvert H, Renvert S (2006a) Nine- to fourteen-year follow-up of implant treatment. Part I: implant loss and associations to various factors. J Clin Periodontol 33(4):283–289

Roos-Jansaker AM, Lindahl C, Renvert H, Renvert S (2006b) Nine- to fourteen-year follow-up of implant treatment. Part II: presence of peri-implant lesions. J Clin Periodontol 33(4):290–295

Roos-Jansaker AM, Renvert H, Lindahl C, Renvert S (2006c) Nine- to fourteen-year follow-up of implant treatment. Part III: factors associated with peri-implant lesions. J Clin Periodontol 33(4):296–301

Roos J, Sennerby L, Albrektsson T (1997) An update on the clinical documentation on currently used bone anchored endosseous oral implants. Dent Updat 24(5):194–200

Sanchez AR, Sheridan PJ, Kupp LI (2003) Is platelet-rich plasma the perfect enhancement factor? A current review. Int J Oral Maxillofac Implants 18(1):93–103

Sato M, Aslani A, Sambito MA, Kalkhoran NM, Slamovich EB, Webster TJ (2007) Nanocrystalline hydroxyapatite/titania coatings on titanium improves osteoblast adhesion. J Biomed Mater Res A 84(1):265–272

Shalabi MM, Gortemaker A, Van't Hof MA, Jansen JA, Creugers NH (2006) Implant surface roughness and bone healing: a systematic review. J Dent Res 85(6):496–500

Sims NA, Gooi JH (2008) Bone remodeling: Multiple cellular interactions required for coupling of bone formation and resorption. Semin Cell Dev Biol 19(5):444–451

Slaets E, Naert I, Carmeliet G, Duyck J (2009) Early cortical bone healing around loaded titanium implants: a histological study in the rabbit. Clin Oral Implants Res 20(2):126–134

Smith DE, Zarb GA (1989) Criteria for success of osseointegrated endosseous implants. J Prosthet Dent 62(5):567–572

Stanford C, Schneider G, Masaki C, Zaharias R, Seabold D, Eckdhal J, Di Paola J (2006) Effects of fluoride-modified titanium dioxide grit blasted implant surfaces on platelet activation and osteoblast differentiation. Appl Osseointegration Res 5:24–30

Stanford CM (1999) Biomechanical and functional behavior of implants. Adv Dent Res 13:88–92

Stanford CM (2010) Surface modification of biomedical and dental implants and the processes of inflammation, wound healing and bone formation. Int J Mol Sci 11(1):354–369

Stanford CM, Brand RA (1999) Toward an understanding of implant occlusion and strain adaptive bone modeling and remodeling. J Prosthet Dent 81(5):553–561

Tan KS, Qian L, Rosado R, Flood PM, Cooper LF (2006) The role of titanium surface topography on J774A.1 macrophage inflammatory cytokines and nitric oxide production. Biomaterials 27(30):5170–5177

Thalji G, Cooper LF (2013) Molecular assessment of osseointegration in vivo: a review of the current literature. Int J Oral Maxillofac Implants 28(6):e521–e534

Thalji G, Cooper LF (2014) Molecular assessment of osseointegration in vitro: a review of current literature. Int J Oral Maxillofac Implants 29(2):e171–e199

Thalji GN, Nares S, Cooper LF (2013) Early molecular assessment of osseointegration in humans. Clin Oral Implants Res. 25(11):1273–1285

Thor A, Rasmusson L, Wennerberg A, Thomsen P, Hirsch JM, Nilsson B, Hong J (2007) The role of whole blood in thrombin generation in contact with various titanium surfaces. Biomaterials 28(6):966–974

Valencia S, Gretzer C, Cooper LF (2009) Surface nanofeature effects on titanium-adherent human mesenchymal stem cells. Int J Oral Maxillofac Implants 24(1):38–46

Veis AA, Papadimitriou S, Trisi P, Tsirlis AT, Parissis NA, Kenealy JN (2007) Osseointegration of Osseotite and machined-surfaced titanium implants in membrane-covered critical-sized defects: a histologic and histometric study in dogs. Clin Oral Implants Res 18(2):153–160

Wang YC, Kan JY, Rungcharassaeng K, Roe P, Lozada JL (2015) Marginal bone response of implants with platform switching and non-platform switching abutments in posterior healed sites: a 1-year prospective study. Clin Oral Implants Res 26(2):220–227

Webster TJ, Ahn ES (2007) Nanostructured biomaterials for tissue engineering bone. Adv Biochem Eng Biotechnol 103:275–308

Webster TJ, Ergun C, Doremus RH, Siegel RW, Bizios R (2000) Specific proteins mediate enhanced osteoblast adhesion on nanophase ceramics. J Biomed Mater Res 51(3):475–483

Webster TJ, Siegel RW, Bizios R (1999) Design and evaluation of nanophase alumina for orthopaedic/dental applications. Nanostruct Mater 12(5–8):983–986

Wennerberg A, Albrektsson T (2000) Suggested guidelines for the topographic evaluation of implant surfaces. Int J Oral Maxillofac Implants 15(3):331–344

Wennerberg A, Ektessabi A, Albrektsson T, Johansson C, Andersson B (1997) A 1-year follow-up of implants of differing surface roughness placed in rabbit bone. Int J Oral Maxillofac Implants 12(4):486–494

Wennstrom JL, Derks J (2012) Is there a need for keratinized mucosa around implants to maintain health and tissue stability? Clin Oral Implants Res 23(Suppl 6):136–146

Widmark G, Andersson B, Carlsson GE, Lindvall AM, Ivanoff CJ (2001) Rehabilitation of patients with severely resorbed maxillae by means of implants with or without bone grafts: a 3-to 5-year follow-up clinical report. Int J Oral Maxillofac Implants 16(1):73–79

Wikesjo UM, Qahash M, Polimeni G, Susin C, Shanaman RH, Rohrer MD, Wozney JM, Hall J (2008) Alveolar ridge augmentation using implants coated with recombinant human bone morphogenetic protein-2: histologic observations. J Clin Periodontol 35(11):1001–1010

Xiao G, Wang D, Benson MD, Karsenty G, Franceschi RT (1998) Role of the alpha2-integrin in osteoblast-specific gene expression and activation of the Osf2 transcription factor. J Biol Chem 273(49):32988–32994

Revisiting the Role of Implant Design and Surgical Instrumentation on Osseointegration

4

Paulo G. Coelho, Estevam A. Bonfante, and Ryo Jimbo

Abstract

Osseointegration of metallic devices has shown to be successful in several biomedical fields. Despite the high success rates, continuous efforts to reduce osseointegration time have been marked by investigations considering a limited number of variables. Recent research has pointed that the interplay between surgical instrumentation and device macrogeometry not only plays a key role on both early and delayed stages of osseointegration but may also be key in how efficient smaller length scale designing (at the micro- and nanogeometrical levels) may be in hastening early stages of osseointegration. The present chapter focuses on how the different metallic device design length scales' interplay (macro, micro, and nano) affects the bone response and how its understanding may affect the next generation of metallic device designing for osseointegration.

P.G. Coelho, DDS, PhD
Department of Biomaterials and Biomimetics,
Hansjörg Wyss Department of Plastic Surgery,
NYU College of Dentistry, NYU Langone Medical Center, 433 1st ave room 844, New York, NY, 10010, USA
e-mail: pgcoelho@nyu.edu

E.A. Bonfante, DDS, MS, PhD (✉)
Department of Prosthodontics and Periodontology,
Bauru School of Dentistry – University of São Paulo,
Al. Otavio Pinheiro Brisola 9-75, Bauru, SP, Brazil, 17.012-901
e-mail: estevamab@gmail.com

R. Jimbo, DDS, PhD
Department of Oral and Maxillofacial Surgery and Oral Medicine, Faculty of Odontology,
Malmö University, Carl Gustafs väg 34,
SE 205 06, Malmo, Sweden
e-mail: ryo.jimbo@mah.se

4.1 Introduction

The healing of bone around metallic devices including titanium was described in 1940 by Bothe et al. (1940). With further results demonstrating minimal soft tissue reaction to titanium in 1951 by Leventhal (1951) who suggested that anchorage to titanium prostheses would be feasible. Several years later, research led by Per-Ingvar Brånemark (Branemark et al. 1977) and his group described it as the formation of a direct interface between an implant and bone without soft tissue interposition at the optical microscopy level. The term osseointegration was suggested in 1981 (Albrektsson et al. 1981; Albrektsson and Johansson 2001) and has operated in modern metallic bone anchor devices utilized in orthopedics, craniomaxillofacial fixation, and in dental implants where biomechanical competence is achieved through their surgical placement, bone healing, and subsequent remodeling (Coelho et al. 2009, 2015; Coelho and Jimbo 2014). Its application has improved the quality of life of millions of patients in the past half century and has been the foundation for multiple implant rehabilitative procedures (Barber et al. 2011).

The continued evolution of implantable devices has allowed significant improvement in the quality and the rate of osseointegration. The potential to increase host-to-implant response has fostered clinical treatment protocols that decrease or eliminate the time allowed between surgical placement and functional loading (De Bruyn et al. 2013; Shigehara et al. 2014; Vervaeke et al. 2013). Although osseointegration in most instances has been hastened by a multitude of individual implant design parameters, we are still far from reaching implant systems (hereon defined as the implant hardware and software altogether) that are atemporally stable (Browaeys et al. 2014; Deporter et al. 2012; Jimbo et al. 2013a, b, c; Yeniyol et al. 2013). An atemporally stable device is a desired target since it would allow clinicians to rehabilitate patients in the shortest treatment time (Jimbo et al. 2014).

The difficulty in designing atemporally stable implant systems primarily lies upon the historical lack of a hierarchical approach concerning the multivariable nature of bone healing around implants, which eventually hinders biomedical engineers to retrospectively address the interaction of the main design parameters such as macrogeometry, microgeometry, nanogeometry, and surgical instrumentation in an objective fashion (Coelho et al. 2009, 2015; Coelho and Jimbo 2014; Jimbo et al.2014). Due to poor baseline knowledge of the contribution of implant main design variables on both early and delayed bone response, a systematic approach that addresses implant design in a multifactorial fashion is warranted.

Currently, a MEDLINE literature search shows that implant surface design investigations outnumber all the other implant design studies by two orders of magnitude. While it is desirable to design surfaces that will hasten osseointegration, its relative contribution when other parameters are involved, such as two different implant systems presenting distinct macrogeometry and surgical instrumentation and the same surface treatment, is seldom reported in the literature (Coelho et al. 2011).

This chapter will present how osseointegration is determined by numerous factors such as surgical drilling protocols, drilling speed, implant macrogeometry, implant micro- and nanotopography, and status of the host bone quality (Albrektsson et al. 1981; Jimbo et al. 2012; Oh et al. 2002).

Given the breadth of the topic, it will attempt to provide a first step toward understanding how bulk device design and related surgical instrumentation dimensions (implant hardware) influence short- and long-term osseointegration. While of extreme importance, the effect of the here defined implant software (micrometer and nanometer design alterations) will be briefly presented in light of how they can be efficiently incorporated in implant systems as a function of implant hardware design.

4.2 Bone Healing Pathway and Long-Term Osseointegration Is Affected by Implant Hardware

After sometime following implantation, an intimate contact between bone and endosteal device (cleaned and sterilized commercially pure Ti and Ti-6Al-4V) will biomechanically stabilize these bone anchors that may be utilized for multiple purposes (Chowdhary et al. 2013; Coelho et al. 2014; Gottlow et al. 2012). Far less reported is how osseointegration temporally varies as a function of two major key parameters: implant macrogeometry and its associated surgical instrumentation dimensions (Coelho et al. 2010; Leonard et al. 2009). While it is obvious that two different parameters are under consideration, their contribution to the healing mode cannot be considered separately, rationalizing the term implant hardware, a factor which will primarily drive bone healing mode around dental implants leading to their ultimate osseointegration, as subsequently presented (Coelho et al. 2010; Leonard et al. 2009).

4.2.1 Interfacial Remodeling Healing Pathway

Arguably, one of the most important aspects with regard to achieving osseointegration clinically is implant initial stability. Initial or primary stability, also known as mechanical stability, is the sole mechanical interlocking between the bone and the implant where there exists no biologic interplay (Halldin et al. 2011; Norton 2013). And once again, initial stability cannot be regarded as osseointegration since osseointegration is the result of the osteoconduction of the implant system. The mechanical interlocking is influenced by the implant geometry and topography at different levels, as well as the implant osteotomy protocols, which all regulate the strain applied to the hard tissue in proximity of the implant (Gottlow et al. 2012; Isidor 2006; Petrie and Williams 2005). Strain is directly related to bone-implant interfacial stress and frictional force, which is expressed clinically as insertion torque (Chowdhary et al. 2013; Halldin et al. 2011; Huang et al. 2011).

In general, higher insertion torque of the implant is intuitively and fallaciously perceived as higher primary stability, which has been clinically regarded as an indication for procedures such as immediate loading (Javed and Romanos 2010; Freitas et al. 2012). The theoretical background to this concept is that the bone is assumed to be an elastic material and that strain and implant stability will have a linear relation (Halldin et al. 2011). However, in reality, the stability of the implant would decrease beyond the yield strain of the bone due to excessive microcrack formation and compression necrosis, which both phenomena trigger bone remodeling (Chamay and Tschantz 1972; Halldin et al. 2011; Verborgt et al. 2000). Although microcrack formation is regarded as an important phenomenon for the intracortical remodeling (Bentolila et al. 1998), the excessive microcrack formation however has the risk of generating a macrocrack (fracture) through interconnection of unrepaired individual microcracks (Burr et al. 1997, 1998). Compression necrosis occurs when the hard tissue around the implant is faced with excessive strain, where the circulation of the capillaries and nerves is severely damaged (Zizic et al. 1985). Both microcracking and compression necrosis are observed to different degrees when a mismatch between implant thread outer diameter and surgical instrumentation inner diameter is present. Thus, depending on the thread design and its related surgical instrumentation dimension, different degrees of friction and interlock between implant and bone will be generated leading to higher or lower degrees of insertion torque, equivocally interpreted by several clinicians as proportional to implant primary stability, despite experimental evidence proving otherwise (Bashutski et al. 2009; Freitas et al. 2012; Jimbo et al. 2014).

High degrees of insertion torque must be questioned since elastic theory predicts that excessive strain leads to a decrease of biomechanical stability and provokes negative biologic responses depending on the implant thread design controlling the compression (Jimbo et al. 2014). Such cell-mediated bone resorption and subsequent bone apposition from the pristine bone wall toward the implant surface are responsible for what has under theoretical (Raghavendra et al. 2005) and experimental (Gomes et al. 2013) basis been coined as implant stability dip, where high degrees of stability (primary stability) obtained through the mismatch between implant macrogeometry and surgical instrumentation dimensions are lost due to the cell-mediated interfacial remodeling to be regained through bone apposition (Jimbo et al. 2007; Raghavendra et al. 2005).

This healing mode scenario is presented in Fig. 4.1. It is imperative to note at this stage that canine bone healing takes place substantially faster (controversy exists in the literature regarding to its magnitude) than humans. Figure 4.1 depicts V-shaped threaded implants placed in sites that were surgically instrumented to

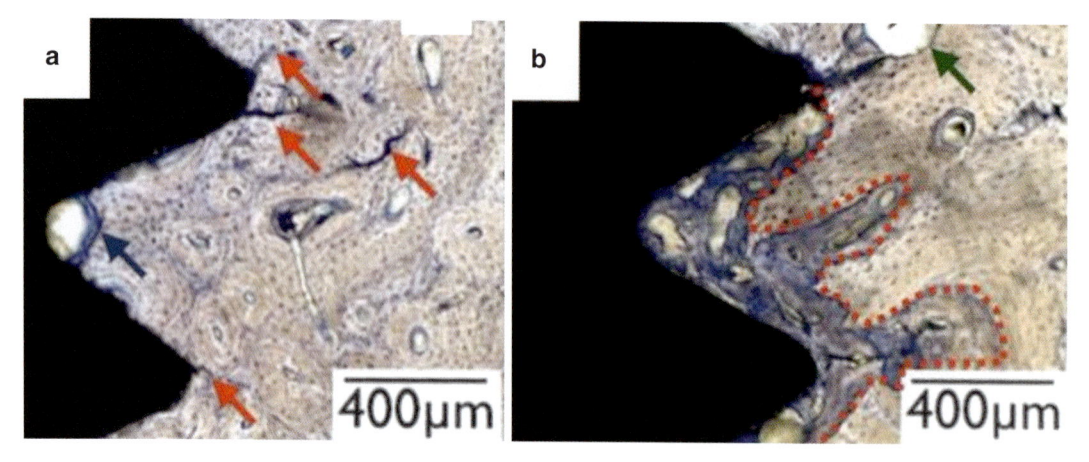

Fig. 4.1 Optical micrographs of V-threaded implants placed in sites surgically instrumented to the inner diameter of the implant thread at (**a**) 2 weeks and (**b**) 4 weeks in vivo in a beagle dog model. (**a**) At 2 weeks in vivo, the almost continuous bone-implant interface reveals mechanical interlocking between components, responsible to the implant primary stability. The *red arrows* depict microcracks at regions where the yield strength of bone has been exceeded due to high stress concentration; the *blue arrow* depicts initial remodeling taking place between the implant threads due to compression necrosis. (**b**) At 4 weeks, substantial remodeling has occurred at the interface where cell-mediated processes resorbed the region encompassed between the *dashed line* and the implant. A remodeling site occurring at the extension of a microcrack is depicted by a *green arrow* (From Coelho and Jimbo (2014). With permission from Elsevier)

dimensions matching the inner diameter of the implant threads (Fig. 4.1) (Bonfante et al. 2013). The optical micrographs presented in Fig. 4.1 were obtained from implants that remained in vivo for 2 (Fig. 4.1a) and 4 weeks (Fig. 4.1b) in a canine laboratory model. At 2 weeks in vivo (Fig. 4.1a), the almost continuous bone-implant interface revealed mechanical interlocking between components, responsible for the implant primary stability. At 2 weeks, microcracks at regions where the yield strength of bone has been exceeded due to high stress concentration are easily depicted along with initial remodeling taking place between the implant threads due to compression necrosis. At 4 weeks (Fig. 4.1b), a substantial remodeling region is evident after compression necrosis and/or microcracking due to the mismatch between implant macrogeometry and drilled osteotomy dimensions. Remodeling sites occurring in the proximity of the microcrack can also be observed along with void spaces partially filled by newly formed bone that occurred between 2 and 4 weeks in vivo following the cell-mediated remodeling (Bonfante et al. 2013).

The panorama depicted in Fig. 4.1 not only histologically confirms the theoretical and experimental basis (Gomes et al. 2013; Raghavendra et al. 2005) for the initial stability rendered by mechanical interlocking between implant and bone that at some point in time decreased due to extensive resorption but also explains the higher clinical failure rates of early (1–2 months) compared to immediate or delayed loaded implants (4–6 months) (Esposito et al. 2009, 2013). In the purely interfacial remodeling pathway, early loading has been associated with increased failure rates likely because it takes place when the stability dip has reached its lowest valley to be succeeded by initial secondary stability gain (osseointegration). Subsequently, the resorbed area will be altered by newly formed woven bone, which eventually reestablishes the contact to the implant interface (secondary stability), and as per a plethora of implant retrieval studies has shown, bone in proximity to the implant has remodeled multiple times to a lamellar configuration that will support the metallic device throughout its lifetime (Coelho et al. 2009,

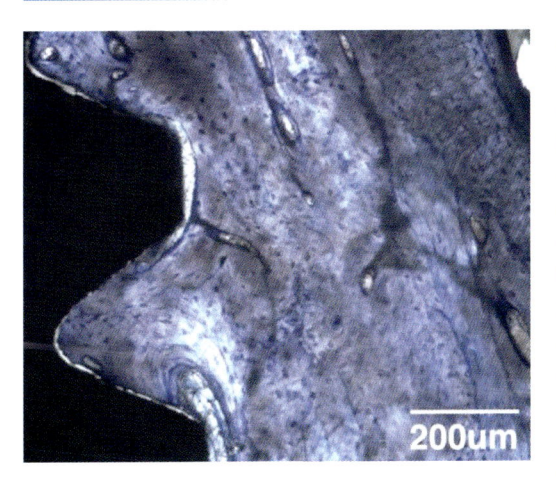

Fig. 4.2 A human retrieved sample at approximately 8 years of functional loading showing direct agreement with other reports for screw-type implants placed in undersized drilled sites. The bone surrounding these implants presents a compact mature lamellar bone with few and small marrow spaces (From Coelho and Jimbo (2014). With permission from Elsevier)

2010; Gil et al. 2014; Iezzi et al. 2012, 2014; Mangano et al. 2013).

Finally, under such implant hardware configuration, bone surrounding these devices has been often described as compact mature lamellar bone with few and small marrow spaces (Iezzi et al. 2014, Mangano et al. 2013) (Fig. 4.2). To date, no human retrieval study concerning implants that primarily heal through this pathway at dense bone regions has presented sufficiently large sample size to determine their time course alteration in histomorphometric and mechanical properties of osseointegration.

4.2.2 Intramembranous-Like Healing Pathway

The intramembranous-like healing pathway concerns the opposite scenario of the tight fit screw-type implant. Here, void spaces between the implant bulk and the surgically instrumented drilled site walls are formed (Berglundh et al. 2003) and are often referred as healing chambers. Such void spaces do not contribute to primary stability, but have been regarded as a key contributor to secondary stability (Coelho et al. 2010; Leonard et al. 2009). Immediately after implant placement, the healing chambers are filled with the blood clot that will evolve toward osteogenic tissue that subsequently ossifies through an intramembranous-like pathway (Berglundh et al. 2003). Therefore, implant healing chambers provide the pathway for direct new bone formation which skips the biologic cleanup process of the necrotic bone by the macrophages (Berglundh et al. 2003; Coelho et al. 2011).

This osseointegration pathway has been temporally characterized in preclinical studies, where independent of species (including humans), bone formation through the intramembranous-like pathway leads to rapid healing chamber filling with woven bone (Fig. 4.3a) (Berglundh et al. 2003; Bosshardt et al. 2011; Buser et al. 2004; Marin et al. 2010). Bone filling occurs from all surfaces bounding the healing chambers (surgically instrumented bone wall and implant surface) through contact osteogenesis, and bone nucleation occurs throughout the chamber volume (Coelho et al. 2010; Leonard et al. 2009; Marin et al. 2010; Suzuki et al. 2010). The woven bone is subsequently replaced by lamellar bone surrounding multiple primary osteonic structures throughout the healing chamber volume (Fig. 4.3b) (Leonard et al. 2009).

Several reports have demonstrated osteocyte lacunae in close proximity with the implant surface without hard or soft interposing tissue at the optical microscopy level demonstrating that bone-forming cells can easily populate the implant surface early after implant placement (Fig. 4.3c) and promote contact osteogenesis (Coelho et al. 2010; Marin et al. 2010). Human retrieval studies concerning the temporal morphology of implants that primarily heal through healing chambers have shown that the primary osteonic structure achieved over the first 6 months to a year after placement (Fig. 4.4a) remodels over time under functional loading evolving toward a haversian-like structure regardless of location in the maxilla or mandible (Coelho et al. 2009, 2010; Gil et al. 2014).

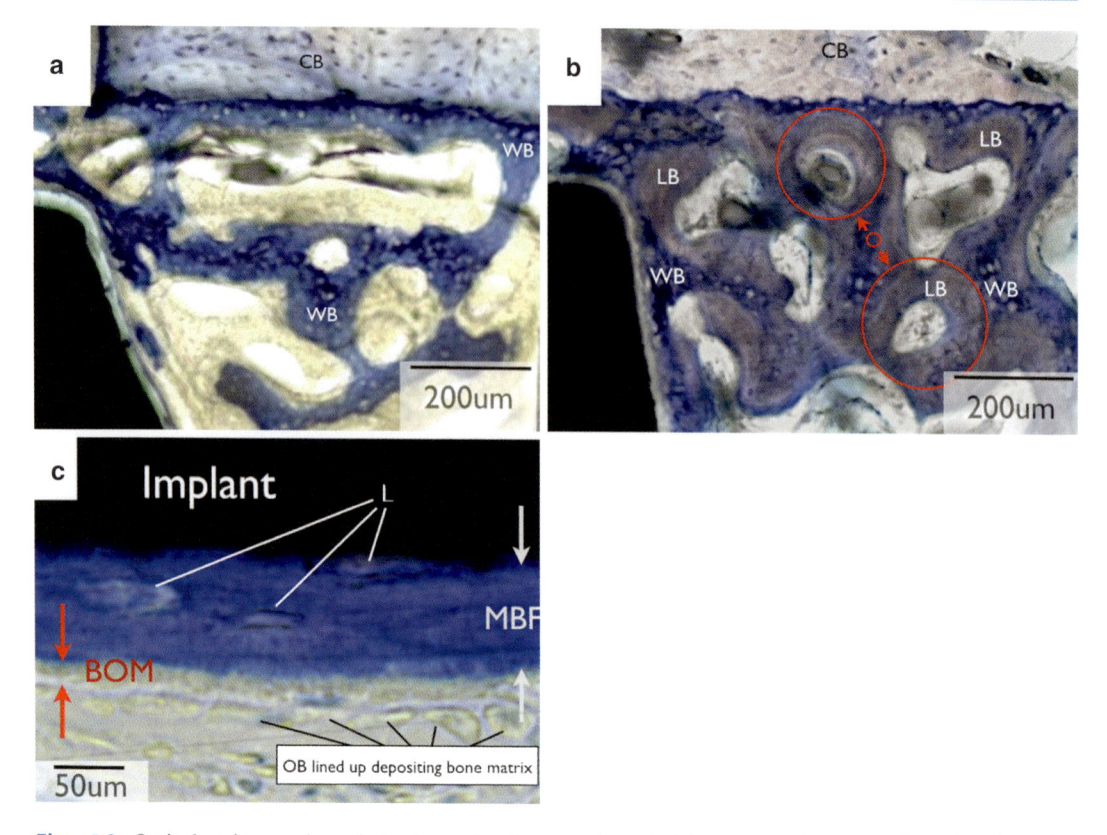

Fig. 4.3 Optical micrographs of healing chamber implants that remained (**a**) 3 weeks and (**b**) 5 weeks in vivo in a beagle dog model. (**a**) At 3 weeks in vivo, woven bone (*WB*) lining the surgically instrumented cortical bone plate (*CB*) and throughout the volume of the healing chamber region. (**b**) At 5 weeks, replacement of woven bone (*WB*) by lamellar bone (*LB*) throughout the healing chamber is depicted along with primary osteonic structures (*O*) which revealed that onset of woven bone remodeling toward lamellar configuration surrounding blood vessels. (**c**) Since immediately after placement, the void region rendered due to the implant macrogeometry and surgical instrumentation outer dimension is readily filled with a blood clot and healing takes place in an intramembranous-like pathway where cells readily migrate throughout the fibrin network, osteoblasts are able to directly populate the implant surface prior to matrix deposition, resulting in lacunae (*L*) directly in contact and in close proximity with the implant surface. *Lines of cube* shaped cells (osteoblasts, *OB*) depositing bone organic matrix (*BOM*) directly over the mineralizing bone front (*MBF*) are readily observed (From Coelho and Jimbo (2014). With permission from Elsevier)

While a haversian-like morphology is achieved 1 year after placement (Fig. 4.4b, c), nanomechanical evaluation of these human retrieved implants has shown that it is not until after approximately 5 years under functional loading that the haversian-like configuration significantly increase in mechanical property (both hardness and elastic modulus) (Baldassarri et al. 2012). Thus, while low levels of insertion torque are achieved when pure healing chamber implants are tapped into surgically instrumented sites drilled to the dimension of the implant outer diameter, the resulting healing mode presents substantial deviation from the classic interfacial remodeling healing pathway. Implants with healing chamber configurations possess sufficient level of primary stability (low micromotion), obtained with the tip of the implant threads or plateaus, stable enough for the blood clot trapped within chambers to enable the development of a highly osteogenic stroma through which osteogenic cells migrate resulting in osseointegration (Baldassarri et al. 2012; Coelho et al. 2009, 2010a, b; Gil et al. 2014; Leonard et al. 2009; Marin et al. 2010; Suzuki et al. 2010).

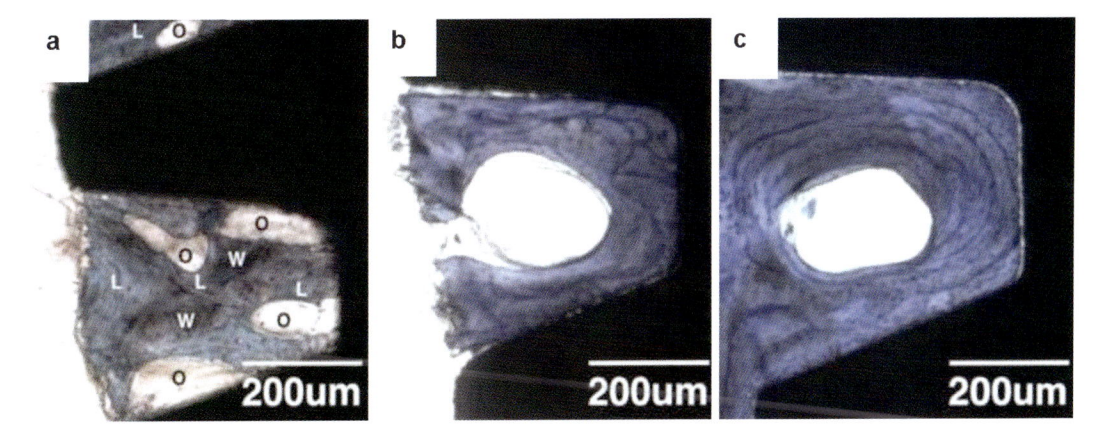

Fig. 4.4 Optical micrographs representative of (**a**) implants that were loaded up to 1 year in vivo that presented a mixed bone morphology with regions of woven (*w*) and lamellar bone surrounding primary osteonic structures (*O*). Implants that remained loaded for longer periods of time such as in (**b**) 5 years and (**c**) 18 years primarily presented a haversian-like lamellar structure (From Coelho and Jimbo (2014). With permission from Elsevier)

4.2.3 Temporal Comparison Between Interfacial Remodeling and Intramembranous-Like Healing Pathways

Whereas at longer healing times, both osseointegrated implants will present bone morphologic evolution toward more organized structures (Figs. 4.2 and 4.4), previous long-term human retrieval studies (Coelho et al. 2009, 2010; Gil et al. 2014) have shown the main differences in bone evolution over time between interfacial compared to intramembranous-like healing pathways. In the latter scenario, primary osteonic structures are present within the healing chambers, possibly due to the higher cellular and vascular content, eventually evolving toward a haversian-like structure (Fig. 4.4). Long-term mechanical properties have been well determined in a human retrieval study (Baldassarri et al. 2012). In contrast, a compact mature lamellar bone with few and small marrow spaces has been observed around implants which osseointegrated through interfacial remodeling (Fig. 4.2) (Iezzi et al. 2014; Mangano et al. 2013), and consistent characterization in human retrieval studies is yet to be performed in this scenario.

4.2.4 The Hybrid Healing Pathway: Merging Interfacial Remodeling and Intramembranous-Like Bone Healing Modes Through Implant Hardware Design

The hybrid healing pathway described in this section occurs when an outer thread design provides immediate device stability, while the inner thread and osteotomy dimensions allow healing chambers (Abrahamsson et al. 2004, 2009; Berglundh et al. 2003; Bonfante et al. 2011) or alterations in osteotomy dimensions in large thread pitch implant designs (Campos et al. 2012; Coelho et al. 2010, 2013) which will temporally maximize stability. The rationale for these alterations lies upon the fact that thread designing may allow for both high degrees of primary stability along with a surgical instrumentation outer diameter that is closer to the outer diameter of the implant allowing healing chamber formation. Since no bone resorption occurs in healing chambers and rapid intramembranous-like rapid woven bone formation occurs (Witek et al. 2013), such rapid bone growth may compensate for the implant stability loss due to compression regions where implant contacts bone for primary stability.

A healing mode shift has been demonstrated when incrementally increasing the final surgical instrumentation dimension from drilling to a dimension lower than the inner implant thread, to the dimension of the implant inner thread diameter, and to the implant outer thread diameter (Fig. 4.5) (Coelho et al. 2013). When the surgical instrumentation dimension was below the size of the implant inner thread, substantial interfacial remodeling occurred over time (Fig. 4.5a, b, e, f). When surgical instrumentation was closer to the implant outer thread dimensions, healing chambers formed and bone healed through the intramembranous-like pathway (Fig. 4.5c, f). These investigations highlighted that while all implants presented adequate primary stability (note that the study was conducted in beagle dogs, higher bone mechanical properties than humans), the higher torque values obtained during placement of the two smaller surgical instrumentation dimensions did not necessarily result in temporal healing panoramas that would maximize the implant-in-bone biomechanical competence (Campos et al. 2012; Coelho et al. 2013).

Different than altering surgical drilling dimension to obtain hybrid healing, implants presenting power thread designs to assure primary stability have been deliberately designed for placement into surgically instrumented sites with dimensions larger than the inner thread aspect of the implant (Fig. 4.6) (Bonfante et al. 2011; Jimbo et al. 2014). Relative to the micrographs presented in Fig. 4.1, a lower extension of bone resorption (interfacial remodeling) takes place at regions where the implant threads engaged bone

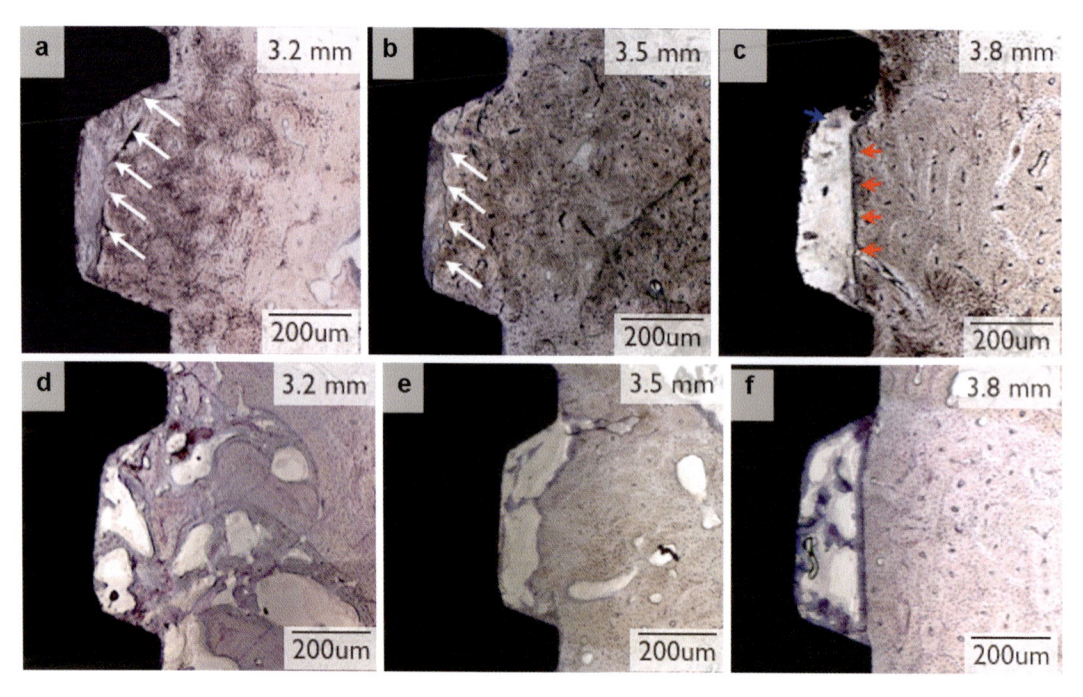

Fig. 4.5 1 Week in vivo optical micrographs of the implant-bone interface showing that implants placed into (**a**) 3.2 mm and (**b**) 3.5 mm drilling sites presented necrotic bone areas in the region between the first three implant threads (*white arrows*). Implants placed into (**c**) 3.8 mm drilling sites presented a chamber (depicted by *red arrows*) filled with osteogenic tissue between the implant inner diameter and the drilled wall. Initial osteoid nucleation was observed in minor amounts within the healing chamber (*blue arrow*). Three weeks in vivo optical micrographs of the implant-bone interface showing that implants placed into (**d**) 3.2 mm and (**e**) 3.5 mm drilling sites presented extensive remodeling along with newly formed bone. At 3 weeks, implants placed into (**f**) 3.8 mm drilling sites presented extensive woven bone formation at the drilled bone walls, implant surface, and within the healing chamber volume (From Coelho and Jimbo (2014). With permission from Elsevier)

4 Revisiting the Role of Implant Design and Surgical Instrumentation on Osseointegration   51

Fig. 4.6 Optical micrographs at (**a**) 2 weeks in vivo and (**b**) 4 weeks in vivo in a beagle model. The *red arrows* depict newly formed bone at the healing chambers regions; *yellow arrows* depict bone remodeling regions (From Coelho and Jimbo (2014). With permission from Elsevier)

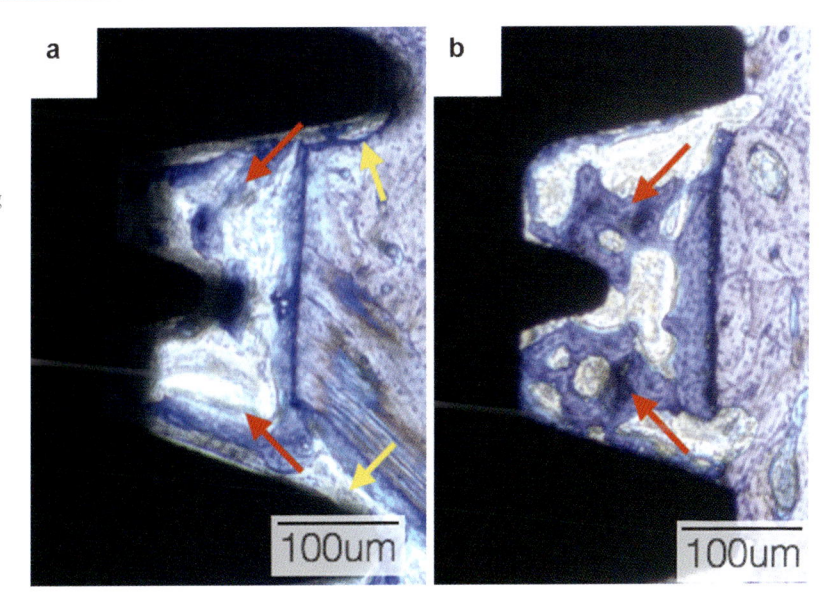

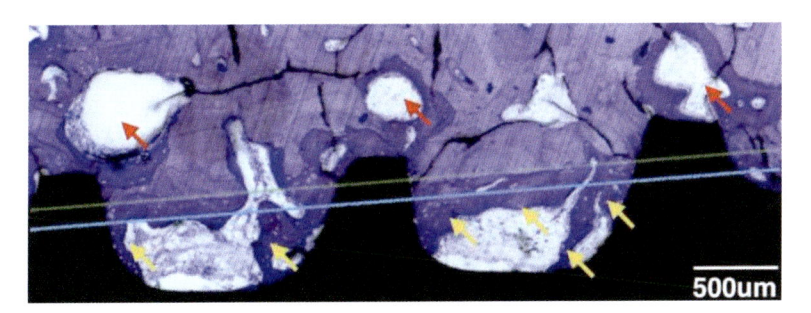

Fig. 4.7 Implant in bone presenting hybrid healing at the time when the regions that engaged bone due to a mismatch between implant thread outer diameter and surgical instrumentation outer diameter (*blue line*) present extensive remodeling (*red arrows*). Note the partial presence of bone replacing the void spaces from remodeling dark stained bone in proximity with the void spaces denoted by the *red arrows*. In tandem, bone growth at the healing chambers took place from all available surfaces (instrumented surface after its dieback due to surgical instrumentation – green line) (From Coelho and Jimbo (2014). With permission from Elsevier)

for primary stability between 2 and 4 weeks (Bonfante et al. 2011, 2013). In tandem with this interfacial remodeling that decreases implant primary stability levels achieved by partial engagement of the implant power threads and bone, woven bone formation occurred within the healing chamber region potentially compensating for the stability loss (Fig. 4.6) (Bonfante et al. 2011, 2013). Figure 4.7 illustrates a time point where implant hardware allowed for healing chamber filling (secondary stability well underway) in tandem with bone resorption at the regions that provided primary stability.

Currently, very few commercially available systems present the hybrid design configuration; thus, the long-term effect of hybrid healing on osseointegration is years from being evaluated. Nonetheless, it is somewhat expected that a combination of a compact lamellar and haversian-like structures will result due to the presence of bone interfacial remodeling and intramembranous-like components during early healing.

4.2.5 Surgical Drilling Technique and Its Effect on the Different Bone Healing Pathways

It is remarkable that surgical instrumentation investigations are clearly the least abundant in the osseointegration literature, given that it is a feature of extreme importance if one is attempting to modulate implant hardware influence in healing mode and the degree of primary and secondary stability (Giro et al. 2011, 2013; Jimbo et al. 2013; Yeniyol et al. 2013).

Unlike for the case which implant hardware results in interfacial remodeling healing mode, where bone damage due to surgical instrumentation is likely to be overcome by the bone damage due to compression osteonecrosis and microcracking, implant hardware leading to intramembranous-like and hybrid healing may have their biomechanical competence over time set back due to surgical instrumentation damage.

In the case of healing chambers (intramembranous-like healing), it is obvious that the lower the damage to the drilled wall, less resorption will occur and lesser the volume to be filled through the intramembranous healing pathway (Giro et al. 2011). A more complex scenario arises in hybrid healing, since a temporal balance between healing modes is required for atemporally stable implant system design. For this hardware design, surgical drilling technique must be carefully accounted since osteotomy line dieback (presented in Fig. 4.7) will invariably occur potentially altering balance of the in tandem relationship of primary and secondary stability. For instance, excessive drilled wall retraction due to dieback will not only decrease primary stability due to lesser engagement between implant thread and pristine bone but also increase the healing chamber component responsible for assuring implant stability when interfacial remodeling occurs at the regions that assured primary stability during placement.

Drilling speed proportionally influences heat generation to the surrounding bone (Iyer et al. 1997a, b). Research has indicated that an overheat exceeding 47 °C for 1 min would provoke an irreversible thermal injury to the bone (Eriksson et al. 1984) with osteoclasts activation due to local surgical instrumentation damage and/or osteocyte death (Yoshida et al. 2009). On the contrary, Yeniyol et al. have demonstrated higher degrees of osseointegration for implants placed in sites prepared under low-speed drilling (Yeniyol et al. 2013). Similarly, Giro et al. (2011) reported lower bone dieback degree when low-speed drilling was used for osteotomy relative to high-speed drilling (Giro et al. 2011). Thus, while studies suggest that slower speeds may result in site overdrilling due to wobbling and higher temperatures that may damage the bone (Iyer et al. 1997a, b; Lindstrom et al. 1981; Sharawy et al. 2002; Yeniyol et al. 2013), a recent experimental study has shown higher osseointegration levels and lower degrees of bone dieback for drilling <400 rpm (Yeniyol et al. 2013).

In tandem with implant hardware designing, it is acknowledged that implant software, briefly described subsequently, comprising micrometer and nanometer length scale designing, may strongly influence early osseointegration.

4.2.6 Implant Software or Hardware Ad Hoc: Surface at Micrometer and Nanometer Length Scale Levels

Implant software, commonly referred to as surface topography designing, results, from a biomechanical standpoint, to expanded surface area of the moderately rough implant surface, which is in contact with the surrounding bone tissue, increasing the friction coefficient and the kinetic friction during implant insertion. Along with implant macrogeometry, the increased kinetic friction naturally provides higher implant primary stability (Richards et al. 2012). The high primary stability of the implant provides a stable host bed, and only after this, the biological effect of the surface microstructure and, recently, the intended nanostructures exerts their osteogenic effects. The high primary stability and the osteoconductive surface in contact to blood clots within the chamber allow growth factors and cells to successfully adhere to the implant surface (Coelho et al. 2014).

Nanotopography, if strategically applied, presents enhanced osteoconductivity (Coelho et al. 2015; Jimbo et al. 2014). It has been demonstrated that the application of nanotopography not only enhances osseointegration but also improves the nanomechanical properties of the surrounding bone (Jimbo et al. 2012). However, this early effect of the nanotopography is only effective where the implant has adequate stability in the bone, allowing the same is faced with enough osteogenic cells to interact with the surface. It must be clearly stated that nanotopography has no correlation on the primary stability and is only effective in achieving secondary (biologic) stability (Coelho and Jimbo 2014; Coelho et al. 2015).

4.2.7 Other Considerations and Final Remarks

Another relevant future consideration is bone quality of the implantation site as it is evident that the implant hardware configuration should be altered based on the quality of the bone, and for the time present, the hardware interplay to maximize implant stability over time in different bone types has not been characterized. It may be speculated that the lower the bone density, the higher the mixed amount of interfacial remodeling and intramembranous-like bone healing modes will be present. However, this must be determined in future studies to obtain sufficient evidence, and such optimization will likely occur through factorial study designs where hardware is first adjusted as a function of bone density for primary stability maximization and adequate software is then adapted to the hardware to maximize secondary stability achievement.

Acknowledgments To Conselho Nacional de Desenvolvimento Científico e Tecnológico (CNPq), grant # 309475/2014-7.

References

Abrahamsson I, Berglundh T, Linder E, Lang NP, Lindhe J (2004) Early bone formation adjacent to rough and turned endosseous implant surfaces. An experimental study in the dog. Clin Oral Implants Res 15:381–392

Abrahamsson I, Linder E, Lang NP (2009) Implant stability in relation to osseointegration: an experimental study in the labrador dog. Clin Oral Implants Res 20:313–318

Albrektsson T, Johansson C (2001) Osteoinduction, osteoconduction and osseointegration. Eur Spine J 10(Suppl 2):S96–101

Albrektsson T, Branemark PI, Hansson HA, Lindstrom J (1981) Osseointegrated titanium implants. Requirements for ensuring a long-lasting, direct bone-to-implant anchorage in man. Acta Orthop Scand 52:155–170

Baldassarri M, Bonfante E, Suzuki M, Marin C, Granato R, Tovar N, Coelho PG (2012) Mechanical properties of human bone surrounding plateau root form implants retrieved after 0.3–24 years of function. J Biomed Mater Res B Appl Biomater 100:2015–2021

Barber AJ, Butterworth CJ, Rogers SN (2011) Systematic review of primary osseointegrated dental implants in head and neck oncology. Br J Oral Maxillofac Surg 49:29–36

Bashutski JD, D'Silva NJ, Wang H-L (2009) Implant compression necrosis: current understanding and case report. J Periodontol 80:700–704

Bentolila V, Boyce TM, Fyhrie DP, Drumb R, Skerry TM, Schaffler MB (1998) Intracortical remodeling in adult rat long bones after fatigue loading. Bone 23:275–281

Berglundh T, Abrahamsson I, Lang NP, Lindhe J (2003) De novo alveolar bone formation adjacent to endosseous implants. Clin Oral Implants Res 14:251–262

Bonfante EA, Granato R, Marin C, Suzuki M, Oliveira SR, Giro G, Coelho PG (2011) Early bone healing and biomechanical fixation of dual acid-etched and as-machined implants with healing chambers: an experimental study in dogs. Int J Oral Maxillofac Implants 26:75–82

Bonfante EA, Granato R, Marin C, Jimbo R, Giro G, Suzuki M, Coelho PG (2013a) Biomechanical testing of microblasted, acid-etched/microblasted, anodized, and discrete crystalline deposition surfaces: an experimental study in beagle dogs. Int J Oral Maxillofac Implants 28:136–142

Bonfante EA, Janal MN, Granato R, Marin C, Suzuki M, Tovar N, Coelho PG (2013b) Buccal and lingual bone level alterations after immediate implantation of four implant surfaces: a study in dogs. Clin Oral Implants Res 24:1375–1380

Bosshardt DD, Salvi GE, Huynh-Ba G, Ivanovski S, Donos N, Lang NP (2011) The role of bone debris in early healing adjacent to hydrophilic and hydrophobic implant surfaces in man. Clin Oral Implants Res 22:357–364

Bothe R, Beaton L, Davenport H (1940) Reaction of bone to multiple metallic implants. Surg Gynecol Obstet 71:598–602

Branemark PI, Hansson BO, Adell R, Breine U, Lindstrom J, Hallen O, Ohman A (1977) Osseointegrated implants in the treatment of the edentulous jaw. Experience from a 10-year period. Scand J Plast Reconstr Surg Suppl 16:1–132

Browaeys H, Dierens M, Ruyffelaert C, Matthijs C, De Bruyn H, Vandeweghe S (2014) Ongoing crestal bone loss around implants subjected to computer-guided flapless surgery and immediate loading using the all-on-4® concept. Clin Implant Dent Relat Res 2015 Oct;17(5):831–843. doi: 10.1111/cid.12197

Burr DB, Forwood MR, Fyhrie DP, Martin RB, Schaffler MB, Turner CH (1997) Bone microdamage and skeletal fragility in osteoporotic and stress fractures. J Bone Miner Res 12:6–15

Burr DB, Turner CH, Naick P, Forwood MR, Ambrosius W, Sayeed Hasan M, Pidaparti R (1998) Does microdamage accumulation affect the mechanical properties of bone? J Biomech 31:337–345

Buser D, Broggini N, Wieland M, Schenk RK, Denzer AJ, Cochran DL, Hoffmann B, Lussi A, Steinemann SG (2004) Enhanced bone apposition to a chemically modified sla titanium surface. J Dent Res 83:529–533

Campos FE, Gomes JB, Marin C, Teixeira HS, Suzuki M, Witek L, Zanetta-Barbosa D, Coelho PG (2012) Effect of drilling dimension on implant placement torque and early osseointegration stages: an experimental study in dogs. J Oral Maxillofac Surg 70:e43–e50

Chamay A, Tschantz P (1972) Mechanical influences in bone remodeling. Experimental research on wolff's law. J Biomech 5:173–180

Chowdhary R, Halldin A, Jimbo R Wennerberg A (2013) Influence of micro threads alteration on osseointegration and primary stability of implants: an fea and in vivo analysis in rabbits. Clin Implant Dent Relat Res 2015 Jun;17(3):562–569. doi: 10.1111/cid.12143

Coelho PG, Jimbo R (2014) Osseointegration of metallic devices: current trends based on implant hardware design. Arch Biochem Biophys 561:99–108

Coelho PG, Takayama T, Yoo D, Jimbo R, Karunagaran S, Tovar N, Janal MN, Yamano S. Bone. (2014) Nanometer-scale features on micrometer-scale surface texturing: a bone histological, gene expression, and nanomechanical study. Aug;65:25–32. doi: 10.1016/j.bone.2014.05.004

Coelho PG, Granjeiro JM, Romanos GE, Suzuki M, Silva NR, Cardaropoli G, Thompson VP, Lemons JE (2009a) Basic research methods and current trends of dental implant surfaces. J Biomed Mater Res B Appl Biomater 88:579–596

Coelho PG, Marin C, Granato R, Suzuki M (2009b) Histomorphologic analysis of 30 plateau root form implants retrieved after 8 to 13 years in function. A human retrieval study. J Biomed Mater Res B Appl Biomater 91:975–979

Coelho PG, Bonfante EA, Marin C, Granato R, Giro G, Suzuki M (2010a) A human retrieval study of plasma-sprayed hydroxyapatite-coated plateau root form implants after 2 months to 13 years in function. J Long Term Eff Med Implants 20:335–342

Coelho PG, Granato R, Marin C, Bonfante EA, Janal MN, Suzuki M (2010b) Biomechanical and bone histomorphologic evaluation of four surfaces on plateau root form implants: an experimental study in dogs. Oral Surg Oral Med Oral Pathol Oral Radiol Endod 109:e39–e45

Coelho PG, Marin C, Granato R, Bonfante EA, Lima CP, Suzuki M (2010c) Surface treatment at the cervical region and its effect on bone maintenance after immediate implantation: an experimental study in dogs. Oral Surg Oral Med Oral Pathol Oral Radiol Endod 110:182–187

Coelho PG, Suzuki M, Guimaraes MV, Marin C, Granato R, Gil JN, Miller RJ (2010d) Early bone healing around different implant bulk designs and surgical techniques: a study in dogs. Clin Implant Dent Relat Res 12:202–208

Coelho PG, Granato R, Marin C, Teixeira HS, Suzuki M, Valverde GB, Janal MN, Lilin T, Bonfante EA (2011) The effect of different implant macrogeometries and surface treatment in early biomechanical fixation: an experimental study in dogs. J Mech Behav Biomed Mater 4:1974–1981

Coelho PG, Marin C, Teixeira HS, Campos FE, Gomes JB, Guastaldi F, Anchieta RB, Silveira L, Bonfante EA (2013) Biomechanical evaluation of undersized drilling on implant biomechanical stability at early implantation times. J Oral Maxillofac Surg 71:e69–e75

Coelho PG, Teixeira HS, Marin C, Witek L, Tovar N, Janal MN, Jimbo R (2014) The in vivo effect of p-15 coating on early osseointegration. J Biomed Mater Res B Appl Biomater 102:430–440

Coelho PG, Jimbo R, Tovar N, Bonfante EA (2015) Osseointegration: hierarchical designing encompassing the macromer, micrometer, and nanometer length scales. Dent Mater 31:37–52

De Bruyn H, Raes F, Cooper LF, Reside G, Garriga JS, Tarrida LG, Wiltfang J, Kern M (2013) Three-years clinical outcome of immediate provisionalization of single osseospeed() implants in extraction sockets and healed ridges. Clin Oral Implants Res 24:217–223

Deporter DA, Kermalli J, Todescan R, Atenafu E (2012) Performance of sintered, porous-surfaced, press-fit implants after 10 years of function in the partially edentulous posterior mandible. Int J Periodontics Restorative Dent 32:563–570

Eriksson RA, Albrektsson T, Magnusson B (1984) Assessment of bone viability after heat trauma. A histological, histochemical and vital microscopic study in the rabbit. Scand J Plast Reconstr Surg 18:261–268

Esposito M, Grusovin MG, Achille H, Coulthard P, Worthington HV (2009) Interventions for replacing missing teeth: different times for loading dental implants. Cochrane Database Syst Rev 2009: CD003878

Esposito M, Grusovin MG, Maghaireh H, Worthington HV (2013) Interventions for replacing missing teeth: different times for loading dental implants. Cochrane Database Syst Rev 3:CD003878

Freitas AC Jr, Bonfante EA, Giro G, Janal MN, Coelho PG (2012) The effect of implant design on insertion torque and immediate micromotion. Clin Oral Implants Res 23:113–118

Gil LF, Suzuki M, Janal MN, Tovar N, Marin C, Granato R, Bonfante EA, Jimbo R, Gil JN, Coelho PG (2014) Progressive plateau root form dental implant osseointegration: a human retrieval study. J Biomed Mater Res B Appl Biomater 103:1328–1332

Giro G, Marin C, Granato R, Bonfante EA, Suzuki M, Janal MN, Coelho PG (2011) Effect of drilling technique on the early integration of plateau root form endosteal implants: an experimental study in dogs. J Oral Maxillofac Surg 69:2158–2163

Giro G, Tovar N, Marin C, Bonfante EA, Jimbo R, Suzuki M, Janal MN, Coelho PG (2013) The effect of simplifying dental implant drilling sequence on osseointegration: an experimental study in dogs. Int J Biomater 2013:230310

Gomes JB, Campos FE, Marin C, Teixeira HS, Bonfante EA, Suzuki M, Witek L, Zanetta-Barbosa D, Coelho PG (2013) Implant biomechanical stability variation at early implantation times in vivo: an experimental study in dogs. Int J Oral Maxillofac Implants 28:e128–e134

Gottlow J, Barkarmo S, Sennerby L (2012) An experimental comparison of two different clinically used implant designs and surfaces. Clin Implant Dent Relat Res 14:e204–e212

Halldin A, Jimbo R, Johansson CB, Wennerberg A, Jacobsson M, Albrektsson T, Hansson S (2011) The effect of static bone strain on implant stability and bone remodeling. Bone 49:783–789

Huang H-L, Chang Y-Y, Lin D-J, Li Y-F, Chen K-T, Hsu J-T (2011) Initial stability and bone strain evaluation of the immediately loaded dental implant: an in vitro model study. Clin Oral Implants Res 22:691–698

Iezzi G, Vantaggiato G, Shibli JA, Fiera E, Falco A, Piattelli A, Perrotti V (2012) Machined and sandblasted human dental implants retrieved after 5 years: a histologic and histomorphometric analysis of three cases. Quintessence Int 43:287–292

Iezzi G, Piattelli A, Mangano C, Shibli JA, Vantaggiato G, Frosecchi M, Di Chiara C, Perrotti V (2014) Peri-implant bone tissues around retrieved human implants after time periods longer than 5 years: a retrospective histologic and histomorphometric evaluation of 8 cases. Odontology 102:116–121

Isidor F (2006) Influence of forces on peri-implant bone. Clin Oral Implants Res 17:8–18

Iyer S, Weiss C, Mehta A (1997a) Effects of drill speed on heat production and the rate and quality of bone formation in dental implant osteotomies. Part I: relationship between drill speed and heat production. Int J Prosthodont 10:411–414

Iyer S, Weiss C, Mehta A (1997b) Effects of drill speed on heat production and the rate and quality of bone formation in dental implant osteotomies. Part II: relationship between drill speed and healing. Int J Prosthodont 10:536–540

Javed F, Romanos GE (2010) The role of primary stability for successful immediate loading of dental implants. A literature review. J Dent 38:612–620

Jimbo R, Sawase T, Shibata Y, Hirata K, Hishikawa Y, Tanaka Y, Bessho K, Ikeda T, Atsuta M (2007) Enhanced osseointegration by the chemotactic activity of plasma fibronectin for cellular fibronectin positive cells. Biomaterials 28:3469–3477

Jimbo R, Coelho PG, Bryington M, Baldassarri M, Tovar N, Currie F, Hayashi M, Janal MN, Andersson M, Ono D, Vandeweghe S, Wennerberg A (2012) Nano hydroxyapatite-coated implants improve bone nanomechanical properties. J Dent Res 91:1172–1177

Jimbo R, Anchieta R, Baldassarri M, Granato R, Marin C, Teixeira HS, Tovar N, Vandeweghe S, Janal MN, Coelho PG (2013a) Histomorphometry and bone mechanical property evolution around different implant systems at early healing stages. Implant Dent 22:596–603

Jimbo R, Giro G, Marin C, Granato R, Suzuki M, Tovar N, Lilin T, Janal M, Coelho PG (2013b) Simplified drilling technique does not decrease dental implant osseointegration: a preliminary report. J Periodontol 84:1599–1605

Jimbo R, Tovar N, Yoo DY, Janal MN, Anchieta RB, Coelho PG (2013c) The effect of different surgical drilling procedures on full laser-etched microgrooves surface-treated implants: an experimental study in sheep. Clin Oral Implants Res 25:1072–1077

Jimbo R, Andersson M, Vandeweghe S (2014a) Nano in implant dentistry. Int J Dent 2014:314819

Jimbo R, Tovar N, Marin C, Teixeira HS, Anchieta RB, Silveira LM, Janal MN, Shibli JA, Coelho PG (2014b) The impact of a modified cutting flute implant design on osseointegration. Int J Oral Maxillofac Surg 43:883–888

Leonard G, Coelho P, Polyzois I, Stassen L, Claffey N (2009) A study of the bone healing kinetics of plateau versus screw root design titanium dental implants. Clin Oral Implants Res 20:232–239

Leventhal GS (1951) Titanium, a metal for surgery. J Bone Joint Surg Am 33-A:473–474

Lindstrom J, Branemark PI, Albrektsson T (1981) Mandibular reconstruction using the preformed autologous bone graft. Scand J Plast Reconstr Surg 15:29–38

Mangano C, Perrotti V, Raspanti M, Mangano F, Luongo G, Piattelli A, Iezzi G (2013) Human dental implants with a sandblasted, acid-etched surface retrieved after 5 and 10 years: a light and scanning electron microscopy evaluation of two cases. Int J Oral Maxillofac Implants 28:917–920

Marin C, Granato R, Suzuki M, Gil JN, Janal MN, Coelho PG (2010) Histomorphologic and histomorphometric evaluation of various endosseous implant healing chamber configurations at early implantation times: a study in dogs. Clin Oral Implants Res 21:577–583

Norton M (2013) Primary stability versus viable constraint – a need to redefine. Int J Oral Maxillofac Implants 28:19–21

Oh TJ, Yoon J, Misch CE, Wang HL (2002) The causes of early implant bone loss: myth or science? J Periodontol 73:322–333

Petrie CS, Williams JL (2005) Comparative evaluation of implant designs: influence of diameter, length, and taper on strains in the alveolar crest. Clin Oral Implants Res 16:486–494

Raghavendra S, Wood MC, Taylor TD (2005) Early wound healing around endosseous implants: a review of the literature. Int J Oral Maxillofac Implants 20:425–431

Richards RG, Moriarty TF, Miclau T, McClellan RT, Grainger DW. Advances in biomaterials and surface technologies. J Orthop Trauma 2012;26:703–707.

Sharawy M, Misch CE, Weller N, Tehemar S (2002) Heat generation during implant drilling: the significance of motor speed. J Oral Maxillofac Surg 60:1160–1169

Shigehara S, Ohba S, Nakashima K, Takanashi Y, Asahina I (2014) Immediate loading of dental implants inserted in edentulous maxillas and mandibles; 5-year results of a clinical study. J Oral Implantol 16:411–415

Suzuki M, Calasans-Maia MD, Marin C, Granato R, Gil JN, Granjeiro JM, Coelho PG (2010) Effect of surface modifications on early bone healing around plateau root form implants: an experimental study in rabbits. J Oral Maxillofac Surg 68:1631–1638

Verborgt O, Gibson GJ, Schaffler MB (2000) Loss of osteocyte integrity in association with microdamage and bone remodeling after fatigue in vivo. J Bone Miner Res 15:60–67

Vervaeke S, Collaert B, De Bruyn H (2013) The effect of implant surface modifications on survival and bone loss of immediately loaded implants in the edentulous mandible. Int J Oral Maxillofac Implants 28:1352–1357

Witek L, Marin C, Granato R, Bonfante EA, Campos FE, Gomes JB, Suzuki M, Coelho PG (2013) Surface characterization, biomechanical, and histologic evaluation of alumina and bioactive resorbable blasting textured surfaces in titanium implant healing chambers: an experimental study in dogs. Int J Oral Maxillofac Implants 28:694–700

Yeniyol S, Jimbo R, Marin C, Tovar N, Janal MN, Coelho PG (2013) The effect of drilling speed on early bone healing to oral implants. Oral Surg Oral Med Oral Pathol Oral Radiol 116:550–555

Yoshida K1, Uoshima K, Oda K, Maeda T. (2009) Influence of heat stress to matrix on bone formation. Clin Oral Implants Res. Aug;20(8):782–90. doi: 10.1111/j.1600-0501.2008.01654.x.

Zizic TM, Marcoux C, Hungerford DS, Dansereau JV, Stevens MB (1985) Corticosteroid therapy associated with ischemic necrosis of bone in systemic lupus erythematosus. Am J Med 79:596–604

Anatomic Considerations in Dental Implant Surgery

5

Mitra Sadrameli

Abstract

Dentate or edentulous sites do not always provide the surgeon with ideal topography and anatomy for dental implant placement. Precise planning and a thorough understanding of the anatomy of the proposed implant site will reduce avoidable and predictable complications. This chapter provides an overview of the anterior maxillofacial anatomy important in anterior implant placement.

5.1 Introduction

Successful surgical placement of dental implants requires careful planning as well as thorough understanding of the limitations provided by the surgical site. Anatomic limitations remain a constant consideration in implant placement. Location of vital structures such as sinus floor, mandibular canal, and bone ridge concavity, in addition to acquired anatomical changes such as moderate to extensively resorbed alveolar process, as well as angulation and size of the implant must be carefully considered and determined prior to the surgical appointment. As a result, detailed evaluation of the osseous, the adjacent structures, the alveolar ridge morphology, as well as the proximity of vital structures is crucial. Until the advent of three-dimensional (3D) techniques, two-dimensional (2D) imaging such as panoramic and intraoral radiographs was commonly used for surgical treatment planning. 2D imaging, however, is subject to significant unpredictable geometric magnifications inherent to the technology and the acquisition techniques (Sarment 2014).

The introduction of computed tomography (CT) provided the surgeon with cross-sectional images from multiplanar-reformatted (MPR) images with considerably greater information compared to the 2D images traditionally used. However, the dose, cost, and general limited access to the CT scanners prohibited widespread use of the technology. The introduction of cone beam computed tomography (CBCT) provided similar osseous information with significantly lower dose, cost, and greater access. CBCT's potential for allowing surgical planning and anatomical and morphological analyses are advantageous in personalizing patient care. In 2012, the American Academy of Oral and

---

M. Sadrameli, DMD, MS, Dipl. ABOMR
Clinical Assistant Professor, University of British Columbia, Vancouver, BC, Canada

Private Practice, 1201 S. Prairie Ave, Suite 4901, Chicago, IL 60605, USA
e-mail: ddximaging@gmail.com

Maxillofacial Radiology (AAOMR) updated its recommendations first published in 2000, reconfirming its position on the role of 3D cross-sectional imaging in dental implant treatment planning. After reviewing the literature, they stated, "the diagnostic phase of dental-implant therapy and, in particular, the appropriate choice of radiographic examination is important to the long-term success of a dental implant…. To optimize implant placement and to avoid surgical complications, the clinician must have full knowledge of oral-bone anatomy so that any osseous-topography, bone-volume excesses/deficiencies can be corrected before implant placement" (Tyndall et al. 2012).

Rehabilitation of the anterior edentulous sites with dental implant restorations has become a mainstay of comprehensive patient treatment (Kumar and Satheesh 2013). The edentulous or traumatized alveolar ridge morphology is often unfavorable for aesthetic-conscious implant treatment. Deficient osseous quantity may render incorrect placement of the implant fixture, improper prosthetic rehabilitation, or unattractive aesthetics. Digital radiographic technology such as 3D imaging is an important tool in thorough assessment of the surgical site (Kumar and Satheesh 2013). While success rate of implant placement is extremely high, as with other surgical procedures, inherent risks if not predicted in advance will progress to postsurgical complications. Specific anatomical features, individual unique variations of anatomy, and characteristics of the edentulous site dictate the morphology of the proposed implant sites. Presurgical identification of the alveolar ridge morphology is paramount in ensuring predictability of the surgical procedure. Proper treatment planning with specific attention paid to identification of critical anatomic landmarks; analysis of the height, width, and shape of the alveolar ridge; and utilization of accurate surgical guides will greatly increase accuracy of implant fixture placement and the prosthetic rehabilitation results.

Various regions of the oral cavity present with unique surgical challenges. The maxillary anterior region known as the aesthetic zone, or informally as the "social 6," is scrutinized in detail by patients for the appearance of their smile. Following loss of dentition, diminished alveolar ridge height and/or width, as well as the concomitant development of the labial concavity, may necessitate bone augmentation, whether prior to or at the same time as the endosseous implant installation procedure (Tyndall et al. 2012). Location, dimensions, and morphology of vital anatomic structures, for example, of the maxillary nasopalatine (incisive) canal and the floor of the nasal fossae in relationship to the alveolar crest may become of surgical importance.

Anterior mandible was long considered a safe location for implant placement. In patients with prominent interforaminal neurovascular structures, knowledge of the anatomy will help avoid complications of postoperative hemorrhage or neurosensory loss due to trauma during osteotomy and fixture placement (Tyndall et al. 2012).

Utilization of CBCT scan with 3D implant planning software programs, presurgical evaluation, and treatment planning of the proposed implant site(s) allows for preoperative fixture diameter and length, prosthetic abutment type, and size determination prior to treatment appointments. Consideration of the bone height and width provides the surgical and prosthetic team with rehabilitation strategies. 3D and specifically CBCT analysis is and should be an integral step in this process.

5.2 Alveolar Ridge Atrophy

After tooth loss, the progressive, irreversible alveolar ridge resorption will uniquely change the morphology as well as the volume of the proposed implant site(s). Horizontal and vertical crestal atrophy diminishes optimum implant recipient site characteristics. Etiology of crestal atrophy is varied and may include frequency, direction, and intensity of forces, as well as the construction and fit of the existing prosthesis (Atwood 1971). Other contributing factors which may hasten this process include systemic diseases, patient's sex and advancing age, as well as hormonal imbalances, metabolic factors, and inflammation (Atwood 1971).

Success in implant placement is influenced by many factors including availability of bone in the proposed implant site. Depending on the prosthetic plan, ideal placement of the implant fixture and the longevity of the functional implant-supported restorations require the presence of adequate volume of bone in specific regions (Block 2014; Araújo et al. 2006).

Atwood early on noticed that resorption of the edentulous alveolar ridge follows a characteristic pattern (Atwood 1971). Fallschüssel's classification was later modified by Cawood and Howell, who posited that there are morphologic differences between the anterior and posterior alveolar ridge pattern of atrophy with the latter authors offering the following commonly referenced classification (Atwood 1971; Von Arx et al. 2013):

Class 1: Dentate.
Class 2: Immediately post-extraction; the alveolar ridge has healed.
Class 3: Well-rounded ridge, adequate in height and width.
Class 4: Knife-edged ridge, adequate in height and inadequate in width.
Class 5: Flat ridge, inadequate in height and width.
Class 6: Depressed ridge with varying degrees of basal bone loss that may be extensive but follows no predictable pattern.

As in all resorptive processes, after tooth loss, the external osteoclastic activity supersedes the internal osteoblastic activity (Chan et al. 2011). Interestingly, in most patients, even in extreme resorbed ridges, in the absence of external local forces, the basal bone does not appear to change shape significantly, while the alveolar bone may change shape in both the vertical and/or horizontal axes (Von Arx et al. 2013). Cadaveric observations recorded by Rogers and Applebaum in 1941 concluded that following teeth loss, maxillary alveolar ridge height is reduced, and its crest shifts palatally (Trikeriotis et al. 2008). Tylman and Tylman in 1960 noticed that with the removal of the teeth, the buccal alveolar bone plates of both anterior maxillary and mandibular arches resorbed at a faster rate than the lingual plates, a conclusion reached based on anecdotal information (Trikeriotis et al. 2008). Pietrovski and Massler in 1967 additionally stated that the amount of resorption is greater along the labial/buccal surface than along the lingual/palatal surface, although the absolute rate and amount varies between individuals and sites (Trikeriotis et al. 2008).

Long-term edentulous sites present with the greatest loss of bone in the labio/buccal-lingual/palatal or horizontal direction (Evian et al. 1982). In the majority of cases, the greatest bone loss is noted on the facial/buccal aspect of the alveolar ridge (Evian et al. 1982).

Patterns of bone loss are site dependent. The anterior maxilla and mandible and the posterior maxilla exhibit vertical as well as horizontal bone loss mainly from the labial aspect, while the posterior mandible exhibits mainly vertical atrophy with some labially directed horizontal bone loss (Von Arx et al. 2013).

Presurgical 3D evaluation of the alveolar ridge should offer assessment of the existing morphology, pattern of alveolar resorption, as well as existing horizontal and vertical osseous dimensions and volumes in the precise site housing the future implant fixture. 3D evaluation of the alveolar ridge is accomplished using the axial and cross-sectional images to assess the presence and morphology of the basilar and the alveolar processes, the direction of atrophy, as well as characteristics of cortication of the labial/buccal and/or lingual/palatal plates, in addition to that of the alveolar crest. True cross-sectional images provide accuracy in vertical and horizontal measurements.

5.3 Lingual Cortical Plate and Adjacent Anatomy

Identification of the lingual cortical plate morphology reduces risk of complications such as perforation and injury of the structures immediately adjacent to the lingual plate by the implant fixture. The proximity of the adjacent neurovascular structures, which are soft tissue in nature, cannot be evaluated utilizing CBCT scans directly.

However, knowledge of the anatomy and the anatomic variations of these soft tissue structures aid with the proper orientation of the fixtures during implant placement to avoid complications such as perforation and life-threatening hemorrhage. CBCT scanners are unable to register soft tissues; as such the presence of neurovascular structures will not be registered on the scanned images. Indirect anatomical signs may be used to approximate and predict the location of vital structures and predict potential future complications; for example, perforation of the lingual plate, acute tear of the lingual periosteum, and/or surgical manipulation of the deep muscles in the floor of the mouth may in turn cause perforation of the arteries causing massive hemorrhage and increase possibility of subsequent fatal airway obstruction (Nowzari et al. 2012; Mraiwa et al. 2003b). In the absence of neurovascular perforation, the piercing implant fixture may increase risk of persistent inflammation or infection, a condition most likely if the oral mucosa is traumatized and communication with the oral cavity is established (Nowzari et al. 2012).

Delayed manifestation of these complications and the severe nature of the consequences render presurgical planning crucial (Nowzari et al. 2012). In the majority of cases, hemorrhage resulted from laceration or perforation of the sublingual or submental arteries (Mraiwa et al. 2003b). A more detailed description of the interforaminal neurovasculature is included later in this chapter.

Thickness of the buccal and lingual cortical plates in cross-sectional images is important when installing implant fixture in a horizontally narrow ridge. Noting the inter-plate dimensions and placing the fixtures such that the thickness of the cortices is maintained will in the absence of other factors prevent life-threatening complications. Preserving the labial bone prevents implant-related buccal cortical plate dehiscence, a major contributor to aesthetic complications not to mention potential osseointegration complications (Block 2014).

Teeth within the alveolar ridge lie oblique to the vertical axis of the cranium (Garg 2010). Apices of maxillary teeth, on a horizontal plane, are closer to each other than their respective crowns (Garg 2010). This results in the maxillary teeth appearing to tilt outward at the coronal level (Garg 2010). The mandibular teeth are inclined lingually with the contralateral crowns placed closer than their respective roots (Garg 2010). These distinctive anatomic characteristics result in thicker mandibular and maxillary lingual cortical plates compared to their labial counterparts (Garg 2010). The height of the labial plate will influence the position of the respective mucosal margin (Lee et al. 2012). The plate thickness will influence the facial convexity of the alveolar process at the emergence profile (Lee et al. 2012). Preservation of the existing labial plate or augmentation of area when needed is necessary to avoid postsurgical resorption, which may result in aesthetic and functional failure (Lee et al. 2012). In the anterior maxillary region, compared to the palatal, the labial plate exhibits naturally narrower width or may be partially absent (Lee et al. 2012). While individual measurements may vary, prevalence of a mean dimension of ≥ 2 mm labial plate thickness has been reported (Lee et al. 2012; Miller et al. 2011). In contrast to the anterior region, posterior sites present with greater labial plate thickness. With advanced age horizontal narrowing of the cortical plate thickness at the crestal level is commonly noted. While the etiology of this finding remains elusive, this may be secondary to external factors such as chronic local infections and/or other systemic or local conditions (Lee et al. 2012). In addition, pre-atrophy anatomy may play an important role in the degree of post-extraction bone loss. Araújo and Lindhe stated that post-extraction resorption of buccal walls is more pronounced in patients with naturally thin buccal plate dimensions (Miller et al. 2011).

5.4 Classification of the Anterior Alveolar Ridge and Basal Bone

The cross-sectional images provide excellent review of the height and width of the proposed implant site, the thickness of the cortical plates, and the overall shape of the alveolar ridge as well as the morphology of the basilar process.

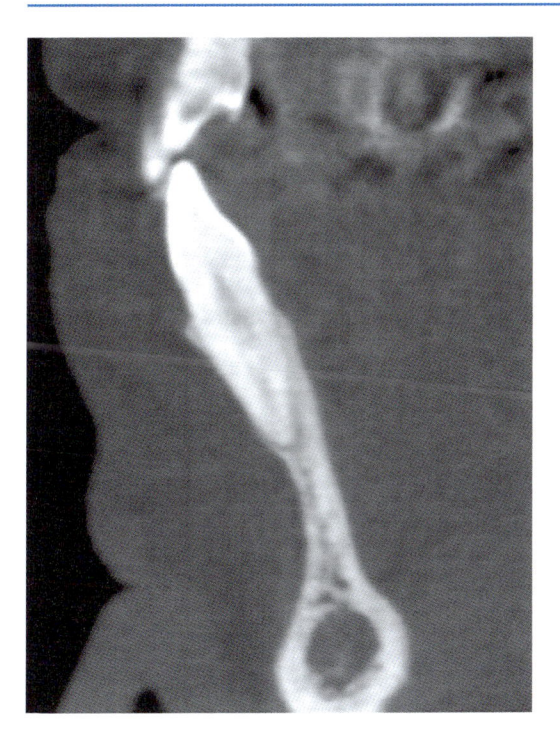

Fig. 5.1 Narrow anteroposterior alveolar process dimension (cross section)

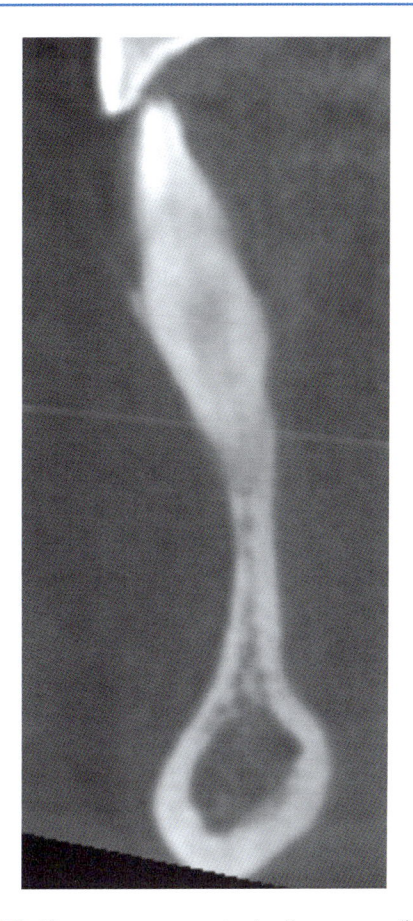

Fig. 5.2 Narrow anteroposterior basilar process dimension (cross section)

The horizontal morphology of the anterior alveolar ridge may be classified as:

1. Narrow buccolingual dimensions: in which the ridge appears as wide as the tooth it houses (Fig. 5.1)
2. Slightly greater buccolingual dimensions: in which the alveolar ridge is slightly larger than the tooth it houses
3. Moderate buccolingual thinning specifically at the level of the alveolar crest: with greater bone loss noted from the labial aspect
4. Significant buccolingual thinning specifically at the level of the alveolar crest

The horizontal morphology of the basilar process may be classified as (Fig. 5.2):

1. Similar width as the alveolar ridge resulting in a fairly uniform somewhat cylindrical shape
2. Naturally narrower width inferior to the odontogenic apices, resulting in a corticated constriction inferior to the existing teeth

5.4.1 Maxillary Anterior Implant Region

Conventionally, the *anterior maxilla* is referred to as the area anterior to the lateral walls of the nasal cavity and the anterior border of the sinus (Block 2014). The *posterior maxilla* is the region posterior to the second premolars and molars (Block 2014).

5.4.2 Nasopalatine Canal (Maxillary Incisive Canal)

Within the anatomic structures present in the anterior maxilla, the maxillary nasopalatine canal which carries the nasopalatine nerves, arteries, and veins from the anteromedial region of the nasal cavities to the primary palate exiting from the incisive foramen is considered the most prominent (Goel and Weerakhody). The terms nasopalatine foramen, and foramen of Stensen are interchangeably used in the literature. So are the terms maxillary nasopalatine canal and incisive canal. For the purposes of this chapter, the term nasopalatine canal is used to refer to this anatomic structure.

The apico-lingual resorption of the alveolar ridge results in the crestal edentulous site assuming a location in the premaxillary region adjacent to the incisive foramen (Jacobs et al. 2004). This acquired morphology often introduces complications in the osteotomy site preparation (Jacobs et al. 2004; Liang et al. 2009). The final rehabilitation of the area is of great significance in the aesthetic, phonetic, as well as surgical outcome (Jacobs et al. 2004).

Placing an implant fixture adjacent to the nasopalatine canal, in an area which when compared to posterior regions is naturally narrower in facio-palatal dimensions, presents the surgeon with significant challenges not encountered in other areas. There is a close anatomic relationship between the nasopalatine canal, the roots of the existing central maxillary incisors, as well as the acquired morphology of the future recipient site of the implant fixture (Tözüm et al. 2012). The shape, size, and dimensions of the canal may radically influence the proposed location and/or osteotomy preparation. Alternatively it may highlight the necessity for presurgical modifications to accommodate the ideal placement of the dental implant (Kan et al. 2012; Kumar and Satheesh 2013; Tözüm et al. 2012; Liang et al. 2009, 2010). In cases where long-term edentulism of the maxillary central incisor sites is reported, the degree of disuse atrophy may negatively influence the osseous morphology at the proposed implant site (Liang et al. 2009). Placement of an implant fixture or removal of a failing implant will as a result require not only careful assessment of the proximity of the canal to the surgical site but also an assurance that the walls of the canal remain intact (Kan et al. 2012).

Presurgical evaluation of the maxillary anterior region should include assessment of the integrity of the nasopalatine canal walls, in all views but specifically in axial views. As alveolar ridge atrophy due to prolonged edentulism increases, the resorption of the buccal ridge becomes more pronounced. The new location of the buccal cortical plate increasingly encroaches toward the nasopalatine canal reducing the quantity of bone for safe, predictable implant placement, resulting in a relative enlargement of the canal compared to the surrounding bone (Liang et al. 2009).

In addition, in the absence of significant alveolar ridge alterations, the presence of large anatomic variations of the canal necessitates a thorough presurgical dimensional as well as positioning assessment (Liang et al. 2009). 3D mapping of their locations and sizes remains a vital presurgical treatment planning step. The presence of neurovascular structures within the canal, given their soft tissue nature, cannot be visualized in CBCT images. Potential complications such as failure of osseointegration of the implant fixture or development of sensory dysfunction arising from contact between the fixture and the neurovascular contents of the canal have been reported (Liang et al. 2009; Jacobs et al. 2004; Tözüm et al. 2012).

The nasopalatine canal connects the roof of the oral cavity with the nasal floor (Theodorou et al. 2007). The canal is a long slender channel located on the median plane of the palatine process of the maxilla, opening inferiorly into the midline, in the incisive foramen posterior to the maxillary central incisors (Tözüm et al. 2012). The canal is located approximately 12–15 mm posterior to the anterior spine (Theodorou et al. 2007). It contains the nasopalatine (incisive) nerves and vessels and the terminal branch of the descending nasopalatine artery (Liang et al. 2009; Alexander 2010; Tözüm et al. 2012). Neurovascular bundles supplying the palatal region of the anterior palate innervate the tissues after exiting the inferiorly placed incisive foramen (Theodorou et al. 2007). The nasopalatine canal has two openings:

5 Anatomic Considerations in Dental Implant Surgery

1. The oval-shaped inferior opening also known as the incisive foramen which is located in the midline of the anterior palate and most often inferior to the incisive papilla is accessible orally and a common place for local anesthetic injections (Alexander 2010; Song et al. 2009).
2. The superior opening, the nasopalatine foramen (foramina Stenson), is located in the anterior aspect of the nasal floor with its openings at either side of the nasal septum (Tözüm et al. 2012; Theodorou et al. 2007; Bornstein et al. 2011).

Two additional canals, accessory minor openings referred to as foramina of Scarpa, are sometimes present (Theodorou et al. 2007). Most variations are found at the most superior foramen at the nasal floor in which the nasopalatine foramina may present as one or up to six separate foramina (Liang et al. 2009).

As with most anatomical sites, morphologic variations compelling multiple classification systems are not uncommon (Kumar and Satheesh 2013; Bornstein et al. 2011; Liang et al. 2009; Tözüm et al. 2012) (Fig. 5.3). Adding to the cadaveric and 2D-based classifications, sagittal views from 3D images provide different anatomical emphasis and provide the basis for new classification systems (Tözüm et al. 2012). The inclusion of other multiplanar reconstruction (MPR) planes, such as coronal or corrected sagittal views, has resulted in other classification systems describing the incisive canal as cylindrical, funnel (conical), hourglass, and banana shape (Tözüm et al. 2012; Theodorou et al. 2007). Understanding variations in canal morphology is essential when in addition to the procedures already mentioned; intentional obliteration of the canal itself or nasal floor augmentation graft to correct significant loss of bucco-palatal width and vertical deficiencies is planned (Raitz et al. 2012; Liang et al. 2009).

Bornstein et al. in 2011 proposed a morphology-related classification system based on the presence of (a) single canal, (b) two parallel canals, and (c) variations of Y-type (shaped) canal (Bornstein et al. 2011). The anatomic variations as mentioned earlier were found at the level of the nasal floor. The authors also postulated that in their study, >50% of the cases were a combination of the parallel and Y-type variations, leaving the single canal presentation the most prevalent (Alexander 2010) (Fig. 5.4).

Small canals (<3 mm) presented mostly as cone-shaped, whereas the larger canals (>4 mm) appeared more often with cylindrical shape (Liang et al. 2009). The mean length between the nasopalatine foramen and the alveolar crest in a dentate person has been reported with the range of 9.4–11.5 mm

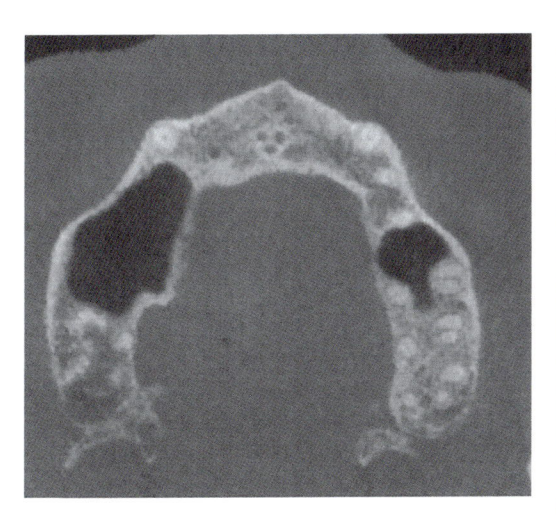

Fig. 5.3 Nasopalatine canal at the level of the nasal floor

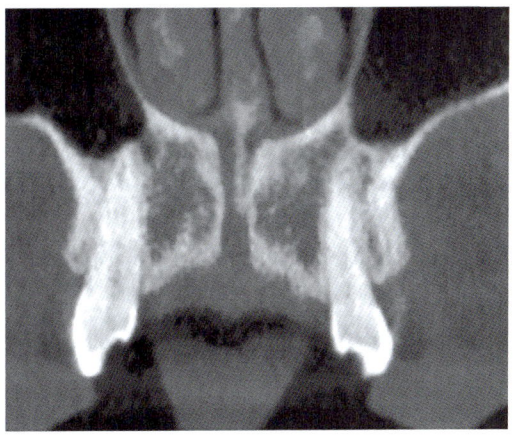

Fig. 5.4 Example of nasopalatine canal with one oral/palatal opening and two nasal opening

(Alexander 2010; Liang et al. 2009). The mean diameter of the nasopalatine foramen reported is in the range of 3.49–6 mm, while the incisive foramen was reported as being wider with a range of 2.80–4.45 mm (Liang et al. 2009; Alexander 2010; Theodorou et al. 2007). In axial views, the mediolateral measurements of the incisive foramen up to 1 cm are considered within normal limits; however, the average diameter of 3.3 mm is reported as the more common finding (Liang et al. 2009; Tözüm et al. 2012; Koenig et al. 2011).

In CBCT axial images, the canal may appear as a round- to heart-shaped radiolucency, ideally surrounded by uniform corticated walls. Influence of age as an absolute factor is a point of much debate, in combination with alveolar ridge atrophy; however, the relative dimensions of the canal may appear larger compared to pre-atrophy conditions (Kumar and Satheesh 2013; Tözüm et al. 2012; Song et al. 2009; Alexander 2010; Theodorou et al. 2007). Studies on the characteristic changes of the nasopalatine canal in the atrophic maxillary arch are scarce and those that are available differ in their findings. Liang et al. and Tözüm et al. found no significant difference between the diameter of the canal in dentate and edentulous populations they studied, whereas Mardinger et al. reported an increase in diameter with ridge resorption (Tözüm et al. 2012; Liang et al. 2009). Whether or not the canal dimensions truly increase in atrophied arches, when pre- and post-atrophy alveolar ridges are compared, there appears to be a relative widening of the canal dimensions compared to the remaining ridge surrounding the canal (Fig. 5.5). Since placing the implant fixture within the triangle of bone (Araújo et al. 2006; Ganz 2006) is considered a vital step for stability and long-term longevity of the restored implant fixture, the dimensions of the bone anterior to the canal are considered a crucial factor in proper implant selection (Araújo et al. 2006; Tözüm et al. 2012). As such careful dimensional analysis will provide the surgeon with invaluable information, preventing unanticipated encroachment on the nasopalatine canal.

Gender-linked differences in the mean length of the canal, suggesting significantly longer and wider canals in males compared to females, have been reported (Liang et al. 2009; Tözüm et al. 2012; Alexander 2010; Theodorou et al. 2007). At the mid-root level of the maxillary central incisors, in females and young adults receiving immediate implant fixtures, the roots may be in close proximity to the canal (Theodorou et al. 2003, 2007; De Santana Santos et al. 2013).

While the neurosensory changes reported after invasive surgical procedures involving the canal appear to be transient (Theodorou et al. 2007; Alexander 2010), the main concern remains contact between neurovascular bundles within the canal and the fixture resulting in failure of osseointegration (Jacobs et al. 2004).

When viewing CBCT images, the number of canals, locations, diameter, length, slope, and morphologic variations of the maxillary incisive canal and its relationship to the alveolar crest should be assessed in detail (Liang et al. 2009). CBCT sagittal views offer anteroposterior, while the axial images provide mediolateral dimensional assessments. There are a great diversity of surgical techniques and augmentation procedures and materials to improve the defects or deficiencies of the alveolar ridge. Most corrective techniques are focused on rehabilitation of the labial wall deficiencies. It is worth consideration that a high palatal resorption rate of the premaxilla in the post-extraction phase may be caused as a result of trauma or a surgical removal of enlarged cystic or tumoral lesions. As such it is imperative that both buccal and cortical plates in the vicinity of the canal be analyzed carefully.

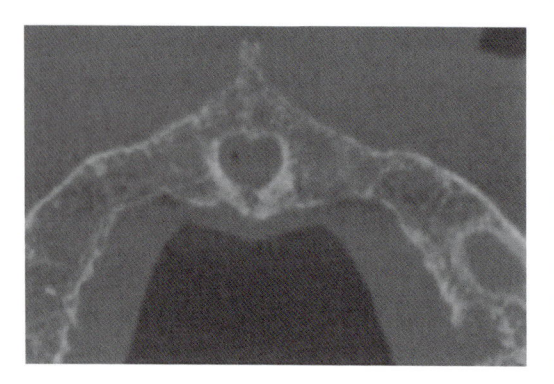

Fig. 5.5 Nasopalatine canal's relative enlargement in comparison to the atrophied anterior maxillary arch

5.4.3 Nasal Cavity/Floor

With dental implant common placement in the anterior maxilla, the alveolar ridge dimensions influence location of the implant, lip position, and free gingival margin architecture. Alveolar ridge resorption pattern in this area contributes to an unfavorable maxillo-mandibular relationship, in addition to insufficient bone volume for implant fixture placement (Serhal et al. 2002). In the absence of augmentation procedures, combination of modified implant and/or abutment position, encroachment or involvement of the adjacent anatomical sites such as the nasal cavity may become unavoidable (Serhal et al. 2002).

Augmentation of the severely atrophic anterior maxillary alveolar ridge may necessitate nasal floor modification to augment the bone height (Kuzmanovic et al. 2003). Post-extraction, disuse atrophy, hormonal-metabolic conditions, trauma, and iatrogenic changes are among many causes which may result in challenging resorptive patterns (Kuzmanovic et al. 2003). Post-resorption augmentation of the anterior maxillary alveolar ridge is limited by the location and the anatomy of the nasal cavity. Thorough understanding of the anterior maxillary alveolar ridge resorptive patterns and the anatomy of the nasal cavity is important in order to predictably avoid complications such as bleeding, infection, swelling, pain, hematoma, and rhinitis to name a few (Kuzmanovic et al. 2003; Serhal et al. 2002).

The nasal mucosa is thicker and more tear resistant than the antral mucosa, resulting in lower prevalence of surgical nasal mucosal tear (Kuzmanovic et al. 2003). While nasal mucosal tear has been reported, unlike maxillary sinus augmentation graft procedures, modifications of the planned surgical or rehabilitation to avoid the tear were not reported (El-Ghareeb et al. 2012).

The nasal cavities are surrounded by frontal sinuses superiorly, the oral cavity inferiorly, and the orbits and the maxillary sinuses laterally. Anteriorly the bony floor is created by the palatine process of the maxilla (Jensen et al. 1994). It is separated into two compartments by the nasal septum, a multicomponent structure partially dividing the cavity into two compartments with fairly similar volumes. Both the palatine process of the maxillary and nasal crest of the palatine bone have small contributions to the nasal septum (Jensen et al. 1994). The cartilage of the septum maintains the position of the columella and nasal tip and is thicker at its margins than at the center. Articulation of the septal cartilage inferiorly with the vomer and the maxilla may form horizontal "premaxillary wings" which could make mucoperiochondrium elevation difficult (Jensen et al. 1994).

There are three turbinates in each compartment of the cavity named after their physical locations and relationships to each other; superoinferiorly they are called the superior, middle, and inferior turbinates. These are vertically positioned and are slightly curved in appearance with the inferior turbinate being the largest and the middle the longest (Jensen et al. 1994). Each of the passages in between the turbinates is referred to as a *nasal meatus*, with the most inferior located between the nasal floor and its respective inferior turbinate. This area may become the future recipient of nasal floor augmentation should alveolar ridge height deficiency correction be required.

The presence of anatomic variations such as pneumatization of the middle turbinates, called *concha bullosa*, may, depending on the size of the pneumatization, reduce the dimensions of the adjacent nasal passages (Fig. 5.6).

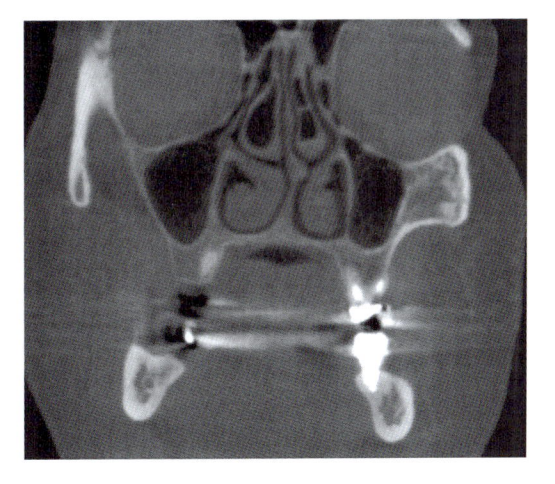

Fig. 5.6 Bilateral pneumatization of the middle turbinates, also known as concha bullosas

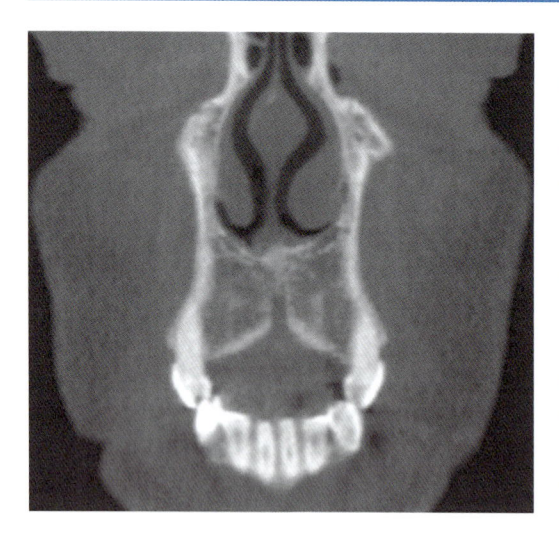

Fig. 5.7 Canalis sinuosus passing in the floor of the nasal cavity toward the midline

The presence of *canalis sinuosus*, a variation of normal anatomy, a tortuous corticated channel traversing in the floor of the nasal cavity toward the midline, should alert the practitioner to the potential presence of neurovascular structures. In CBCT images this structure is best viewed in coronal views (Frederico Sampaio Neves et al. 2012). The anterior superior alveolar nerve (ASAN), a branch of the infraorbital nerve, creates a neural plexus in the alveolar process, supplying the canines and the incisors (Frederico Sampaio Neves et al. 2012). The ASAN in conjunction with its artery innervate the maxilla through a bony canal named *canalis sinuosus*, which when present supplies the soft tissues, as well as the maxillary anterior teeth (Goel and Weerakhody) (Fig. 5.7).

Recent publications have highlighted other accessory canals extending or communicating with the canalis sinuosus and are referred to by various terms including lateral incisive canal or accessory canals (Cawood and Howell 1988; Von Arx et al. 2013). It has been suggested that there is higher incidence of accessory canals in the older population (Von Arx et al. 2013).

5.4.4 Paranasal Sinuses

When visible within the field of view (FOV) of the acquired scan, the paranasal sinuses which consist of the ethmoid air cells, frontal, sphenoid, and maxillary sinuses should be evaluated. If present, sino-nasal polyps, moderate to significant opacifications, or other pathologies are easily identified and may need to be treated prior to installation of implant fixtures.

5.4.5 Maxillary Sinuses

A pyramidal cavity with a quadrangular base forming the lateral wall of the nose and its apex extending into the zygoma, the maxillary sinus is an important structure due to both its anatomy and its location (Watzek 2012).

The four walls of the maxillary sinuses are made up of the anterior (buccal), posterior (intratemporal), superior (orbital), and medial (nasal) sections. The antral floor is formed partly by the maxillary alveolar process and partly by the hard palate (Chan et al. 2011; Watzek 2012). It is normally approximately 1 cm inferior to the floor of the nasal cavity (Watzek 2012).

Maxillary sinus pneumatization into the alveolar ridge in the posterior maxillary arch is common and easily noticed on panoramic radiographs. Anterior pneumatization of the maxillary sinuses inferior to the nasal floor creating alveolar recesses is also considered a common variation of normal anatomy (Fig. 5.8). Generally bilateral, these alveolar recesses are similar in size and location and only of significance if surgical procedures involving this area are contemplated. Surgical procedures involving the maxillary sinuses demand detailed evaluation of the antral anatomy and possible pathologies present. In anterior implant surgical procedures however, the entire maxillary sinuses may not be fully visible within the field of view

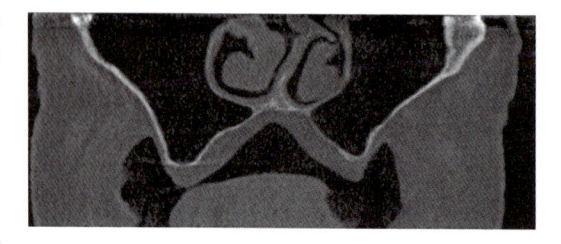

Fig. 5.8 Bilateral pneumatization of the maxillary sinuses inferior to the nasal floor and palate resulting in recesses

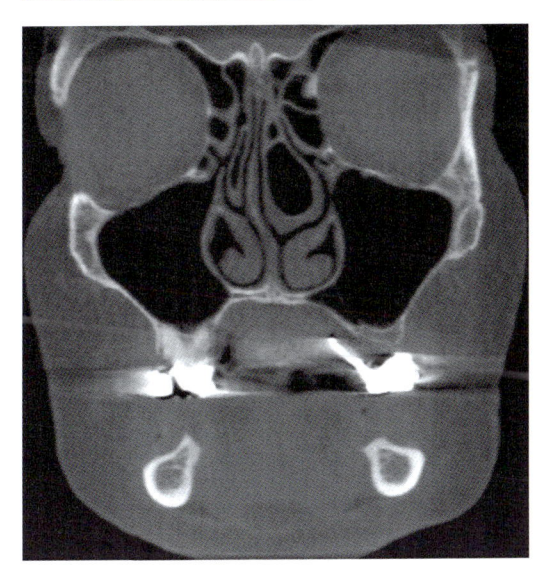

5 Anatomic Considerations in Dental Implant Surgery

Fig. 5.9 Anterior pneumatization of the maxillary sinuses inferior to the nasal floor, as well as bilateral concha bullosa of the middle turbinates

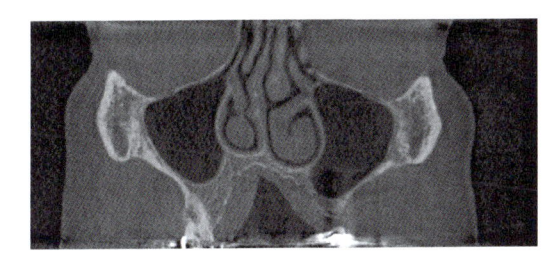

Fig. 5.10 Hypoplasia of the right maxillary sinus

of the scan. When recesses inferior to the nasal floor are present and contain mucosal thickening, nature of the thickening may be of importance and must be diagnosed. If necessary, treatment may have to be rendered prior to the surgical appointment (Fig. 5.9).

Morphologic anomalies such as aplasia or hypoplasia of the maxillary sinuses may increase the volume of bone present (Watzek 2012). While aplasia is rare, unilateral or bilateral reduction in vertical and/or horizontal dimensions of the maxillary sinuses is more common (Watzek 2012) (Fig. 5.10).

5.4.6 Mandible

The mandible is "the largest and strongest of the facial bones" (Garg 2010). It consists of a horseshoe-shaped body which houses the teeth and the rami, which appear as bilateral processes projecting superiorly from the posterior aspect of the mandibular body (Garg 2010). The body of the mandible is further divided into the anterior and posterior regions.

At the facial midline, the external surface is marked by the *symphysis menti* (Garg 2010). Inferiorly adjacent to the midline, the anterior surface projects to form triangular prominences on either side of the symphysis referred to as the mental protuberance. A depression, the *mental fossa*, lies laterally on either side of the chin (Garg 2010).

A detailed understanding of the anatomic variations of the anterior mandible, the interforaminal neurovascular bundle, and the location of the anterior loop when present is vital to successful surgery.

5.4.7 Mandibular Canal

The inferior alveolar nerve (IAN) enters the mandible through the mandibular foramen located on the medial surface of the ramus and runs anteriorly through the mandibular canal, progressively traveling from the lingual to the labial side of the mandible (Pires et al. 2012; Juodzbalys et al. 2010).

The IAN, which is itself a branch of the posterior trunk of V3 (mandibular) of the CN V (trigeminal nerve), has an intraosseous course within the mandibular canal until it reaches the mandibular foramen. The inferior alveolar artery, a branch of the maxillary artery, accompanies the IAN. Together they innervate the teeth and periodontium on the ipsilateral side of the mandibular arch, respectively. Exiting from the mental foramen, the IAN and the artery innervate the adjacent soft tissues. A variation of normal anatomy, the mandibular incisive canal containing the mandibular incisive nerve, has been identified as a terminal branch of the IAN, extending intraosseously anterior to the mental foramen (Raitz et al. 2012). For a more detailed discussion on the mandibular incisive canal, see later sections.

The mandibular canal's position and location vary in different individuals (Juodzbalys et al. 2010). Gender, age, race, and imaging techniques such as 2D vs 3D imaging will produce different presentations of the canal. Determination of the location and depth of osteotomies is directly influenced by the location of the canal (Juodzbalys et al. 2010). Neurosensory alterations and/or excessive bleeding are complications to be concerned about when the integrity of the canal and its contents are violated.

Cadaveric studies of the canal diameter in the mandibular body have been reported in the range of 2.6–3.4 mm (Mraiwa et al. 2003a; Rajchel et al. 1986). The vertical diameter in cadaveric studies in the Japanese population measured approximately 5 mm (Obradovic et al. 1993).

There are a number of classifications detailing the vertical location of the mandibular canal (Juodzbalys et al. 2010): (1) high mandibular canal (within 2 mm of the apices of the first and second molars), (2) intermediate mandibular canal, (3) low mandibular canal, and (4) other less common variations, such as duplication, division of the canal, or lack of left and right symmetry (Juodzbalys et al. 2010). Mandibular canals are generally bilaterally symmetrical; however, hemi-mandibles presenting with only one major canal have also been reported (Juodzbalys et al. 2010).

Bifurcation of the canal, a variation of normal anatomy, is reported in 1–3% of the population. Langlais et al. evaluated 6,000 panoramic radiographs and found 0.95% bifid inferior mandibular canal (Sato et al. 2005). Considering the limitations of panoramic imaging, the actual prevalence of bifid canals may be higher. Naitoh et al. reviewing three-dimensional images observed branched mandibular canal in 65% of patients (Langlais et al. 1985). They classified the mandibular branched canal into four distinct groups: (1) retromolar, (2) dental, (3) forward, and (4) buccolingual canals (Langlais et al. 1985).

The horizontal course and its buccolingual location were used by Kim et al. to classify the canal into three types: type 1 canal (follows the lingual cortical plate, the mandibular ramus, and the body (70%)), type 2 canal (follows the middle ramus behind the second molar and the lingual plate passing through the second and first molars (15%)), and type 3 canal (follows the middle or the lingual one third of the mandible from the ramus to the body (15%)) (Juodzbalys et al. 2010; Naitoh et al. 2009).

5.4.8 Mental Foramen, the Anterior Loop, and the Mandibular Incisive Canals

Identification of vital structures with the increase in the anterior mandible utilized as donor sites for graft procedures and/or placement of implant fixtures in the interforaminal region is crucial. To avoid perforation of the neurovascular structures recognizing the presence, morphology, and location of the neurovascular structures is imperative (Pires et al. 2012). The anatomic landmarks of interest in this region are the mental foramina, mental canal, mandibular incisive canal, and their neurovascular bundle, as well as the lingual foramen and its contents (Pires et al. 2012). The mental foramina are generally considered the terminal boundary of the mandibular canal and the IAN. In panoramic radiographs, it is traditionally visualized between the first and second mandibular premolars.

An important consideration during implant surgery is the location of the mental nerve associated with the mental foramen which innervates the soft tissues. The mental nerve is a somatic afferent nerve providing sensation to the skin of the mental area, lower lip, mucous membrane, and gingiva as posteriorly as the second premolars (Pires et al. 2012; Ogle et al. 2012).

Utilizing CBCT imaging the location of each mental foramen in the proposed implant site must be evaluated carefully to avoid postsurgical complications. Location of each foramen is referenced by its relationship to the closest neighboring teeth. If more than one mental foramen on each side exists, determination of the location of each foramen in relation to the adjacent teeth and the proposed implant site must be noted. When installing the implant fixture in close proximity to the mental foramen, the shape and size of the foramen may become of surgical importance.

5 Anatomic Considerations in Dental Implant Surgery

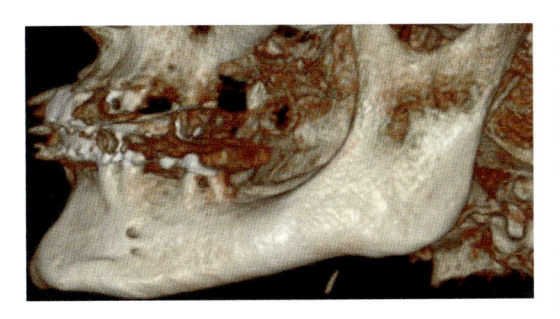

Fig. 5.11 Double mental foramina

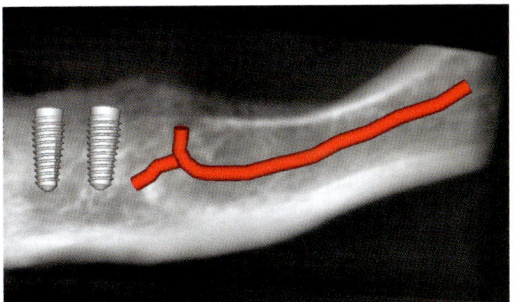

Fig. 5.12 Anterior loop

The mental foramen located on each side of the mandible is ordinarily a singular structure. However ipsilateral double foramina are not uncommon, while rare multiple (3%) or absences of ipsilateral foramina have also been reported (Pires et al. 2012; Kim et al. 2009; Raitz et al. 2012; Fujita and Suzuki 2014). When additional foramina are present, they are referred to as accessory mental foramen/foramina (Pires et al. 2012) (Fig. 5.11).

Location of the mental foramen is also varied, ranging from inferior to the first and second premolars to more posterior locations inferior to the first and less commonly second molar. Anteriorly it may be present as far anteriorly as the canine (Pires et al. 2012).

The mandibular canal near to the mental foramen divides into the mental and incisive branches.

The course of the mandibular canal containing the inferior alveolar bundle "swerves upward, backward, and laterally" to reach the mental foramen (Mraiwa et al. 2003b; Apostolakis and Brown 2012). The mental foramina, as a result, are placed superior to the level of the mandibular canal. This allows for the mental canal to deviate toward the mental foramen and the incisive canal to continue toward the midline at a level inferior to the apices of the incisor teeth (Pires et al. 2012; Parnia et al. 2012). Anatomic presentation of the mandibular incisive canal is considered a variation of normal anatomy which may present in a distinctive but smaller canal or as an incisive plexus supplying innervation to the mandibular anterior teeth (Pires et al. 2012; Mazor et al. 2012; Parnia et al. 2012). The section of the canal between the mental foramen and just before its ramification to the incisive nerve may be defined as the *anterior loop* (Pires et al. 2012; Apostolakis and Brown 2012; Bou Serhal et al. 2002; Ogle et al. 2012; Mazor et al. 2012) (Fig. 5.12).

Implant placement in the interforaminal region, symphyseal bone harvesting, or genioplasty in orthognathic procedures may disturb the anterior loop and result in potential postoperative neurosensory disturbances (Apostolakis and Brown 2012). Accurate preoperative identification of the anterior loop will assist the surgeon to avoid potential postoperative complications of altered lip and chin sensations. In addition to direct trauma, postsurgical edema and retrograde pressure on the mental nerve may also cause neurosensory deficiencies (Apostolakis and Brown 2012; Parnia et al. 2012).

The anterior loop's visibility on panoramic radiographs is limited at best (Apostolakis and Brown 2012). While identification of the mental foramina on panoramic imaging is fairly reliable, assessment of the anterior loop and/or the incisive mandibular canal is not recommended (Apostolakis and Brown 2012). Panoramic images consistently underestimate the presence of these structures.

5.4.9 Mandibular Incisive Canal

Mardinger et al. studying cadaveric specimen classified the mandibular incisive canal into:

1. Complete bony cortical walls throughout the canal

2. Partial cortical bony borders and areas of the medullary bone in part of the canal
3. No cortical walls, with the bundle traveling through the medullar bone
4. Large incisive bundles and fascia attached to the inferior alveolar nerve creating a delta-shaped structure

Radiographically classifications with no cortical walls will not be visible.

Jacobs et al. reported that while CT scan studies demonstrate the presence of incisive canal in 93% of the cases reviewed, panoramic studies were only able to identify 15% of cases (Fujita and Suzuki 2014). The small size of the canal, the two dimensionality, and inherent geometric distortions of the panoramic imaging may explain the low incidence in their study (Fig. 5.13).

Radiographically, structures with higher cortication of the canals were better visualized. In general, even when utilizing three-dimensional imaging such as CT or CBCT scans, the mandibular incisive canal because of its smaller size and possibility of partial or absence of cortication is more challenging to identify (Sahman et al. 2014). The dimensions of the mandibular incisive canal are largest closest to the mental foramen (Raitz et al. 2012). The canal may

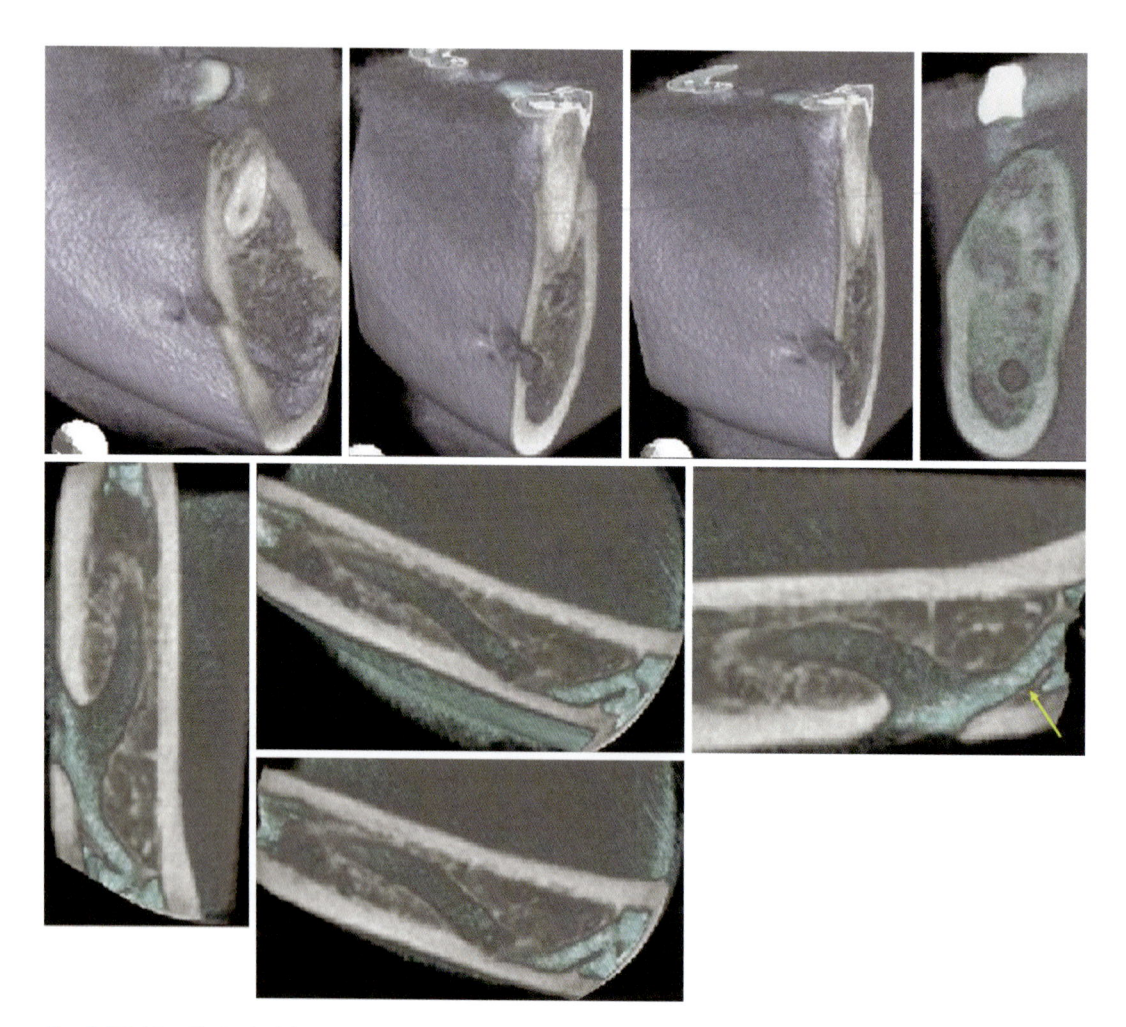

Fig. 5.13 Mandibular incisive canal (*yellow arrow*), extending anterior to the mental foramen (Courtesy of Dr. Silvio Diego Bianchi (Turin, Italy))

progressively narrow until the neurovascular bundle enters a labyrinth of medullary spaces (plexus) without evidence of containment within a canal. Equally problematic is lack of visualization of canals smaller than the spatial resolution of the scanner.

When surgical procedures are planned for areas in close proximity of the mental foramina, when possible, the average diameter as well as the length of the mandibular incisive canal should be noted.

5.4.10 Anterior Loop

The anterior extension of the mandibular canal when located in the surgical site is of significant importance (Mazor et al. 2012). The mean prevalence of the anterior loop varies in the literature and is reported in the range of 11% (Fujita and Suzuki 2014) to 97.3% (Gómez-Roman et al. 2015). Not surprisingly, 3D studies compared to panoramic studies provide higher incidences of identification of the loop. The distance between the mental foramen and the most anterior extension of the anterior loop exhibits great variety in length but is commonly reported as ranging from 0.4 to 2.19 mm (Apostolakis and Brown 2012; Mazor et al. 2012; Kuzmanovic et al. 2003). While in most studies, the anterior extension of the loop is not reported to be greater than 1 mm, extreme cases of the extension reaching 5–6.95 mm have been reported (Kuzmanovic et al. 2003).

Significant variations in morphology, as well as imaging modalities utilized to study the loop, have resulted in contradictory conclusions, with a few authors going as far as to refute its existence (Yildirim et al. 2014). However, among authors verifying the presence of the anterior loop, there is no reported right- or left-side preference (Apostolakis and Brown 2012; Uchida et al. 2009; Mardinger et al. 2000; Mazor et al. 2012; Uchida et al. 2007). In terms of prevalence, the anterior loop is commonly bilateral, followed by unilateral loops which appear to have a predilection for the right side (Ngeow et al. 2009). When bilaterally present, the right loop, in some patients, has been reported as possessing a slightly longer extension (Ngeow et al. 2009; Gómez-Roman et al. 2015).

Advancing age negatively affects the visibility of the anterior loop (Juodzbalys et al. 2010; Ngeow et al. 2009). The reduced visibility may be the result of reduced calcification of the cortical borders undergoing aging-related quantitative and qualitative changes.

Ideally implants are placed superior to the level of the mental foramen. However, increasingly when implants are placed in a long-term edentulous interforaminal area with limited bone height, modifications such as alternative locations, lengths, or dimensions of implants are sought. When surgical procedures are performed in close proximity of the mental foramina, such modifications may force the implant apex to be partially or completely placed medio-inferior to the level of the mental foramen increasing the risk of traumatizing the anterior loop.

Utilizing CBCT, the axial views allow visualization of the narrowing of the mandibular canal anterior to the mental foramen. This point, while difficult to visualize, may correlate with the approximate location of the branching of the mandibular incisive canal. The diameter of the incisive canal is suggested to be maximum of 3 mm. Canals larger than 3 mm are considered to be part of the anterior loop of the mandibular canal. Once located, these findings must be verified on cross-sectional views, where on the same slice, two mandibular canals appear to be present (Apostolakis and Brown 2012; Kim et al. 2009).

5.4.11 Accessory Foramina of the Mandible

Accessory foramina are located on the lingual aspect of the mandibular symphysis (Pires et al. 2012). Not only the accessory foramina of the mandible, as a result of their location, may cause complications in a multitude of dental procedures, but they remain of critical importance with respect to installation of dental implant fixtures. Life-threatening hemorrhage and sensory impairment as a direct result of the surgical procedure have been reported (Przystańska and Bruska 2010).

Contents of the foramina remain for the most part elusive. Przystańska et al. reported that the neurovascular bundle consisted of a branch of the mylohyoid nerve, the sublingual artery, and accompanying veins. However, the artery, they reported, had the greatest diameter (Przystańska and Bruska 2010). In a series of dissections, neurovascular bundles branching from the mylohyoid nerve, with accompanying branches of the sublingual artery, leave the muscles and continue to travel medially to the anterior aspect of the sublingual gland and subsequently medially to the symphysis. From the symphyseal region, the incoming left and right nerves and blood vessels form one neurovascular bundle and enter the accessory foramen (Przystańska and Bruska 2010).

It has been opined that the neurovascular bundles within the mandibular foramina may provide supplementary innervation for mandibular incisors (Przystańska and Bruska 2010; Dubois et al. 2010). Lack of profound anesthesia following mandibular block injections has been taken as confirmation that the mylohyoid branch innervates the mandibular teeth (Przystańska and Bruska 2010). The vascular component, an extension of the sublingual artery, provides blood supply which when traumatized during implant fixture placement may cause intraosseous hemorrhages (Przystańska and Bruska 2010).

Preoperative treatment planning and identification of the accessory mandibular foramina and its normal anatomic variations are essential in preventing complications such as sensory loss or life-threatening hemorrhage as a result of the surgical intervention.

5.4.12 Surgical Considerations Associated with the Lingual Aspect of the Anterior Mandible

The lingual aspect of the anterior mandible consists of rich anastomosing blood supply from many arteries such as the sublingual artery (a branch of the lingual artery), submental artery (a branch of the facial artery), and incisive artery (Sahman et al. 2014). There is paucity of information on the precise anatomy, the anatomic variations, as well as the contents of the neurovascular canals, rendering conclusions concerning this important region controversial.

Vascular complication may arise as a result of damage to the lingual periosteum iatrogenically caused by perforations of the lingual cortical plate. Bleeding may then spread to the soft tissues of the floor of the mouth, the sublingual space, and other areas it can travel to. In the cases of uncontrolled profuse bleeding, loss of life has been reported.

Traditionally anatomy textbooks identify two major vessels, the submental and the sublingual artery supplying blood supply to the floor of the mouth, with the primary blood supply provided by the sublingual branch of the lingual artery (Lana et al. 2011). Recent cadaveric studies have added a variation in which a submental branch of the facial artery penetrates through the mylohyoid muscle to supply the floor of the mouth (Lana et al. 2011).

Atrophic edentulous ridge may alter the anatomy such that arteries typically located in safe distances are placed closer to the surgical site, increasing their risk of vascular perforation.

5.4.13 Mandibular Lingual Canals and Foramina

Radiographically the lingual canals and foramina are typically presented in the midline and the canine – premolar regions (Ganz 2015). Mraiwa et al. in their cadaveric study found 32% of their samples contained two or more midline lingual foramina, while the majority, 64%, exhibited single lingual foramina (Raitz et al. 2012).

Midline lingual canal is situated in the midline of the mandible, at the level of or superior to the mental spines, and is present in 85–99% of reported radiographic cases studied (Pires et al. 2012). In intraoral radiographs it appears as a circular radiolucency surrounded by a peripheral corticated border. However, acquisition technique errors and

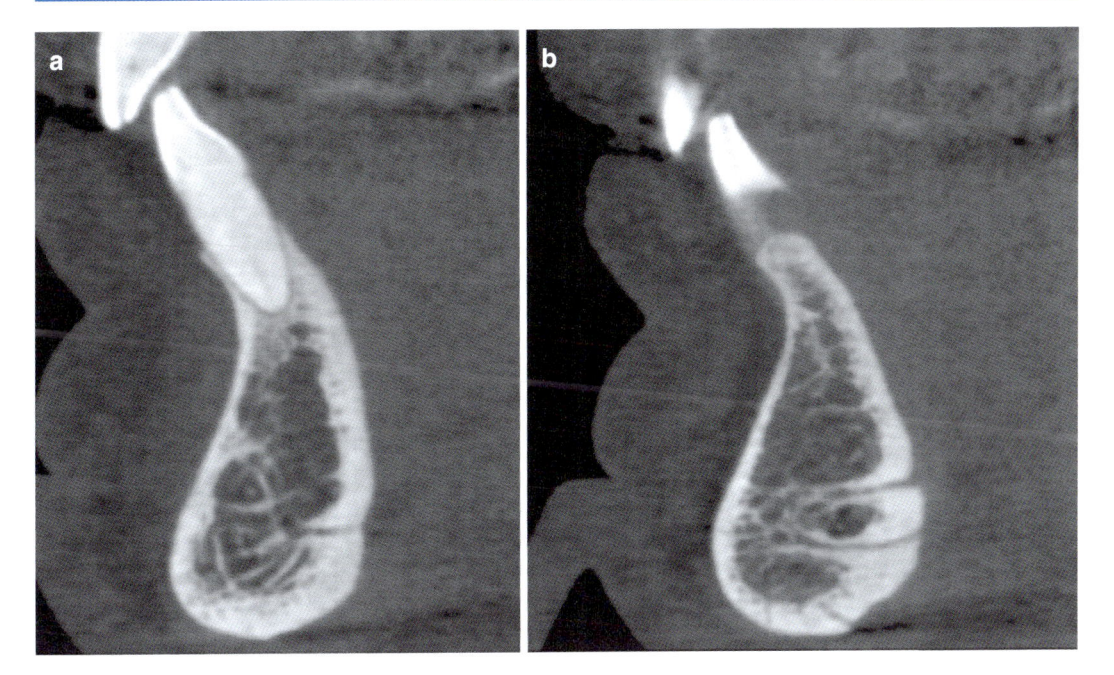

5 Anatomic Considerations in Dental Implant Surgery

Fig. 5.14 (**a**) Mandibular midline lingual canal. (**b**) Double mandibular midline lingual canal, considered a variation of normal anatomy

absence of parallelism between the foramen and the x-ray beam may prevent clear observation. In 3D cross-sectional images, it appears as a canal extending from the lingual plate partway toward the buccal plate (Fig. 5.14a, b).

The dimensions of the midline foramina and canal are generally believed to be larger than the canals and foramina located more laterally.

The contents of the canals may consist of neurovascular bundles, arising from the anastomosis of some or all of the following: submental branch of the facial artery, sublingual branches of the lingual arteries, lingual nerves, incisive arteries, and branches of the mylohyoid nerve (Pires et al. 2012; Jacobs et al. 2007). Arterial anastomoses are formed between sublingual and submental arteries and between sublingual and incisive arteries through multiple accessory lingual foramina (Jacobs et al. 2007). To add to the complexity of this region, there are reported cases of the mental artery, a branch of the inferior alveolar artery communicating with the sublingual artery in the mental region (Jacobs et al. 2007).

A concern in surgical procedures in which the integrity of the anterior mandibular lingual cortical plate is violated, whether by surgical instruments or the implant fixture, is perforation of the sublingual artery followed by the perforation of other arteries mentioned. Arterial perforation increases the potential risk of hemorrhage in the floor of the mouth with subsequent life-threatening complications.

During 3D evaluations, location of the foramina and canals as well as the relationship to the adjacent structures and existing teeth should be noted. The vertical distance from the alveolar crest to the canal provides safety zone guidelines. As mentioned before, CBCT is not the imaging modality of choice for soft tissue evaluations; however, location of the canals and foramina will provide indirect information.

5.5 Quantification of Bone in the Implant Site

While 3D analysis of the proposed implant sites will provide significant amount of information, true quantification of the bone using CBCT images is not possible at this time. This is due to inherent technical limitations stemming from manufacturing to software design.

In 3D digital radiology, the radiographic density (x-ray attenuation) in each voxel of the volume of interest is expressed by a single number called the CT number (sometimes also referred to as the grayscale value) (Ganz 2015). CT numbers are calculated utilizing the relative density of the body tissue according to a calibrated gray-level scale, based on values for air (−1,000 HU), water (0 HU), and bone density (+1,000 HU) (Ganz 2006). The scale of CT numbers is specific to the imaging equipment and to the modality used. In their purest form, CT numbers describe the anatomy of interest by using Arabic numbers which are understandable to the computer. In order to display the same images on monitors, the CT numbers are correlated to gray levels or gray shades which provide us with a visually understandable anatomy (Artzi et al. 2000).

Hounsfield units (HU), a concept used widely in CT units, provide standardization for scaling of the reconstructed attenuation coefficients to provide a quantifiable means of measurements (Reeves et al. 2010; Artzi et al. 2000). Without HU bone quality cannot be assessed (Katsumata et al. 2007). To date, dental CBCT manufacturers have not implemented a standardized system for scaling the gray levels representing the reconstructed values (Reeves et al. 2010). Published reports of the calculated density (HU) on CBCT scans vary widely from a range of −1,500 to over +3,000 for different types and locations of bones (Katsumata et al. 2007).

Although CBCT units display grayscale units, these cannot be treated as true Hounsfield units. The grayscale numbers assigned to the voxels are relative HU values and do not reflect the precise bone density as HU values in CT units do (Molteni 2013). For the implant surgeon, preoperative understanding of the bone quality and grading the bone within the proposed implant site may have significant relevance on the outcome. Misch's bone type to HU value correlation chart was derived utilizing CT units and not CBCT (Misch). It is worth the consideration that overestimation of HU values derived from CBCT compared to that of classic CT has been reported (Lagravère et al. 2008; Ganz 2006). As such, CBCT-generated HU numbers are imprecise in bone density quantification and should not be used for definitive treatment planning purposes.

Technical limitations preventing the use of CBCT's HU values are plentiful, and while some may be easily addressed, others require different software logarithms or major modifications to the CBCT units themselves. Nonstandardization of the x-ray beam spectrum used in the CBCT units is a major barrier in measuring accurate HU numbers (Artzi et al. 2000; Molteni 2013). In CBCT, the CT numbers throughout the volume of interest are not consistent, and may be influenced by the location within the scanner of the anatomical site of interest, although other authors have suggested no such influence (Artzi et al. 2000; Ganz 2015b; Lagravère et al. 2008). This inconsistency may be attributed to the nonideal geometry (cone shape of the beam), scatter radiation, beam hardening, and/or metal artifacts, among other inherent limitations of the technology itself, not to mention the density and atomic characteristics of the area of interest undergoing imaging (Artzi et al. 2000; Ganz 2015b). In addition, software programs utilizing varying algorithms to reconstruct the images may calculate different HU values (Lagravère et al. 2008). The greater propensity of CBCT images for artifacts in comparison to classic CT units affects the consistency of CBCT's CT numbers and as a result the accuracy of the mathematical conversion of these numbers into Hounsfield units (Artzi et al. 2000).

5.6 Dose

While the advantages of 3D imaging is plentiful, and it is an integral part of treatment planning especially in complicated restorative rehabilitation procedures, the risk-benefit ratio of information received by the dental team and the radiation dose received by the patient must be balanced. Even though the risks involved are generally assumed to be low, they are not nonexistent. Development of new cancers in the population receiving radiation dose is the potential risk assumed by the patient. The pediatric and adolescent population has lower tolerance for radiation dose and assumes greater potential risk. There is controversy as to the extent of dental radiation's ability to cause new cancer; however, in the absence of proof that it does not, dental radiation dose must be prescribed with care and only in situations in which the information received outweighs the potential risks involved.

5.7 Artifacts

The presence of artifacts is inherent to certain technologies such as CT and CBCT. They are unavoidable and inherent to the technology or caused by patient's existing metallic or other high-density restorations, jewelry, or anatomy. Familiarity with and profound understanding of these artifacts and their contribution to reducing the quality of the image are vital.

5.7.1 Partial Volume Averaging Artifact

This artifact is commonly seen in areas where multiple small (thin) anatomic structures are, simultaneously, imaged within a voxel (three-dimensional pixel). Each voxel will represent one tissue density. The density that is captured by the scanner and reconstructed by the computer is a mathematical average of all the anatomic structures within that voxel. The density of a voxel containing multiple anatomic structures of different densities is a mathematical average of all the tissue densities within the voxel, since each voxel can only display one density. The average value is not a true representative of the individual tissues it has registered, and is not a true representation of any of the densities (tissues) it has registered.

In clinical terms the presence of partial volume averaging artifact means very thin structures with similar densities will lose some or complete delineation, rendering them partially or entirely difficult to visualize. To minimize the effect of this artifact and increase visibility of the thin buccal plate, for example, separation of the soft tissue of the lip during image acquisition with cotton roll will introduce air density (black) adjacent to the thin cortical plate and gingiva, which in turn may highlight these structures and allow better visibility (Oliveira et al. 2013).

5.7.2 Beam-Hardening Artifact

In the presence of metallic object within the area of interest, x-ray imaging techniques such as CT and CBCT are prone to produce artifacts. When extensive, these artifacts may render a scan non-diagnostic. A thorough understanding of the radiographic appearance, shape, and direction of artifacts is helpful in identifying useful from meaningless information (Schulze et al. 2010).

Beam hardening occurs when with the absorption of lower-energy x-ray photons by the object being imaged the original polychromatic x-ray beam "hardens" resulting in a beam containing more wavelengths of higher energy. As a consequence, the reconstruction process is disturbed because the sensor records greater concentration of beams with higher energy (Schulze et al. 2010). Dental implants, for example, may absorb lower-energy photons, selectively creating higher-energy beams. Subsequently, reconstruction results in higher gray values, therefore appearing as dark air density areas compared to the rest of the scan, which may be interpreted as areas devoid of bone.

When evaluating CBCT scans containing multiple high-density or metallic objects within the field of view, especially evaluating osseointegration of existing implant fixtures, not all air density areas surrounding the implants are "true" bone loss. Beam-hardening artifact may appear as circumferential lytic areas surrounding one or multiple implant fixtures mimicking loss of bone in areas where clinically and histologically bone may be present.

The discussion on artifacts is an important and complex topic, one which is beyond the scope of this chapter. It is important to remember that all artifacts diminish the quality of the images viewed.

Summary

1. 3D treatment planning allows for consideration of greater specific patient-related information, resulting in surgical plans that are personalized for the patient and the surgical sites. 3D treatment planning allows for inclusion of patient's variations of anatomy as well as alterations due to trauma, pathology, or edentulism.
2. Unlike 2D images, when utilizing 3-D images, all findings noted on one of the views (axial, coronal, sagittal) must be verified on other views. A finding on axial views must be confirmed on one or all of the remaining views.
3. Osseous structural visualization among other factors is directly related to the degree of mineralization or cortication of the structure of interest. Voxel size and the scanner spatial resolution will also affect visualization of various anatomic structures. The smaller the voxel size and the higher the resolution theoretically, the better the visualization of the thin anatomic structures will be.
4. Location of the vital anatomic structures adjacent and within the proposed implant sites must be carefully mapped.

References

Alexander K (2010) Reducing error in radiographic interpretation. Can Vet J 51:533–536

Apostolakis D, Brown JE (2012) The anterior loop of the inferior alveolar nerve: prevalence, measurement of its length and a recommendation for interforaminal implant installation based on cone beam CT imaging. Clin Oral Implants Res 23:2012

Araújo MG, Wennström JL, Lindhe J (2006) Modeling of the buccal and lingual bone walls of fresh extraction sites following implant installations. Clin Oral Implants Res 17:606–614

Artzi Z, Nemcovsky CE, Bitlitum I, Segal P (2000) Displacement of the incisive foramen in conjunction with implant placement in the anterior maxilla without jeopardizing vitality of nasopalatine nerve and vessels: a novel surgical approach. Clin Oral Implants Res 11:505–510

Atwood DA (1971) Reduction of residual ridges: a major oral disease entity. Prosthet Dental 26:266–279

Block M (2014) Color atlas of denal implant surgery. Color Atlas of Dental Implant Surgery, 4th edition, 2017. Elsevier Saunders- St. Louis, Missouri

Bornstein MM, Balsiger R, Sendi P, Von Arx T (2011) Morphology of the nasopalatine canal and dental implant surgery: a radiographic analysis of 100 consecutive patients using limited cone-beam computed tomography. Clin Oral Implants Res 22:295–301

Bou Serhal C, Jacobs R, Flygare L, Quirynen M, Van Steenberghe D (2002) Perioperative validation of localisation of the mental foramen. Dento Maxillo Facial Radiol 31:39–43

Cawood JI, Howell RA (1988) A classification of the edentulous jaws. Int J Oral Maxillofac Surg 17:232–236

Chan H-L, Brooks SL, Fu J-H, Yeh C-Y, Rudek I, Wang H-L (2011) Cross-sectional analysis of the mandibular lingual concavity using CBCT. Clin Oral Implants Res 22:201–206

De Santana Santos T, De Carvalho Raimundo R, Martins-Filho PRS, De Souza de Andrade ES, De Oliveira E, Silva ED, Gomes ACA (2013) Destruction aneurysmal bone cyst of the mandible. J Cranio Fac Surg 24:e123–e124

Dubois L, De Lange J, Baas E, Van Ingen J (2010) Excessive bleeding in the floor of the mouth after endosseus implant placement: a report of two cases. Int J Oral Maxillofac Surg 39:412–415

El-Ghareeb M, Pi-Anfruns J, Khosousi M, Aghaloo T, Moy P (2012) Nasal floor augmentation for the reconstruction of the atrophic maxilla: a case series. J Oral Maxillofac Surg 70:e235–e241

Evian CI, Rosenberg ES, Coslet JG, Corn H (1982) The osteogenic activity of bone removed from healing extraction sockets in humans. J Periodontol 53:81–85

Frederico Sampaio Neves, et al, Canalis sinuosus: a rare anatomical variation, Surg Radiol Anat (2012):34; 563–566

Fujita A, Suzuki T (2014) Computed tomographic analysis of the mental foramen and nerve in Japanese patients. Implant Dent 23:471–476

Ganz SD (2006) The reality of Anatomy and the triangle of bone. Inside Dent 2:72–77

Ganz SD (2015) Improved CBCT diagnostic acuity with the 'Lip-Lift' technique. Cone Beam 1:6–9

Garg AK (2010) Implant dentistry a practical approach. Mosby Inc, an affiliate of Elsevier inc. 2nd edition. St. Louis, Missouri

Gómez-Roman G, Lautner NV, Goldammer C, McCoy M (2015) Anterior loop of the manibular canal- A source of possible complications. Implant Dent 24(5):578–585

Jacobs R, Mraiwa N, Van Steenberghe D, Sanderink G, Quirynen M (2004) Appearance of the mandibular incisive canal on panoramic radiographs. Surg Radiol Anat 26:329–333

Jacobs R, Lambrichts I, Liang X, Martens W, Mraiwa N, Adraemsens P, Gelan J (2007) Neurovascularization of the anterior jaw bones revisited using high-resolution magnetic resonance imaging. Oral Surg Oral Med Oral Pathol Oral Radiol Endod 103(5):683–693

Jensen J, Sindet-Pedersen S, Oliver AJ (1994) Varying treatment strategies for reconstruction of maxillary atrophy with implants: results in 98 patients. J Oral Maxillofac Surg 52:210

Juodzbalys G, Wang H-L, Sabalys G (2010) Anatomy of mandibular vital structures. Part I: mandibular canal and inferior Alveolar neurovascular bundle in relation with dental implantology. J Maxillofac Res 1(1):e2

Kan JYK, Rungcharassaeng K, Roe P, Chatriyanuyoke P, Caruso JM (2012) Maxillary central incisor-incisive canal relationship: a cone beam computed tomography study. Am J Esthet Dent 2:180–187

Katsumata A, Hirukawa A, Okumura S, Naitoh M, Fujishita M, Ariji E, Langlais RP (2007) Effects of image artifacts on gray-value density in limited-volume con-beam computerized tomography. Oral Surg Oral Med Oral Pathol Oral Radiol Endod 104:829–836

Kim ST, Hu KS, Song WC, Kang MK, Park HD, Kim HJ (2009) Location of the mandibular canal and the topography of its neurovascular structures. J Craniomaxillofac Surg 20:936–939

Koenig L, Tamimi D, Petrikowski G, Harnsberger HR, Ruprecht A, Benson BW, Van Dis ML, Hatcher DC, Perschbacher S (2011) Diagnostic imaging oral & maxillofacial

Kumar V, Satheesh K (2013) Applications of Cone Beam Computed Tomography (CBCT) in implant treatment planning. JSM Dent 1:1008–1001

Kuzmanovic DV, Payne AG, Kieser JA, Al E (2003) Anterior loop of the mental nerve: a morphological and radiographic study. Clin Oral Implants Res 14:464–471

Lagravère MO, Carey J, Ben-Zvi M, Packota GV, Major PW (2008) Effect of object location on the density measurement and Hounsfield conversion in a NewTom 3G cone beam computed tomography unit. Dentomaxillofac Radiol 37:305–308

Lana JP, Rodrigues PM, De Carvalho CV, De Souza PEA, Manzi RF, Horta MCR (2011) Anatomic variations and lesions of the maxillary sinus detected in cone beam computed tomography for dental implants. Clin Oral Implants Res 23(12):1398–1403

Langlais RP, Broadus R, Glass BJ (1985) Bifid mandibular canals in panoramic radiographs. J Am Dent Assoc 110:923–926

Lee CYS, Yanagihara LC, Suzuki JB (2012) Brisk, pulsatile bleeding from the anterior mandibular incisive canal during implant surgery: a case report and use of an active hemostatic matrix to terminate acute bleeding. Implant Dent 21:368–373

Liang X, Jacobs R, Martens W, Hu Y, Adriaensens P, Quirynen M, Lambrichts I (2009) Macro-and microanatomical, histological and computed tomography scan characterization of the nasopalatine canal. J Clin Periodontol 36:598–603

Liang X, Lambrichts I, Sun Y, Denis K, Hassan B, Li L, Pauwels R, Jacobs R (2010) A comparative evaluation of cone beam computed tomography (CBCT) and Multi-Slice CT (MSCT). Part II: on 3D model accuracy. Eur J Radiol 75:270–274

Mardinger O, Chaushu G, Arensburg B, Taicher S, Kaffe I (2000) Anterior loop of the mental canal: an anatomical-radiologic study. Implant Dent 9:120–122

Mazor Z, Lorean A, Mijiritsky E, Levin L (2012) Nasal floor elevation combined with dental implant placement. Clin Implant Dent Relat Res 14:768–771

Miller RJ, Edwards WC, Boudet C, Cohen JH (2011) Maxillofacial anatomy: the mandibular symphysis. J Oral Implantol 37:745–751

Misch CE Bone density a key determinant for clinical success

Molteni R (2013) Prospects and Challenges of rendering tissue density in Hounsefield units for cone beam computed tomography, Elsevier. Oral and Maxillofacial Radiol 116(1)

Mraiwa N, Jacobs R, Moerman P, Lambrichts I, Van Steenberghe D, Quirynen M (2003) Presence and course of the incisive canal in the human mandibular interforaminal region: two-dimensional imaging versus anatomical observations. Surg Radiol Anat 25:416–423

Mraiwa N, Jacobs R, Van Steenberghe D (2003) Clinical assessment and surgical implications of anatomic challenges in the anterior mandible. Clin Implant Dent Relat Res 5:219–225

Naitoh M, Hiraiwa Y, Aimiya H, Ariji E (2009) Observation of bifid mandibular canal using cone-beam computerized tomography. Int J Oral Maxillofac Implants 24:155–159

Ngeow CW, Dionysius DD, Ishak H, Nambiar P (2009) A radiographic study on the visualization of the anterior loop in dentate subjects of different age groups. J Oral Sci 51:231–237

Nowzari H, Molayem S, Chiu CHK, Rich SK (2012) Cone beam computed tomographic measurement of maxillary central incisors to determine prevalence of facial alveolar bone with ≥2 mm. Clin Implant Dent Relat Res 14:595–602

Obradovic O, Todorovic L, Pesic V, Pejkovic B, Vitanovic V (1993) Morphometric analysis of mandibular canal: clinical aspects. Bull Group Int Rech Sci Stomatol Odontol 36:109–113

Ogle OE, Weinstock RJ, Friedman E (2012) Surgical anatomy of the nasal cavity and paranasal sinuses. Oral Maxillofac Surg Clin N Am 24:155–166

Oliveira M, Tosoni GM, Lindsey DH, Mendoza K, Tetradis S, Mallya SM (2013) Influence of anatomical location on CT numbers in cone beam computed tomography. Oral Surg Oral Med Oral Pathol Oral Radiol 115:558–564

Parnia F, Moslehifard E, Hafezeqoran A, Mahboub F, Mojaver-Kahnamoui H (2012) Characteristics of anatomical landmarks in the mandibular interforaminal region: a cone-beam computed tomography study. Med Oral Patol Oral Cir Bucal 17:e4290–e4295

Pires CA, Bissada NF, Becker JJ, Kanawati A, Landers MA (2012) Mandibular incisive canal: cone beam computed tomography. Clin Implant Dent Relat Res 14:67–73

Przystańska A, Bruska M (2010) Accessory mandibular foramina: histological and immunohistochemical studies of their contents. Arch Oral Biol 55:77–80

Raitz R, Shimura E, Chilvarquer I, Fenyo-Pereira M (2012) Assessment of the mandibular incisive canal by panoramic radiograph and cone-beam computed tomography. Clin Implant Dent Relat Res 14:67–73

Rajchel J, Ellis ER, Fonseca RJ (1986) The anatomical location of the mandibular canal: its relationship to the sagittal ramus osteotomy. Int J Adult Orthodon Orthognath Surg 1:37–47

Reeves TE, Mah P, McDavid WD (2010) Deriving Hounsfield units using grey levels in cone beam computed tomography. Dentomaxillofac Radiol 39(6):323–335

Sahman H, Sekerci E, Ertas ET (2014) Lateral lingual vascular canals of the mandible: a CBCT study of 500 cases. Surg Radiol Anat 36:865–870

Sarment D (2014) Cone beam computed tomography: oral and maxillofacial diagnosis and applications. Wiley, Ames

Sato I, Ueno R, Kawai T, Yosue T (2005) Rare courses of the mandibular canal in the molar regions of the human mandible: a cadaveric study. Okajimas Folia Anat Jpn 82:95–101

Schulze RKW, Berndt D, D'Hoedt B (2010) On cone-beam computed tomography artifacts induced by titanium implants. Clin Oral Implants Res 21:100–107

Serhal BC, Jacobs R, Flygare L (2002) Perioperative validation of localisation of the mental foramen. Dentomaxillofac Radiol 31:39–43

Song W-C, Jo D-I, Lee J-Y, Kim J-N, Shin C, Koh K-S (2009) Microanatomy of the incisive canal using three-dimensional reconstruction of microCT images: an ex vivo study. Oral Surg Oral Med Oral Pathol Oral Radiol Endod 108:583–590

Theodorou DJ, Theodorou SJ, Sartoris D (2003) Primary non-odontogenic tumors of the jaw bones an overview of essential radiographic findings. J Clin Imaging 27:59–70

Theodorou SJ, Theodorou DJ, Sartoris D (2007) Imaging characteristics of neoplasms and other lesions of the jawbones Part 2. Odontogenic tumor-mimickers and tumor-like lesions. J Clin Imaging 31:120–126

Tözüm TF, Güncü GN, Yildirim YD, Yilmaz HG, Galindo-Moreno P, Velasco-Torres M, Al-Hezaimi K, Al-Sadhan R, Karabulut E, Wang H-L (2012) Evaluation of maxillary incisive canal characteristics related to dental implant treatment with computerized tomography: a clinical multicenter study. J Periodontol 83:337–343

Trikeriotis D, Paravalou E, Diamantopoulos P, Nikolaou D (2008) Anterior mandible canal communications: a potential portal of entry for tumour spread. Dentomaxillofac Radiol 37:125–129

Tyndall DA, Price JB, Tetradis S, Ganz SD, Hildebolt CF, Scarfe WC, Radiology, A. A. O. O. A. M (2012) Position statement of the American Academy of Oral and Maxillofacial Radiology on selection criteria for the use of radiology in dental implantology with emphasis on cone beam computed tomography. Oral Surg Oral Med Oral Pathol Oral Radiol 113:817–876

Uchida Y, Yamashita Y, Goto M (2007) Measurement of anterior loop length for the mandibular canal and diameter of the mandibular incisive canal to avoid nerve damage when installing endosseous implants in the interforaminal region. J Oral Maxillofac Surg 65:1772–1779

Uchida Y, Noguchi N, Goto M, Yamashita Y, Hanihara T, Takamori H, Sato I, Kawai T, Yosue T (2009) Measurement of anterior loop length for the mandibular canal and diameter of the mandibular incisive canal to avoid nerve damage when installing endosseous implants in the interforaminal region: a second attempt introducing cone beam computed tomography. J Oral Maxillofac Surg 67:744

Von Arx T, Lozanoff S, Sendi P, Bornstein MM (2013) Assessment of bone channels other than the nasopalatine canal in the anterior maxilla using limited cone beam computed tomography. Surg Radiol Anat 35:783–790

Watzek G (2012) The Percrestal sinuslift from illusion to reality. Quintessence Publishing, London

Yildirim YD, Güncü GN, Galindo-Moreno P, Velasco-Torres M, Juodzbalys G, Kubilius M, Gervickas A, Al-Hezaimi K, Al-Sadhan RE, Yilmaz HG, Asar NV, Karabulut E, Wang H-L, Tözüum TF (2014) Evaluation of mandibular lingual foramina related to dental implant treatment with computerized tomography: a multicenter clinical study. Implant Dent 23:57–63

The Aesthetic Challenge: Three-Dimensional Planning Concepts for the Anterior Maxillary Aesthetic Zone

Scott D. Ganz

Abstract

Patients who are missing teeth in the anterior maxillary aesthetic zone present difficult challenges for both the surgical and restorative clinician due to the fact that every patient presents with a unique and individual anatomical condition. The diagnostic information necessary to properly plan a surgical and restorative treatment should include, but not limited to, (1) intraoral periapical radiographs, (2) maxillary and mandibular impressions, (3) bite relationship/occlusion, (4) lip position/lip support, (5) smile-line, (6) soft tissue volume and biotype, and (7) three-dimensional imaging modalities such as computed tomography (CT) and the rapidly evolving cone beam CT (CBCT). Three-dimensional imaging and interactive treatment planning software is proving to be the modality of choice providing an increased number of diagnostic tools which can dramatically improve the ability for clinicians to assess the issues that present with each patient, especially in the aesthetic zone of the maxillary arch. These new tools have helped to redefine the workflow required to assess and plan each case and have created new paradigms and treatment protocols that will continue to be refined as the technology evolves. The ability to combine digital optical and intraoral scanning technologies with 3-D imaging helps to refine the process and increase accuracy when surgical guides are indicated. As technology improves, so will the clinician's ability to provide enhanced treatment for patients in need.

Patients who are missing teeth or who require tooth extraction in the anterior maxillary aesthetic zone present difficult challenges for both the surgical and restorative clinician. Perhaps the most critical aspect for accurate treatment planning in this region is the underlying concept that every patient presents with a unique and individual anatomical condition. When there are missing or

S.D. Ganz, DMD
Department of Restorative Dentistry,
Rutgers School of Dental Medicine,
Fort Lee, NJ, USA

Private Practice, 158 Linwood Plaza, Suite 204,
Fort Lee, NJ 07024, USA
e-mail: drganz@drganz.com

hopeless teeth in the anterior maxilla, the diagnostic information necessary to properly plan a surgical and restorative treatment should include, but not limited to, (1) intraoral periapical radiographs, (2) maxillary and mandibular impressions, (3) bite relationship/occlusion, (4) lip position/lip support, (5) smile-line, (6) soft tissue volume and biotype, and (7) three-dimensional imaging modalities such as computed tomography (CT) and the rapidly evolving cone beam CT (CBCT). Two-dimensional imaging has inherent limitations and lacks interactivity, while three-dimensional imaging provides an increasing number of diagnostic tools when combined with interactive treatment planning software (Rothman 1998; Sonick 1994; Ganz 2001, 2005a, c). The use of these tools can dramatically improve the ability for clinicians to assess the issues that present with each patient and especially in the aesthetic zone of the maxillary arch. These new tools have helped to redefine the workflow required to assess and plan each case and have created new paradigms and treatment protocols that will continue to be refined as the technology evolves (Rosenfeld and Mecall 1996, 1998; Rosenfeld et al. 2006; Rugani et al. 2009; Verstreken et al. 1998; Mischkowski et al. 2007; Angelopoulos and Aghaloo 2011; Araryarachkul et al. 2005; Berco et al. 2009; Benington et al. 2010; De Vos et al. 2009; Ganz 2009a, b; Guerrero et al. 2006; Haney et al. 2010; Klein et al. 1993; Harris et al. 2002; Jacobs et al. 1999; Mol and Balasundaram 2008).

The relationship between the existing teeth, bone, and various anatomical features of the maxilla is difficult at best to determine by clinical examination alone or the use of two-dimensional imaging. The retracted view of a patient who exhibited congenitally missing maxillary lateral incisors can be seen in Fig. 6.1. The bilateral concave appearance of the bone and mucogingival junction resulted from the lack of tooth and root eminence (Fig. 6.2a, b). Conventional two-dimensional imaging would not reveal the lack of bone volume or the presence of such a concavity. Three-dimensional imaging modalities, however, provide clinicians with a series of important

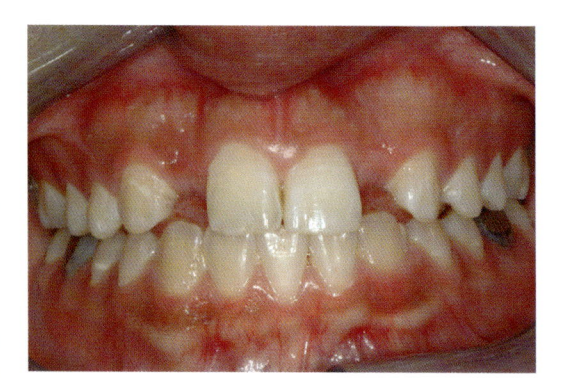

Fig. 6.1 Retracted view of a patient who exhibited congenitally missing maxillary lateral incisors

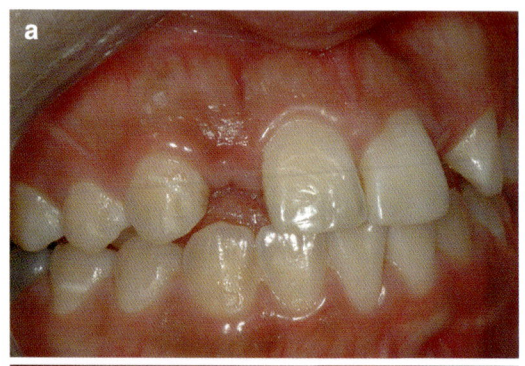

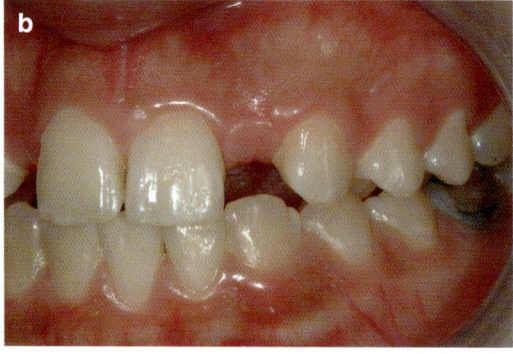

Fig. 6.2 (**a, b**) The bilateral concave appearance of the bone and mucogingival junction resulted from the lack of teeth and lack of a root eminence

views that reveal what the author has termed as the "reality of anatomy" (Ganz 2006b, c, 2008b, c; Lam et al. 1995). The 3-D volumetric reconstructed volume clearly demonstrates the actual bone and tooth anatomy from an occlusal perspective (Fig. 6.3). The diagnostic capabilities

6 The Aesthetic Challenge

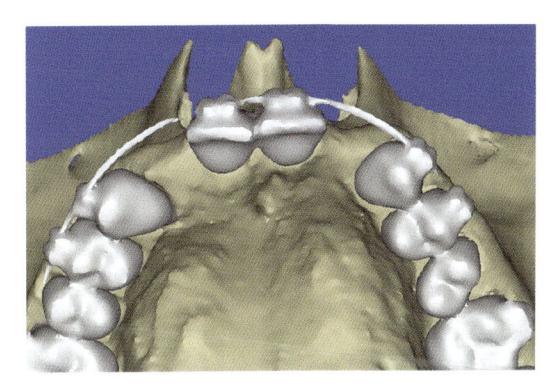

Fig. 6.3 The 3-D volumetric reconstructed volume clearly demonstrates the actual bone and tooth anatomy from an occlusal perspective

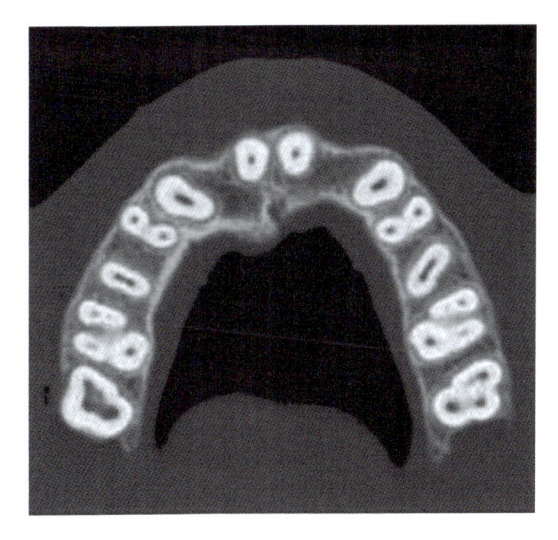

Fig. 6.4 Inspection of the root morphology in the axial view examined layer by layer aids in the diagnostic phase

allow for inspection of the root morphology when the axial view is examined layer by layer (Fig. 6.4). The axial view of the maxilla represents an "occlusal view" helping clinicians to determine the spatial relationship and rotational position of the teeth and surrounding bone. When software zooming features and grayscale values are manipulated, the thickness of the facial and palatal cortical plates and the lamina dura can be appreciated in the various levels of the axial slices. The individual root morphology can also be readily visualized, providing for the author's concept of the "restorative dilemma" (Ganz 2008b, 2010b). When root morphology is seen in the axial slice, it is apparent that tooth roots are not "round" creating a challenge to the restorative dentist when implants are placed. Figure 6.5 illustrates five different shapes for the (1) maxillary central incisor, (2) cuspid, (3, 4) bicuspid, and (5) molar teeth at the level of the cementoenamel junction (CEJ).

Perhaps one of the most striking examples of the power of digital imaging is the ability to separate objects based upon their density or grayscale appearance. The process is called "segmentation" and can vary depending upon the sophistication and depth of the software application (Lam et al. 1995). The segmentation process is used to refine the 3-D images and also can reduce the effects of metal artifacts which cause "scatter" of dense white, preventing accurate assessment of the surrounding anatomy. The 3-D reconstructed volume seen in Fig. 6.3 represented the teeth, roots, and bone. That same volume can be reconstructed without the teeth and the roots, allowing for a unique view of the existing thickness of the cortical bone and alveolar housing (Fig. 6.5b). By virtually "extracting" the teeth from the alveolus, the relationship between the socket shape and the round shape of implants of various diameters can be fully appreciated. Figure 6.5c illustrated realistic virtual implants placed within the sockets of the teeth seen in the axial view of Fig. 6.5a. The "gap" differences are apparent for each of the five examples of standard 3.75 mm diameter (3 and 4) in the bicuspid sockets, 5.0 mm diameter for the central incisor and cuspid teeth (1 and 2), and perhaps most dramatic for a 6.0 mm diameter implant placed within the maxillary first molar site (5). Therefore, the "restorative dilemma" is a real challenge for clinicians each time a round implant emerges from the bone, and the desired prosthetic tooth morphology needs to be fabricated with the proper aesthetic and biologically acceptable emergence profile. The illustration assumes that there would be sufficient bone volume apically and that the implants would be placed in an ideal position to support the desired restoration.

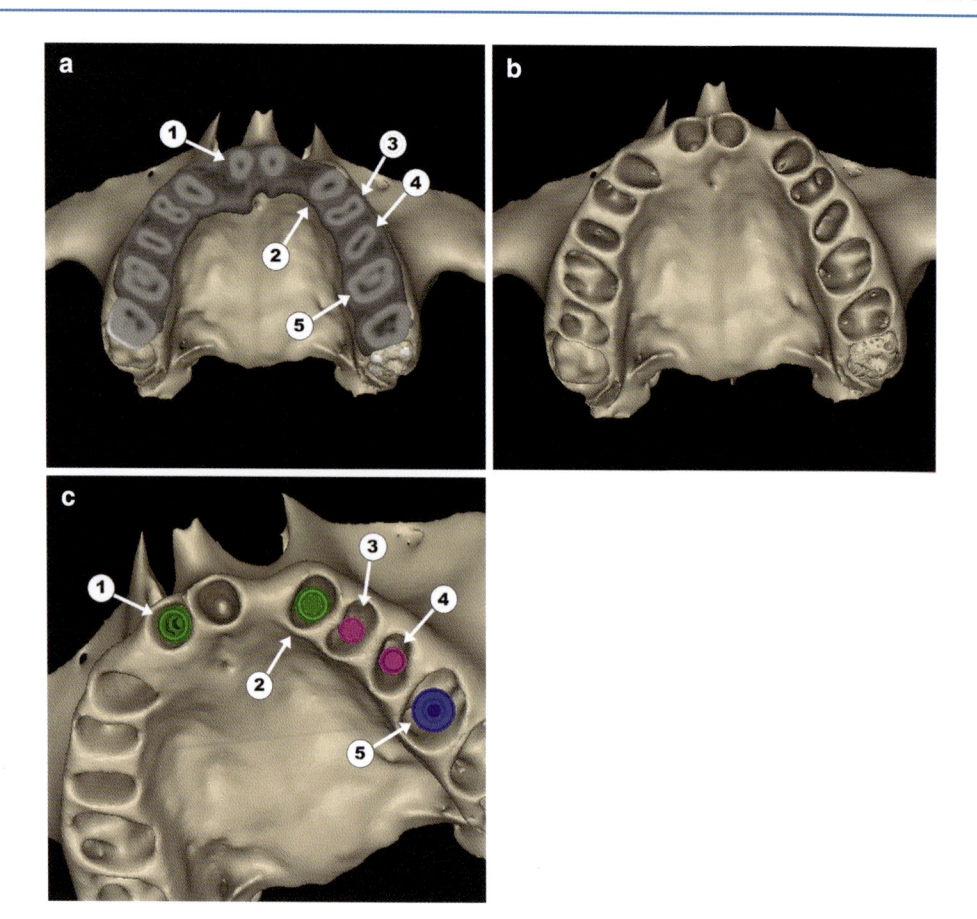

Fig. 6.5 (**a**) Five different shapes for the (1) maxillary central incisor, (2) cuspid, (3 and 4) bicuspid, and (5) molar teeth at the level of the cementoenamel junction (CEJ). (**b**) The reconstructed volume without the teeth and the roots, allowing for a unique view of the existing thickness of the cortical bone and alveolar housing. (**c**) Realistic virtual implants placed within the sockets of the teeth seen in the 3-D volume reveal the potential "gap" differences in the five examples shown

6.1 Case Presentation: 3-D Planning Concepts

6.1.1 Traumatic Injury to Anterior Maxillary Fixed Prosthesis

A 38-year-old male patient presented post-trauma to a preexisting anterior three-unit ceramo-metal fixed bridge supported by natural teeth (Fig. 6.6). The maxillary right lateral incisor and left central incisor were the terminal abutments, with the right central serving as the pontic. The original bridge was necessitated when the right central was lost in a sports-related traumatic event. The left central was most recently damaged by a similar trauma resulting in mobility, root resorption, and possible root fracture. The patient was referred to investigate the potential for an implant reconstruction to replace the failing restoration. The periapical radiograph revealed the presence of preexisting root canal therapy, a post, and radiolucent areas representing root resorption. A CBCT was indicated to determine the extent of the bone loss and the integrity of the remaining maxillary alveolar bone in the region of interest.

The initial CBCT view revealed the preexisting bridge and the surrounding dentition in several views (Fig. 6.7) (Invivo5, Anatomage Inc., San Jose, Califorina). Placing a cotton roll under the lip, described by the author as the "lip-lift" technique,

6 The Aesthetic Challenge

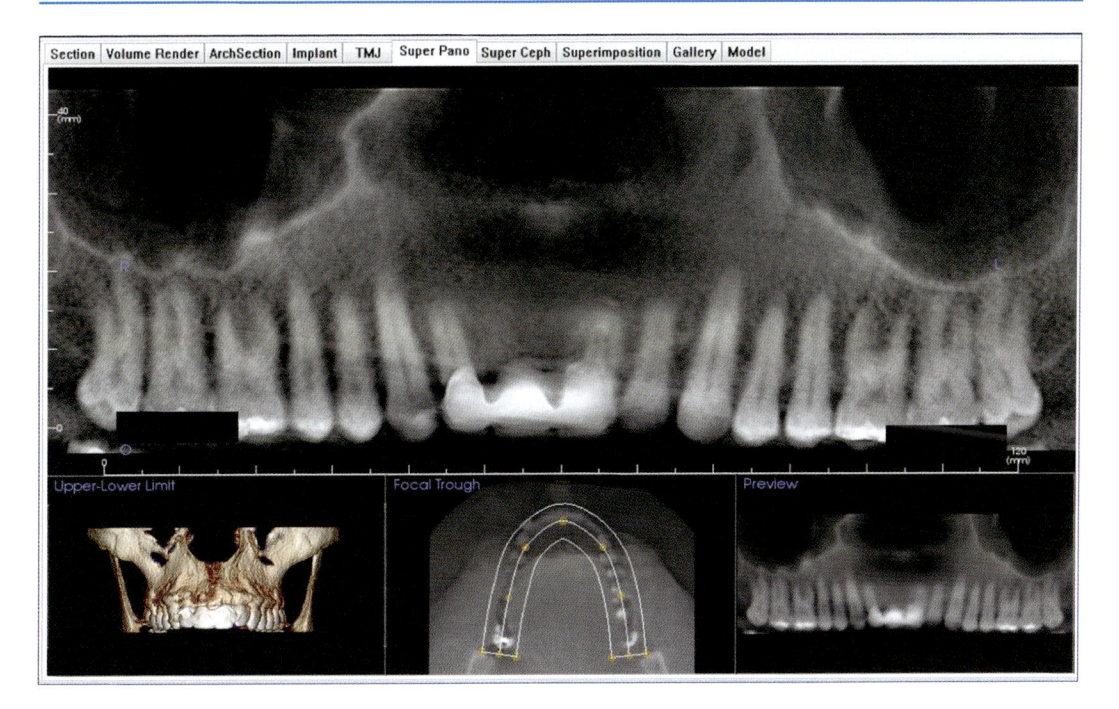

Fig. 6.6 The patient presented post-trauma to a preexisting anterior three-unit ceramo-metal fixed bridge supported by natural teeth

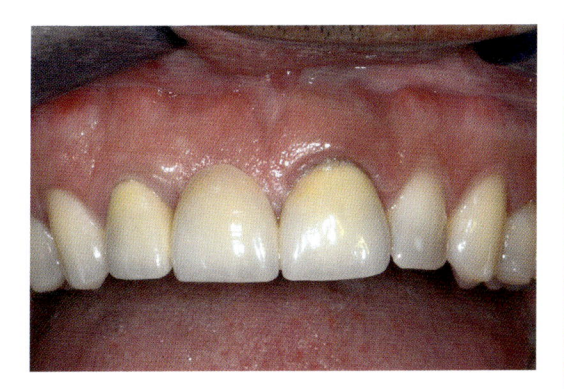

Fig. 6.7 A CBCT was indicated to determine the extent of the bone loss and the integrity of the remaining maxillary alveolar bone in the region of interest. The panoramic CBCT view revealed the preexisting bridge and the surrounding dentition

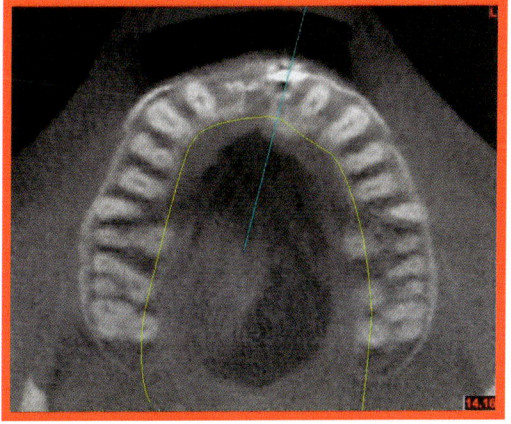

Fig. 6.8 Placing a cotton roll under the lip, described by the author as the "lip-lift" technique, allows for improved inspection of the facial soft tissue and thickness of the facial cortical plate as seen in the axial view

allows for improved inspection of the facial soft tissue and thickness of the facial cortical plate as seen in the axial view (Fig. 6.8) (Ganz 2005a, 2008d, 2010b, 2012, 2015a; Benavides et al. 2012). Note the scatter artifact from the preexisting post and core in the maxillary left central incisor (red arrow). The cross-sectional images enhanced with the "lip lift" (yellow arrows) revealed the extent of the facial bone loss associated with the left central incisor (green arrows) (Fig 6.9a). The lip lift helps to define the vestibule and allow inspection of the soft tissue covering the facial plate and the shape of the vestibule as seen in the area of the pontic site

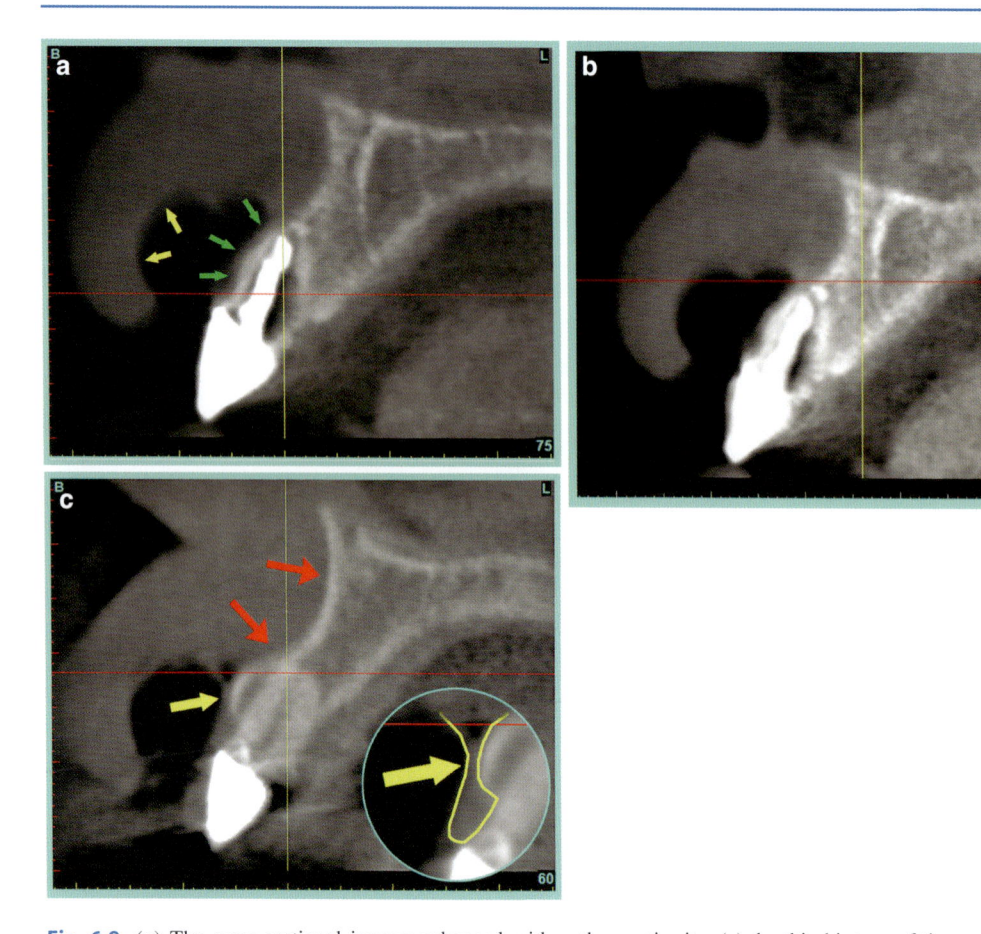

Fig. 6.9 (**a**) The cross-sectional images enhanced with the "lip lift" (*yellow arrows*) revealed the extent of the facial bone loss associated with the left central incisor (*green arrows*); (**b**) the lip lift helps to define the vestibule and allow inspection of the soft tissue covering the facial plate and the shape of the vestibule as seen in the area of the pontic site; (**c**) the thin biotype of tissue covering the natural tooth (*yellow arrow*) can be evaluated as seen in the circular callout (**c**). It is important to evaluate the extent of the vestibule when planning the flap reflection within the facial concavity to the floor of the nose (*red arrows*)

(Fig. 6.9b). The thin biotype of tissue covering the natural tooth (yellow arrow) can be evaluated as seen in the circular callout (Fig. 6.9c). It is important to evaluate the extent of the vestibule when planning the flap reflection within the facial concavity to the floor of the nose (red arrows) (Fig. 6.9c). Using interactive treatment planning software, virtual implants were simulated and placed within two potential implant receptor sites, the right and left central incisor teeth (Fig. 6.10a, b). Simulated components represent realistic manufacturer-specific implant with the exact diameter, lengths, thread design, and connection to aid in the digital planning process.

It is important to note that there is no one image that should be used to plan implant positioning. CBCT data allows clinicians to visualize the panoramic, cross-sectional, coronal, sagittal, axial, and the 3-D reconstructed volumes which all should be carefully assimilated until the final plan is complete (Rothman 1998; Ganz 2005b, c, 2006a, 2007b, 2010b, 2013, 2015b; Rosenfeld and Mecall 1996; Dreiseidler et al. 2009; Dula et al. 2001; Jamali et al. 2007; Amet and Ganz 1997; Orentlicher et al. 2009, 2010). Two implants as positioned within the axial slice reveal proximity to the incisal canal, the adjacent tooth roots, and an implant placed within the proposed extraction site

6 The Aesthetic Challenge

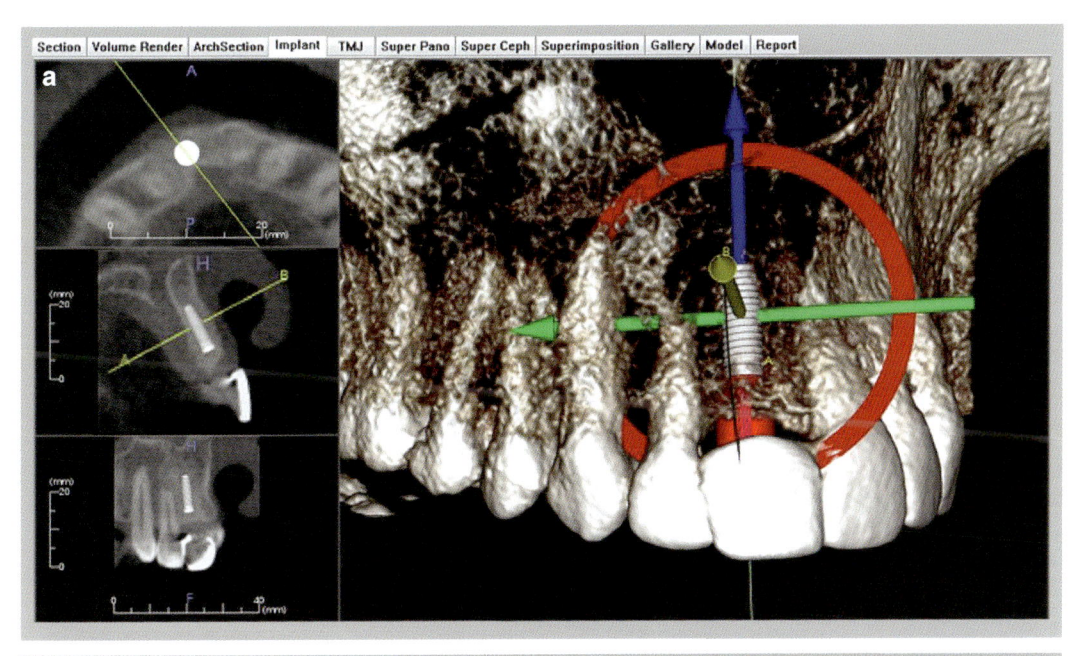

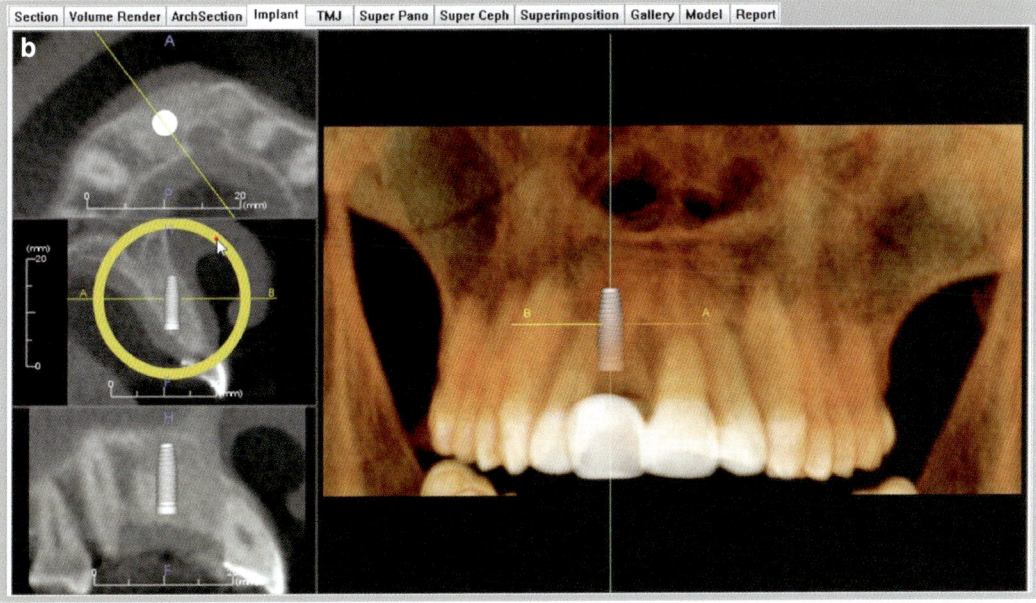

Fig. 6.10 (**a, b**) Using interactive treatment planning software, virtual implants were simulated and placed within two potential implant receptor sites, the right and left central incisor teeth

of the hopeless left maxillary central incisor (Fig. 6.11). Although the cross-sectional revealed significant loss of bone support within the alveolar socket, sufficient bone volume did exist to allow fixation of the implant within the author's concept of the "triangle of bone" extending well beyond the apex of the natural tooth root with an abutment extension in yellow (Fig. 6.12). The implant was positioned so as to take advantage of the palatal cortical bone height aiding in fixation, but the coronal-facial aspect would be within the socket requiring bone grafting to fill the residual gap.

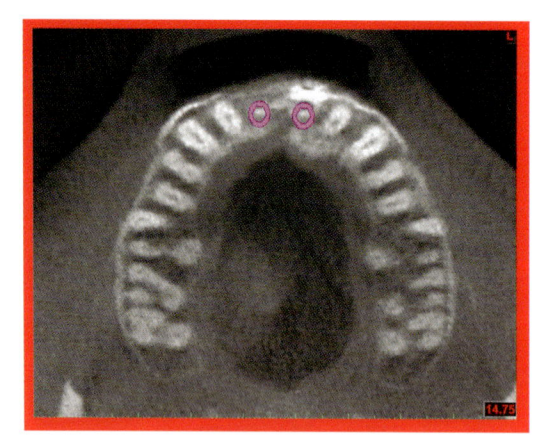

Fig. 6.11 Two implants as positioned within the axial slice reveal proximity to the incisal canal, the adjacent tooth roots, and an implant placed within the proposed extraction site of the hopeless left maxillary central incisor

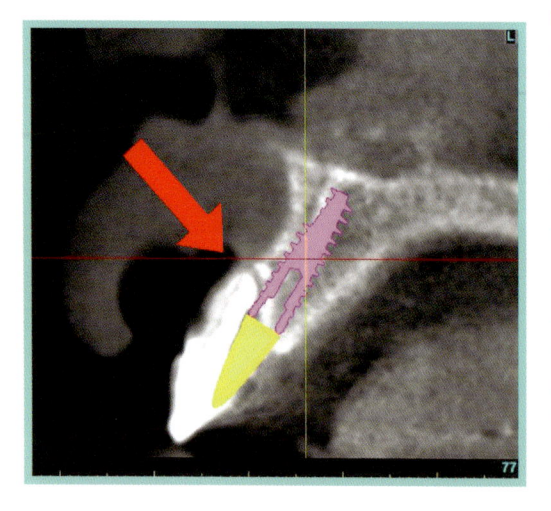

Fig. 6.12 Sufficient bone volume was present to allow fixation of the implant within the author's concept of the "triangle of bone" extending well beyond the apex of the natural tooth root with an abutment extension (*yellow*)

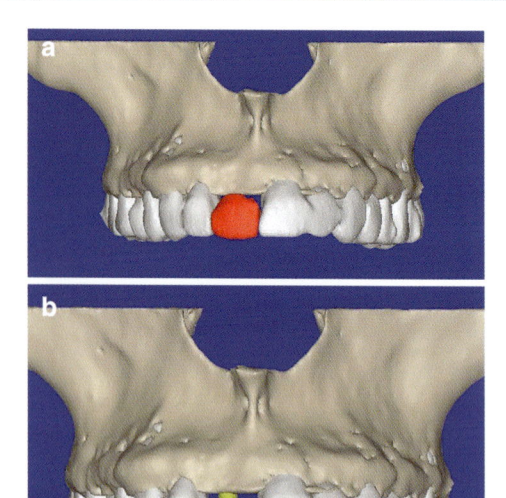

Fig. 6.13 (**a**) The entire maxilla after the segmentation process to remove artifact and separate the pontic tooth (*red*) from the preexisting three-unit fixed bridge to aid in the virtual planning; (**b**) the maxillary anatomy revealing the facial positioning of the tooth roots, and the deep anterior bony concavities with an abutment projecting from the implant (represented *in yellow*) to appreciate the tilt, and trajectory of the emergence from the coronal aspect of the implant

To further explore the power of interactive treatment planning software tools, increased definition is accomplished with a thorough evaluation of the reconstructed 3-D volumetric rendering. The entire maxilla after the segmentation process to remove artifact and separate the pontic tooth (red) from the preexisting three-unit fixed bridge to aid in the virtual planning (Fig. 6.13a). The maxillary anatomy exemplifies the concept of the "reality of anatomy" by revealing the facial positioning of the tooth roots and the deep anterior bony concavities. The author contends that it is essential to have an abutment projecting from the implant (represented in yellow) to appreciate the tilt and trajectory of the emergence from the coronal aspect of the implant (Fig. 6.13b) (Ganz 2005b, 2006a, b, c, 2007b, 2008b). The abutment projections ideally should extend above the occlusal plane or the incisal edge of the teeth to maximize diagnostic planning by relating the implant position to the envelope of the proposed restoration. Depending upon the specific capabilities of the software, the 3-D reconstructed volumes can be modified by varying the object's opacity, defined by the author as "selective transparency" (Ganz 2008d, 2009a, 2012, 2015a; Lam et al. 1995; Norton et al. 2010). "Selective transparency" combined with segmentation or separation of anatomic entities based upon an object's density can create layers used to visualize what would ordinarily be hidden from view. Once the existing teeth and roots have been separated from

6 The Aesthetic Challenge

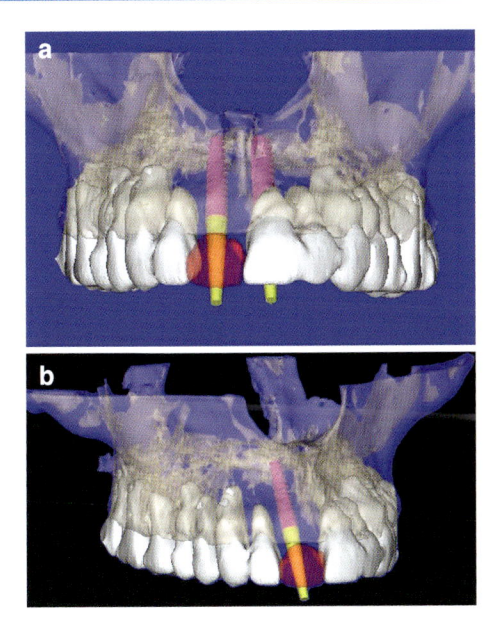

Fig. 6.14 (**a**, **b**) The existing teeth and roots separated from the bony housing through segmentation, allowing for adjacent structures to be better appreciated in relation to the proposed implant location in various views

the bony housing through the process of segmentation, and the opacity of the maxilla is adjusted to a translucent state, the effect allows for adjacent structures to be better appreciated in relation to the proposed implant location in various views (Fig. 6.14a, b).

Further refinement of the diagnostic undertaking includes the ability to slice through the 3-D reconstructed volumes termed, "clipping." The location similar to the cross-sectional slice seen in Fig. 6.12 can be amplified by clipping through the 3-D maxillary left central incisor region (Fig. 6.15a). The careful virtual extraction of the left central incisor through segmentation helps to define the shape of the socket and the "gap" that would potentially exist if the thin facial cortical bone could be preserved after extraction and implant placement (Fig. 6.15b). The gap can be quantified, and a decision can be made as to how to manage this important region to maintain the vertical height of the bone and support the soft tissue for the eventual emergence profile of the abutment and crown (red) (Fig. 6.15c). In the author's opinion, the final position of the proposed implants should not be confirmed without

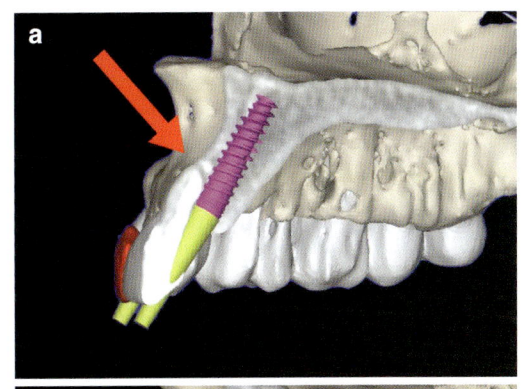

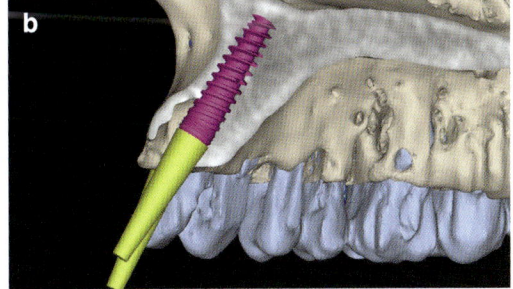

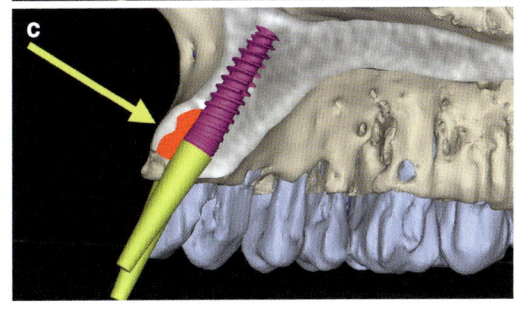

Fig. 6.15 (**a**) "Clipping" through the 3-D maxillary *left central* incisor region. (**b**) The virtual extraction of the left central incisor defines the "gap" that would potentially exist if the thin facial cortical bone could be preserved. (**c**) Treatment can then be determined to maintain the vertical height of the bone, support the soft tissue for the eventual emergence profile of the abutment and crown (*red*)

an indication of the size and shape of the desired restorations (Ganz 2005b, 2006a, b, c, 2008b, c, d, 2010b, 2012, 2015a, b; Benavides et al. 2012; Amet and Ganz 1997; Lee et al. 2012, 2015; Lanis and Álvarez Del Canto 2015; Scherer 2014; Chan et al. 2010; Kang et al. 2014a, b; Eggers et al. 2009; Farley et al. 2013; Arisan et al. 2010; Ganz 2003; Ersoy et al. 2008; Klein and Abrams 2001; Lal et al. 2006).

The morphology of the restorations can be virtually simulated by tools provided within the software application, through a diagnostic wax-up or from the original position of the fixed restoration superimposed/merged to the CBCT dataset. An optical scan of the preoperative stone cast represented the morphology of the original bridge which was acceptable to the patient (Fig. 6.16a). The optical scan is converted into a standard triangulation (STL) file which can be merged and registered to the 3-D reconstructed volume (Fig. 6.16b). If the existing bridge aesthetics and morphology of the teeth were unacceptable, then a diagnostic wax-up would serve to bring the desired restorative information to the treatment planning software application. When the software has the ability to render virtual teeth, it adds another dimension to the planning process (Lam et al. 1995; Benavides et al. 2012; Ganz 2015a; Orentlicher et al. 2009, 2010; Tahmaseb et al. 2014; Lee et al. 2012, 2015; Lanis and Álvarez Del Canto 2015; Scherer 2014; Chan et al. 2010). The virtual tooth creation process as seen overlaying the 3-D reconstructed volume (Fig. 6.16c) and overlaying the STL model (Fig. 6.16d). The incorporation of additional data and new software tools helps define the new digital workflow and aids in increasing accuracy and consistency of the treatment planning process and provides a path to template fabrication and potential CAD-CAM applications.

The positioning of the implants should be appreciated in all views to avoid potential complications and proximity to vital structures such as the incisal canal (yellow arrow) as visualized in the occlusal view with and without the virtual teeth (Fig. 6.17a, b) (Ganz 2010a). The implant placement within the virtual extraction socket can be adjusted based upon the restorative requirements as well as the size of the facial cortical gap (Fig. 6.17c). Software tools are available which can move implants in designated increments to help minimize the facial gap (Fig. 6.17d). The final implant positioning should be determined by the need to fabricate a screw-retained or cement-retained restoration within the envelope of the teeth (Fig. 6.18).

It was the patient's desire to retain the right lateral incisor if possible, and therefore the bridge was sectioned on the mesial aspect with care not to fracture the porcelain (Fig. 6.19). The clinical crown immediately separated from the root of the

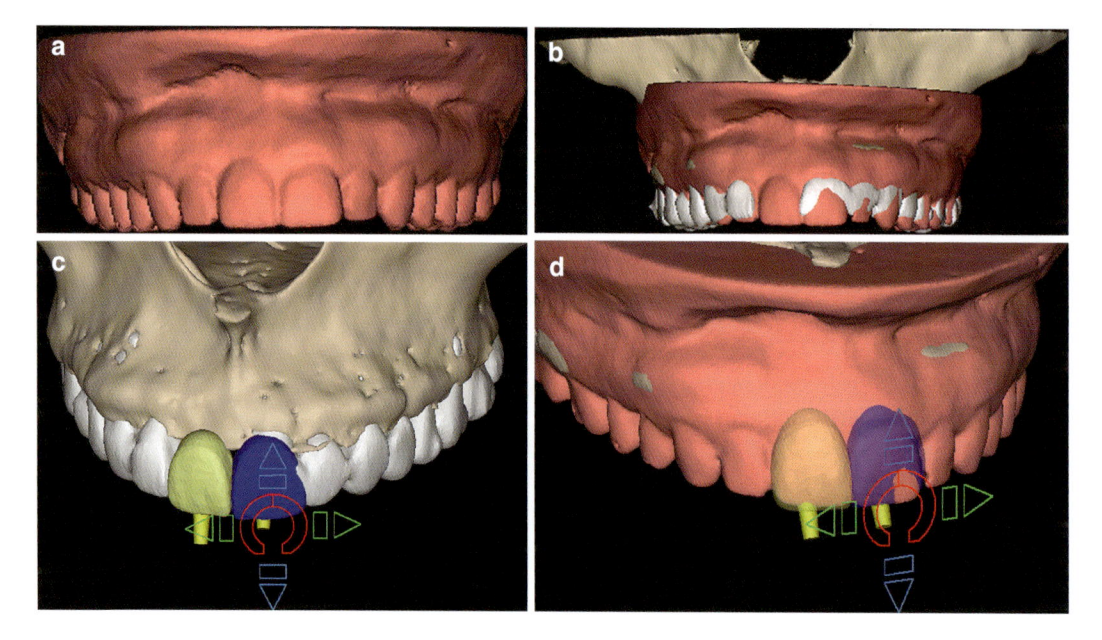

Fig. 6.16 (**a**) An optical scan of the preoperative stone cast represented the morphology of the original bridge. (**b**) The optical scan converted to an STL file merged and registered to the 3-D reconstructed volume. (**c**) The virtual tooth creation process overlaying the 3-D reconstructed volume. (**d**) Overlaying the STL model and the 3-D volumetric reconstruction

maxillary left central incisor, documenting the need for the procedure. The residual root was carefully extracted, preserving the fragile facial cortical plate. The Ganz-Rinaldi Protocol for Guided Surgery procedures defined three different categories for guided surgery procedures based on CT or CBCT imaging and 3-D Planning (Rinaldi et al. 2015). The first category is "diagnostic-freehand" providing only the diagnostic information from the scan data, measurements, bone density, etc., and the surgical intervention is done freehand. The second category is described as "template assisted" which provides template guidance fabricated either by the dental laboratory, CAD-CAM, or rapid prototyping such as stereolithography (Ozan et al. 2009; Di Giacomo et al. 2005; Danza et al. 2009; Borrow and Smith Justin 1996; Jabero and Sarment 2006). The template provides guidance for the drills and may control depth with either pilot or sequential drilling protocols. The final category is termed "full-template guidance" which is possible only with the collaboration with specific manufacturer drills and implant carriers to drill the osteotomies, control depth, and then to place the

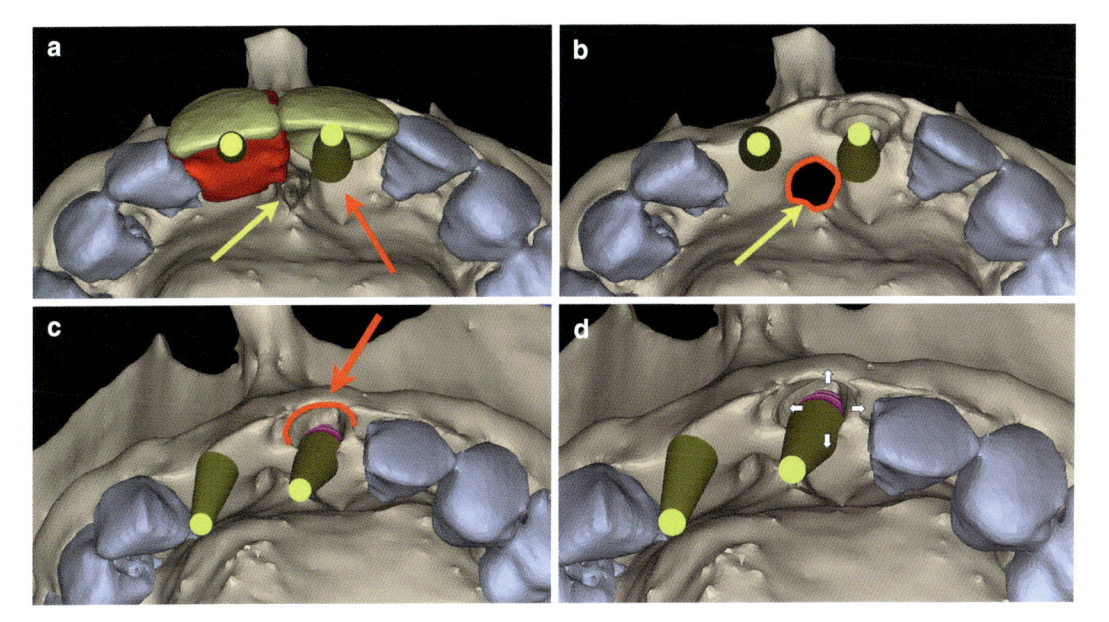

Fig. 6.17 (**a, b**) Positioning of the implants in all views helps to avoid potential complications and proximity to vital structures such as the incisal canal (*yellow arrow*) as visualized in the occlusal view with and without the virtual teeth. (**c, d**) Implant placement can be adjusted based upon the restorative requirements and the facial cortical gap; (**d**) software tools can move implants in designated increments to help minimize the facial gap

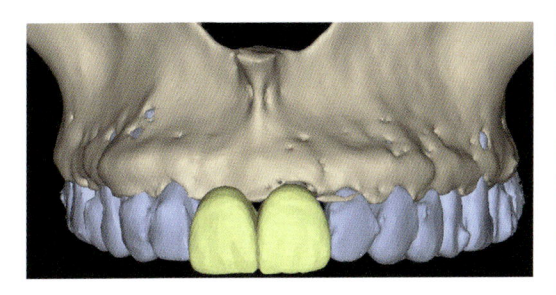

Fig. 6.18 The final implant positioning determined by either a screw-retained or cement-retained design for the restoration

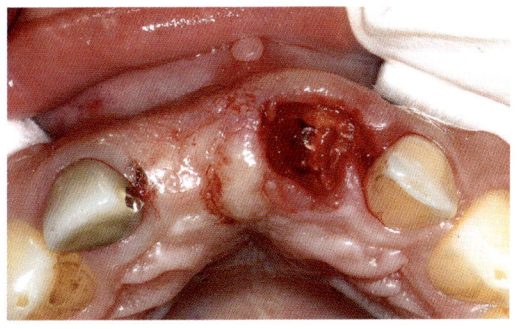

Fig. 6.19 The preexisting bridge was sectioned on the mesial aspect with care not to fracture the porcelain

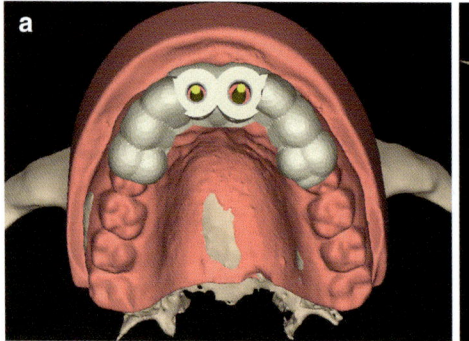

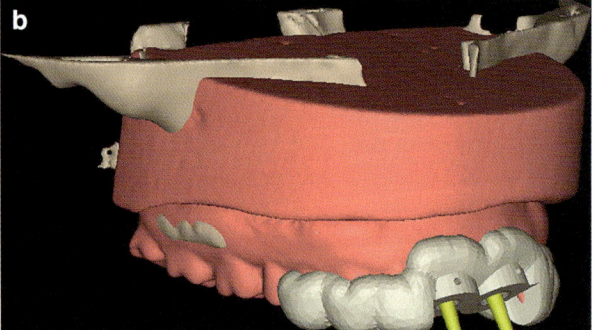

Fig. 6.20 (**a, b**) A tooth-borne template, with a "template-assisted" procedure allowed for the preparation of the sequential osteotomies with a universal drilling system

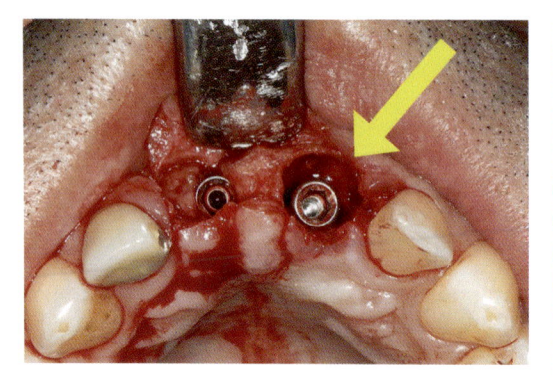

Fig. 6.21 A full-flap design was necessary to expose the underlying bone, and the preexisting facial concavities requiring grafting, after the two implants, were well fixated, with the fragile facial place still intact (*yellow arrow*)

implants through the templates to maximize accuracy. A tooth-borne template with a "template-assisted" procedure allowed for the preparation of the sequential osteotomies with a universal drilling system (Fig. 6.20a, b). A full-thickness mucoperiosteal flap design was necessary to expose the underlying bone and the preexisting facial concavities requiring grafting (Fig. 6.21). The two implants were well fixated, with the fragile facial place still intact (yellow arrow).

It should be noted that the rotational position of the internal hexagonal connection was an important consideration. The author has termed the rotational aspect of the implant connection as the "fifth dimension." For each implant, the flat of the internal hexagon was positioned to the facial to correspond stock abutments that will subsequently be used to support the transitional restoration (Ganz 2006a, 2007b, 2008b, c; Lam

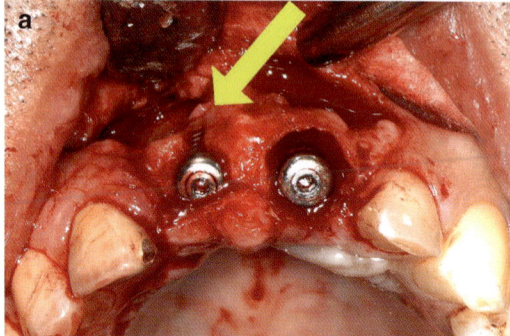

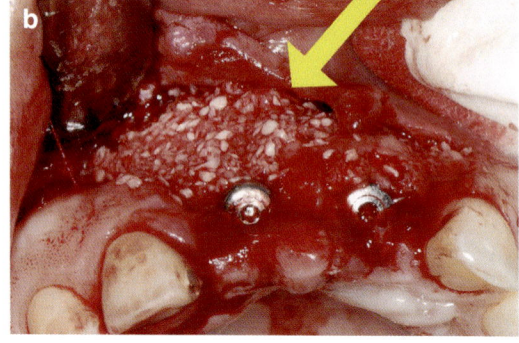

Fig. 6.22 (**a, b**) As originally planned, the implant placed within the *right central* incisor or pontic area exhibited thread exposure which was to be covered with the graft material (*yellow arrow*)

et al. 1995; Benavides et al. 2012). As originally planned, the implant placed within the right central incisor or pontic area exhibited thread exposure which was to be covered with the graft material (yellow arrow) (Fig. 6.22a, b). Mineralized bone was used to cover the implants and fill the extraction gap and the concavities to help support the soft tissue (Aghaloo and Moy

6 The Aesthetic Challenge

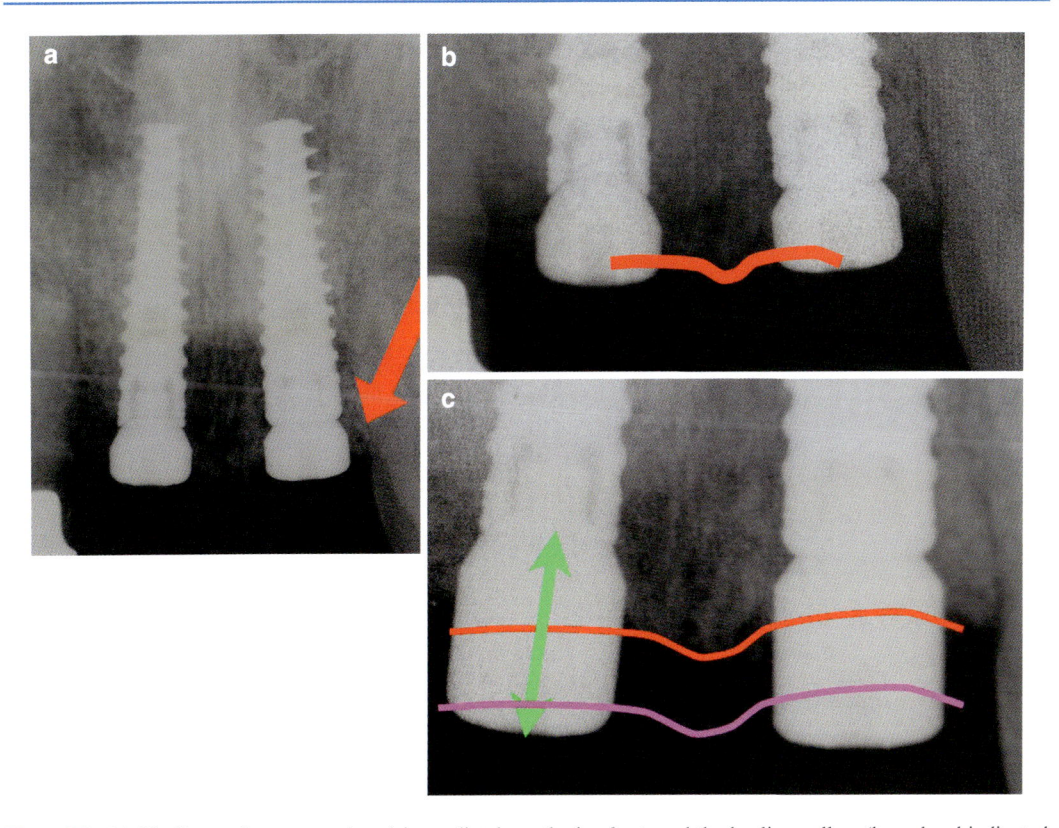

Fig. 6.23 (**a**) Healing collars were placed immediately (*red arrow*) as seen in the postoperative periapical radiograph, and (**b**) tension-free closure was achieved covering the implants and the healing collars (bone level indicated by the *red line*)

2007; Chiapasco et al. 2006, 2009; Ganz 2009c). To aid in the soft tissue support, and to help maintain the vertical height, healing collars were placed immediately (red arrow) as seen in the postoperative periapical radiograph (Fig. 6.23a). Tension-free closure was achieved covering the implants and the healing collars. The level of the bone was indicated by the red line (Fig. 6.23b). A prefabricated removable partial denture served as the transitional restoration during the healing phase. Care was taken to relieve the intaglio surface to avoid pressure on the surgical site.

Four months post-implant placement, the follow-up radiograph showed the height of the soft tissue (pink line), the bone levels preserved above the coronal aspect of the implant (red line), and the soft tissue depth shown by the green line (Fig. 6.23c). At 5 months, the healing was complete (Fig. 6.24). The restorative planning aspect included the positioning of stock abutments which were to be used during the initial soft tissue healing phase (Fig. 6.25). The treatment planning software provided a library of realistic stock abutments which helped confirm the parallel condition of the implants and the restorative components (Fig. 6.26). The implants were uncovered with small incisions, and stock, 15° degree angulated abutments were placed to support a temporary acrylic restoration (Fig. 6.27). Over a period

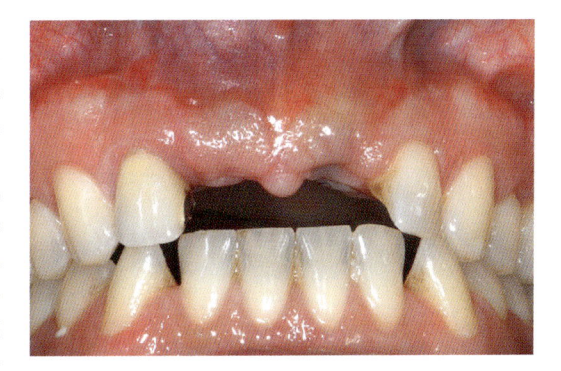

Fig. 6.24 At 5 months, the healing was complete

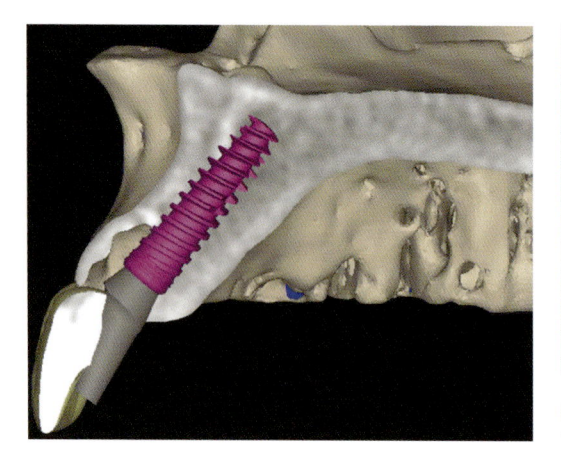

Fig. 6.25 The restorative planning aspect included the positioning of stock abutments which were to be used during the initial soft tissue healing phase

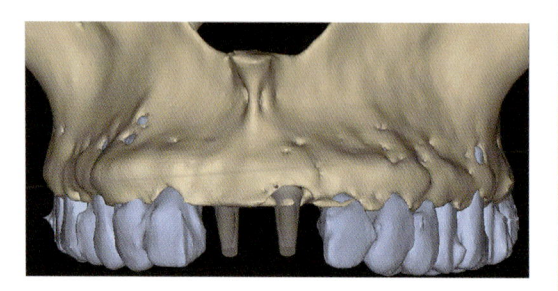

Fig. 6.26 The treatment planning software provided a library of realistic stock abutments which helped confirm the parallel condition of the implants and the restorative components

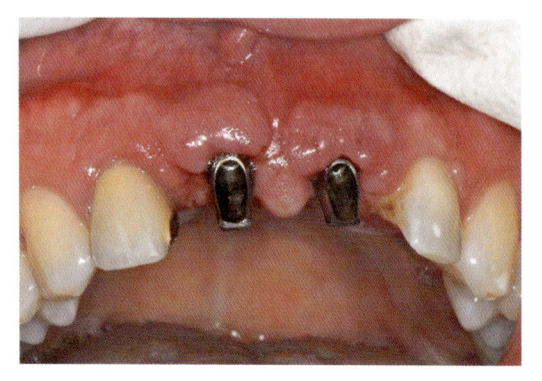

Fig. 6.27 The implants were uncovered with small incisions, and stock, 15° angulated abutments were placed to support a temporary acrylic restoration

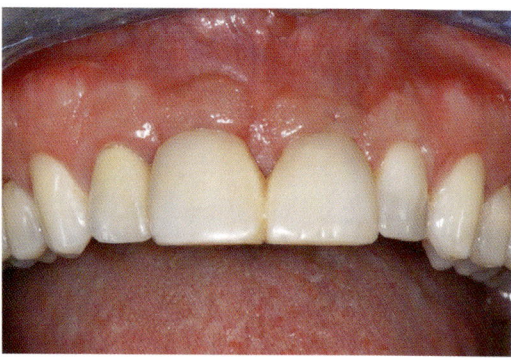

Fig. 6.28 The transitional restorations were used to help "sculpt" the soft tissue sulcus and the emergence profile for the definitive prosthetic result

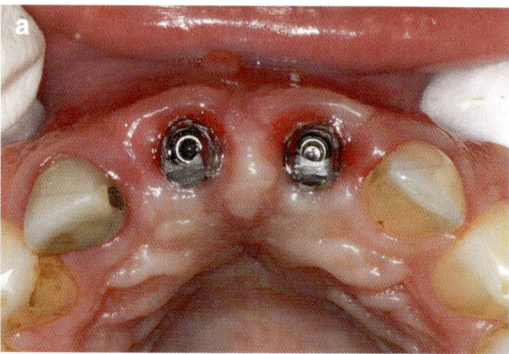

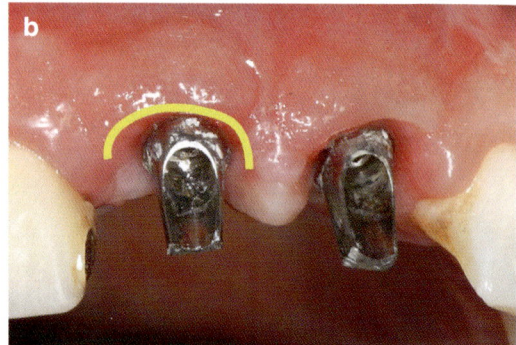

Fig. 6.29 (**a**, **b**) Within weeks, the soft tissue sulcus was formed to preserve the interdental papilla and emergence profile

of 2 months, the transitional restorations were then used to help "sculpt" the soft tissue sulcus and the emergence profile for the definitive prosthetic result (Fig. 6.28) (Roe et al. 2012). Within weeks the soft tissue sulcus was formed to preserve the interdental papilla and emergence profile (Fig. 6.29a, b). Once satisfied with the maturity of the tissue, fixture level impression transfer copings were placed and resin pattern used to preserve the framework of the sulcus (Fig. 6.30). A polyether impression material was

6 The Aesthetic Challenge

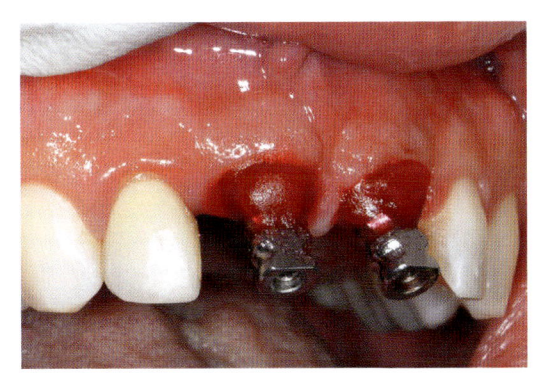

Fig. 6.30 Fixture level impression transfer copings were placed and resin pattern used to preserve the framework of the sulcus

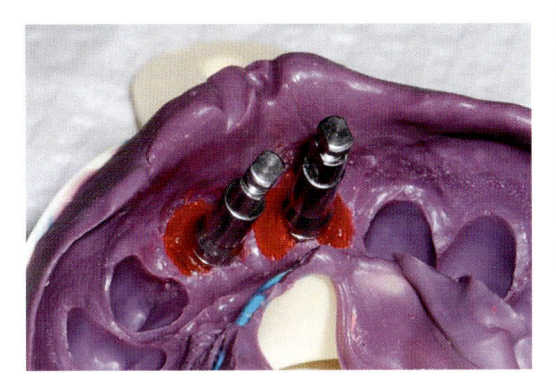

Fig. 6.31 A polyether impression material was injected around the closed-tray transfers in a stock tray. After the material was set, the transfer posts were then connected to implant-specific analogs

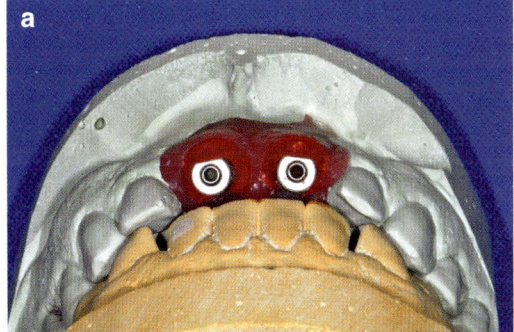

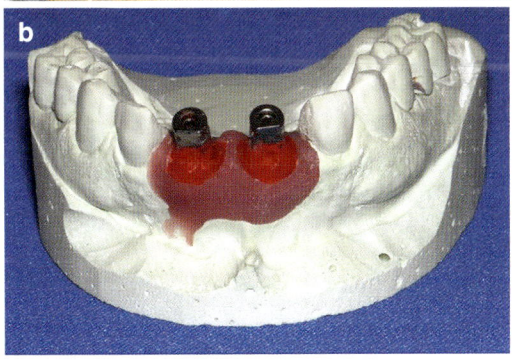

Fig. 6.32 (**a**) To facilitate the laboratory phase, a soft tissue model material was first placed around the analogs, followed by the stone resulting in (**b**) a soft tissue cast with the fixture mount transfer copings in place

injected around the closed-tray transfers in a stock tray. After the material had set and the tray removed from the mouth, the transfer posts were then connected to implant-specific analogs (Fig. 6.31).

To facilitate the laboratory phase, a soft tissue model material was first placed around the analogs, followed by the stone. The resulting soft tissue cast with the fixture mount transfer copings in place is seen in Fig. 6.32a, b. Hand articulating the maxillary and mandibular casts revealed the inter-arch space (Fig. 6.33a) and the desired trajectory of the transfer copings for two cement-retained restorations (Fig. 6.33b). The soft tissue cast provided information about the depth and morphology of the sulcus that was carefully expanded by the acrylic transitional restorations (yellow) (Fig. 6.34a, b). Two custom CAD-CAM gold-hued anodized titanium abutments were then fabricated to match the emergence profile as established with the soft tissue cast (Fig. 6.35). Cement-retained restorations were planned to help correct the angulation of the abutment needed to fill the envelope of each individual tooth. Two separate ceramo-metal restorations were fabricated and the marginal fit and smooth emergence profile evaluated on separate analogs (Fig. 6.36a–d). The margin was designed to be approximately 1 mm below the soft tissue margin to allow for ease of cement removal and to prevent cement from migrating into the sulcus as seen on the soft tissue cast (Fig. 6.37a) and intraorally (Fig. 6.37b, c). The final restoration exhibited excellent emergence profile (Fig. 6.38) and an emulation of root eminence for both right and left central incisors (Fig. 6.39). Postoperative radiograph at 18 months reveals a stabile relationship between implants, abutments, and surrounding bone (Fig. 6.40).

In order to determine the accuracy of the planning process, a noninvasive method was chosen. The working cast with the fixture level transfer copings which represents the actual position of the implants was scanned with an intraoral scanner. The subsequent data was exported as an STL file and imported into the original preoperative CBCT scan data (Fig. 6.41a–c). The merged STL file revealed the postoperative location of the implants. The yellow abutment projections from the original plan could then be compared with the fixture level transfer copings. Using "selective transparency," the yellow abutment projections can be clearly visualized within the body of the transfer copings (outlined in red), confirming that the original plan was executed with great accuracy and precision (Fig. 6.42). This noninvasive verification method helped to corroborate or confirm that the actual intraoral implant position matched the preoperative plan, without the need for a second postoperative CBCT scan, therefore meeting the "aesthetic challenge" in the anterior maxillary arch (Chen and Buser 2014; Cosyn et al. 2011).

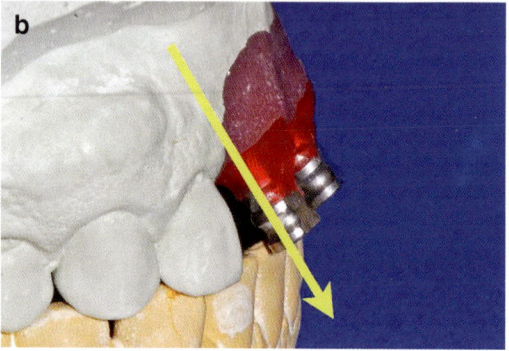

Fig. 6.33 (**a**) The articulation of the maxillary and mandibular casts revealed the inter-arch space and (**b**) the desired trajectory of the transfer copings for two cement-retained restorations

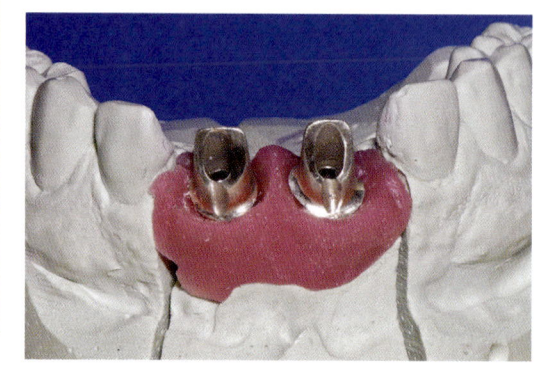

Fig. 6.35 Two custom CAD-CAM gold-hued anodized titanium abutments were then fabricated to match the emergence profile as established with the soft tissue cast

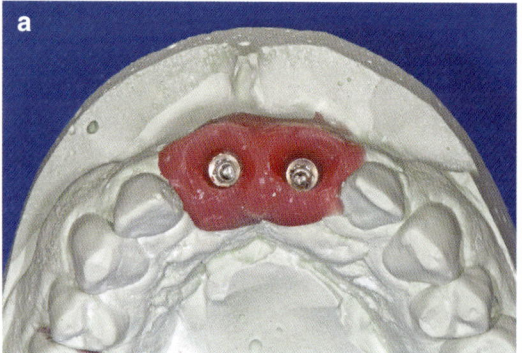

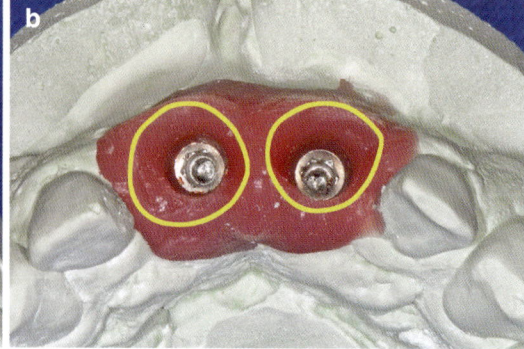

Fig. 6.34 (**a**) The soft tissue cast provided information about the depth and morphology of the sulcus that was carefully expanded by the (**b**) acrylic transitional restorations (*yellow*)

6 The Aesthetic Challenge

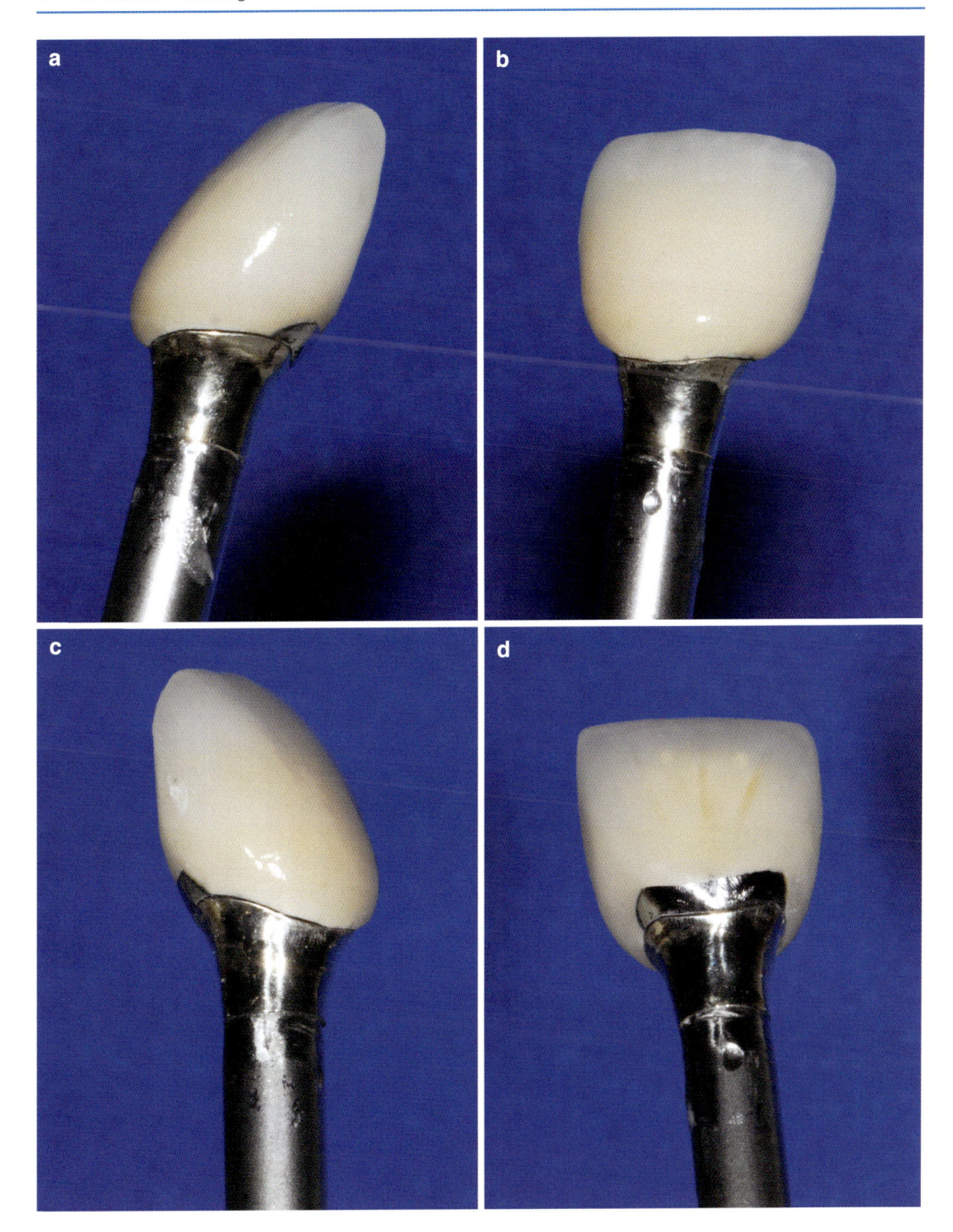

Fig. 6.36 (**a–d**) Two separate ceramo-metal restorations were fabricated and the marginal fit and smooth emergence profile evaluated on separate analogs

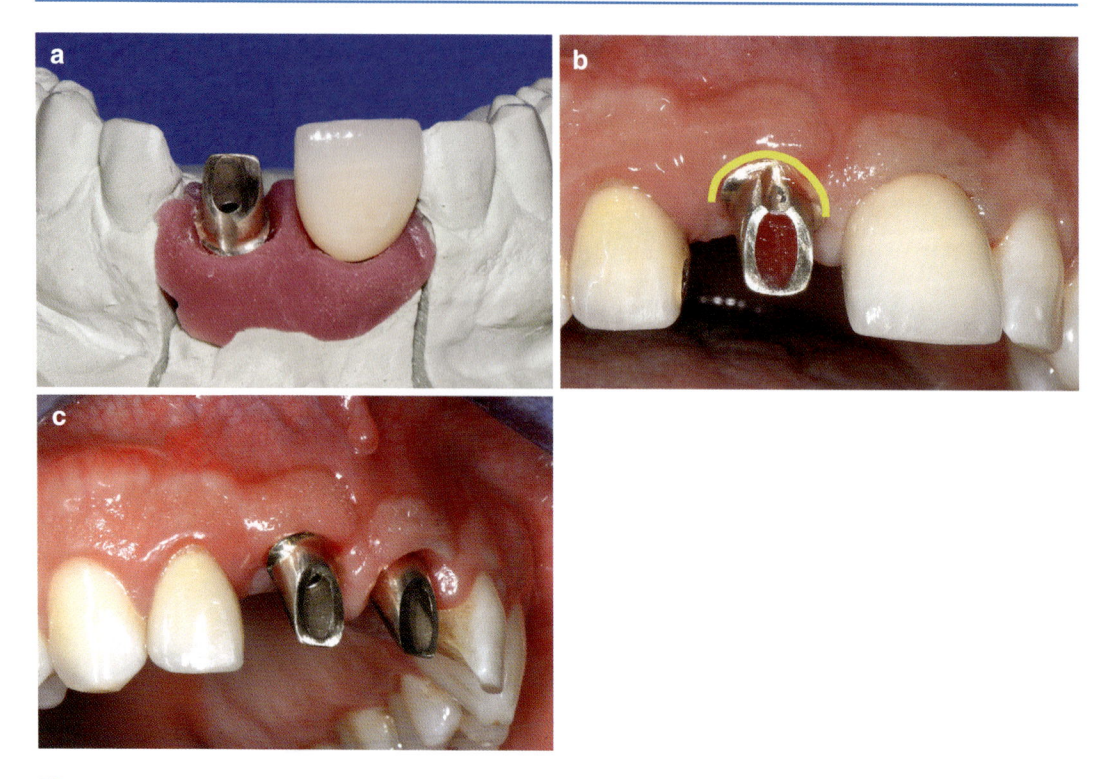

Fig. 6.37 (**a**) The abutment margin was designed to be approximately 1 mm below the soft tissue margin to prevent cement from migrating into the sulcus, seen on the soft tissue cast, and (**b, c**) intraorally

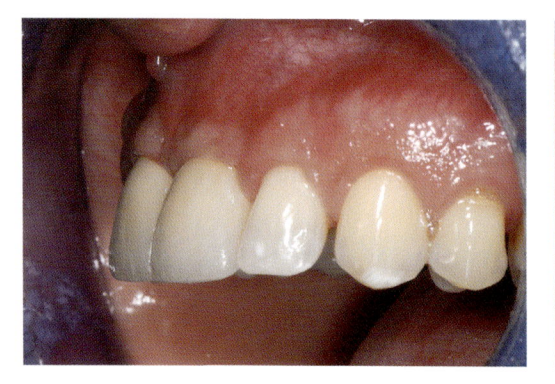

Fig. 6.38 The final restoration exhibited excellent emergence profile

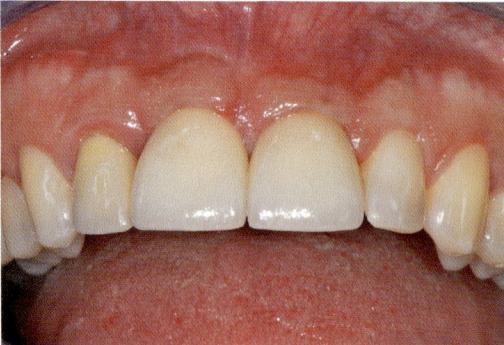

Fig. 6.39 An emulation of the root eminence was seen for both right and left central incisor restorations

6 The Aesthetic Challenge

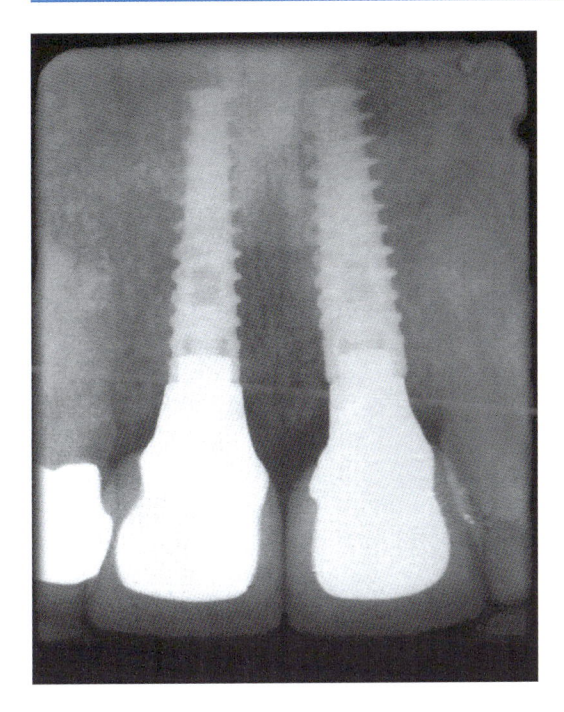

Fig. 6.40 Postoperative radiograph at 18 months reveals a stabile relationship between implants, abutments, and surrounding bone

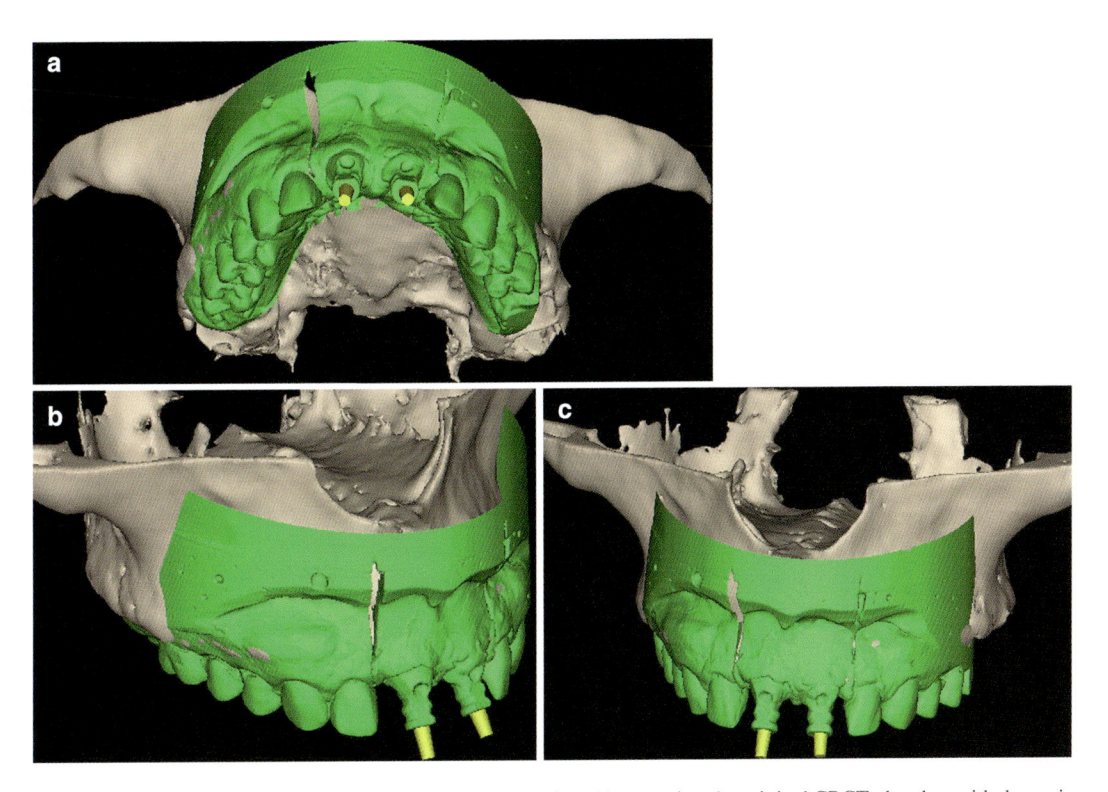

Fig. 6.41 (**a–c**) A noninvasive verification method was achieved by merging the original CBCT plan data with the optical scan of the actual position of the implants from the working cast (*yellow* abutment projections)

Fig. 6.42 Using "selective transparency," the yellow abutment projections can be clearly visualized within the body of the transfer copings (outlined in *red*), confirming that the original plan was executed with great accuracy and precision

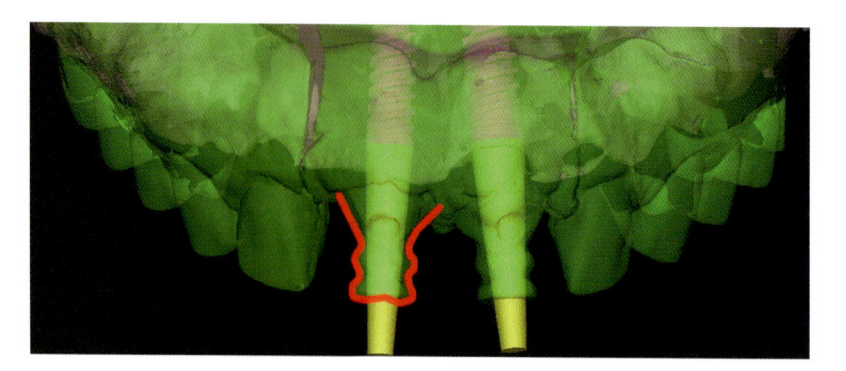

Conclusion

The maxillary anterior aesthetic zone presents many challenges for the clinician when teeth are missing or when teeth are to be extracted and replaced with implant-supported restorations. This chapter presented a step-by-step process of the diagnostic, surgical, and restorative phase of an immediate extraction and implant placement, followed by bone grafting, and recontouring of the soft tissue with stock abutments and acrylic transitional restorations. The foundation for the treatment plan was based on the use of three-dimensional imaging modalities which have provided clinicians with new tools to improve the diagnostic capabilities and to avoid potential surgical and restorative complications (Behneke et al. 2012; Moreira et al. 2009; Nairn et al. 2013; Nickenig and Eitner 2007; Valente et al. 2009; Hof et al. 2015; Kan et al. 2010, 2011, 2015; Tyndall et al. 2012). The use of CT and CBCT, when combined with interactive treatment planning software applications, can help clinicians understand that each patient presents with individual anatomical realities, requiring unique treatment plans that will meet the surgical and restorative needs of the region of interest (Ganz 2007a, 2008a). The concept of the "restorative dilemma" as presented in this chapter confirms that the relationship between round implants and the actual tooth/root morphology is often incongruent and offers challenges for the clinician to replicate nature with an implant-supported restorative solution. The "lip-lift" technique provides a simple means of moving the lip away from the soft tissue coverage of the tooth, helps to define the vestibule, and improves the ability to determine the soft tissue biotype and diagnose the thickness of the facial cortical plate of bone.

Finally, the diagnostic phase has been greatly improved with advances in 3-D imaging, interactive treatment planning software, and the ability to combine digital optical and intraoral scanning technologies. It is possible to identify implant receptor sites and plan with realistic implants and realistic abutments from a software library of manufacturer-specific components. The need for bone grafting or soft tissue grafting can be predicted in advance of touching the scalpel to the patient, and the resulting images provide an excellent communication tool to describe the procedure and improve case acceptance. Three-dimensional reconstructive volumes are useful in both the presurgical prosthetic planning and also in confirming that the surgical intervention went as planned. As technology improves, so will the clinician's ability to provide enhanced treatment for patients in need.

References

Aghaloo TL, Moy PK (2007) Which hard tissue augmentation techniques are the most successful in furnishing bony support for implant placement? Int J Oral Maxillofac Implants 22(Suppl):49–70

Amet EM, Ganz SD (1997) Functional and aesthetic acceptance prior to computerized tomography or implant placement. Implant Dent 6(3., Fall): 193–197

Angelopoulos C, Aghaloo T (2011) Imaging technology in implant diagnosis. Dent Clin N Am 55(1):141–158

Araryarachkul P, Caruso J, Gantes B, Schulz E, Riggs M, Dus I, Yamada J, Crigger M (2005) Bone density assessments of dental implant sites: 2. Quantitative cone-beam computerized tomography. Int J Oral Maxillofac Implants 20:416–424

Arisan V, Karabuda ZC, Ozdemir T (2010) Accuracy of two stereolithographic guide systems for computer-aided implant placement: a computed tomography-based clinical comparative study. J Periodontol 81(1):43–51

Behneke A, Burwinkel M, Behneke N (2012) Factors influencing transfer accuracy of cone beam CT-derived template-based implant placement. Clin Oral Implants Res 23(4):416–423

Benavides E, Rios HF, Ganz SD, An CH, Resnik R, Reardon GT, Feldman SJ, Mah JK, Hatcher D, Kim MJ, Sohn DS, Palti A, Perel ML, Judy KW, Misch CE, Wang HL (2012) Use of cone beam computed tomography in implant dentistry: the International Congress of Oral Implantologists consensus report. Implant Dent 21(2):78–86

Benington PC, Khambay BS, Ayoub AF (2010) An overview of three-dimensional imaging in dentistry. Dent Update 37(8):494–496. 499–500, 503–4

Berco M, Rigali PH Jr, Miner RM, DeLuca S, Anderson NK, Will LA (2009) Accuracy and reliability of linear cephalometric measurements from cone-beam computed tomography scans of a dry human skull. Am J Orthod Dentofac Orthop 136(1):17. e1-9; discussion 17-8

Borrow W, Smith Justin P (1996) Stent marker materials for computerized tomograph-assisted implant planning. Int J Periodontics Restor Dent 16:61–67

Chan HL, Misch K, Wang HL (2010) Dental imaging in implant treatment planning. Implant Dent 19(4):288–298

Chen ST, Buser D (2014) Esthetic outcomes following immediate and early implant placement in the anterior maxilla – a systematic review. Int J Oral Maxillofac Implants 29(Suppl):186–215

Chiapasco M, Zaniboni M, Boisco M (2006) Augmentation procedures for the rehabilitation of deficient edentulous ridges with oral implants. Clin Oral Implants Res 17(Suppl 2):136–159. Review

Chiapasco M, Casentini P, Zaniboni M (2009) Bone augmentation procedures in implant dentistry. Int J Oral Maxillofac Implants 24(Suppl):237–259

Cosyn J, Eghbali A, De Bruyn H, Collys K, Cleymaet R, De Rouck T (2011) Immediate single-tooth implants in the anterior maxilla: 3-year results of a case series on hard and soft tissue response and aesthetics. J Clin Periodontol 38(8):746–753

Danza M, Zollino I, Carinci F (2009) Comparison between implants inserted with and without computer planning and custom model coordination. J Craniofac Surg 20(4):1086–1092

De Vos W, Casselman J, Swennen GR (2009) Cone-beam computerized tomography (CBCT) imaging of the oral and maxillofacial region: a systematic review of the literature. Int J Oral Maxillofac Surg 38(6):609–625. Epub 2009 May 21. Review

Di Giacomo GA, Cury PR, de Araujo NS, Sendyk WR, Sendyk CL (2005) Clinical application of stereolithographic surgical guides for implant placement: preliminary results. J Periodontol 76(4):503–507

Dreiseidler T, Mischkowski RA, Neugebauer J, Ritter L, Zöller JE (2009) Comparison of cone-beam imaging with orthopantomography and computerized tomography for assessment in presurgical implant dentistry. Int J Oral Maxillofac Implants 24(2):216–225

Dula K, Mini R, van der Stelt PF, Buser D (2001) The radiographic assessment of implant patients: decision-making criteria. Int J Oral Maxillofac Implants 16(1):80–89

Eggers G, Patellis E, Mühling J (2009) Accuracy of template-based dental implant placement. Int J Oral Maxillofac Implants 24(3):447–454

Ersoy AE, Turkyilmaz I, Ozan O, McGlumphy EA (2008) Reliability of implant placement with stereolithographic surgical guides generated from computed tomography: clinical data from 94 implants. J Periodontol 79(8):1339–1345

Farley NE, Kennedy K, McGlumphy EA, Clelland NL (2013) Split-mouth comparison of the accuracy of computer-generated and conventional surgical guides. Int J Oral Maxillofac Implants 28(2):563–572

Ganz SD (2001) CT scan technology – an evolving tool for predictable implant placement and restoration. Int Mag Oral Implantol Vol. 1:6–13

Ganz SD (2003) Use of stereolithographic models as diagnostic and restorative aids for predictable immediate loading of implants. Pract Proced Aesthet Dent 15(10):763–771

Ganz SD (2005a) Use of conventional CT and cone beam for improved dental diagnostics and implant planning. AADMRT Newsletter, Spring Issue. (AADMRT)

Ganz SD (2005b) Presurgical planning with CT-derived fabrication of surgical guides. J Oral Maxillofac Surg 63((9), Supplement 2):59–71

Ganz SD (2005c) Conventional CT and cone beam CT for improved dental diagnostics and implant planning. Dent Implantol Updat 16(12):85

Ganz SD (2006a) Techniques for the use of CT imaging for the fabrication of surgical guides. Atlas Oral Maxillofac Surg Clin North Am., Elsevier Saunders 14:75–97

Ganz SD (2006b) The reality of anatomy and the triangle of bone. Inside Dent 2(5):72–77

Ganz SD (2006c) The reality of anatomy and the triangle of bone. Inside dentistry. Proceedings of ICOI World Congress XXIV. Suppl Implant Dent 14:182–191

Ganz SD (2007a) 3-D imaging and cone beam CT is "Where the Action is!" inside. Dentistry 2007:102–103

Ganz SD (2007b) CT-derived model-based surgery for immediate loading of maxillary anterior implants. Pract Proced Aesthet Dent 19(5):311–318

Ganz SD (2008a) Using interactive technology: "In the Zone with the Triangle of Bone.". Dent Implantol Updat 19(5):33–38. quiz p1

Ganz SD (2008b) Defining new paradigms for assessment of implant receptor sites – The use of CT/CBCT and interactive virtual treatment planning for congenitally missing lateral incisors. Compend Cont Educ Dent 29(5):256–267

Ganz SD (2008c) Restoratively driven implant dentistry utilizing advanced software and CBCT: realistic abutments and virtual teeth. Dent Today 27(7):122. 124, 126–7

Ganz SD (2008d) Computer-aided design/computer-aided manufacturing applications using CT and cone beam CT scanning technology. Dent Clin N Am 52(4):777–808

Ganz SD (2009a) Advances in diagnosis and treatment planning utilizing CT scan technology for improving surgical and restorative implant reconstruction: tools of empowerment. In: Jokstad A (ed) Osseointegration and dental implants. Wiley-Blackwell, Iowa, pp 88–116

Ganz SD (2009b) Advanced case planning with SimPlant. In: Tardieu P, Al R (eds) The art of computer-guided implantology. Quintessence Publishing, Chicago

Ganz SD (2009c) Bone grafting assessment: focus on the anterior and posterior maxilla utilizing advanced 3-D imaging technologies. Dent Implantol Updat 20(6):41–48

Ganz SD (2010a) Implant complications associated with two- and three dimensional diagnostic imaging technologies. In: Froum SJ (ed) Dental implant complications – etiology, prevention, and treatment. Wiley-Blackwell, Chichester, pp 71–99

Ganz SD (2010b) The use of CT/CBCT and interactive virtual treatment planning and the triangle of bone: defining new paradigms for assessment of implant receptor sites. In: Babbush CHJ, Krauser J, Rosenlicht J (eds) Dental implants – The art and science. Saunders Maryland Heights, Missouri, pp 146–166

Ganz SD (2012) Utilization of three-dimensional imaging technology to enhance maxillofacial surgical applications. In: Miloro M, Ghali GE, Larsen P, Waite P (eds) Peterson's principles of oral and maxillofacial surgery. People's Medical House-USA, Shelton, pp 179–200

Ganz SD (2013) Dental implantology: an evolving treatment modality. Compend Contin Educ Dent 34(8):628–629

Ganz SD (2015a) Three-dimensional imaging and guided surgery for dental implants. Dent Clin N Am 59(2):265–290

Ganz SD (2015b) Diagnostic imaging for patient evaluation and minimally invasive treatment planning. In: Cullum D, Deporter D (eds) Minimally invasive dental implant surgery. Wilessy-Blackwell, Hoboken

Guerrero ME, Jacobs R, Loubele M, Schutyser F, Suetens P, van Steenberghe D (2006) State-of-the-art on cone beam CT imaging for preoperative planning of implant placement. Clin Oral Investig 10:1–7

Haney E, Gansky SA, Lee JS, Johnson E, Maki K, Miller AJ, Huang JC (2010) Comparative analysis of traditional radiographs and cone-beam computed tomography volumetric images in the diagnosis and treatment planning of maxillary impacted canines. Am J Orthod Dentofac Orthop 137(5):590–597

Harris D, Buser D, Dula K et al (2002) E.A.O. guidelines for the use of diagnostic imaging in implant dentistry. A consensus work-shop organized by the European Association for Osseointegration in Trinity College Dublin. Clin Oral Implants Res 13:566–570

Hof M, Pommer B, Ambros H, Jesch P, Vogl S, Zechner W (2015) Does timing of implant placement affect implant therapy outcome in the aesthetic zone? A clinical, radiological, aesthetic, and patient-based evaluation. Clin Implant Dent Relat Res 17(6):1188–1199

Jabero M, Sarment DP (2006) Advanced surgical guidance technology: a review. Implant Dent 15(2):135–142. Review

Jacobs R, Adriansens A, Verstreken K, Suetens P, van Steenberghe D (1999) Predictability of a three-dimensional planning system for oral implant surgery. Dentomaxillofac Radiol 28(2):105–111

Jamali AA, Deuel C, Perreira A, Salgado CJ, Hunter JC, Strong EB (2007) Linear and angular measurements of computer-generated models: are they accurate, valid, and reliable? Comput Aided Surg 12(5):278–285

Kan JY, Morimoto T, Rungcharassaeng K, Roe P, Smith DH (2010) Gingival biotype assessment in the esthetic zone: visual versus direct measurement. Int J Periodontics Restorative Dent 30(3):237–243

Kan JY, Roe P, Rungcharassaeng K, Patel RD, Waki T, Lozada JL, Zimmerman G (2011) Classification of sagittal root position in relation to the anterior maxillary osseous housing for immediate implant placement: a cone beam computed tomography study. Int J Oral Maxillofac Implants 26(4):873–876

Kan JY, Roe P, Rungcharassaeng K (2015) Effects of implant morphology on rotational stability during immediate implant placement in the esthetic zone. Int J Oral Maxillofac Implants 30(3):667–670

Kang SH, Kim MK, Kim HJ, Zhengguo P, Lee SH (2014a) Accuracy assessment of image-based surface meshing for volumetric computed tomography images in the craniofacial region. J Craniofac Surg 25(6):2051–2055

Kang SH, Lee JW, Lim SH, Kim YH, Kim MK (2014b) Dental image replacement on cone beam computed tomography with three-dimensional optical scanning of a dental cast, occlusal bite, or bite tray impression. Int J Oral Maxillofac Surg 43(10):1293–1301

Klein M, Abrams M (2001) Computer-guided surgery utilizing a computer-milled surgical template. Pract Proced Aesthet Dent 13(2):165–169. quiz 170

Klein M, Cranin AN, Sirakian A (1993) A Computerized Tomographic (CT) scan appliance for optimal presurgical and pre-prosthetic planning of the implant patient. Prac Periodont Asethet Dent 5:33–39

Lal K, White GS, Morea DN, Wright RF (2006) Use of stereolithographic templates for surgical and prosthodontic implant planning and placement. Part I. The concept. J Prosthodont 15(1):51–58

Lam EW, Ruprecht A, Yang J (1995) Comparison of two-dimensional orthoradially reformatted computed tomography and panoramic radiography for dental implant treatment planning. J Prosthet Dent 74:42–46

Lanis A, Álvarez Del Canto O (2015) The combination of digital surface scanners and cone beam computed tomography technology for guided implant surgery using 3Shape implant studio software: a case history report. Int J Prosthodont 28(2):169–178

Lee CY, Ganz SD, Wong N, Suzuki JB (2012) Use of cone beam computed tomography and a laser intraoral scanner in virtual dental implant surgery: part 1. Implant Dent 21(4):265–271

Lee CY, Wong N, Ganz SD, Mursic J, Suzuki JB (2015) Use of an intraoral laser scanner during the prosthetic phase of implant dentistry: a pilot study. J Oral Implantol 41(4):e126–e132

Mischkowski RA, Ritter L, Neugebauer J, Dreiseidler T, Keeve E, Zöller JE (2007) Diagnostic quality of panoramic views obtained by a newly developed digital volume tomography device for maxillofacial imaging. Quintessence Int 38(9):763–772

Mol A, Balasundaram A (2008) In vitro cone beam computed tomography imaging of periodontal bone. Dentomaxillofac Radiol 37(6):319–324

Moreira CR, Sales MA, Lopes PM, Cavalcanti MG (2009) Assessment of linear and angular measurements on three-dimensional cone-beam computed tomographic images. Oral Surg Oral Med Oral Pathol Oral Radiol Endod 108(3):430–436

Nairn NJ, Ayoub AF, Barbenel J, Moos K, Naudi K, Ju X, Khambay BS (2013) Digital replacement of the distorted dentition acquired by cone beam computed tomography (CBCT): a pilot study. Int J Oral Maxillofac Surg 42(11):1488–1493

Nickenig HJ, Eitner S (2007) Reliability of implant placement after virtual planning of implant positions using cone beam CT data and surgical (guide) templates. J Craniomaxillofac Surg 35(4–5):207–211. Epub 2007 Jun 18

Norton MR, Ganeles J, Ganz SD, Stumpel LJ, Schmidt JM (2010) 2010 Guidelines of the Academy of Osseointegration for the provision of dental implants and associated patient care. Int J Oral Maxillofac Implants 25(3):620–627

Orentlicher G, Goldsmith D, Horowitz A (2009) Computer-generated implant planning and surgery: case select. Compend Contin Educ Dent 30(3):162–166. 168–73

Orentlicher G, Goldsmith D, Horowitz A (2010) Applications of 3-dimensional virtual computerized tomography technology in oral and maxillofacial surgery: current therapy. J Oral Maxillofac Surg 68(8):1933–1959

Ozan O, Turkyilmaz I, Ersoy AE, McGlumphy EA, Rosenstiel SF (2009) Clinical accuracy of 3 different types of computed tomography-derived stereolithographic surgical guides in implant placement. J Oral Maxillofac Surg 67(2):394–401

Rinaldi M, Ganz SD, Mottola A (2015) Computer-guided applications for dental implants, bone grafting, and reconstructive surgery. Elsevier, St. Louis

Roe P, Kan JY, Rungcharassaeng K, Caruso JM, Zimmerman G, Mesquida J (2012) Horizontal and vertical dimensional changes of peri-implant facial bone following immediate placement and provisionalization of maxillary anterior single implants: a 1-year cone beam computed tomography study. Int J Oral Maxillofac Implants 27(2):393–400

Rosenfeld AL, Mecall RA (1996) Use of interactive computed tomography to predict the esthetic and functional demands of implant-supported prostheses. Compend Contin Educ Dent 17:1125–1146

Rosenfeld AL, Mecall RA (1998) Use of prosthesis-generated computed tomographic information for diagnostic and surgical treatment planning. J Esthet Dent 10:132–148

Rosenfeld A, Mandelaris G, Tardieu P (2006) Prosthetically directed placement using computer software to insure precise placement and predictable prosthetic outcomes. Part1: diagnostics, imaging, and collaborative accountability. Int J Periodontics Restorative Dent 26:215–221

Rothman SLG (1998) Computerized tomography of the enhanced alveolar ridge. In: Dental applications of computerized tomography. Quintessence Publishing Co, Chicago, pp 87–112

Rugani P, Kirnbauer B, Arnetzl GV, Jakse N (2009) Cone beam computerized tomography: basics for digital planning in oral surgery and implantology. Int J Comput Dent 12(2):131–145

Scherer MD (2014) Presurgical implant-site assessment and restoratively driven digital planning. Dent Clin N Am 58(3):561–595

Sonick M (1994) A comparison of the accuracy of periapical, panoramic, and computed tomographic radiographs in locating the mandibular canal. JOMI 9:455–460

Tahmaseb A, De Clerck R, Wismeijer D (2009) Computer-guided implant placement: 3D planning software, fixed intraoral reference points, and CAD/CAM technology. A case report. Int J Oral Maxillofac Implants 24(3):541–546

Tahmaseb A, Wismeijer D, Coucke W, Derksen W (2014) Computer technology applications in surgical implant dentistry: a systematic review. Int J Oral Maxillofac Implants 29(Suppl):25–42

Tyndall DA, Price JB, Tetradis S, Ganz SD, Hildebolt C, Scarfe WC (2012) American Academy of Oral and Maxillofacial Radiology. Position statement of the American Academy of Oral and Maxillofacial Radiology on selection criteria for the use of radiology in dental implantology with emphasis on cone beam computed tomography. Oral Surg Oral Med Oral Pathol Oral Radiol 113(6):817–826

Valente F, Schiroli G, Sbrenna A (2009) Accuracy of computer-aided oral implant surgery: a clinical and radiographic study. Int J Oral Maxillofac Implants 24(2):234–242

Verstreken K, Van Cleynenbreugel J, Martens K, Marchal G, van Steenberghe D, Suetens P (1998) An image-guided planning system for endosseous oral implants. IEEE Trans Med Imaging 17(5):842–852

Clinical Assessment of the Gingiva and Alveolus

Yung-Ting Hsu and Hom-Lay Wang

Abstract

The first step heading to successful implant outcomes is a meticulous clinical examination. It provides implantologists a clear picture for diagnosis, treatment plan, and prevention of possible complications. This chapter suggests a guideline for comprehensive clinical evaluation on both gingiva and alveolus as well as general checking via palpation, probing, and visual perception. Prior to evaluation of future implant sites, an overall investigation is mandatory to verify the locations of anatomic structures, occlusion, esthetic, and pathologic conditions. Periodontal charting is of the essence in recording current soft tissue conditions to analyze periodontal/peri-implant health. Clinicians should also be aware of individual tissue biotype, keratinized mucosa, and biologic width for better soft tissue management. In addition to soft tissue, ridge dimension and ridge deformities should be entailed. With the aids of both clinical and radiographic examinations, these data found the basis for the precise diagnosis and comprehensive treatments, leading to uneventful outcomes and successful implant therapy.

7.1 Introduction

In the past decades, the advent of dental implants has ushered in a new era of dentistry. With dental implants, clinicians now can provide more treatment options for replacing the missing teeth both functionally and esthetically with high predictability and success rate. Serving as an analog of tooth, the dental implant offers another tooth substitution without sacrificing structures of adjacent teeth. With the popularity of dental implantation, it also brings the challenge of rising implant complications. The consequences of these complications lead to disastrous predicaments which may end up

Y.-T. Hsu, DDS, MDSc, MS
Department of Periodontology and Dental Hygiene, School of Dentistry, University of Detroit Mercy, 2700 Martin Luther King Jr. Blvd., Detroit, MI 48208-2576, USA

H.-L. Wang, DDS, MSD, PhD (✉)
Department of Periodontics and Oral Medicine, School of Dentistry, University of Michigan, 1011 North University Avenue, Ann Arbor, MI 48109-1078, USA
e-mail: homlay@umich.edu

with removal of implants or even fatal incidents. Minimizing the incidence of implant complications, undoubtedly, is now the focus of many implantologists.

As the first step to achieve successful treatment outcomes, thorough clinical assessments are definitely paving the path for an accurate diagnosis, comprehensive treatment plan, and precise surgical approach. Clinicians should carefully evaluate both soft and hard tissues prior to implant treatment. For example, awareness and detection of the dimensional ridge alteration following dentition loss are essential to avoid possible injuries during surgeries and to plan better implant positioning. Without prudent assessments, implants are at higher risk of developing complications due to implant malpositioning, occlusal overload or placement in the sites with insufficient soft and hard tissue support, or uncontrolled inflammation.

To set up foundation for successful implant therapy, careful clinical assessments of the gingiva and alveolus are essential elements. Hence, this chapter provides a guideline to assess both the soft and hard tissues surrounding implant site for ideal implant placement and good long-term stability.

7.2 The Purposes of Clinical Assessment

In addition to candidate selection, careful analysis of implant sites is essential to achieve ideal treatment outcomes. Like searching for the clues of the puzzle, accurate assessments help clinicians to verify current situations, obtaining correct diagnosis and precise treatment plans. The purposes of clinical assessments include:

- To update the current status of implant sites for diagnosis
- To identify the anatomic structures or tissue deformities for prevention of surgical injuries or postoperative complications
- To collect information for a comprehensive treatment plan of implant surgeries and related correction procedures
- To monitor implant clinical conditions in order to establish implant long-term stability

7.3 General Assessments

A comprehensive evaluation should concentrate on but not limit to current status of hard and soft tissue. The entirety of situation would not be disclosed without general assessments, inclusive of anatomic structures, occlusion, esthetic, and pathologic conditions.

7.3.1 Anatomic Landmarks

Like preparation for other surgeries, recognition of important anatomic structures and their possible variations is beneficial to prevent surgical complications. Damages of these vital structures during implant surgeries often lead to temporary or permanent damages, such as hemorrhages, paresthesia, and even life-threatening events (Goodacre et al. 2003; Juodzbalys et al. 2013).

In the maxilla, the maxillary sinus or the antrum is a significant structure. As the largest compartment of paranasal sinuses, the maxillary sinus located at the posterior maxilla of which the size has direct effects on implant lengths and positions. With 20–40% of prevalence (Neugebauer et al. 2010; Park et al. 2011), the presence of antral septum may hamper the sinus elevation procedure in different degrees depending on its size, location, and orientation (Wen et al. 2013). Moreover, of great importance are positions of the greater palatine foramen (GPF) and the greater palatine neurovascular bundle (GPB) for not only maxillary hemianesthesia but also manipulation of the flap elevation and soft tissue grafting during surgeries. From personal communication, Reiser and coworkers manifested that the distances between the cementoenamel junction (CEJ) of maxillary molars and the greater palatine foramen were 7 mm, 12 mm, and 17 mm in the low, medium, and high vault, respectively (Reiser et al. 1996). Nevertheless, a recent autopsy study pointed out the actual positions of GPB were up to 4 mm closer to CEJ of molars than where clinicians palpated, regardless of experience levels (Fu et al. 2011). In esthetic zones, the incisive canal carries the nasopalatine nerve, and vessels may be an issue during implant reconstruction. In addition to the risk of imperiling neurovascular structures, morphologic variation of incisive canals which related to gender and edentulous status may affect the implant stability when placing immediate implants in the anterior maxilla (Mardinger et al. 2008; Tözüm et al. 2012).

In the mandible, inferior alveolar nerves (IAN) and vessels traverse the mandibular foramen, run in the mandibular canal, and give off the mental nerve via mental foramen. At molar area, the mandibular canal runs its course following the lingual plate and makes a gradual change to buccal side at the level of premolars. Related to the anteroposterior position of mental foramen, the course of the mandibular canal varies in horizontal plane (Pyun et al. 2013). Unlike the mandibular canal, the lingual nerve makes its "turn off" at the molar sites, especially in the level of first molar (Chan et al. 2010). Mental foramina and anterior loops of IAN are also critical structures when implantation at premolar sites. Mental foramina are most commonly found below the apices of mandibular premolars (58%), followed by the apex of second premolars (42%) (Neiva et al. 2004). As the most anterior portion of IAN, the presence of anterior loops is high but not always (48–88%). They are frequently found bilaterally. The various extent of anterior loops makes them difficult to identify and easy to be violated (Neiva et al. 2004; Apostolakis and Brown 2012). Located in the posterior mandible, the lingual concavity is another common finding which clinician should pay great attention to minimize the risk of lingual plate perforation during implantation. In spite of the low incidence reported in an earlier study, higher prevalence (36–66%) has been suggested by recent research using cone beam computed tomography (CBCT) scan (Watanabe et al. 2010; Chan et al. 2011). In addition, recognition of the lingual foramen is recommended for the prevention of life-threatening hemorrhage. Recent studies showed it was commonly located at the midline of the symphysis and had high chance of anastomoses with other anatomic structures (von Arx et al. 2011; Yildirim et al. 2014).

In general, the concept of the safety margin has been recommended to keep implants placed away from nerve and blood vessels (Worthington 2004; Apostolakis and Brown 2012). Cautions should be taken to avoid invading lingual cavities or anatomic spaces/fossa. Further surgical procedures may be needed with the presence of sinus at the implant sites.

7.3.2 Occlusion/Prosthesis Considerations

In spite of serving as analogs of natural teeth, dental implants connect with living bone directly, called osseointegration. For lack of the cushion of periodontal ligament (PDL), dental implants present their load-bearing characteristics with stress concentration on crestal bone. To accommodate the disadvantageous kinetics, therefore, occlusion should be taken into consideration for future implant-supported prosthesis. Overall, the occlusal assessments entail occlusal stability, jaw relation (e.g., the Angle's classification), the discrepancy between centric occlusion (CO) and centric relation (CR), and occlusal pattern (e.g., canine guidance or group function). For implant sites, the dimension of edentulous space and vertical dimension assessments (e.g., the interocclusal or interarch space) play an important role on the implant treatment plan (Fig. 7.1). In general, the minimal vertical dimension requirement for the implant-supported prostheses is 8 mm for

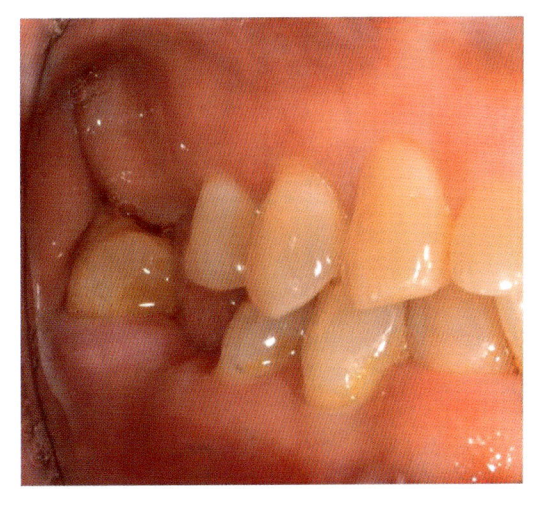

Fig. 7.1 The interocclusal or interarch space. The interocclusal or interarch space should be taken into consideration during assessments to avoid improper crown/implant ratio

posterior implant, 8 mm for the anterior implant crown, and 12 mm for implant-supported removable prosthesis (Misch 2008). Vertical and horizontal overlap, i.e., overbite and overjet, should be recorded for implant rehabilitation in the esthetic zone. The sizes and the positions of tongues may affect designs of implant-supported dentures. In addition, clinicians should keep an eye on the signs of parafunction, including clenching and bruxism, as well as the presence of occlusal interferences or premature contacts during working or nonworking movements since these activities may trigger late implant failure (Miyata et al. 2000; Fu et al. 2012; Hsu et al. 2012).

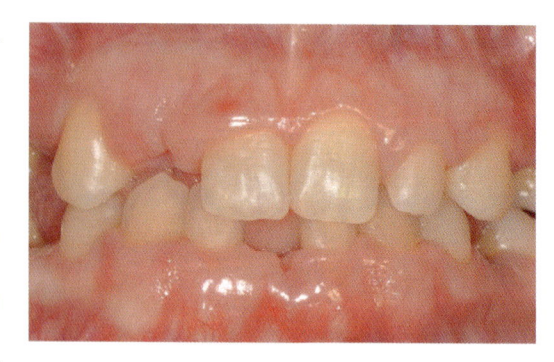

Fig. 7.2 Gingival disharmony. Gingival harmony was impaired due to passive altered eruption and dentition misalignment

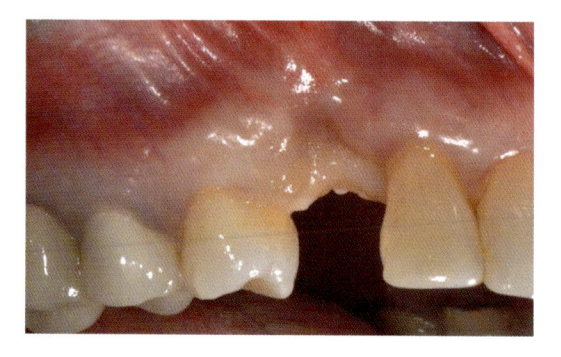

Fig. 7.3 Gingival disharmony. Esthetics was compromised due to localized ridge deformity and gingival recession

7.3.3 Esthetics

Esthetic is subjective and complex. In modern dentistry, it is also part of the essence of optical long-term outcomes. The terms of "macro-," "mini-," and "microesthetic" have been created for the components of modern esthetic analysis, referring to the analysis of the whole face, the smile framework, and tooth and gingival architectures, respectively (Sarver and Jacobson 2007). Clinically, comprehensive assessments for microesthetic analysis on future implant sites encompass gingival features and tooth composition. The elements of tooth composition are the color, shape, dimension, width/length ratio, inclination, and tooth proportion. In regard to soft tissue, quantity and quality of gingiva/peri-implant mucosa also play a significant role on esthetic. The measurable components include keratinized mucosa (KM) width (will be described later in this chapter), papillae height, and gingival position in both horizontal and vertical dimension. In addition, some qualified characters consisting of gingival color, contour, consistency, and surface texture are not countable but essential to identify both the health status of soft tissue and gingival harmony. Gingival harmony may be impaired by several factors, such as gingival recession/gingival enlargement and alignment of adjacent teeth (Figs. 7.2 and 7.3). Dark triangles were enhanced by the occurrences of papilla loss, leading to unpleasant smile. As an important indicator of esthetics, the amounts of papillary loss (Fig. 7.4) have been classified by many researchers which are associated with different prognosis (Jemt 1997; Nordland and Tarnow 1998; Cardaropoli et al. 2004). The classifications of papillary loss were summarized in Table 7.1. In fact, it is critical to have an implant site with appearances and dimension resembling to adjacent natural dentition. Otherwise, correcting procedures are expected before or during implant therapy to achieve esthetic outcomes.

7.3.4 Pathologies

Clinical assessments should entail the screening of pathologic conditions on hard and soft tissues by visual examination and palpation. Soft pathologies may display colors or surface textures deviated from normal tissue, such as candidiasis, lichen

7 Clinical Assessment of the Gingiva and Alveolus

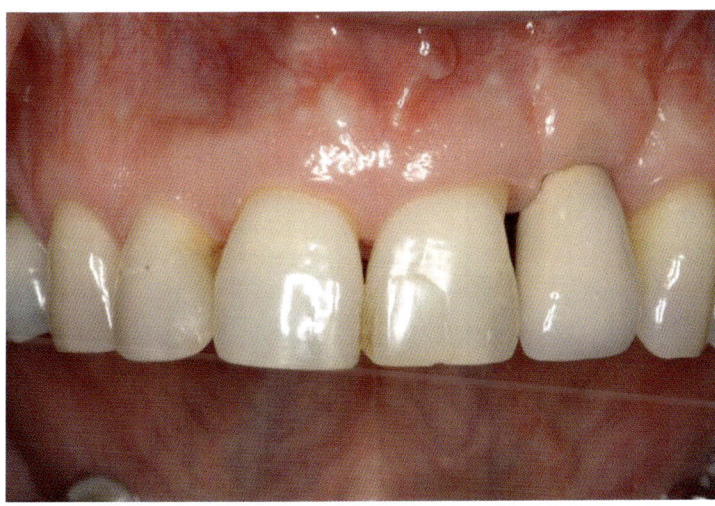

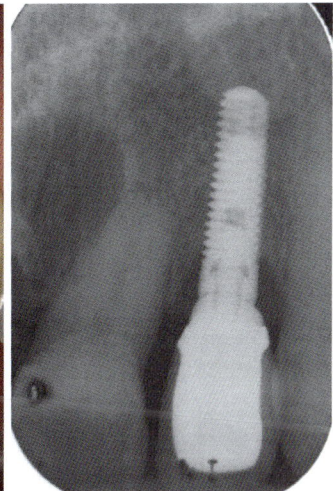

Fig. 7.4 Papillary loss. There was absence of papillae in both mesial and distal areas

Table 7.1 Classifications of papillary loss

Jemt (1997)	0	No papilla
	1	The presence of <50% of papilla height
	2	The presence of 50–99% of the papilla height
	3	100% of the entire proximal space without the signs of hyperplasia
	4	Hyperplasic papillae, covering too much of the restoration and/or adjacent tooth
Nordland and Tarnow (1998)	Normal	Interdental papilla fills the entire embrasure space
	Class I	Partial loss of papilla height, interproximal CEJ is not visible
	Class II	Partial loss of papilla height, interproximal CEJ is visible
	Class III	Total loss of interproximal papillae, of which the tip is equal or apical to the CEJ at the labial aspect
		The tip of the interdental papilla lies level with or apical to the fCEJ
Cardaropoli et al. (2004)	PPI 1	No papillary loss and the papilla height is equal to adjacent papillae
	PPI 2	Partial papillary loss. The papilla height is not equal to adjacent papillae but still cover interproximal CEJ
	PPI 3	The height of papilla is between interproximal CEJ and facial CEJ
	PPI 4	The papilla is apical to both the interproximal CEJ and labial CEJ

planus, mucous membrane pemphigoid, pyogenic granuloma, tumors, etc. In hard tissue, pathologic lesions are more difficult to identify by visible signs. They include cysts, residual roots, benign or malignant tumors, and congenital defects. Some infective lesions may originate from endodontic problems of adjacent teeth (Figs. 7.5 and 7.6). Differential diagnosis may need radiographic examination, biopsy, and further laboratory tests. Generally speaking, most of these lesions should be managed before implant placement.

7.4 Assessments of Soft Tissue

Charting is an efficient way to seize the current dental and periodontal status. Providing a large amount of information, the periodontal charting facilitates accurate diagnosis and treatment planning (Fig. 7.7). It contains the presence of tooth, clinical attachment level (CAL), probing depth (PD), gingival recession (GR), furcation involvement (FI), and tooth mobility (TM). The sites with bleeding on probing (BOP) and suppuration must be marked in the chart. For a comprehensive record, clinicians should also measure the amount of keratinized gingiva/mucosa (KG/KM) and record the presence of mucogingival defects.

7.4.1 Periodontal/Peri-implant Health

Periodontal health has strong influences on long-term stability of implant therapy. It has been shown that previous history of periodontitis is a major risk factor for developing peri-implantitis (AAP 2013 position paper). Hence, it is very important to achieve periodontal health/stability prior to implant therapy; otherwise, periodontal inflammation may cause hard and soft tissue destruction around dental implants. The signs of tissue inflammation include color alternation, tissue swelling/ recession, the presence of BOP, and exudate discharge. In addition, the severity of periodontal/peri-implant diseases has been categorized by the measurement of CAL and PD (Eke et al. 2012). Generally speaking, the inflammation should be controlled before initiating implant therapy.

7.4.2 Tissue Biotype

Tissue biotype was first defined by Claffey and Shanley (1986). Gingival tissue with thickness less than 1.5 mm was classified as "thin biotype," whereas gingival thickness with "thick biotype" was more than 2 mm. Kois listed tissue biotype as one of the five diagnostic keys, in which thin biotype was prone to gingival recession, whereas thick biotype leads to pocket formation during inflammation (Kois 2004). Despite the relationship between tissue biotype and peri-implant gingival recession remains unclear, studies using CBCT scan suggested tissue biotype may correlate with the thickness of underlying bone (Evans and Chen 2008; Fu et al. 2010; Nisapakultorn et al. 2010; Cook et al. 2011). In addition to direct measurements and visual inspection, several researchers have advocated using the transparency of the periodontal probe to perform the assessment (Kan et al. 2003;

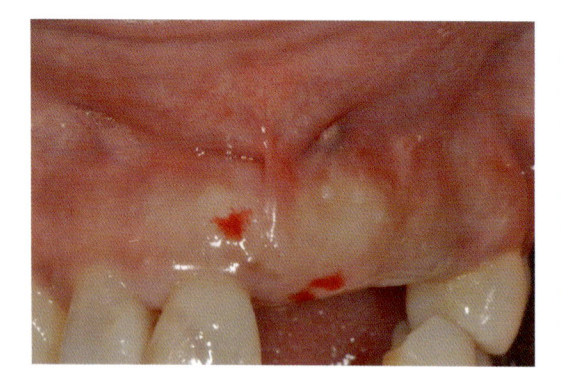

Fig. 7.5 The presence of pathologies. A symptomless, bluish lesion with fluctuation was found on the buccal mucosa of edentulous ridge

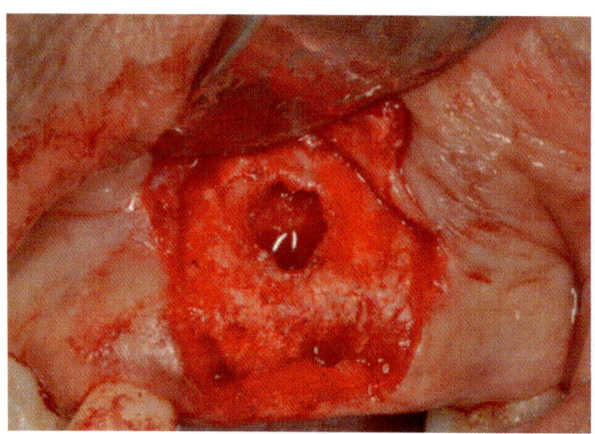

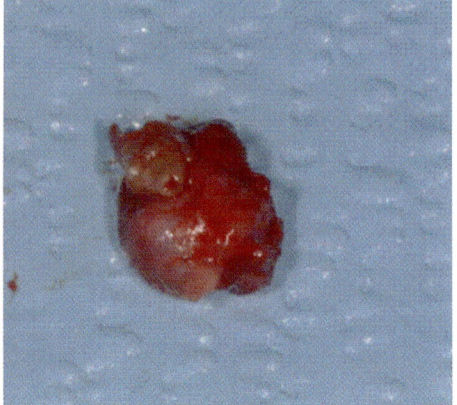

Fig. 7.6 The presence of pathologies. The entire cyst was enucleated after flap reflection

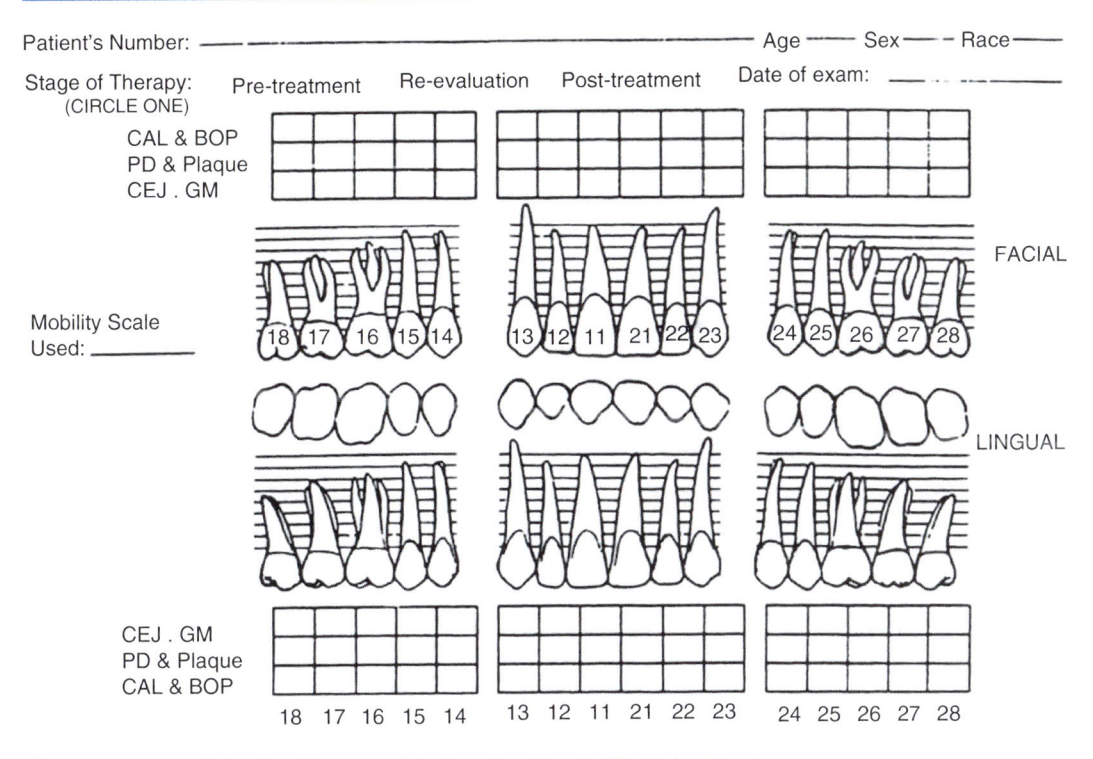

7 Clinical Assessment of the Gingiva and Alveolus

Fig. 7.7 Periodontal charting (Courtesy of the American Board of Periodontology)

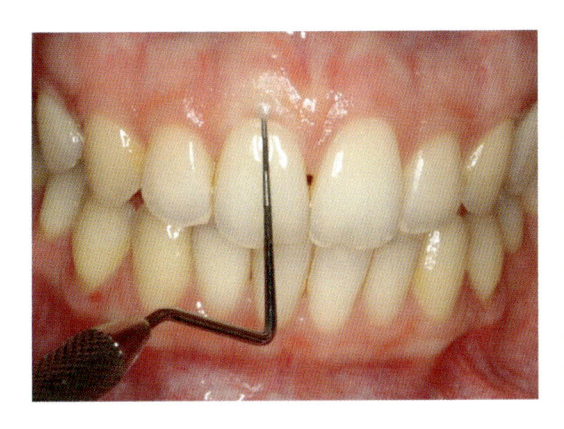

Fig. 7.8 Assessments of tissue biotype. Tissue biotype was evaluated by the transparency of the periodontal probe

De Rouck et al. 2009). Compared with gold standard, i.e., direct measurements, tissue biotype was able to be accurately identified by the placement of the probe into the labial gingiva (Kan et al. 2010). On the contrary, the reliability of visual assessments was pessimistic regardless of examiners' experience levels (Eghbali et al. 2009) (Fig. 7.8).

7.4.3 Keratinized Mucosa

The amount of KM should also be evaluated because of its potential effects on plaque control in periodontal or peri-implant tissue (Lang and Loe 1972; Ericsson and Lindhe 1984; Chung et al. 2006). Remaining inconclusive (Wennstrom et al. 1994; Bragger et al. 1997) due to heterogeneity of experimental designs, the positive relationship between KM width and peri-implant health has been advocated (Chung et al. 2006; Bouri et al. 2008; Lin et al. 2013). In a canine model with 3 months of experimental period, Benqazi and coworkers found that the alveolar level adjacent to implants with no KM had significantly apical position than implants with KM (Bengazi et al. 2013). A human study with 12 months follow-up also supported the need of adequate band of peri-implant KM to prevent plaque accumulation and induced tissue inflammation (Boynueğri et al. 2013). Clinically, there are several methods that can be used to determine the location of mucogingival junction: (1) visual inspection of color differences from

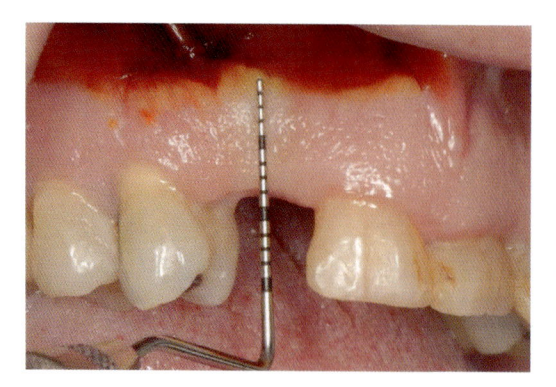

Fig. 7.9 Assessments of keratinized mucosa width. With the application of Schiller's iodine solution, MGJ was located. The width of keratinized mucosa was measured using a periodontal probe

nonkeratinized mucosa to keratinized gingiva, (2) stretching examination by pulling the tissue to distinguish attached and movable tissue, and (3) the application of Schiller's iodine solution (Fig. 7.9): As a temporary staining for glycogen-containing tissues, Schiller's solution leaves dark-brown stains on the mucosa and therefore has been used to identify the mucogingival junction (MGJ) bounding keratinized and nonkeratinized mucosa (Maurer et al. 2000).

7.4.4 Biologic Width

The existence of biologic width in peri-implant tissue is equally important as those noted in the periodontal tissue. Similar with the phenomenon found on periodontium, a soft tissue barrier attached to the implant abutment was first emphasized by Berglundh and colleagues in a canine model. A cuff-like barrier which was almost free of inflammatory cells was found around the dental implant (Berglundh et al. 1991). The concept of "peri-implant biologic width" was further advocated in 1996. In this later study, they found that a certain minimum width of the peri-implant mucosa was always formed following implantation even in the sites where the epithelium was intentionally excised (Berglundh and Lindhe 1996). Consisting of an epithelial attachment and a zone of connective tissue attachment, biologic width aims to establish the soft tissue seal which protects osseointergrated implants against pathogen invasion. Violation of biologic width may lead to the occurrence of bone remodeling process/ bone loss around the implant (Berglundh and Lindhe 1996). In addition, repeated dislodgement and reconnection of abutments may also compromise the healing process, resulting in an apical migration of marginal bone (Abrahamsson et al. 1997).

7.5 Assessments of Hard Tissue

As a part of nature courses, changes of alveolar ridges have been observed immediately following teeth loss. This dynamic process, so-called wound healing, includes several stages and ended with tissue maturation/ tissue remodeling. From a clinical point of view, this remodeling alters not only the volume but also the shape of alveolar ridges. The unavoidable dimensional changes and correction of these ridge deficiencies should be taken into account for implant treatment planning (Wang and Al-Shammari 2002).

Several things should be considered prior to actual clinical evaluation. First of all, the amounts of tissue changes recorded from hard tissue only may not be equal to the combined hard and soft tissue changes (Tan et al. 2012). In other words, bone resorption may be underestimated because the thickness of soft tissue may compensate the change of bone volume and cover up the ridge deformities, leading to implant malpositioning. Second, this healing process may last from several months to years following teeth extraction. Several researchers demonstrated the occurrence of rapid ridge resorption in first 3 months of socket healing (Johnson 1969; Schropp et al. 2003; Tan et al. 2012).

7 Clinical Assessment of the Gingiva and Alveolus

However, a slight but gradual bone remodeling may continue for several years (Carlsson and Persson 1967). Indeed, the reduction of the residual ridges continues in denture wearers even after edentulism for 25 years (Tallgren 1972). The magnitude of ridge resorption varies from jaws and from prosthesis (Tallgren 1972; Jacobs et al. 1992). Therefore, it is of great importance for a clinician to have a full picture of tissue alteration at edentulous sites.

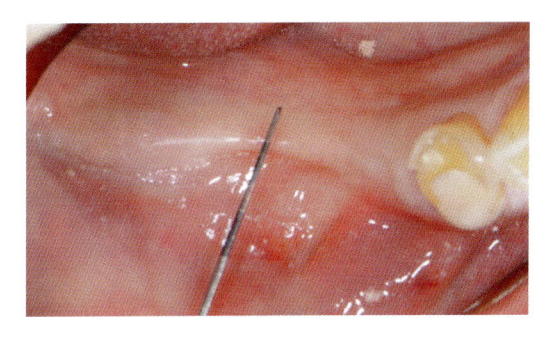

Fig. 7.10 Measurement of ridge dimension. Michigan O probe was used to measure the ridge width

7.5.1 Ridge Dimension

For ideal implantation, ridge dimension plays an important role in treatment planning. In general, the minimal of bone around implant should be at least 0.5–1 mm and in anterior will be 2 mm facial bone (Spray et al. 2000). In partial edentulism, the distance between adjacent teeth is vital to determine implant numbers and positions. The buccolingual distance of ridge, i.e., ridge width, should also be assessed not only to clarify the implant position but also to verify the demand of bone regeneration. In esthetic zone, implant placement at the site with insufficient width of labial plate (≤2 mm) risks esthetics in developing midfacial mucosal recession by accidental fenestration or dehiscence (Spray 2000 article). Moreover, approximation of alveolar height is equally vital in clinical evaluation. Ridge resorption may compromise the implant length, leading to inappropriate crown/implant ratio which may trigger peri-implant marginal bone loss and also cause implant failure if exceeding the threshold (Garaicoa-Pazmino et al. 2014; Malchiodi et al. 2014) (Fig. 7.10.). Also, the minimal distance from adjacent tooth should be at least 1.5 mm. Nonetheless, this is often true for the anterior implants, but for the posterior implants, it should be 3 mm instead because of the restoration's emergence profile (Grunder et al. 2005; Zetu and Wang 2005).

7.5.2 Classifications of Edentulous Ridge Deformities

Following tooth loss, ridge alteration is a long-lasting and dynamic process. With apical migration of the edentulous ridge, bone resorption occurred in both maxilla and mandible in a reverse manner horizontally (Pietrokovski et al. 2007). Based on the severity of ridge atrophy, Lekholm and Zarb illustrated the residual bone morphology of both jaws from the ridge resorption to basal bone loss (Brånemark et al. 1985). Several classifications of ridge deformities have been proposed according to tissue contour in the 1980s (Kent et al. 1983; Brånemark et al. 1985; Cawood and Howell 1988; Misch 1990). In the meantime, other researchers stood on the defect regions to categorize the ridge deficiency (Seibert 1983; Allen et al. 1985; Wang and Al-Shammari 2002). In 2002, Wang and Al-Shammari proposed HVC classification, a modification of Seibert's classification with three subclassifications and corresponding treatment options for fixed prosthesis and implant therapy. Considering both soft tissue and hard tissue, this classification offered multiple treatment modalities for the correction of ridge insufficiencies (Wang and Al-Shammari 2002). Classifications of ridge deformities are summarized in Table 7.2, (Figs. 7.11 and 7.12).

Table 7.2 Classifications of ridge deformities

Authors	Classifications	Subclassifications/divisions
Ridge deficiencies		
Seibert (1983)	I: Buccolingual loss of tissue with adequate height	
	II: Apicocoronal loss of tissue with adequate width	
	III: Combination of type I and II	
Allen et al. (1985)	A: Loss of tissue contour in apicocoronal dimension	Mild: <3 mm
	B: Loss of tissue contour in buccolingual dimension	Medium: 3–6 mm
	C: Combination of type A and B	Severe: >6 mm
Wang and Al-Shammari (2002)	H: Horizontal tissue loss	S: small ≤3 mm
	V: Vertical tissue loss	M: medium 4–6 mm
	C: Combination	L: large ≥7 mm
Jaw shapes and contours		
Kent et al. (1983)	I: Ridge resorption, inadequate in width or undercut regions	
	II: Ridge resorption with knife-edge appearance, inadequate in both height and width	
	III: Resorption of basal bone, with concaved form of the mandible and sharp-edge form of the maxilla. Mobile soft tissue was presented in the maxilla	
	IV: Resorption of basal bone, flat appearance in both jaws	
Lekholm and Zarb (1985)	A: Most of the ridge remains intact	
	B: Moderate ridge atrophy, with inadequate ridge height and/or ridge width	
	C: Severe ridge atrophy toward the arch base with the integrity of basal bone	
	D: Advanced ridge atrophy with initiation of basal bone loss	
	E: Extreme atrophy of basal bone	
Cawood and Howell (1988)	I: Dentate	
	II: Post-extraction sockets	
	III: Well-rounded ridge form with sufficient ridge height and width	
	IV: Knife-edge ridge form with sufficient height but insufficient width	
	V: Flat ridge form with insufficient ridge height and width	
	VI: Depressed ridge form with evidence of basilar loss	
Misch (1990)	I: Same division shown in the all sections	Division
	II: Different divisions between posterior and anterior sections	A: >5 mm width, >8–12 mm height, >5 mm length, <30°trajectory
	III: Different divisions among each section	B: 2.5–5 mm width, >10 mm height, >15 mm length, <20°trajectory
		C: Inadequate width, height, length, trajectory
		D: Severe atrophy with basal bone loss

7 Clinical Assessment of the Gingiva and Alveolus

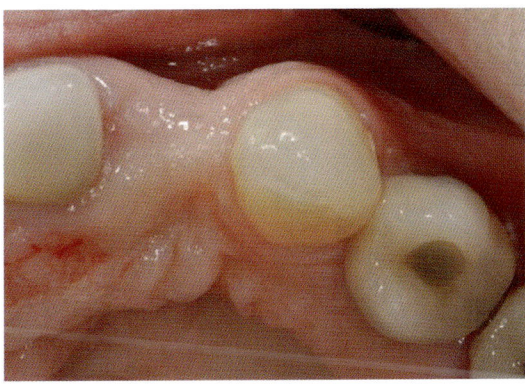

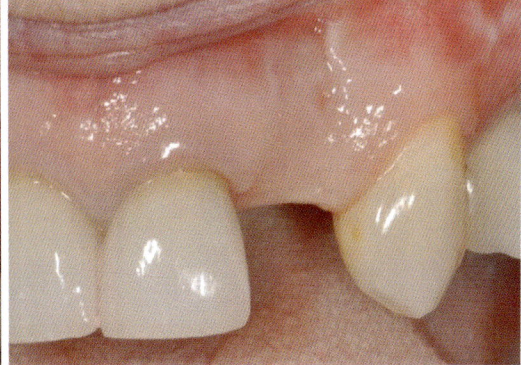

Fig. 7.11 Ridge deformities. The edentulous ridge displayed with buccolingual loss of tissue but adequate height

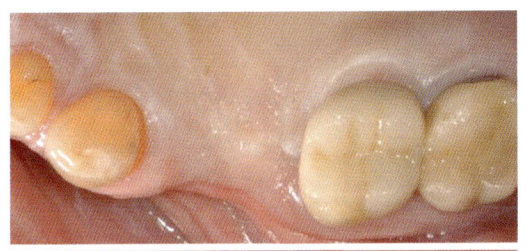

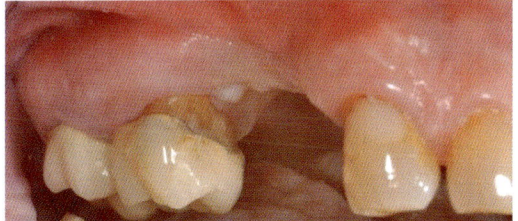

Fig. 7.12 Ridge deformities. An edentulous ridge with both vertical and horizontal tissue loss. Additional correcting procedure was required

Conclusion

Meticulous assessments should be taken prior to any treatments. Clinical evaluation of the gingiva and alveolus entails three components: soft tissue, hard tissue, and general inspection by palpation, probing, and visual perception. With the aids of both clinical and radiographic examinations, these data found the basis for the precise diagnosis and comprehensive treatments, leading to uneventful outcomes and successful implant therapy. Figure 7.13 is a flowchart that summarized the abovementioned assessments.

Clinical Assessments of Gingiva and Alveolus

General Assessments	*Anatomic landmarks* Maxilla Mandible	☐ Sinus: location, size, the presence of septa or pathologies ☐ Positions of the greater palatine foramen and the greater palatine neurovascular bundle ☐ Positions of incisive canal ☐ Inferior alveolar canal, including vessels and nerve ☐ Mental foramen and anterior loop of inferior alveolar nerve ☐ The presence of lingual concavity ☐ Lingual foramen
	Occlusion/ prosthesis consideration	☐ Occlusal stability ☐ Jaw relation (e.g., the Angle's classification) ☐ Discrepancy between centric occlusion and centric relation ☐ Occlusal pattern: canine guidance or group function ☐ Interocclusal or interarch space ☐ Vertical and horizontal overlap ☐ The signs of parafunction
	Esthetics Tooth components Gingival components	☐ Color ☐ Shape ☐ Dimension ☐ Inclination ☐ Width/ length ratio ☐ Tooth proportion ☐ Width of keratinized mucosa/ gingiva ☐ Papillae height ☐ Gingival position ☐ Color ☐ Contour ☐ Consistency ☐ Surface texture ☐ Gingival harmony
	Pathologies	The presence of pathologies: Yes or No
Soft Tissue	*Periodontal/ peri-implant health*	Clinical attachment level, probing depth, gingival recession, furcation involvement, tooth mobility, bleeding on probing, suppuration
	Tissue biotype	☐ Thin or ☐ Thick
	Keratinized mucosa	☐ The presence of keratinized mucosa/ gingiva: YES or NO ☐ Width of keratinized mucosa/ gingiva
	Biological width	
Hard Tissue	*Ridge dimension*	☐ Ridge height ☐ Ridge width (bucco-lingual distance of ridge) ☐ Length of space (distance between adjacent teeth)
	Ridge deformities	☐ Severity ☐ Orientation

Fig. 7.13 Flowchart of clinical assessments

References

Abrahamsson I, Berglundh T et al (1997) The mucosal barrier following abutment dis/reconnection. An experimental study in dogs. J Clin Periodontol 24(8):568–572

Allen EP, Gainza CS et al (1985) Improved technique for localized ridge augmentation. A report of 21 cases. J Periodontol 56(4):195–199

Apostolakis D, Brown JE (2012) The anterior loop of the inferior alveolar nerve: prevalence, measurement of its length and a recommendation for interforaminal implant installation based on cone beam CT imaging. Clin Oral Implants Res 23(9):1022–1030

Bengazi F, Botticelli D et al (2013) Influence of presence or absence of keratinized mucosa on the alveolar bony crest level as it relates to different buccal marginal bone thicknesses. An experimental study in dogs. Clin Oral Implants Res. 25(9):1065–1071

Berglundh T, Lindhe J (1996) Dimension of the periimplant mucosa. Biological width revisited. J Clin Periodontol 23(10):971–973

Berglundh T, Lindhe J et al (1991) The soft tissue barrier at implants and teeth. Clin Oral Implants Res 2(2):81–90

Bouri A Jr, Bissada N et al (2008) Width of keratinized gingiva and the health status of the supporting tissues around dental implants. Int J Oral Maxillofac Implants 23(2):323–326

Boynueğri D, Nemli SK et al (2013) Significance of keratinized mucosa around dental implants: a prospective comparative study. Clin Oral Implants Res 24(8):928–933

Brånemark P-I, Zarb GA et al (1985) Tissue-integrated prostheses: osseointegration in clinical dentistry. Quintessence, Chicago

Bragger U, Burgin WB et al (1997) Associations between clinical parameters assessed around implants and teeth. Clin Oral Implants Res 8(5):412–421

Cardaropoli D, Re S et al (2004) The Papilla Presence Index (PPI): a new system to assess interproximal papillary levels. Int J Periodontics Restor Dent 24(5):488–492

Carlsson GE, Persson G (1967) Morphologic changes of the mandible after extraction and wearing of dentures. A longitudinal, clinical, and x-ray cephalometric study covering 5 years. Odontol Revy 18(1):27–54

Cawood JI, Howell RA (1988) A classification of the edentulous jaws. Int J Oral Maxillofac Surg 17(4):232–236

Chan HL, Brooks SL et al (2011) Cross-sectional analysis of the mandibular lingual concavity using cone beam computed tomography. Clin Oral Implants Res 22(2):201–206

Chan HL, Leong DJ et al (2010) The significance of the lingual nerve during periodontal/implant surgery. J Periodontol 81(3):372–377

Chung DM, Oh TJ et al (2006) Significance of keratinized mucosa in maintenance of dental implants with different surfaces. J Periodontol 77(8):1410–1420

Claffey N, Shanley D (1986) Relationship of gingival thickness and bleeding to loss of probing attachment in shallow sites following nonsurgical periodontal therapy. J Clin Periodontol 13(7):654–657

Cook DR, Mealey BL et al (2011) Relationship between clinical periodontal biotype and labial plate thickness: an in vivo study. Int J Periodontics Restorative Dent 31(4):345–354

De Rouck T, Eghbali R et al (2009) The gingival biotype revisited: transparency of the periodontal probe through the gingival margin as a method to discriminate thin from thick gingiva. J Clin Periodontol 36(5):428–433

Eghbali A, De Rouck T et al (2009) The gingival biotype assessed by experienced and inexperienced clinicians. J Clin Periodontol 36(11):958–963

Eke PI, Page RC et al (2012) Update of the case definitions for population-based surveillance of periodontitis. J Periodontol 83(12):1449–1454

Ericsson I, Lindhe J (1984) Recession in sites with inadequate width of the keratinized gingiva. An experimental study in the dog. J Clin Periodontol 11(2):95–103

Evans CD, Chen ST (2008) Esthetic outcomes of immediate implant placements. Clin Oral Implants Res 19(1):73–80

Fu JH, Hasso DG et al (2011) The accuracy of identifying the greater palatine neurovascular bundle: a cadaver study. J Periodontol 82(7):1000–1006

Fu JH, Hsu YT et al (2012) Identifying occlusal overload and how to deal with it to avoid marginal bone loss around implants. Eur J Oral Implantol 5(Suppl):S91–103

Fu JH, Yeh CY et al (2010) Tissue biotype and its relation to the underlying bone morphology. J Periodontol 81(4):569–574

Garaicoa-Pazmino C, Suarez F et al (2014) Influence of crown-implant ratio upon marginal bone loss. A systematic review. J Periodontol 85:1214

Goodacre CJ, Bernal G et al (2003) Clinical complications with implants and implant prostheses. J Prosthet Dent 90(2):121–132

Grunder U, Gracis S et al (2005) Influence of the 3-D bone-to-implant relationship on esthetics. Int J Periodontics Restor Dent 25(2):113–119

Hsu YT, Fu JH et al (2012) Biomechanical implant treatment complications: a systematic review of clinical studies of implants with at least 1 year of functional loading. Int J Oral Maxillofac Implants 27(4):894–904

Jacobs R, Schotte A et al (1992) Posterior jaw bone resorption in osseointegrated implant-supported overdentures. Clin Oral Implants Res 3(2):63–70

Jemt T (1997) Regeneration of gingival papillae after single-implant treatment. Int J Periodontics Restor Dent 17(4):326–333

Johnson K (1969) A study of the dimensional changes occurring in the maxilla following tooth extraction. Aust Dent J 14(4):241–244

Juodzbalys G, Wang HL et al (2013) Inferior alveolar nerve injury associated with implant surgery. Clin Oral Implants Res 24(2):183–190

Kan JY, Morimoto T et al (2010) Gingival biotype assessment in the esthetic zone: visual versus direct measurement. Int J Periodontics Restor Dent 30(3):237–243

Kan JY, Rungcharassaeng K et al (2003) Dimensions of peri-implant mucosa: an evaluation of maxillary anterior single implants in humans. J Periodontol 74(4):557–562

Kent JN, Quinn JH et al (1983) Alveolar ridge augmentation using nonresorbable hydroxylapatite with or without autogenous cancellous bone. J Oral Maxillofac Surg 41(10):629–642

Kois JC (2004) Predictable single-tooth peri-implant esthetics: five diagnostic keys. Compend Contin Educ Dent 25(11):895–896 898, 900 passim; quiz 906–897

Lang NP, Loe H (1972) The relationship between the width of keratinized gingiva and gingival health. J Periodontol 43(10):623–627

Lekholm U, Zarb G (1985) Patient selection and preparation. In: Brånemark P-I (ed). Tissue-Integrated Prostheses: Osseointegration in Clinical Dentistry. Quintessence, Chicago 199–209

Lin GH, Chan HL et al (2013) The significance of keratinized mucosa on implant health: a systematic review. J Periodontol 84(12):1755–1767

Malchiodi L, Cucchi A et al (2014) Influence of crown-implant ratio on implant success rates and crestal bone levels: a 36-month follow-up prospective study. Clin Oral Implants Res 25(2):240–251

Mardinger O, Namani-Sadan N et al (2008) Morphologic changes of the nasopalatine canal related to dental implantation: a radiologic study in different degrees of absorbed maxillae. J Periodontol 79(9):1659–1662

Maurer S, Hayes C et al (2000) Width of keratinized tissue after gingivoplasty of healed subepithelial connective tissue grafts. J Periodontol 71(11):1729–1736

Misch C (1990) Classifications and treatment options of the completely edentulous arch in implant dentistry. Dent Today 9(8):26 28-30

Misch CE (2008) Contemporary implant dentistry. Mosby/Elsevier, St. Louis

Miyata T, Kobayashi Y et al (2000) The influence of controlled occlusal overload on peri-implant tissue. Part 3: a histologic study in monkeys. Int J Oral Maxillofac Implants 15(3):425–431

Neiva RF, Gapski R et al (2004) Morphometric analysis of implant-related anatomy in Caucasian skulls. J Periodontol 75(8):1061–1067

Neugebauer J, Ritter L et al (2010) Evaluation of maxillary sinus anatomy by cone-beam CT prior to sinus floor elevation. Int J Oral Maxillofac Implants 25(2):258–265

Nisapakultorn K, Suphanantachat S et al (2010) Factors affecting soft tissue level around anterior maxillary single-tooth implants. Clin Oral Implants Res 21(6):662–670

Nordland WP, Tarnow DP (1998) A classification system for loss of papillary height. J Periodontol 69(10):1124–1126

Park YB, Jeon HS et al (2011) Analysis of the anatomy of the maxillary sinus septum using 3-dimensional computed tomography. J Oral Maxillofac Surg 69(4):1070–1078

Pietrokovski J, Starinsky R et al (2007) Morphologic characteristics of bony edentulous jaws. J Prosthodont 16(2):141–147

Pyun JH, Lim YJ et al (2013) Position of the mental foramen on panoramic radiographs and its relation to the horizontal course of the mandibular canal: a computed tomographic analysis. Clin Oral Implants Res 24(8):890–895

Reiser GM, Bruno JF et al (1996) The subepithelial connective tissue graft palatal donor site: anatomic considerations for surgeons. Int J Periodontics Restor Dent 16(2):130–137

Sarver D, Jacobson RS (2007) The aesthetic dentofacial analysis. Clin Plast Surg 34(3):369–394

Schropp L, Wenzel A et al (2003) Bone healing and soft tissue contour changes following single-tooth extraction: a clinical and radiographic 12-month prospective study. Int J Periodontics Restor Dent 23(4):313–323

Seibert JS (1983) Reconstruction of deformed, partially edentulous ridges, using full thickness onlay grafts. Part I. Technique and wound healing. Compend Contin Educ Dent 4(5):437–453

Spray JR, Black CG et al (2000) The influence of bone thickness on facial marginal bone response: stage 1 placement through stage 2 uncovering. Ann Periodontol 5(1):119–128

Tallgren A (1972) The continuing reduction of the residual alveolar ridges in complete denture wearers: a mixed-longitudinal study covering 25 years. J Prosthet Dent 27(2):120–132

Tan WL, Wong TL et al (2012) A systematic review of post-extractional alveolar hard and soft tissue dimensional changes in humans. Clin Oral Implants Res 23(Suppl 5):1–21

Tozum TF, Guncu GN et al (2012) Evaluation of maxillary incisive canal characteristics related to dental implant treatment with computerized tomography: a clinical multicenter study. J Periodontol 83(3):337–343

von Arx T, Matter D et al (2011) Evaluation of location and dimensions of lingual foramina using limited cone-beam computed tomography. J Oral Maxillofac Surg 69(11):2777–2785

Wang HL, Al-Shammari K (2002) HVC ridge deficiency classification: a therapeutically oriented classification. Int J Periodontics Restor Dent 22(4):335–343

Watanabe H, Mohammad Abdul M et al (2010) Mandible size and morphology determined with CT on a premise of dental implant operation. Surg Radiol Anat 32(4):343–349

Wen SC, Chan HL et al (2013) Classification and management of antral septa for maxillary sinus augmentation. Int J Periodontics Restor Dent 33(4):509–517

Wennstrom JL, Bengazi F et al (1994) The influence of the masticatory mucosa on the peri-implant soft tissue condition. Clin Oral Implants Res 5(1):1–8

Worthington P (2004) Injury to the inferior alveolar nerve during implant placement: a formula for protection of the patient and clinician. Int J Oral Maxillofac Implants 19(5):731–734

Yildirim YD, Guncu GN et al (2014) Evaluation of mandibular lingual foramina related to dental implant treatment with computerized tomography: a multicenter clinical study. Implant Dent 23:57

Zetu L, Wang HL (2005) Management of inter-dental/inter-implant papilla. J Clin Periodontol 32(7):831–839

Interdisciplinary Planning, Development, and Treatment

Keith M. Phillips

Abstract

Interdisciplinary treatment planning in dentistry has become both more complicated and facilitated with the advent of dental implants. The use of dental implants allows the practitioner to make their therapies more predictable by removing biomechanical issues, minimizing the need for tooth preparation, minimizing the use of compromised teeth, and allowing for more simplified planning. This, along with the use of digital workflows, allows for more efficient therapies for our patients. This digital world can help in the proper planning for implant placement to be in harmony with all components of the stomatognathic system. Combining the tools available from both the analog and digital worlds is key to contemporary interdisciplinary treatment planning from the initial visit through the actual fabrication of the definitive prostheses.

The use of dental implants has arguably become the more traditional approach to restoring partially and fully edentulous patients. Because of their predictable nature, incorporating them into everyday treatment planning has now become commonplace. This is due to the increasing understanding of the experimental science and body of clinical experience which has led us to a low morbidity of the surgical procedures, a high success rate of osseointegration, a better understanding of the surgical/restorative requirements, the impact of immediate loading protocols, and their ability to be used in multiple disciplines to secure an efficient and predictable outcome. There has been a significant evolution in the use of dental implants from the initial full-arch tissue-integrated prostheses (Brånemark et al. 1969, 1977), which gave severely debilitated patients the ability to function remarkably well, to anterior single tooth replacement which many times requires the need for detailed planning to ensure an esthetic and functional outcome (Chen and Buser 2014).

Even though dental implants may be planned for support of a restoration, the remaining teeth and overall stomatognathic system need to be evaluated. This is critical as the placement of the dental implants may be dependent on the overall

K.M. Phillips, DMD, MSD, CDT, FACP
Department of Restorative Dentistry,
University of Washington School of Dentistry,
Private Practice, 5619 Valley Ave E,
Fife, WA 98424, USA
e-mail: kphil5@comcast.net

restorability of the remaining dentition and vice versa (Ploumaki et al. 2013). It is a prerequisite to determine patient desires, esthetic determinants, tooth position, periodontal conditions, structural compromises, and anatomic compromises.

Interdisciplinary treatment planning for advanced dental therapies can be difficult to plan and sequence. Treatment planning must start from the outside-in. Lip dynamics, ideal incisal edge position, occlusal plane, occlusal vertical dimension, and midline all need to be determined for that particular patient. Determining the existing parameters for the particular patient must be accomplished in order to see what the differences are from the desired outcome. Incorporating one or more of the different dental specialties to get from the existing situation to the ideal one efficiently then needs to be determined. Either the specialty can be assisted with the use of dental implants or the therapy must be completed with the knowledge that a dental implant will be placed for the definitive prosthesis.

When first evaluating a patient, the presence of edentulous areas would certainly indicate the need for tooth replacement. However, as simple as this might seem, there are many considerations for determining which prosthodontic mode should be utilized. If there are issues with the residual tissues regarding volume and quality, then pre-prosthetic procedures may be required to make a better foundation for the prosthodontic restoration. If there are esthetic concerns regarding the position of teeth or of facial esthetic determinants, then a plan would be required to facilitate correcting these issues as part of the overall therapy.

The use of an interdisciplinary approach to dentistry originated with the philosophies of periodontal prosthodontics. This philosophy utilizes the therapeutic modalities of the various disciplines of dentistry in order to maintain as much of the dentition to support artificial dental prostheses (Amsterdam 1974). Therapeutic concepts used include the use of endodontics, periodontics, orthodontics, and oral surgery in order to retain residual roots for various prosthodontic options including fixed partial dentures, cantilever prostheses, and coping prostheses. Many of these same modalities can be used in order to maintain or rebuild bone volumes in order to place dental implants for prosthetic support (Salama et al. 1998a; Wadhwani et al. 2015.).

The dilemma in treatment planning comes when the decision needs to be made whether to keep a potentially compromised tooth or remove it in favor of implant support. During the data collection in the diagnostic phase of patient treatment, it is necessary to determine the potential risk factors for that particular patient (Kois and Kois 2015). Evaluating the functional, periodontal, biomechanical, and esthetic risks is quite important in developing the long-term prognosis for the patient (Kois and Kois 2015). This risk assessment can help guide the dentist toward the most efficient, cost-effective, long-term therapy for the patient. For example, Figs. 8.1 and 8.2 show a patient who traumatically lost the maxillary right central incisor. Fabricating a three-unit fixed partial denture would increase the long-term biomechanical risk for that patient by removing sound tooth structure on the adjacent teeth. In order to maintain a low biomechanical risk, a dental implant was placed to

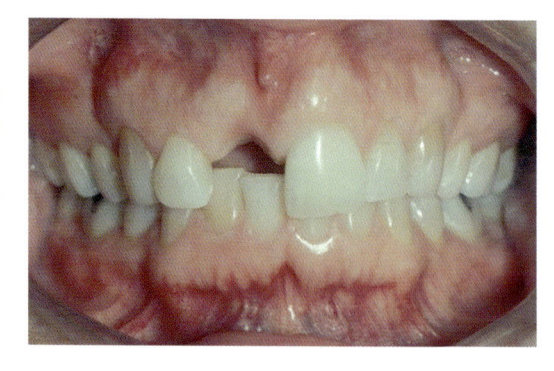

Fig. 8.1 Patient with traumatically lost right central incisor

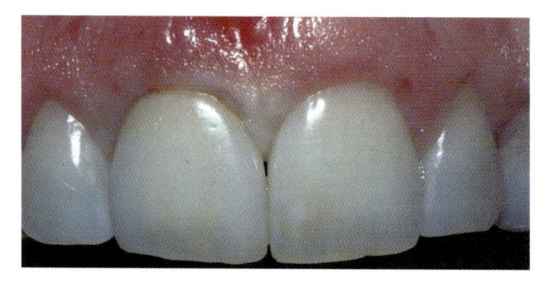

Fig. 8.2 Single-tooth implant-retained crown at day of insertion

support the prosthetic crown. Figure 8.3 shows the same implant-retained crown 21 years after insertion. This brings up the question as to whether to choose conventional prosthodontics or implant prosthodontics. Looking at the literature evaluating the success rates of fixed dental prostheses on teeth, we see that the success rates can vary widely with up to 32% failure after 15 years (Scurria et al. 1998). The implant literature shows consistently high success rates for implant and prosthetic success (Jimbo and Albrektsson 2015). The literature along with the practitioner's experience level helps in deciding whether to move more toward implant support rather than utilizing teeth when the risk factors warrant a more predictable long-term prognosis.

For many patients, the esthetic risk factor may be exacerbated by a high lip dynamic range (Tjan et al. 1984) (Fig. 8.4). This 18-year-old healthy patient underwent orthodontic therapy to correct the space appropriation issues due to a congenitally missing left lateral incisor. The undersized right lateral incisor was provisionally built up with composite resin in order to help the orthodontist visualize the correct space requirements to complete the orthodontic therapy (Fig. 8.5). Reevaluation of the patient's situation at completion of the orthodontic therapy shows that the space appropriation of teeth is corrected; there is a gingival margin discrepancy between the right anterior teeth and the left and a defect causing an unesthetic shadowing on the facial tissue of the left lateral incisor edentulous site (Figs. 8.6 and 8.7). The question arises as to whether there is enough bone for implant placement. The use of a CBCT scan will allow visualization in different planes to evaluate this (Fig. 8.8). If not, then an osseous graft would be indicated in order to have

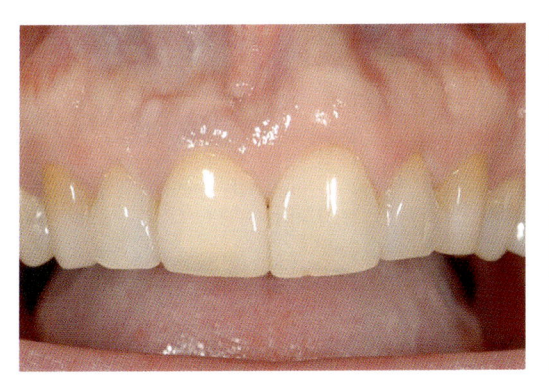

Fig. 8.3 The same implant restoration 21 years after insertion

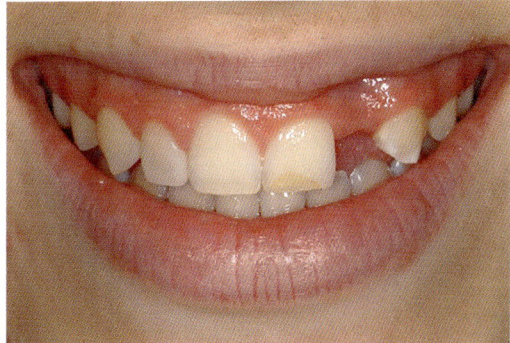

Fig. 8.5 Orthodontic therapy completed. Note high lip dynamics

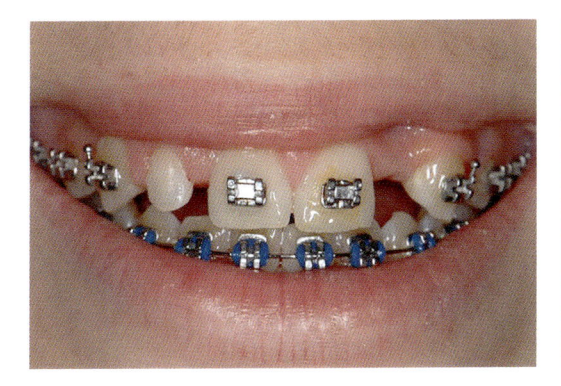

Fig. 8.4 Patient evaluated for space appropriation during orthodontic treatment

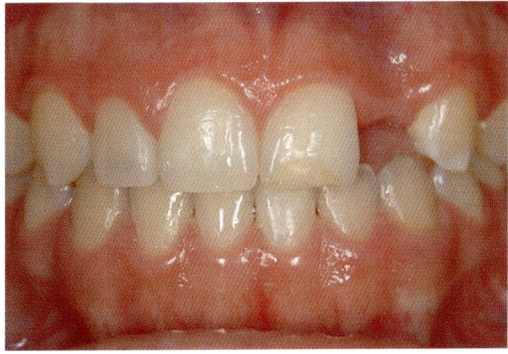

Fig. 8.6 Note facial defect of left lateral incisor tissue and unharmonious gingival levels

adequate bone volume to house the dental implant with at least 1 mm of bone. If there is adequate bone, then the facial defect can be treated with soft tissue grafting alone which would expedite therapy since this procedure can be done at the time of implant placement without the need to wait for a bone graft to mature (Poskevicius et al. 2015). The slice from the CBCT scan in the region of the left lateral incisor shows there is greater than 5 mm of bone width and greater than 15 mm of height which would allow for a 3 mm two-piece dental implant (Fig. 8.9). Restoratively, a diagnostic wax up is completed in order to evaluate proper positioning for the dental implant. Also, gingival levels can be evaluated for harmony between the contralateral sides (Fig. 8.10).

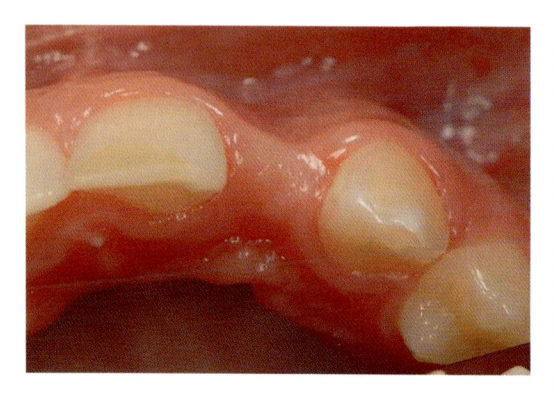

Fig. 8.7 Incisal view showing extent of facial defect

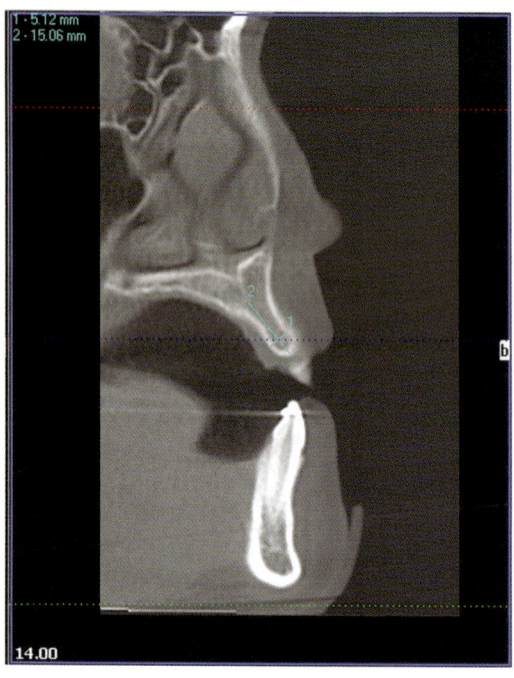

Fig. 8.9 A slice from the CBCT showing bone dimensions of 5.12 width and greater than 15 mm height

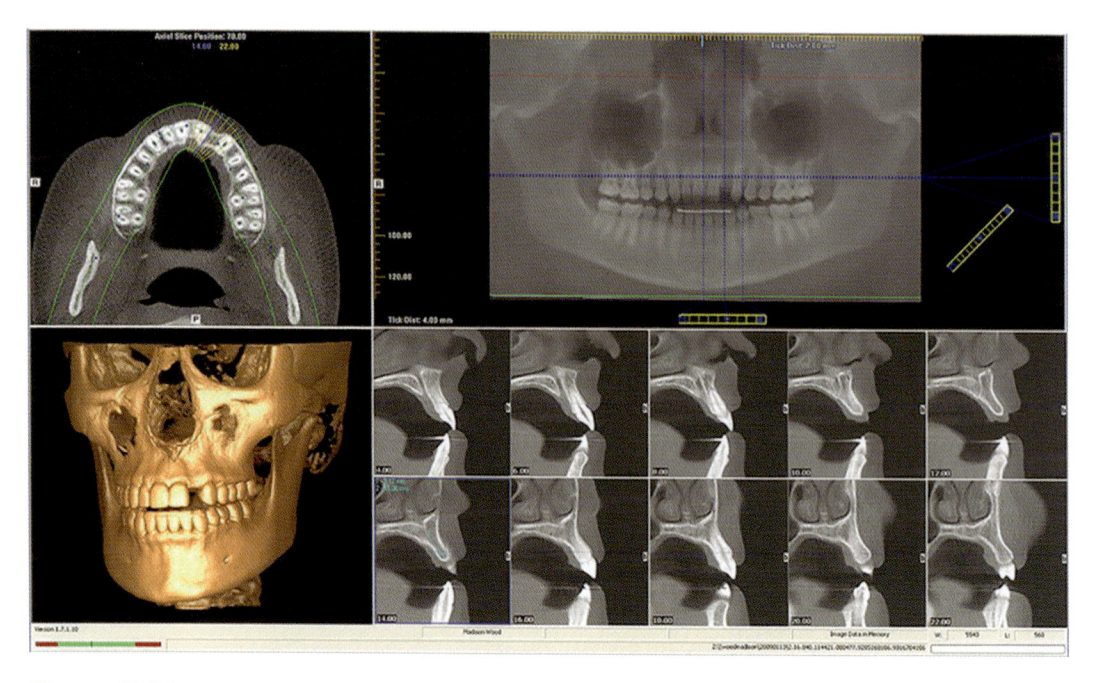

Fig. 8.8 CBCT scan evaluating bone dimensions of defect of maxillary left lateral incisor

8 Interdisciplinary Planning, Development, and Treatment   121

With all the diagnostic information at hand, the surgical treatment plan can be made to be as efficient as possible. For this patient, the clinical crown lengthening procedure, implant placement, and connective tissue graft will be performed at one time. First, the teeth that will have clinical crown lengthening are bone sounded in order to get a measurement of their particular biologic width dimension (Fig. 8.11). Measurements from the diagnostic cast are transferred to the mouth with a caliper and an internal bevel gingivectomy performed (Figs 8.12 and 8.13). Incisions are extended in order to properly expose the osseous structures in order to perform osteoplasty and ostectomy in order to regain the patient's proper biologic width dimension as well as to gain access to harvest connective tissue from the palatal extension of the flap (Figs. 8.14, 8.15, and 8.16).

The next component of the surgery is the placement of the dental implant. A surgical template is fabricated from the diagnostic wax up. The main rationale for a guide in this instance is to show the

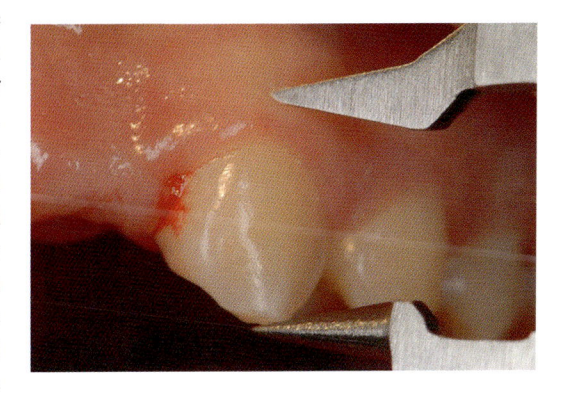

Fig. 8.12 Calipers transferring the gingival margin measurement from the diagnostic cast

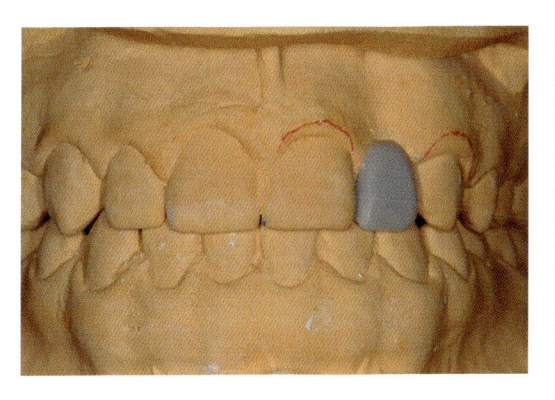

Fig. 8.10 Diagnostic wax up determining implant position and gingival margin levels

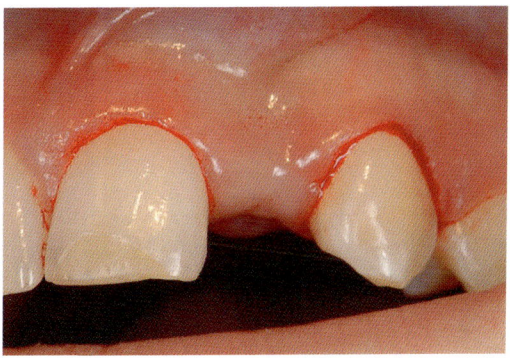

Fig. 8.13 Internal bevel gingivectomy to level the gingival margins to the contralateral side

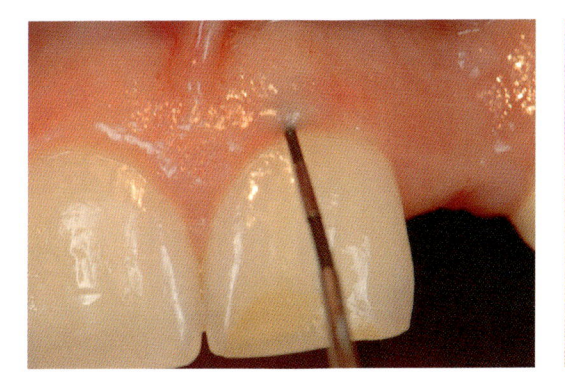

Fig. 8.11 Bone sounding to determine the patient's biologic width dimension

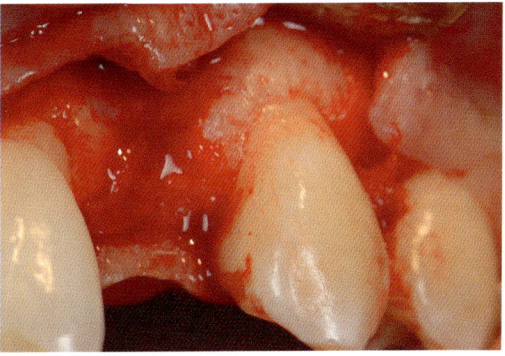

Fig. 8.14 Flap is reflected to perform ostectomy and osteoplasty to regain proper biologic width

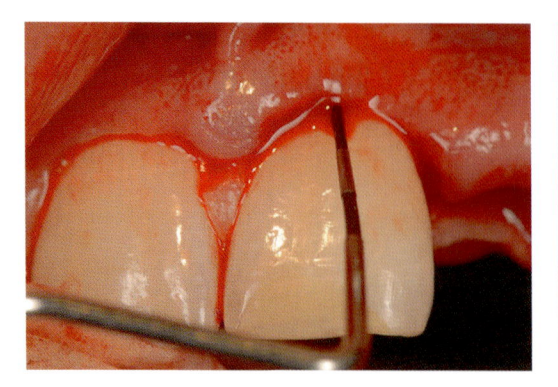

Fig. 8.15 Osseous crest is measured relative to the gingival margin to verify adequate ostectomy was performed

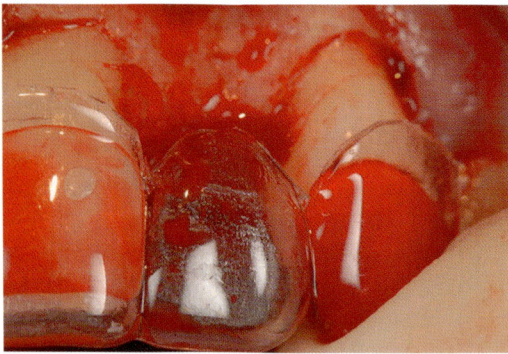

Fig. 8.17 Surgical template in place to evaluate vertical placement of the dental implant. Note the excess bone relative to the apical extent of the template

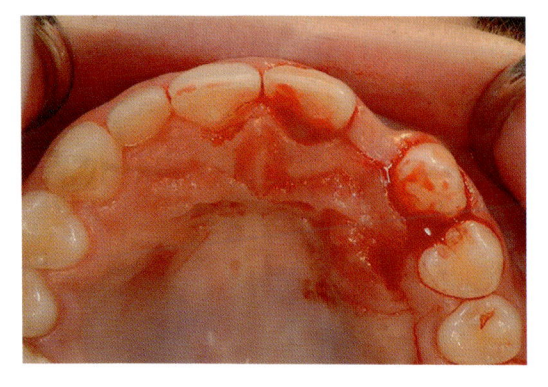

Fig. 8.16 The incision is extended on the palate to allow access for harvesting connective tissue

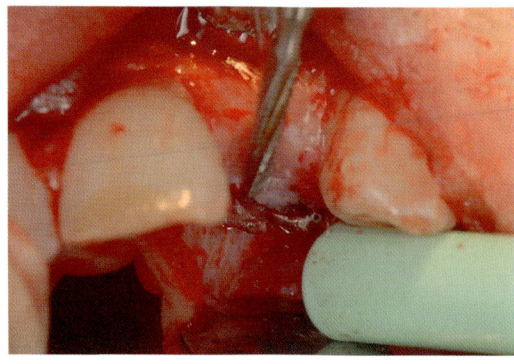

Fig. 8.18 Osteoplasty of the crestal bone for proper vertical placement of the implant

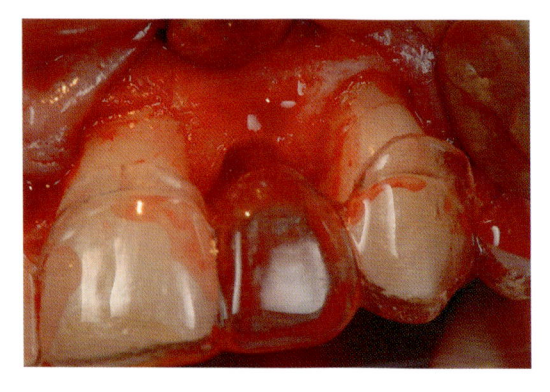

Fig. 8.19 Adequate osteoplasty of 3 mm from apical extent of guide. Note proximal bone was maintained

vertical placement of the implant as the mesiodistal and facio-palatal position is dictated by the adjacent teeth (Phillips and Wong 2001, 2002). When spaces are opened laterally orthodontically, many times the vertical amount of bone is relatively coronal compared to the adjacent teeth (Fig. 8.17). From the gingival extent of the surgical template, 3 mm of alveoloplasty is performed to allow for the correct vertical placement of the implant. This will allow for proper emergence of the restoration from the coronal portion of the implant. Care is taken not to remove the proximal bone of the adjacent teeth in order to maintain support for the papillae (Figs. 8.18, 8.19, and 8.20). The final part of the surgery is to perform the connective tissue graft to augment where the facial defect is. Connective tissue is removed from the palatal aspect of the flap and sutured into the area of the defect, and the rest of the flap is sutured for primary closure (Figs. 8.21, 8.22, and 8.23).

Six weeks of healing is allowed prior to the restorative phase (Schliephake et al. 2012) at which time the implant is uncovered and an impression made for a provisional restoration (Phillips and Kois 1998) (Figs. 8.24 and 8.25).

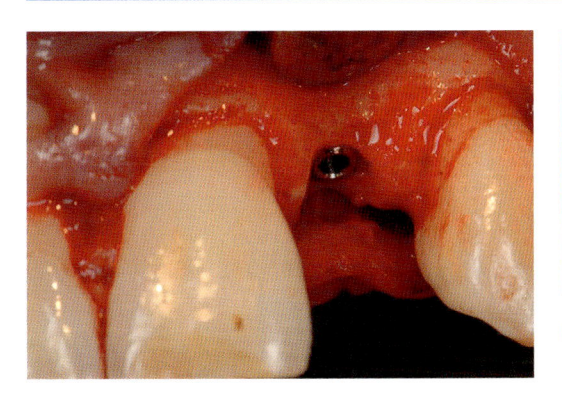

8 Interdisciplinary Planning, Development, and Treatment   123

Fig. 8.20 Dental implant in place in proper three-dimensional positioning

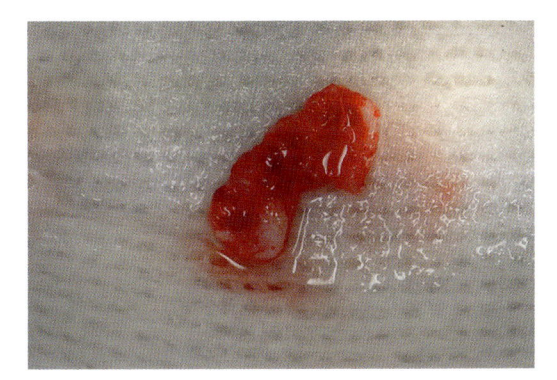

Fig. 8.21 Connective tissue harvested from the palatal flap

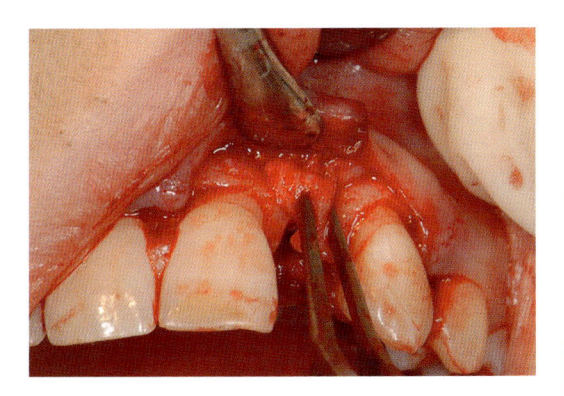

Fig. 8.22 Connective tissue being placed into the facial defect

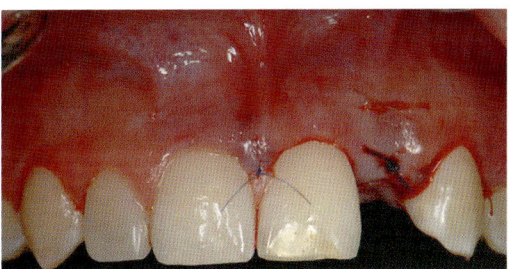

Fig. 8.23 Graft and flaps sutured in place

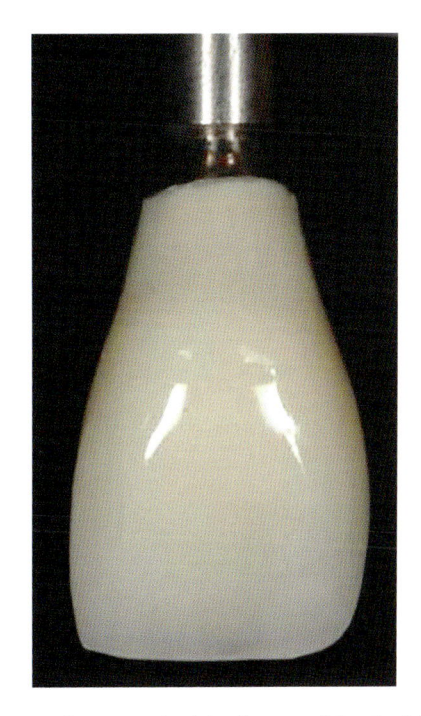

Fig. 8.24 Screw-retained implant provisional with flat subgingival contours

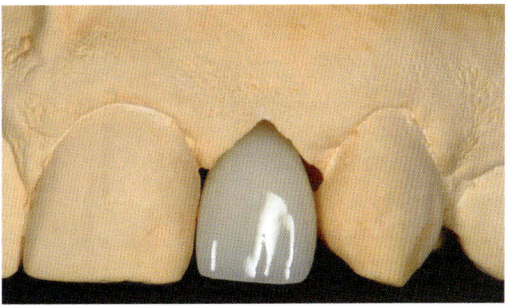

Fig. 8.25 Provisional designed in harmony with the adjacent teeth

This allows the restoring dentist to evaluate the tissue contours surrounding the restoration for the need of any additional procedures prior to fabricating the definitive prosthesis. In this situation there was too much tissue, and an internal bevel gingivectomy was performed in order to gain

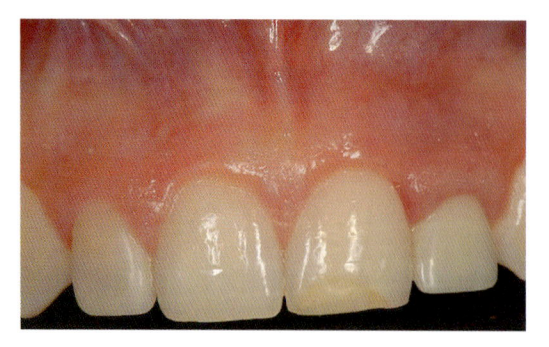

Fig. 8.26 Provisional in situ. Note excess bulk of tissue

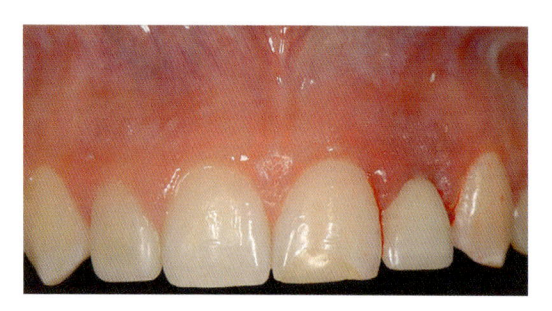

Fig. 8.27 Tissue is removed to level the gingival margin and to thin the tissue

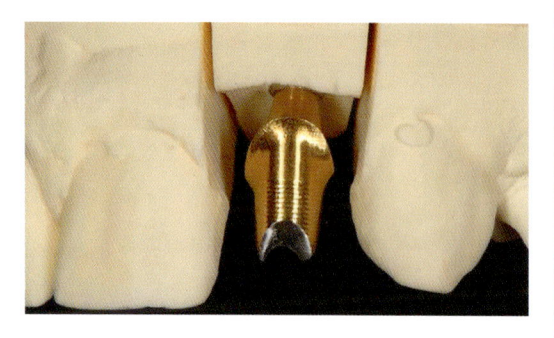

Fig. 8.28 CAD/CAM gold hue titanium custom abutment. Note scallop of the finish line

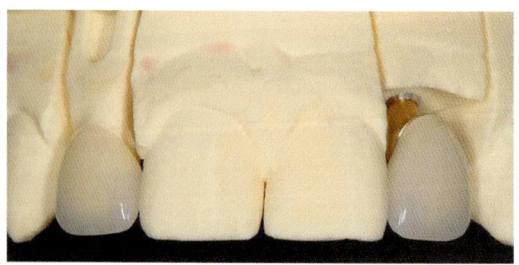

Fig. 8.29 Restorations for the lateral incisors. Porcelain veneer on the right and PFM crown on the *left*

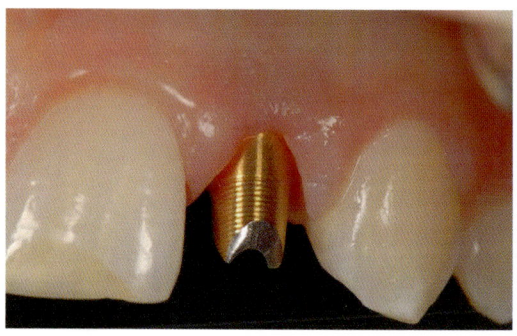

Fig. 8.30 Custom abutment in situ

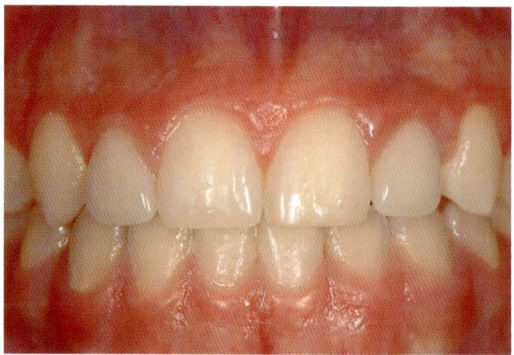

Fig. 8.31 The final restorations 1 year after insertion

adequate height of the restoration for anterior gingival margin harmony (Figs. 8.26 and 8.27). For the definitive prosthesis, a custom CAD/CAM titanium abutment was fabricated for a cement-retained porcelain fused to metal crown. The contralateral tooth was treated with a feldspathic porcelain veneer (Figs 8.28, 8.29, 8.30, and 8.31).

For patients with edentulous arches, Therapies are limited to complete removable prostheses or prostheses that are retained or supported by dental implants. The use of dental implants is always precedent on the availability of adequate osseous structures to house the dental implant. With severe loss of alveolar and basal components of the residual dental arches, the ability to place implants many times can only be accomplished with bone grafting procedures. The 54-year-old healthy patient depicted in Figs. 8.32 and 8.33 has severe resorption of her maxillae making it difficult to function with a conventional complete

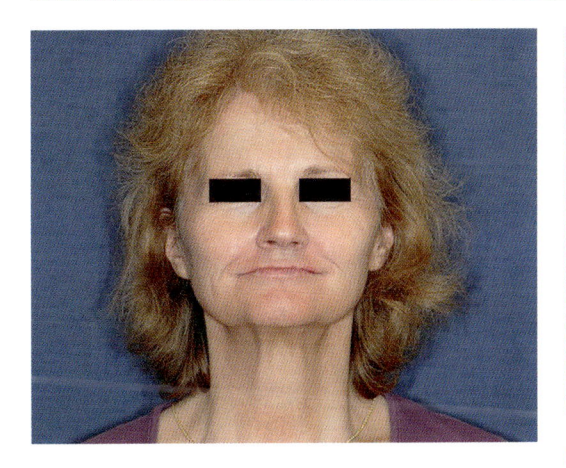

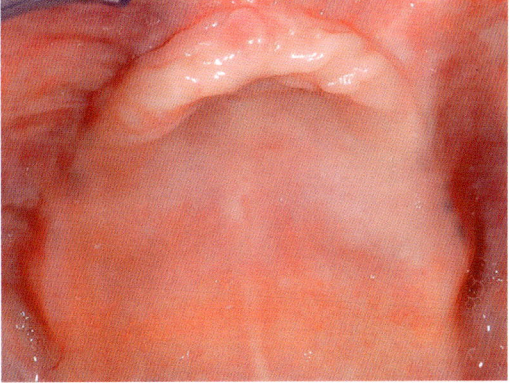

8 Interdisciplinary Planning, Development, and Treatment

Fig. 8.32 Patient showing collapse of the lower third of her face due to severe ridge atrophy

Fig. 8.33 Maxilla with severe ridge resorption

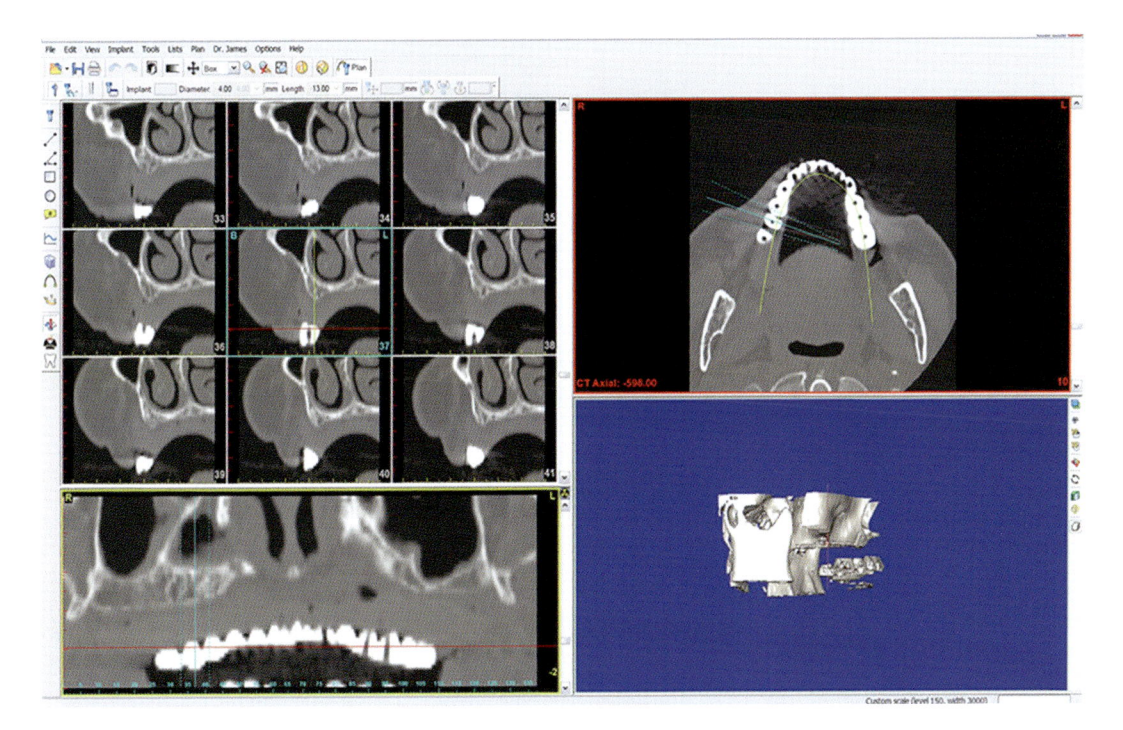

Fig. 8.34 CBCT of maxilla. Note lack of bone and lateralization of the nasal cavity

removable denture. A CBCT scan was made with a radiographic template and showed a minimal amount of alveolar and basal bone (Fig. 8.34). Also, the nasal cavity extended distally toward the first molars making the ability to gain bone volume through maxillary sinus augmentation impossible. The other option for bone grafting in a situation like this is to perform a LeFort I osteotomy with interpositional bone graft harvested from the hip (Soehardi et al. 2015). A diagnostic setup was completed and a surgical stent made in order to place the maxillae in the correct position during fixation (Figs 8.35 and 8.36). During the surgery, the bone graft is harvested from the anterior iliac crest to minimize morbidity (Baqain et al. 2009) (Fig. 8.37). The

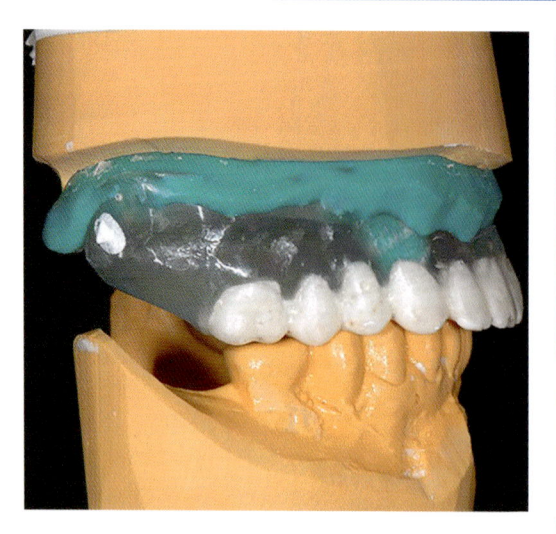

Fig. 8.35 Diagnostic setup for LeFort I osteotomy with advancement

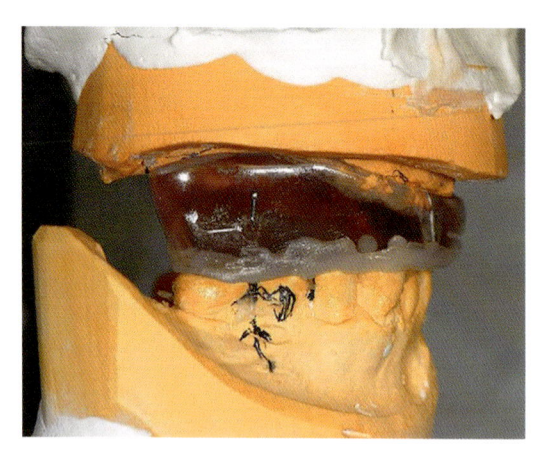

Fig. 8.36 Intra-surgical stent to fixate the maxilla in the predetermined position

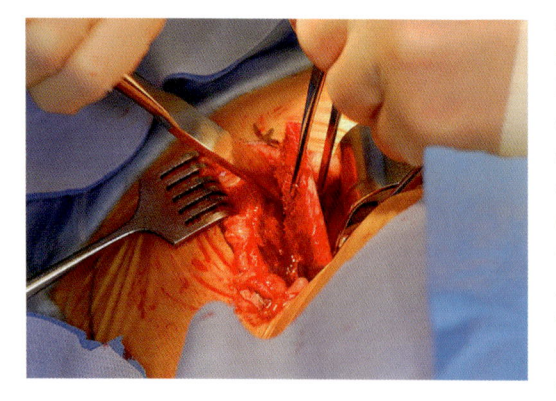

Fig. 8.37 Bone harvested from the anterior iliac crest

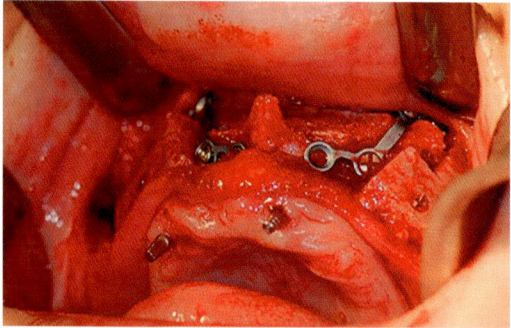

Fig. 8.38 Rigid fixation of the maxilla and interpositional hip graft (Surgery by Dr. Douglas Trimble. Bellevue, WA)

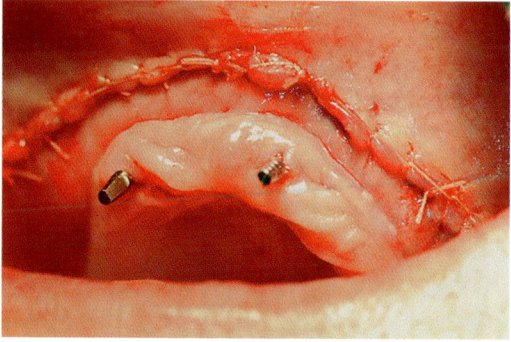

Fig. 8.39 Primary closure of the surgical site

LeFort I osteotomy is completed and the hip graft materials placed between the down fractured maxilla and the base of the nose. Rigid fixation with plates and screws is used to fixate all bony components and the flaps approximated for primary closure (Figs. 8.38 and 8.39).

After 6 months of healing, a CBCT is taken to evaluate the new bone volume for implant placement with a radiographic template (Fig. 8.40). Implant placement is planned with the DICOM data and used to fabricate a computer-generated surgical template in order to accurately and efficiently place the dental implants (Ozan et al. 2009) (Figs. 8.41, 8.42, 8.43, and 8.44). After healing of the implants, impressions and jaw relation records are made in order to fabricate the definitive prosthesis. CAD/CAM custom titanium abutments are fabricated to hold the porcelain fused to metal restoration which is cemented in place (Figs. 8.45, 8.46, 8.47, 8.48, and 8.49). These procedures

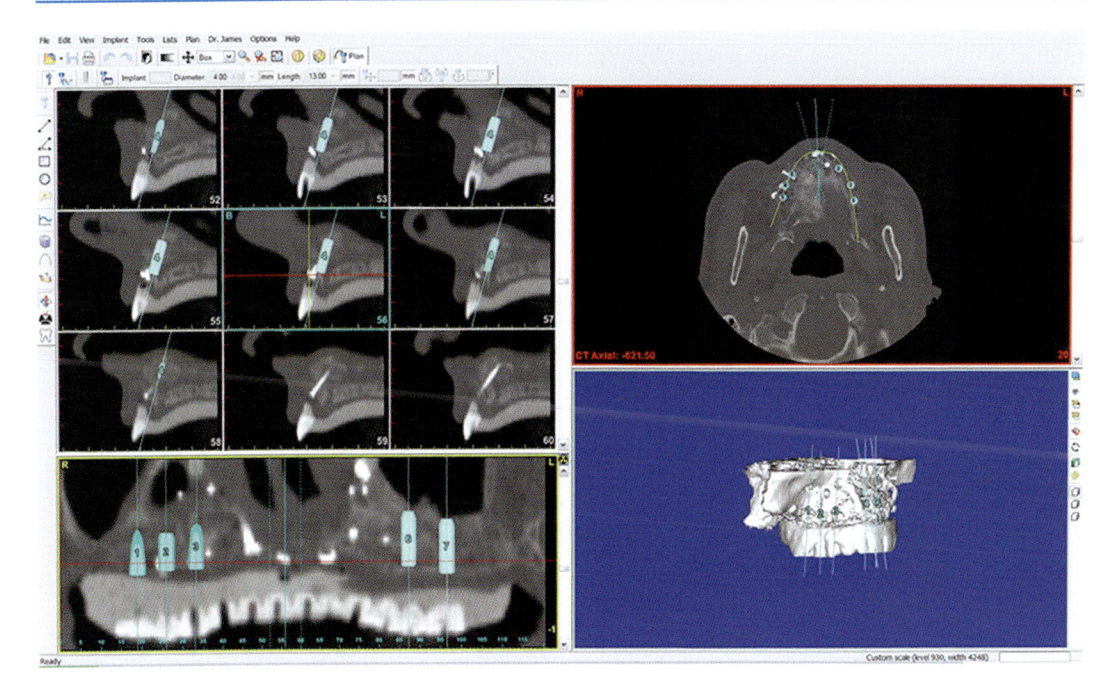

8 Interdisciplinary Planning, Development, and Treatment

Fig. 8.40 CBCT to plan the implant placement after healing of the hip graft

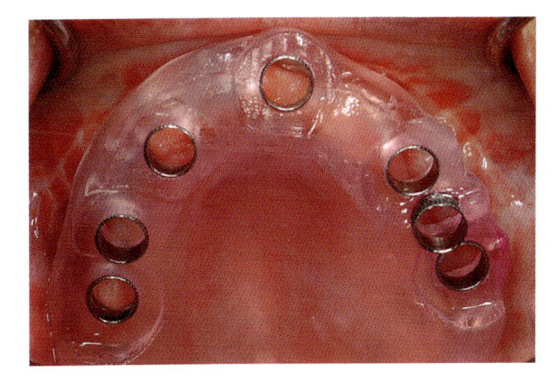

Fig. 8.41 Computer-generated surgical guide evaluated for fit

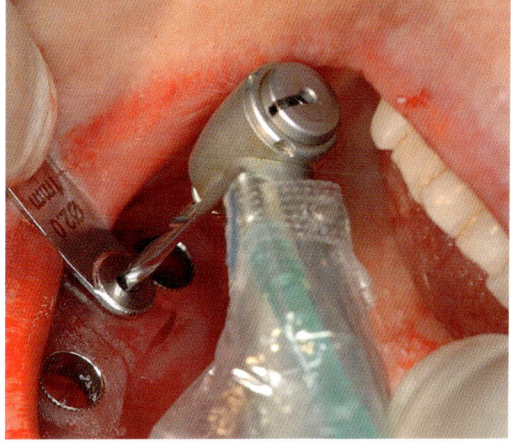

Fig. 8.42 Osteotomies for implant placement through the surgical template

made it possible to take a patient who was crippled dentally to one who is able to function very well from a masticatory as well as a quality of life standpoint (Becker et al. 2015).

Periodontal disease and its associated loss of attachment to the affected teeth can make for a situation that makes it uncomfortable for a patient from a masticatory standpoint. When the affected teeth are in the anterior region, then there can also be an esthetic concern by the patient. The 47-year-old healthy patient depicted in Figs. 8.50 and 8.51 has severe attachment loss to her maxillary incisors and is concerned with the unesthetic recession of the gingival tissues. The panoramic radiograph shows that there is greater than 50% horizontal bone loss around the maxillary incisors (Fig. 8.52). Removal of the teeth would cause additional recession of the residual ridge (Schropp et al. 2003). There are many types of

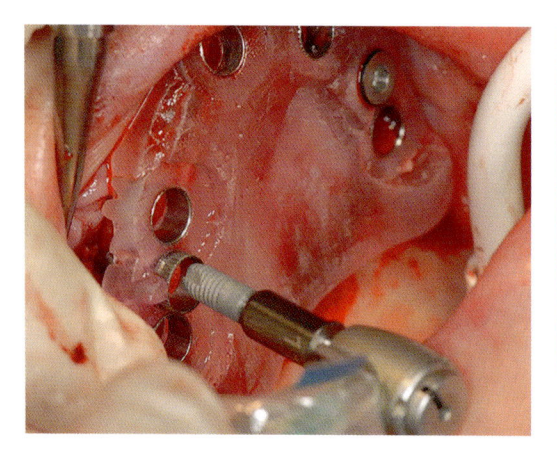

Fig. 8.43 Implant being placed through the surgical template

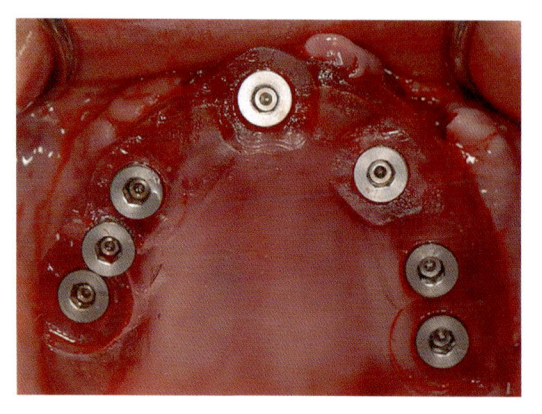

Fig. 8.44 Completion of implant placement with the surgical template

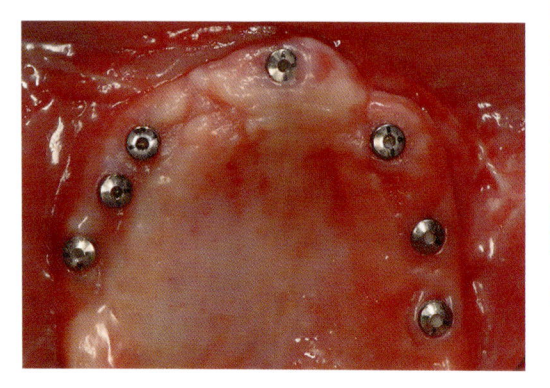

Fig. 8.45 Healing after second-stage surgery

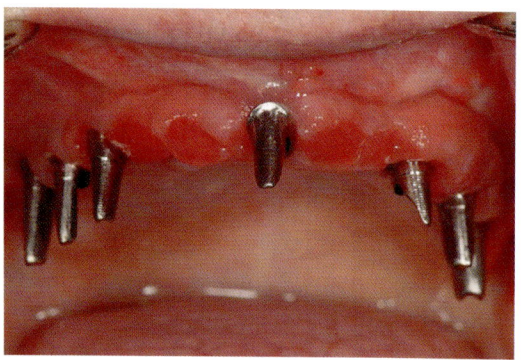

Fig. 8.46 CAD/CAM titanium custom abutments in situ

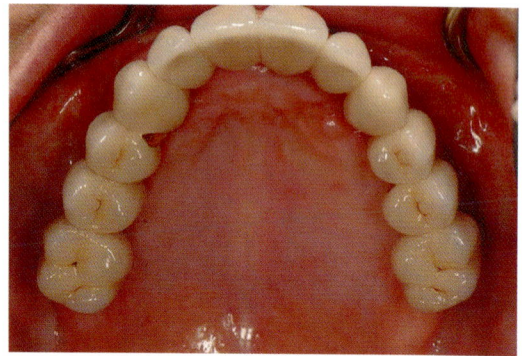

Fig. 8.47 Occlusal view of definitive PFM restoration after cementation

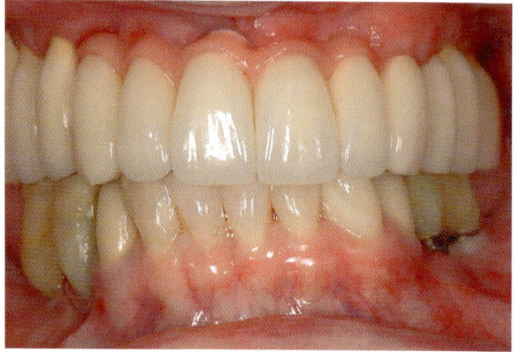

Fig. 8.48 Facial view of the PFM restoration

bone grafting procedures that could be utilized with autogenous, allogeneic, or xenografts, but the ability to get the patient to a normal esthetic situation is not predictable (Esposito et al. 2009). Orthodontic extrusion has been shown to be a highly predictable modality to augment ridges and repair defects when inflammation-controlled teeth are moved through these defects (Ingber 1989). The eruption can be quite useful whether

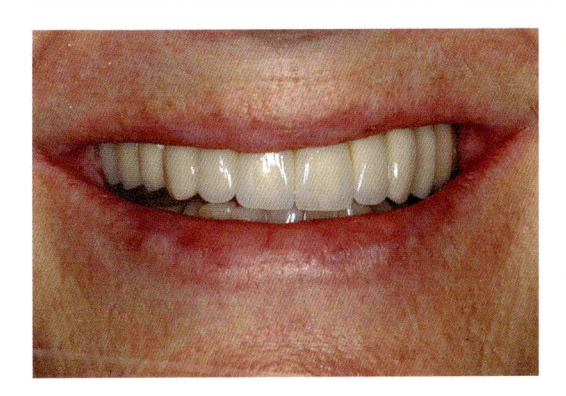

8   Interdisciplinary Planning, Development, and Treatment

Fig. 8.49 Patient's smile after cementation

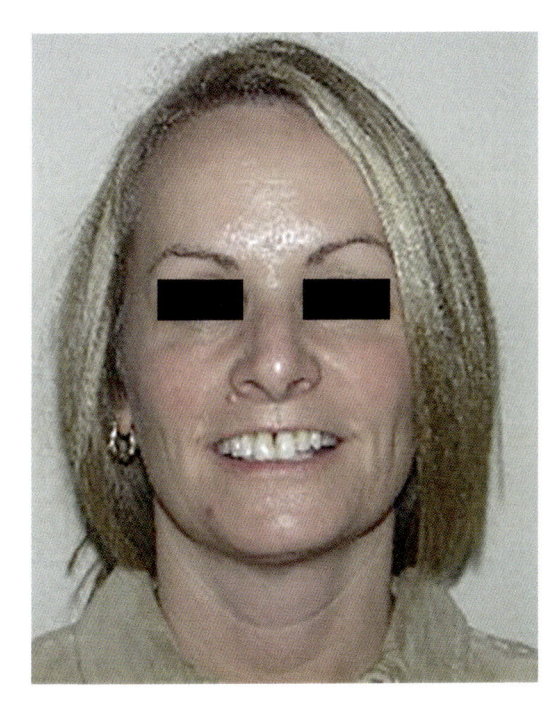

Fig. 8.50 Initial presentation to orthodontist. Patient unhappy with unesthetic *black spaces*

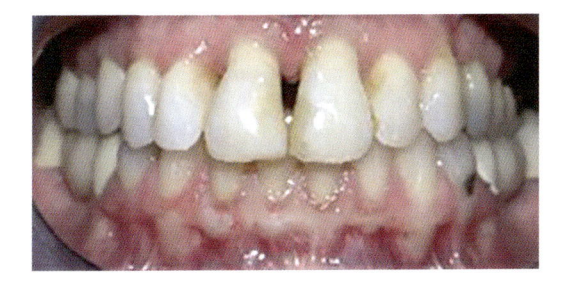

Fig. 8.51 Facial view showing attachment loss causing recession with *black triangles*

the site is to be used for a pontic or an implant site (Kois 1994). The teeth are slowly erupted (Minsk 2000) in order to allow the bone and soft tissue to follow the movement. In the anterior it is essential that the torque on the root angulation is maintained to the palatal so as not to perforate the facial plate of bone (Fig. 8.53). To facilitate the movement, the incisal edges and palatal contours of the teeth need to be adjusted in order to allow for continued eruption. Depending on the amount of eruption needed, the pulpal tissue may also need to be extirpated. Overcompensation of the eruption by about 3 mm is suggested since one can expect this amount of resorption after removal of the teeth (Schropp et al. 2003) (Fig. 8.54). The final position is maintained for 3 months to allow the new osseous structures to mineralize prior to removal (Fig. 8.55).

The prosthetic and surgical planning can be further developed with a diagnostic wax up to determine the esthetic and functional parameters (Fig. 8.56). From this information a vacuum-formed surgical template can be fabricated as well as the provisional restoration. The surgical plan is to place the dental implants in the extraction sockets of the two lateral incisors and to perform ridge preservation in the sockets of the central incisors (Horowitz et al. 2012) (Figs 8.57, 8.58, 8.59, 8.60, 8.61, 8.62, 8.63, and 8.64). The goal is to keep from having adjacent implants which may compromise interproximal bone which is helpful in papillae maintenance (Tarnow et al. 2003; Ishikawa et al. 2010). Also, treating the central incisors as pontics has been shown to better the esthetic tissue contours in comparison to adjacent implants (Salama et al. 1998b). The osteotomies for the immediately placed implants need to take into account the present and proposed gingival levels as shown in Figs. 8.58, 8.59, and 8.60. The implants need to be placed 3 mm apical to the proposed gingival margin, and since there is 3 mm of excess tissue, 6 mm needs to be added to the length measured on the implant drill. Therefore, for an 11 mm long implant to be placed in the right position vertically, we need to measure 17 mm on the drill at the level of the existing gingival margin. After 6–12 weeks of healing, an impression was

Fig. 8.52 Panoramic radiograph showing greater than 50% bone loss to the maxillary incisors

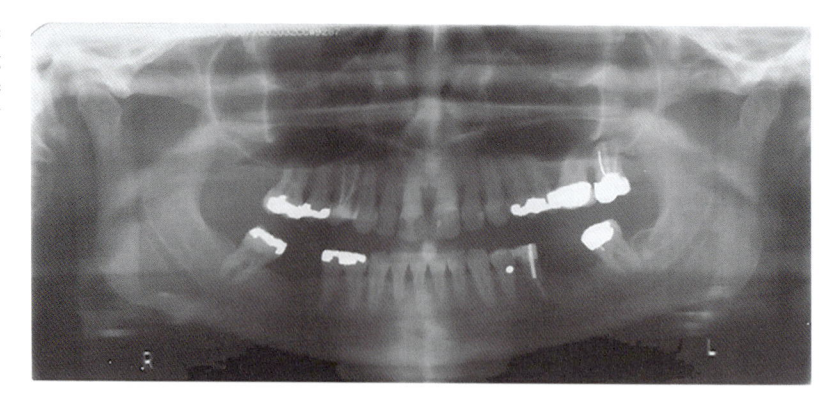

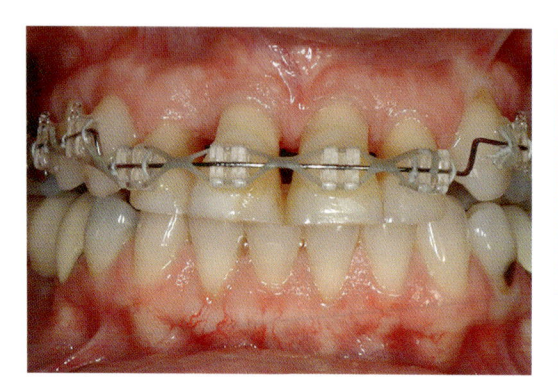

Fig. 8.53 Initial orthodontic extrusion to bring hard and soft tissues coronally

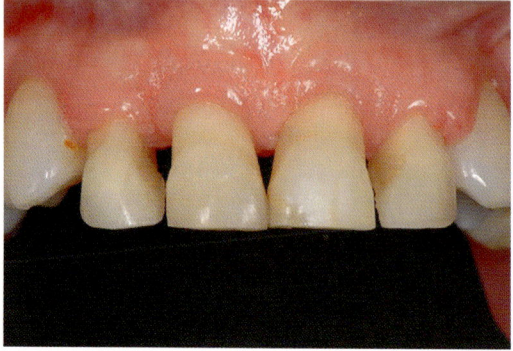

Fig. 8.55 After 3 months of stabilization, the appliances are removed to begin the surgical/restorative phase

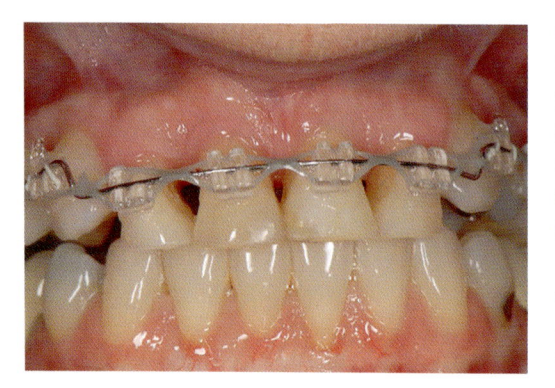

Fig. 8.54 Final eruption of tissues. Note overcompensation of at least 3 mm

v and a screw-retained provisional restoration fabricated to determine that the esthetic and functional requirements have been addressed (Fig. 8.65). In this case, the provisional restoration was used as anchorage to refine the tooth position of the rest of the maxillary arch (Fig. 8.66). The final restoration follows the provisional restoration and is supported by two CAD/CAM-fabricated custom abutments (Figs. 8.67, 8.68, and 8.69).

The use of the different disciplines of dentistry is an invaluable aid in the treatment planning and subsequent therapeutic procedures in implant dentistry. The use of periodontics, oral surgery, and orthodontics as an adjunct to the dilemmas found in the debilitated dentitions of many of our patients is necessary in formulating the correct diagnosis. Knowing the risk factors for a particular patient helps to best form a prognosis that can lead to a long-term functional and esthetic restoration.

8   Interdisciplinary Planning, Development, and Treatment   131

Fig. 8.56 Diagnostic wax up to develop the plan for the definitive restoration which in turn dictates implant placement

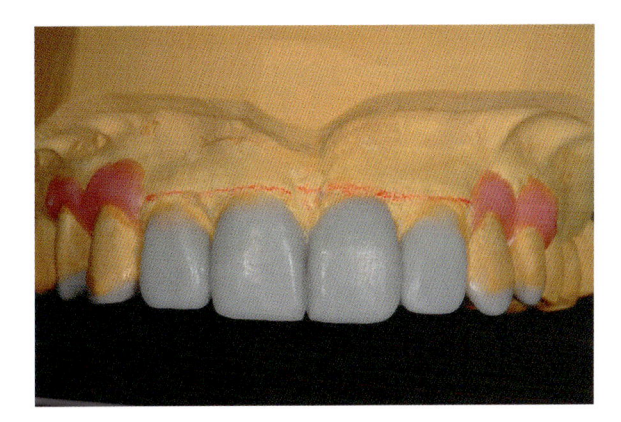

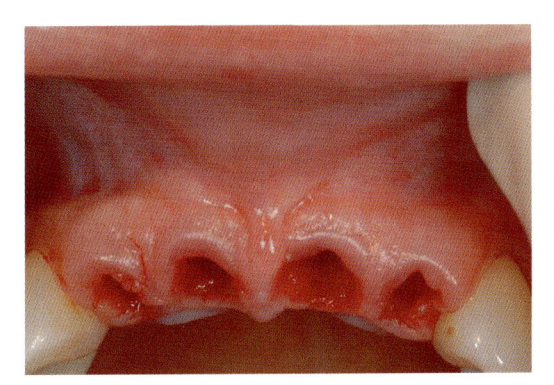

Fig. 8.57 Extraction of the maxillary incisors

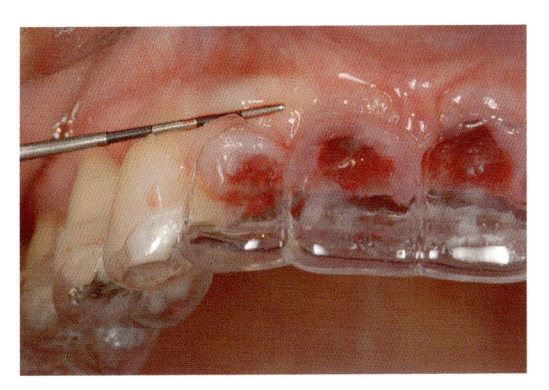

Fig. 8.58 Vacuum-formed surgical template in place. The probe is marking the proposed gingival margin level

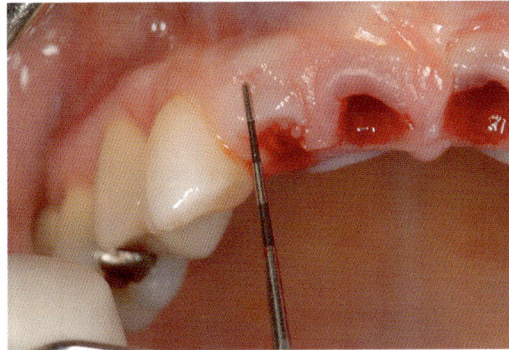

Fig. 8.59 The present gingival margin is about 3 mm coronal to the proposed gingival margin. This needs to be taken into account for the vertical placement of the dental implant

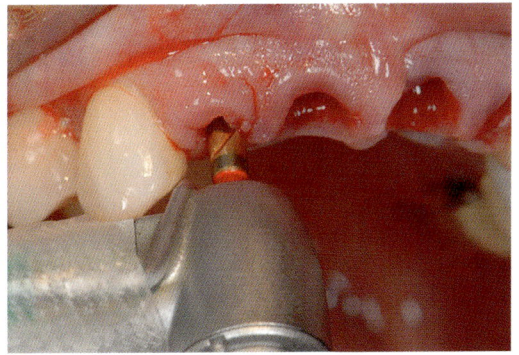

Fig. 8.60 Osteotomy for the immediately placed implant taking into account the present and proposed gingival levels. The osteotomy goes to the 17 mm line on the drill to get the implant at the right vertical placement for the final restoration

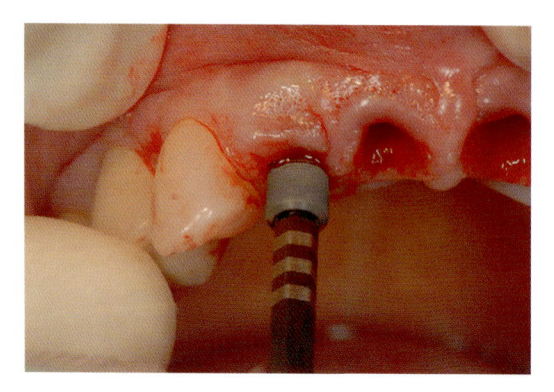

Fig. 8.61 The implant being placed into the osteotomy

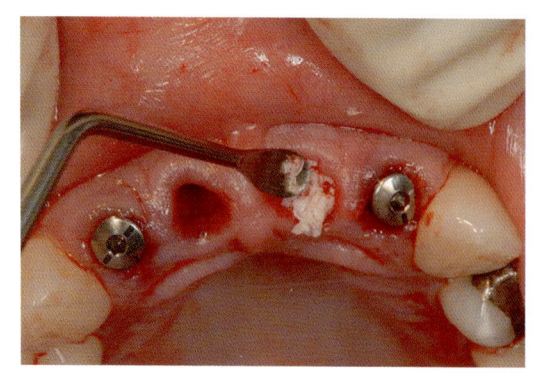

Fig. 8.62 Ridge preservation procedure with xenograft

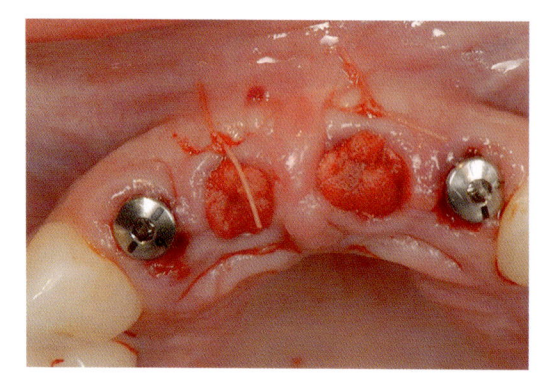

Fig. 8.63 Collagen plug placed over the graft and horizontal mattress suture to keep it in place. Note 6 mm healing abutments verifying correct vertical placement of the implants

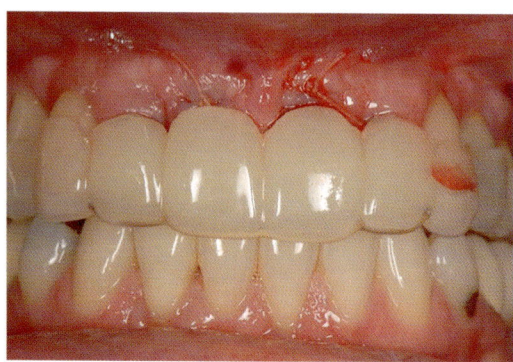

Fig. 8.64 Essix retainer provisional placed postoperatively

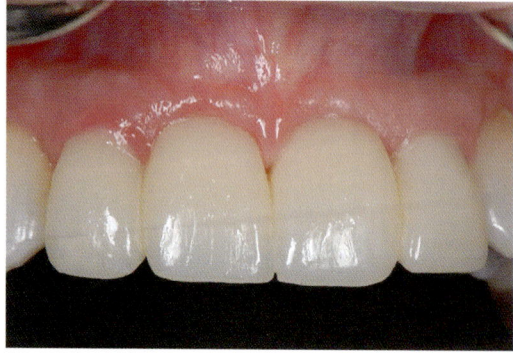

Fig. 8.65 Screw-retained composite resin provisional placed after osseointegration to develop tissue contours

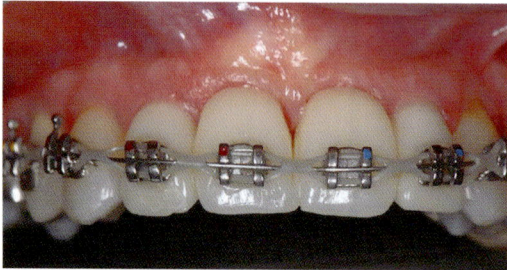

Fig. 8.66 Provisional used for orthodontic anchorage to finalize tooth position and occlusion

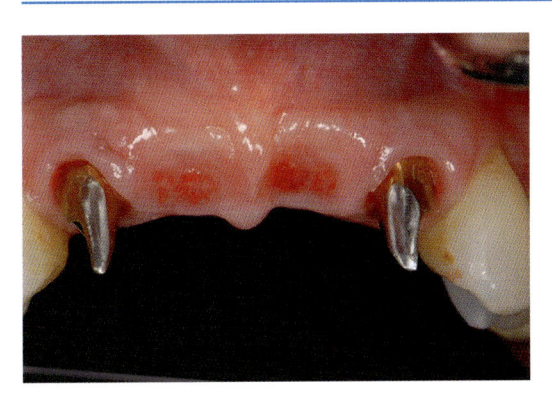

Fig. 8.67 CAD/CAM gold hue titanium custom abutments in situ

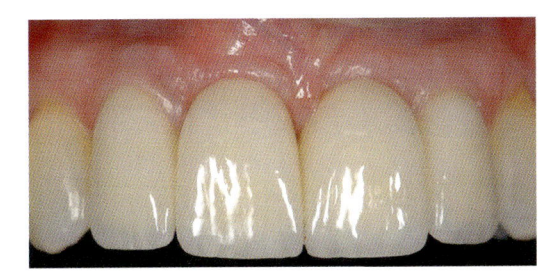

Fig. 8.68 Intraoral view of definitive PFM implant bridge

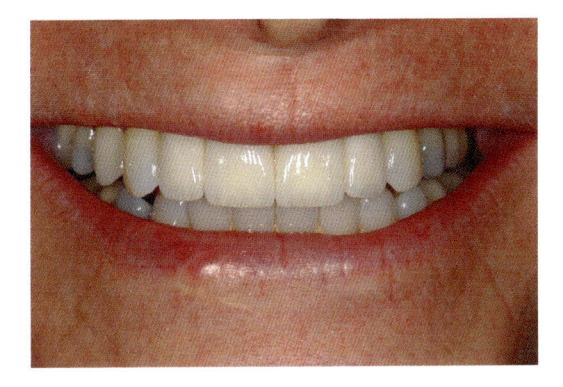

Fig. 8.69 Patient's smile

References

Amsterdam M (1974) Periodontal prosthesis. Twenty-five years in retrospect. Alpha Omegan 67(3):8–52

Baqain ZH, Anabtawi M, Karaky AA, Malkawi Z (2009) Morbidity from anterior iliac crest bone harvesting for secondary alveolar bone grafting: an outcome assessment study. J Oral Maxillofac Surg 67(3):570–575

Becker W, Hujoel P, Becker BE, Wohrle P (2015) Dental implants in an aged population: evaluation of periodontal health, bone loss, implant survival, and quality of life. Clin Implant Dent Relat Res. doi:10.1111/cid.12340

Brånemark PI, Adell R, Breine U, Hansson BO, Lindström J, Ohlsson A (1969) Intra-osseous anchorage of dental prostheses. I. Experimental studies. Scand J Plast Reconstr Surg 3(2):81–10

Brånemark PI, Hansson BO, Adell R, Breine U, Lindström J, Hallén O, Ohman A (1977) Osseointegrated implants in the treatment of the edentulous jaw. Experience from a 10-year period. Scand J Plast Reconstr Surg 16:1–132

Chen ST, Buser D (2014) Esthetic outcomes following immediate and early implant placement in the anterior maxilla – a systematic review. Int J Oral Maxillofac Implants 29:186–215

Esposito M, Grusovin MG, Felice P, Karatzopoulos G, Worthington HV, Coulthard P (2009) The efficacy of horizontal and vertical bone augmentation procedures for dental implants – a Cochrane systematic review. Eur J Oral Implantol 2(3):167–184

Horowitz R, Holtzclaw D, Rosen PS (2012) A review on alveolar ridge preservation following tooth extraction. J Evid Based Dent Pract 12(3):149–160

Ingber JS (1989) Forced eruption: alteration of soft tissue cosmetic deformities. Int J Periodontics Restor Dent 9(6):416–425

Ishikawa T, Salama M, Funato A, Kitajima H, Moroi H, Salama H, Garber D (2010) Three-dimensional bone and soft tissue requirements for optimizing esthetic results in compromised cases with multiple implants. Int J Periodontics Restor Dent 30(5):503–511

Jimbo R, Albrektsson T (2015) Long-term clinical success of minimally and moderately rough oral implants: a review of 71 studies with 5 years or more of follow-up. Implant Dent 24(1):62–69

Kois JC (1994) Altering gingival levels: The restorative connection. Part I. Biological variables. J Esthet Dent 6:3–9

Kois DE, Kois JC (2015) Comprehensive risk-based diagnostically driven treatment planning: developing sequentially generated treatment. Dent Clin N Am 59(3):593–608

Minsk L (2000) Orthodontic tooth extrusion as an adjunct to periodontal therapy. Compend Contin Educ Dent 21(9):768–770 772, 774

Ozan O, Turkyilmaz I, Ersoy AE, McGlumphy EA, Rosenstiel SF (2009) Clinical accuracy of 3 different types of computed tomography-derived stereolithographic surgical guides in implant placement. J Oral Maxillofac Surg 67(2):394–401

Phillips K, Kois JC (1998) Aesthetic peri-implant site development. The restorative connection. Dent Clin N Am 42(1):57–70

Phillips K, Wong KM (2001) Space requirements for implant-retained bar-and-clip overdentures. Compend Contin Educ Dent 22(6):516–518 520, 522

Phillips K, Wong KM (2002) Vertical space requirement for the fixed-detachable, implant-supported prosthesis. Compend Contin Educ Dent 23(8): 750–752 754, 756

Ploumaki A, Bilkhair A, Tuna T, Stampf S, Strub JR (2013) Success rates of prosthetic restorations on endodontically treated teeth; a systematic review after 6 years. J Oral Rehabil 40(8):618–630

Poskevicius L, Sidlauskas A, Galindo-Moreno P, Juodzbalys G (2015) Dimensional soft tissue changes following soft tissue grafting in conjunction with implant placement or around present dental implants: a systematic review. Clin Oral Implants Res. doi:10.1111/clr.12606

Salama H, Garber DA, Salama MA, Adar P, Rosenberg ES (1998a) Fifty years of interdisciplinary site development: lessons and guidelines from periodontal prosthesis. J Esthet Dent 10(3):149–156

Salama H, Salama MA, Garber D, Adar P (1998b) The interproximal height of bone: a guidepost to predictable aesthetic strategies and soft tissue contours in anterior tooth replacement. Pract Periodontics Aesthet Dent 10(9):1131–1141

Schliephake H, Rödiger M, Phillips K, McGlumphy EA, Chacon GE, Larsen P (2012) Early loading of surface modified implants in the posterior mandible – 5 year results of an open prospective non-controlled study. J Clin Periodontol 39(2):188–195

Schropp L, Wenzel A, Kostopoulos L et al (2003) Bone healing and soft tissue contour changes following single-tooth extraction: a clinical and radiographic 12-month prospective study. Int J Periodontics Restor Dent 23:313–323

Scurria MS, Bader JD, Shugars DA (1998) Meta-analysis of fixed partial denture survival: prostheses and abutments. J Prosthet Dent 79(4):459–464

Soehardi A, Meijer GJ, Hoppenreijs TJ, Brouns JJ, de Koning M, Stoelinga PJ (2015) Stability, complications, implant survival, and patient satisfaction after Le Fort I osteotomy and interposed bone grafts: follow-up of 5–18 years. Int J Oral Maxillofac Surg 44(1):97–103

Tarnow D, Elian N, Fletcher P, Froum S, Magner A, Cho SC, Salama M, Salama H, Garber DA (2003) Vertical distance from the crest of bone to the height of the interproximal papilla between adjacent implants. J Periodontol 74(12):1785–1788

Tjan AH, Miller GD, The JG (1984) Some esthetic factors in a smile. J Prosthet Dent 51(1):24–28

Wadhwani C, Akimoto K, Yousefian J (2015) Solving the challenge of the severely compromised implant in the esthetic zone: an interdisciplinary care case. Compend Contin Educ Dent 36(7):484–495

Flap Design, Suturing, and Healing

9

Praveen Gajendrareddy, Sivaraman Prakasam, and Satheesh Elangovan

Abstract

Tissue management is an integral and essential component of implant care. With the evolution of implant dentistry, the functional osteointegration of the implant to the recipient site is no longer considered an adequate measure of a successful outcome of therapy. The restoration of health, function, comfort, and aesthetics are parameters to be considered in the outcome of care. This becomes particularly significant in the anterior maxillary area where the expectation is that reconstructions must be indistinguishable from natural teeth. Different materials and surgical and restorative techniques are continuously being developed and tested to achieve this objective. Surgical tissue management, including soft tissue management, incision design, and suturing, and knowledge of anticipated healing outcomes are essential for a successful aesthetic outcome. This chapter describes flap design, papilla reconstruction techniques, management of soft tissue toward enhancement of attached gingiva, suturing materials, types of needles, types of knots, suturing techniques, and the various phases of soft tissue healing. A well thought-out surgical plan of flap design at every stage of implant surgery is critical to preserve and/or enhance the aesthetics and health of anterior implant restorations. Knowledge of the factors that affect flap design, suturing techniques, and the principles of healing are paramount in obtaining an ideal aesthetic result of an implant restoration that is indistinguishable from adjacent natural dentition.

P. Gajendrareddy, BDS, PhD (✉)
Department of Periodontics, University of Illinois,
801 S. Paulina Street, MC 859, Chicago,
IL 60612, USA
e-mail: Praveen@uic.edu

S. Prakasam, BDS, MSD, PhD
Oregon Health and Science University,
2730 SW Moody Ave,
Portland, OR 97201, USA
e-mail: Prakasam@ohsu.edu

S. Elangovan, BDS, ScD, DMSc
The University of Iowa College of Dentistry
801 Newton Road, Iowa City, IA, 52242, USA
e-mail: satheesh-elangovan@uiowa.edu

The practice of implant dentistry has evolved to a point where just functional osseointegration is considered inadequate, with an increased expectation of a perfect aesthetic result (Paolantoni et al. 2013). Particularly, in the anterior maxillary area, the expectation is that reconstructions must be indistinguishable from natural teeth (Paolantoni et al. 2013). Different materials and surgical and restorative techniques are continuously being developed and tested to achieve this objective. For example, timing of implant placement and restoration (Hürzeler and Weng 1995), palatal position of implant placement, design of the abutment collar, platform switching (Bichacho and Landsberg 1997), and peri-implant soft tissue augmentations have been explored as possible ways to preserve and enhance aesthetics (Belser et al. 2004). Understanding flap design, suturing, and healing is critical for their role in preserving and/or enhancing aesthetics.

9.1 Flap Design Consideration for Implants in the Aesthetic Zone

Basic flap design elements that have been used in traditional periodontal and oral surgical procedures are still relevant when designing flaps for implant-related procedures. Some basic considerations include the effect of incision design on vascular supply of the healing flap, consideration of anatomical landmarks, effect of flap procedures on underlying bone (Vohra et al. 2015), and elevation of intact flap especially in areas with scarring or thin gingival biotype (Suchetha et al. 2014). In general, wider apical base of flaps compared to the coronal area is recommended.

When designing flaps for implant-related procedures in the aesthetic zone, particular attention is given to preserving or reconstructing the interdental papilla and the attached gingiva. Consequently, flap design considerations vary depending on staging of the implant surgery, i.e., immediate implant placement in an extraction socket, delayed implant placement after ridge preservation procedures, and uncovering of a submerged implant. The following sections will address design consideration for each of those stages and the respective objectives in each of the stages. The emphasis in the following section is for single-tooth replacement in the maxillary anterior aesthetic zone.

9.1.1 Immediate Implant Placement

Immediate implant placement procedures for anterior aesthetic areas are advocated on the premise that it preserves the alveolar bone particularly vertical bone height and consequently provides a better aesthetic outcome. Studies have largely confirmed this theory at least in the short term, while in the long term this advantage appears to disappear when compared with delayed implant placement (Chen and Buser 2014). One systematic review reported an elevated risk of midfacial recession with immediate implants (Chen and Buser 2014).

9.1.1.1 Immediate Implant Placement: Two Stages

Newer techniques and materials have simplified placement of immediate submerged implants. After extraction of involved tooth with procedures that preserve the alveolus (minimum trauma extraction) and immediate implant placement, the so-called jump gap, i.e., the gap between implant and socket wall or any buccal dehiscence or fenestrations, was often grafted with bone graft materials. Traditionally, a flap had to be advanced to obtain primary closure of the submerged implant and graft particles. Membranes like the resorbable amnion-chorion allograft membranes (ACM) or alloplastic PLGA membranes and the non-resorbable alloplastic dense polytetrafluoroethylene (d-PTFE) (Luongo et al. 2014) membranes can be used to cover the top of implant and any graft material with minimal flap elevation. About 2–3 mm of buccal and palatal gingiva with the underlying periosteum attached is elevated and is tunneled along with the additional tunneling of the interdental papilla. This is followed by insertion of the ACM (no trimming necessary) or PLGA/d-PTFE membranes (with trimming) into the elevated area over the implant and graft particles (Fig. 9.1). Crisscross sutures or interrupted sutures are then placed over the membrane to retain the mem-

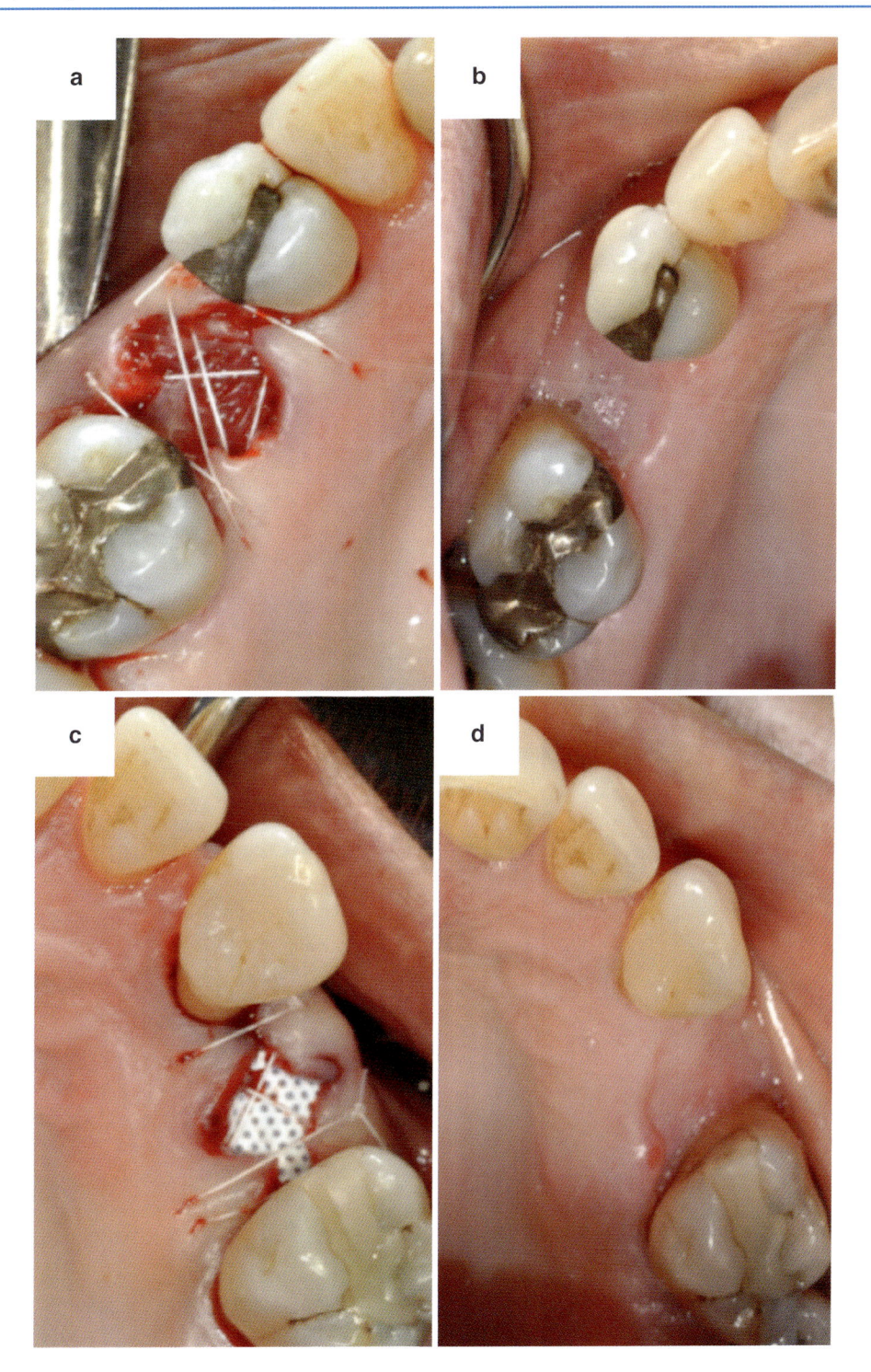

Fig. 9.1 ACM and cytoplast, left intentionally exposed to gain attached gingiva during two-stage immediate implant procedures: (**a**) ACM membrane placed with minimal flap elevation over socket and graft particles and secured with suture; (**b**) after 3 months, the site had wide zone of attached gingiva; (**c**, **d**) PTFE membrane trimmed and placed with minimal flap elevation over socket and graft particles and secured with sutures; (**d**) after 3 months the site had wide zone of attached gingiva (Photos are courtesy of Dr. Muyeenul Hassan, Department of Periodontics, School of Dentistry, Indiana University)

branes in place. With the d-PTFE membranes, it is important to ensure that the membranes are trimmed to be at least 1 mm away from the root surface of adjacent teeth to prevent loss of interdental papilla.

Alternative techniques can also be used to obtain primary closure, for example, a rotated connective tissue pedicle palatal flap or, in the presence of adequate thickness, a rotated connective tissue pedicle buccal flap. When such techniques are used, the incisions must not involve the interdental papilla.

9.1.1.2 One-Stage Immediate Implant Placement

One-stage immediate implant placements typically do not involve flap elevation. In cases with thin gingival biotype, tunneling of the buccal flap with subsequent insertion of a connective tissue graft or dermal allografts may help prevent facial recession/implant bone loss. The flap and the connective tissue are then secured in place with sutures either to the palatal tissue or with a sling suture around the implant depending on the need for coronal advancement of the buccal tissue.

9.1.2 Delayed Implant Placement

With delayed implant placement, the first consideration is whether a flap is necessary or not. If careful and thorough three-dimensional assessment of implant site, oftentimes with the help of cone beam CT scan, reveals that sufficient bone is present and implant placement would be uncomplicated, then a flapless procedure is recommended with the aid of a surgical stent. Nevertheless, a recent systematic review did not find any differences between flapless and flapped techniques in terms of crestal bone loss (Vohra et al. 2015).

Two basic methods have been described to elevate flaps for single delayed implant placements. Gomez-Roman describes these two techniques as widely mobilized flap and limited flap design (Gomez-Roman 2001) (Fig. 9.2). Misch recommends the use of the limited flap design in situations where mesial and/or distal papilla is in

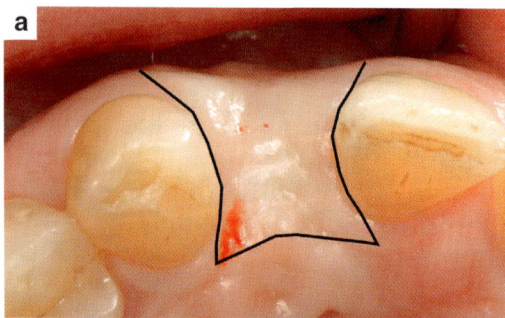

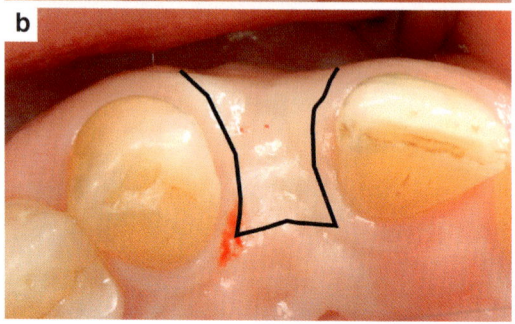

Fig. 9.2 Narrowly mobilized and widely mobilized flap for delayed implant placement as described by Gomez-Roman: (**a**) Widely mobilized flap incisions are placed on the proximal surfaces of adjacent teeth, and a full-thickness flap is elevated. (**b**) Incisions are placed sparing 1–2 mm of the proximal gingiva in an attempt to preserve the papilla (Photos are courtesy of Dr. Colin Graser, Department of Periodontology, School of Dentistry, Oregon Health & Science University)

the ideal positions. In this situation, the papillae are left intact, and adjacent facial vertical release incisions are made which are joined then with a crestal incision. After implant placement, the tissue is displaced toward the buccal if the need to augment keratinized tissue is determined. If the clinical plan requires the implant to be submerged, the flap is replaced and sutured.

The widely mobilized flap may be used if the papilla is already depressed or if the space for implant placement is limited. In these situations, a crestal incision is placed on the palatal aspect, and sulcular incisions are carried out on the proximal surface of the adjacent teeth. After implant placement the tissue is replaced and underlying soft tissue may be augmented with a connective tissue. At the time of second-stage surgery, papilla development may be carried out as described in later sections of this chapter. Gomez-

Roman compared the bone loss subsequent to use of widely mobilized flap versus limited flap and reported that limited flap performed superior in preserving interproximal crestal bone (Gomez-Roman 2001). Therefore, under ideal circumstances, the use of a limited flap may be advisable.

9.1.3 Flap Designs for Second-Stage Implant Surgery

The objective of implant uncovering procedures in the aesthetic zone is not only to expose the implant platform for restorative purposes but also to develop the soft tissue aesthetics around the implant abutment (e.g., preserve/enhance interproximal papilla) and to create healthy peri-implant mucosa (e.g., increase attached gingiva).

Several techniques have been described to achieve the objectives of implant exposure procedures. Bichacho and Landsberg classified it into two categories, i.e., additive procedures, where soft tissue augmentation was desired, and subtractive when simple exposure is desired and more than adequate soft tissue is available to preserve health and aesthetics around the implant (Bichacho and Landsberg 1997). Hertel et al. described these two types of procedures as destructive (excisional) techniques versus incisional (reconstructive) techniques (Hertel et al. 1994). They advocated excisional techniques (e.g., excision with surgical blade, monopole electrotome, lasers, and tissue punches) should be used only in situations with greater than 4 mm of attached gingiva. They recommended incisional/reconstructive techniques (e.g., free gingival grafts) when there is reduced or inadequate attached tissue.

9.1.3.1 Excisional Techniques

These techniques primarily involve the removal of soft tissue overlying the implant platform. Different instruments can be utilized to achieve the same; for example, scalpels, laser, and circular tissue punches can be used to excise and remove the overlying soft tissue. One technique for exposure, when using a scalpel, is to place a vertical incision on the soft tissue above the anticipated cover screw location (Bernhart et al. 1998). Once the cover screw is located, 1–3 mm of circular tissue is excised out, the tissue is then stretched with a blunt instrument, and the cover screw is removed and replaced with healing abutment (Bernhart et al. 1998). Happe et al. recommended just excising 1 mm^2 of overlying tissue, followed by slow stretching of the access hole with a microraspatory until the cover screw can be replaced with the healing abutment (Happe et al. 2010).

A simple technique of "+"- or "×"-shaped incisions may be sufficient in certain cases to expose the cover screw and replace it with the healing abutment (Suchetha et al. 2014). All of these techniques can be done with lasers as well. A tissue punch (Fig. 9.3) allows for precise removal of soft tissue especially when original surgical stent is available for accurately locating the cover screw. Care must be exercised in accurately locating the cover screw prior to punch excision so as not to remove excessive tissue.

9.1.3.2 Incisional/Reconstructive Techniques

Various reconstructive techniques can be used in areas where there is inadequate attached gingiva or where papilla is deficient. The following sections describe a selection of these various techniques.

Papilla Reconstructing Procedures
Nemcovsky et al. Papilla Reconstruction
Nemcovsky et al. described a second-stage procedure that would simultaneously reconstruct interproximal papilla for maxillary implants (Nemcovsky et al. 2000). The design of the flap is similar to narrowly mobilized flap described by Gomez-Roman (2001). Once the full-thickness flap is elevated, the adjacent papilla and the outer edges of the flap are de-epithelialized. The flap is split into mesial and distal halves. Cover screw is then replaced with abutment. The split halves are then placed over the interproximal papillary area and secured with vertical mattress sutures (Fig. 9.4).

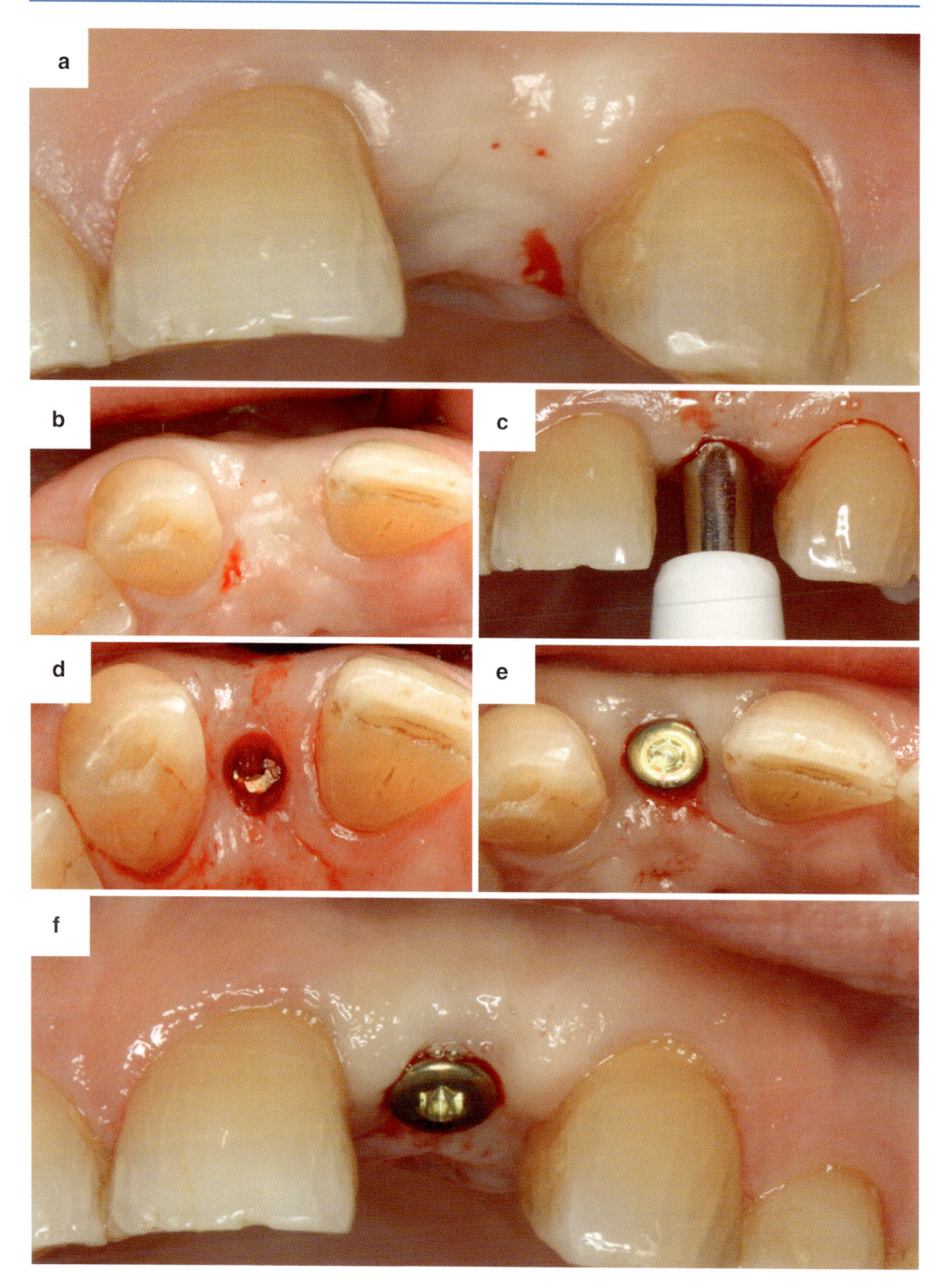

Fig. 9.3 Tissue punch excisional technique: (**a**) presence of wide abundant attached gingival zone (buccal view); (**b**) presence of wide abundant attached gingival zone (occlusal view); (**c**) tissue punch over implant platform; (**d**) tissue over implant platform removed and implant exposed; (**e**) abutment in place (occlusal view); (**f**) abutment in place (buccal view) (Photos are courtesy of Dr. Colin Graser, Department of Periodontology, School of Dentistry, Oregon Health & Science University)

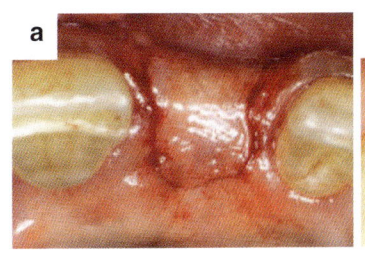

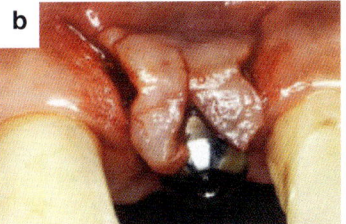

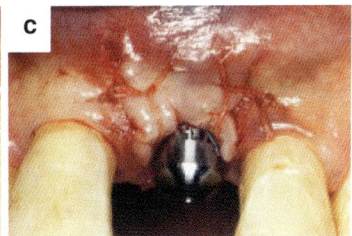

Fig. 9.4 Nemcovsky papilla reconstruction technique: (**a**) Initial incision, proximal papilla left in place. Outer edges of incision and approximal papillae are de-epithelialized. (**b**) Healing abutment is placed, and flap is split in its center separating into mesial and distal halves; (**c**) the two halves are placed over de-epithelialized proximal papilla and secure with sutures

Misch et al. Split-Finger Technique
(Misch et al. 2004)
This technique is similar to the Nemcovsky et al. technique with the key difference being the flap is elevated on the palatal aspect of the implant. Intrasulcular incisions are placed on the proximal surfaces of adjacent teeth and then extended 2–3 mm into the palate at slight angle away from the line angle of the proximal teeth toward the implant. The incision is then looped back with "s"-shaped incisions, which are then joined from both sides at the buccal aspect, right at the buccal margin of the implant platform. Full-thickness flap is elevated; adjacent papilla area and edges of the flap are de-epithelialized. The flap is split into two halves. Cover screw is then replaced with healing abutment. The split halves are then sutured over the de-epithelialized distal interproximal surfaces augmenting the papilla (Fig. 9.5).

Palacci and Nowzari Technique
(Palacci and Nowzari 2008)
This technique reconstructs papilla-like tissue between implants. A full-thickness labial flap is elevated. Healing abutments are placed, and semilunar beveled incisions are placed to create scalloped tissue, which are then rotated to fill inter-abutment or abutment tooth interproximal areas (Fig. 9.6).

Lee et al. "I"-Shaped Incision for Papilla Reconstruction (Lee et al. 2010)
"I"-shaped incision technique involves labial horizontal incision that is given about 1 mm palatal to the buccal border of the implant, followed by a bucco-palatal straight line incision along the middle of the implant till the palatal border of the implant platform. Another horizontal incision is then placed at this border. The flaps are carefully reflected and healing abutments are placed. The flaps are now folded alongside the healing abutment and no sutures are placed.

Techniques to Increase Buccal Attached Gingiva
Nemcovsky Rotated Flap (Nemcovsky and Moses 2002)
Here the crestal incision is placed palatal to the implants with buccal releasing incisions that do not involve the papilla. The full-thickness flap is then displaced buccally and healing abutment is placed. The palatal connective tissue pedicle is then rotated from the palate and adapted in close approximation to the healing abutments, covering the exposed palatal bone near the implants. The two flaps are then sutured in place with appropriate sutures.

Pouch Roll Technique/Modified Roll Flap Technique by Park et al. (Park and Wang 2012)
Buccal mini pedicle flap, 1 mm wider than diameter of implant platform, is raised and de-epithelialized for this technique. This mini pedicle is then rolled underneath the buccal pouch augmenting the buccal attached gingiva. This technique is a recent adaptation/modification, for the purposes of increased implant aesthetics, of the "Abrams roll" first described by Leonard

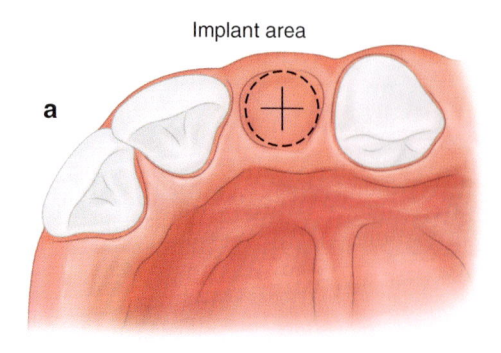

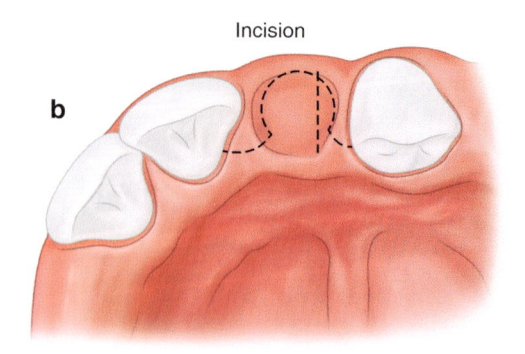

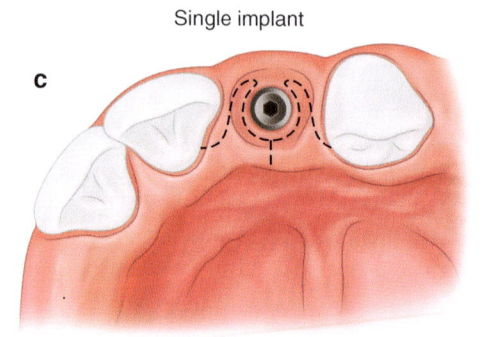

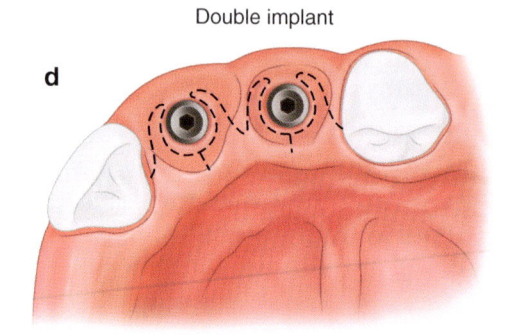

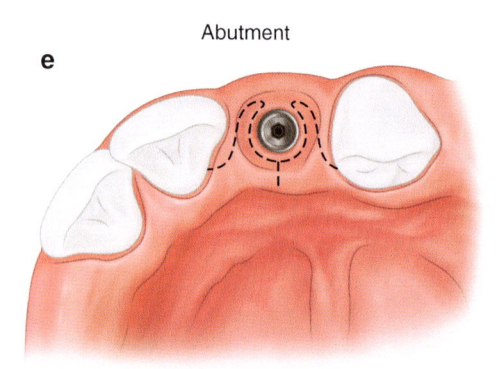

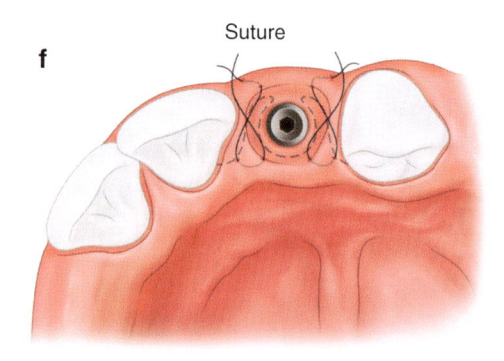

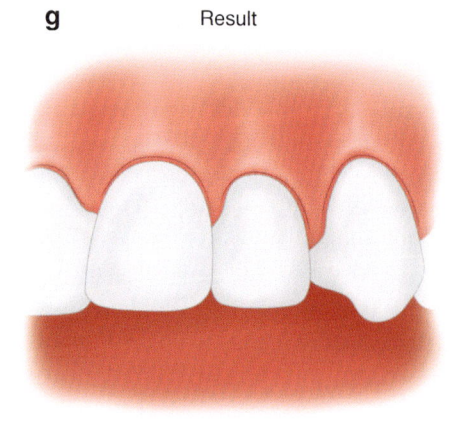

a Implant area
b Incision
c Single implant
d Double implant
e Abutment
f Suture
g Result

Fig. 9.5 Misch split-finger technique. (**a**) Initial implant area. (**b**) Incision design. (**c**) Split-finger flap design for the single implant. (**d**) Split-finger flap design for two implants. (**e**) Abutment (or permucosal extension) connection. (**f**) Modified vertical mattress suture. (**g**) Final clinical appearance (From Misch et al., Creation of Interimplant Papillae Through a SplitFinger Technique, *Implant Dentistry*, vol 13, issues 1, Jan 1, 2004, with permission)

used to connect the vertical incisions to release the flap and expose the implant head. Healing abutment is then placed. The flap is then stabilized, by suturing it at the gingival papilla (Fig. 9.7).

9.2 Suturing

The major objective of suturing in implant dentistry as in any other surgical field is to approximate the wounds created by the surgeon in order to achieve the goals of a specific clinical procedure (Silverstein and Kurtzman 2005). By approximating the surgical flap margins, the size and extent of the surgical wound is minimized to encourage healing by primary intention. Apart from facilitating soft tissue healing, proper execution of suturing allows the surgeon to control flap positioning (apical, coronal, or lateral), in relation to the dental implant, and, most of all, play prevent postoperative infections.

Bringing the wound margin together and holding the wound margins without tension is an important aspect of the suturing process. Tension-free closure can be accomplished by carefully planning the incision designs and also by additional techniques such as a periosteal releasing incision into the suturing flap. Equally important is the need to minimize trauma while suturing in order to avoid compromising the blood supply to the healing site. By placing an adequate number of sutures and by using the appropriate suture diameter, one can reduce the trauma to the tissues significantly. The size of the surgical knot is also important as they can become a food or plaque trap during early healing.

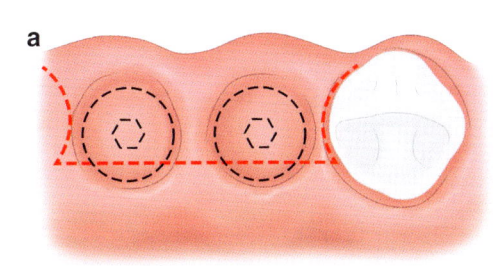

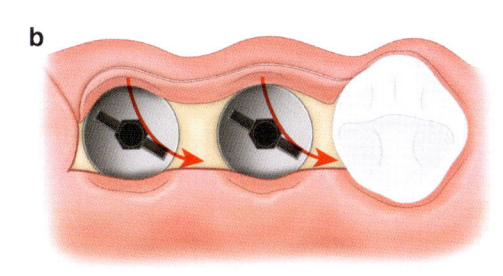

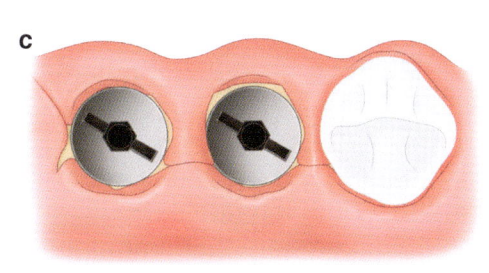

Fig. 9.6 Palacci and Nowzari technique: (**a–c**) occlusal view of horizontal and vertical incisions (Figure courtesy of Palacci and Nowzari and is reproduced with minor modification from Palacci and Nowzari, Soft tissue enhancement around dental implants, *Periodontology 2000*, April 14, 2008, with permission)

Abrams for the enhancement of the ovate pontics in a FPD.

Paolantoni et al. "M" Flap (Paolantoni et al. 2013)
In this technique a full-thickness "M"-shaped flap is mobilized by using intrasulcular beveled incisions around the proximal aspects of the adjacent teeth rounding buccally and palatally. A horizontal slightly palatal "M"-shaped incision is then

9.2.1 Important Variables in Suturing

There are several critical components in suturing. These include but are not limited to the suture

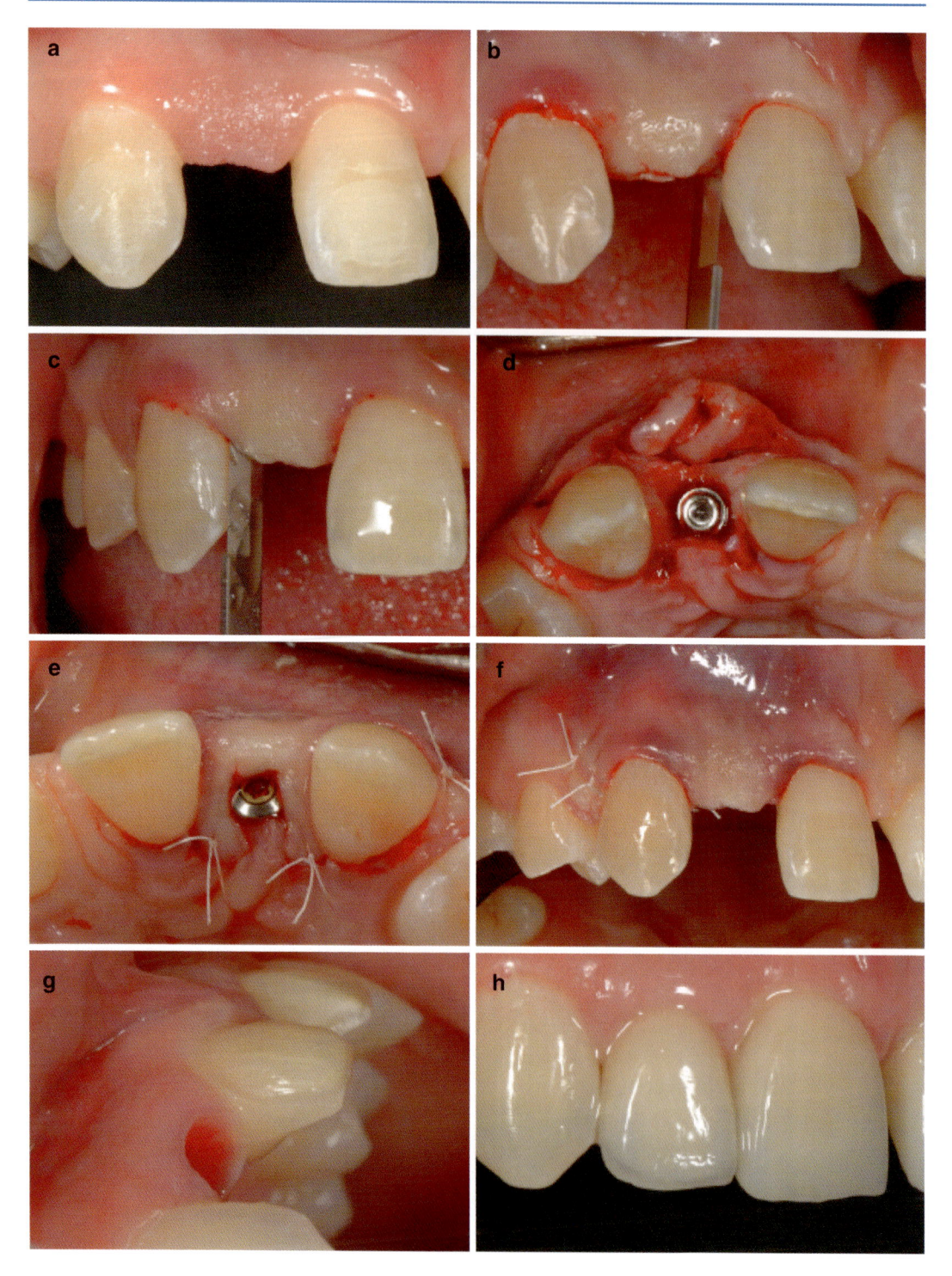

Fig. 9.7 Paolantoni M flap technique. (**a**) Preoperative view: the *right* maxillary lateral incisor was missing, in a thick gingival biotype case. (**b**, **c**) An intrasulcular inner beveled incision was performed around the distal aspect of the adjacent teeth, rounding buccally and palatally and connecting with an M-shaped incision. (**d**) The full-thickness "M" flap was raised to visualize the bone surface and connect the implant abutment. (**e**, **f**) The flap was closed and sutured with a mattress monofilament suture at the gingival papilla to stabilize the flap around the healing cap. Single knots were used to assure a tension-free wound closure. (**g**) After 6 weeks, a complete soft tissue healing was apparently achieved. (**h**) The final zirconia-based implant-supported crown offered an excellent aesthetic outcome (From Paolantoni et al. 2013, with permission)

material utilized and design or technique of the retaining suture. These will all have an influence, either major or minor, on the resultant outcome of the soft tissue healing. Following are the components of suturing that the surgeon has to be familiar with, prior to selecting a particular suture or a suturing technique for a specific clinical situation in implant dentistry.

9.2.1.1 Suture Thread Diameter

The suture materials are available in ten different diameters numbered from 1-0 to 10-0 with 1-0 being the thickest and 10-0 being the thinnest. In dentistry, the most commonly used suture thread diameter ranges from 4-0 to 6-0 (Sharif and Coulthard 2011; Silverstein and Kurtzman 2005). For suturing following conventional dental implant placement, sutures in 4-0 to 5-0 diameter range are commonly employed, whereas, for adjunctive periodontal plastic procedures such as connective tissue grafting at the time of implant placement or during implant uncovery, thinner suture materials (such as 6-0) are commonly employed. As mentioned earlier, thread diameter will have an influence on the amount of trauma induced to a flap, will affect the blood supply, and will also impact the suture characteristics like tensile strength or absorption rate.

9.2.1.2 Suture Material

Based on the absorbability of the suture thread, suture materials are classified into resorbable and non-resorbable types (Table 9.1). As the name suggests, resorbable sutures degrade in the oral cavity over time. They do so primarily by two mechanisms – the effect of intraoral enzymes and the impact of low intraoral pH (Silverstein 2005). Suture materials such as gut and chromic gut that are synthesized from animal tissues undergo resorption by enzymatic degradation, while acidic pH in the oral cavity enhances resorption of synthetic resorbable sutures. Several conditions such as bulimia, gastric reflux, or consumption of certain medications such as steroid inhalers can all lead to lowering of pH in the oral cavity (Silverstein and Kurtzman 2005).

Based on the number of filaments that constitutes the suture material, the suture thread can be further classified into monofilament or multifilament (braided) (O'Neal and Alleyn 1997). Monofilament sutures are smooth, made out of single thread, whereas, as the name implies,

Table 9.1 The list of most commonly used suture materials, their characteristic features and their common indications in implant dentistry

Suture thread material	Ease of handling	Tensile strength	Absorption duration	Common indications in implant dentistry
Resorbable				
Plain gut	Low	Low	70 days	Suturing vertical incisions and for suturing soft tissue grafts surrounding dental implants
Chromic gut	Low	Low	90 days	Suturing vertical incisions and for suturing soft tissue grafts surrounding dental implants
Poliglecaprone (Monocryl)	Very high	Very high	91–119 days	Suturing the flaps after implant placement with or without simultaneous bone grafting
Polyglactin (Vicryl)	High	High	42 days	Suturing the flaps after implant placement with or without simultaneous bone grafting
Polyglactin coated (resolute)	High	High	56–70 days	Suturing the flaps after implant placement with or without simultaneous bone grafting
Non-resorbable				
e-PTFE (Gore-Tex or cytoplast)	Very high	Very high	Non-resorbable	Suturing flaps after ridge augmentation prior to dental implant placement or simultaneously with implant placement
Silk	Very high	Moderate	1 year	Not commonly used but can be used to suture flaps after implant placement
Polydioxanone (PDS plus)	Moderate	Very high	182–238 days	Not commonly used but can be used to suture flaps after implant placement

Sources: http://www.ecatalog.ethicon.com/sutures-absorbable and O'Neal and Alleyn (1997)

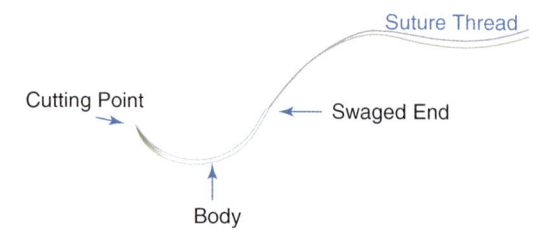

Fig. 9.8 Parts of a suture needle

multifilament suture materials are synthesized by braiding many single threads together. There are pros and cons associated with each category of suture material. Multifilament sutures in general have better handling characteristics than monofilaments, but they do exhibit "wicking effect," which is the process by which they attract oral fluids and bacteria to travel along the suture into the wound site. This is due to the multi-stranded nature and rough surface characteristics of these suture threads.

9.2.1.3 Suture Needle

A typical suture needle consists of three parts, cutting point, body, and swaged end that connect the needle to the thread (Fig. 9.8). Needles can be straight, half curved, or completely curved. Curved needles are commonly employed in dentistry, and among curved needles, 3/8 of a circle or ½ circle needles are commonly employed in implant dentistry. Curved needles allow for quick needle turnout from the tissues, and longer curved needles such as ½ circle needles allow the clinician to pass the needle from buccal to lingual/palatal flap in one motion, whereas smaller curved needles such as 1/4 or 3/8 circle needles are traditionally used for mucogingival procedures around implants and require multiple passings (Silverstein and Kurtzman 2005).

9.2.1.4 Suture Knots

Suture knots are an important component of the suturing process that keeps the suture from untying. The three commonly used suture knots in dentistry are square knot, slipknot, and surgeon's knot (Garg 2012). In order to perform a square knot, two overhand knots should be completed in the opposite direction, whereas for a slipknot, two single overhand knots are made in the same direction (to secure) and the third overhand knot made in the opposite direction. For surgeon's knot, which is a commonly employed knot, two overhand knots are made in the opposite directions, but the first overhand knot is a double overhand knot. Based on the handling characteristics, it is generally recommended that a slipknot be used when using silk, e-PTFE, or gut sutures and a surgeon's knot be used for synthetic resorbable and non-resorbable sutures (Kurtzman 2005).

9.2.1.5 Suturing Techniques

The most commonly employed suturing techniques around dental implants include single interrupted sutures, sling sutures, and mattress (horizontal and vertical) sutures (Fig. 9.9). Horizontal mattress suturing is the technique of choice to approximate flaps as it everts the buccal and lingual flaps and promotes and maintains intimacy of the underlying connective tissues (CT), after ridge augmentation (with or without implant placement). The indications and technique details for each of these suturing techniques and few others with relevance to implant dentistry are given in Table 9.2.

The required suturing instruments include a standard needle holder or a Castroviejo to grasp the suture needle and a scissor (Fig. 9.10). For sutures with longer suture needles with a thread diameter in the range of 4-0 to 5-0, a standard needle holder with possible variants such as with or without ratchet or toothed or non-toothed is used. For microsurgical procedures that utilize shorter needle and suture threads with 5-0 or 6-0 diameters, a Castroviejo needle holder is commonly employed. After placing the knot, a straight or curved Iris scissor is utilized to cut the ends of the sutures to complete suturing.

9.3 Principles of Healing

Healing of a surgical wound is a complex phenomenon that can be broadly categorized into three overlapping phases: an inflammatory phase, a proliferative phase, and a remodeling phase (Cohen et al. 1975). These interdependent phases last from hours to days, days to weeks, and weeks to months, respectively. Cytokines and growth factors released

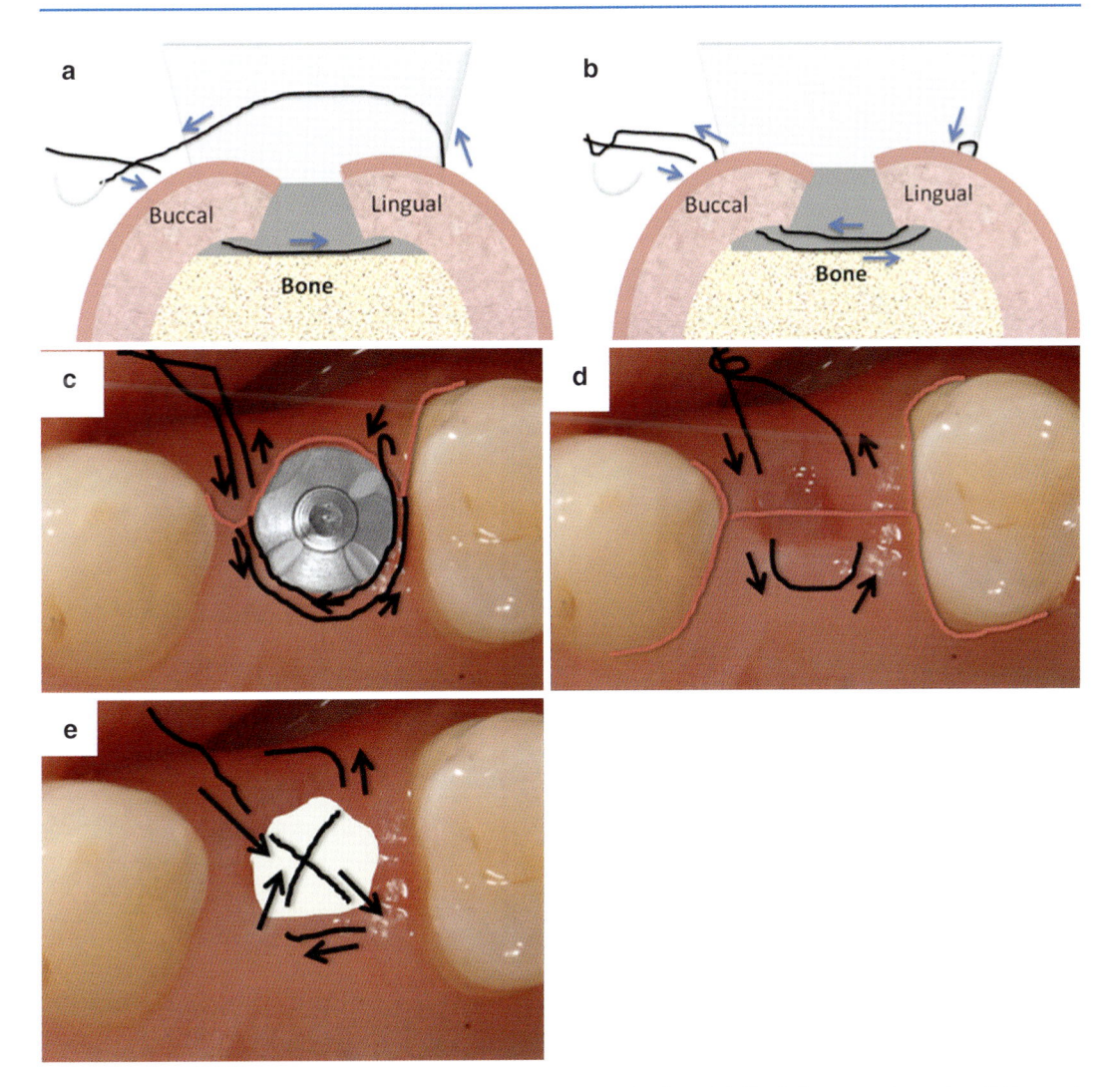

Fig. 9.9 The commonly employed suturing techniques in implant dentistry. (**a**) Single interrupted suturing, (**b**) internal vertical mattress suturing, (**c**) sling suturing, (**d**) horizontal mattress suturing, and (**e**) crisscross suturing

during early inflammation are essential for the proliferative phase. In turn, resolution of inflammation is mediated by elements from the advancing epithelium. Since the timing and activity of each phase depends on the resolution of the previous phase (Hubner et al. 1996), a dysregulation of any phase impairs multiple facets of healing.

9.3.1 Inflammatory Phase

This phase involves minimizing damage, protection from infection, debris removal, and facilitation of downstream events related to repair. The blood clot serves as a provisional matrix and as a scaffold for repair. Several mediators including complement products, kinins, fibrin, and prostaglandins are released by platelets, white blood cells, and other blood elements in response to injury (Hart 2002). This in turn stimulates the expression of adhesion molecules on endothelial cells and chemokines from various immune cells. Thus the migration of immune cells from the circulation to the peripheral tissues is regulated in this phase. Inflammation is mediated by neutrophils that arrive at the site within minutes, macro-

Table 9.2 The commonly utilized suturing techniques, their indications and technique details

Suturing technique	Common indications	Technique
Single interrupted (Fig. YA)	To suture papillae adjacent to implant placed To suture vertical incisions Used (in addition to horizontal mattress suture) to reinforce flap closure following ridge augmentation (with or without implant placement)	From the buccal side, the suture needle goes from outside to inside of the buccal papilla, and then the needle is passed from the inside to outside of the palatal papilla. Suture is then brought to the buccal side, and a knot is tied. The same is applicable when suturing vertical incisions except that instead of papillae, it will be wound margins
Internal vertical mattress (Fig. YB)	To suture papillae adjacent to implant placed in the aesthetic zone Can be used when implant placement is combined with soft tissue augmentation	From the buccal side, the suture penetrates the buccal flap from outside to inside about 5–6 mm apical to the incision. The suture needle is brought to the palatal side and will pierce the palatal flap and will be passed from inside to outside 5–6 mm apical to the palatal wound margin (almost at the same level as buccal piercing). The suture needle is passed from outside to inside of the palatal flap, but this time the point of entry is about 2–3 mm from the incision/flap margin and right above the first piercing. The suture needle is brought to the buccal side, and the needle is passed through the buccal papilla from inside to outside, about 3 mm from the flap margin right above the first piercing. Then the suture knot is made. This flap allows the flaps to be brought together and pushed coronally (eversion)
Sling (Fig. YC)	Can be used when implant placement is combined with soft tissue augmentation Used during soft tissue augmentation around existing dental implant	From the buccal side, the suture goes from outside to inside of the first buccal papilla adjoining the implant, and then the suture thread is looped encircling the implant neck (first sling) and is brought to second buccal papilla adjoining the implant. In this papilla, the needle goes from the inside to outside and is then brought back palatally to encircle the implant again (second sling). The needle then passes through the first buccal papilla from inside to outside where suturing will be completed with a knot
Horizontal mattress (Fig. YD)	To approximate the flaps after ridge augmentation procedures done as a separate procedure or along with implant placement	From the buccal side, the suture needle goes from outside to inside of the flap, and the needle is passed from the inside to outside of the palatal flap. Then the suture needle is passed from outside to inside of the palatal flap at a point that is lateral to the previous point of exit. The suture is passed from inside to outside of the buccal flap at a point that is lateral to the previous point of entry. Then the suturing is completed with a surgical knot
Crisscross (Fig. YE)	Commonly employed in the extraction sockets (after ridge preservation)	From the buccal side, the suture needle is passed from outside to inside of one buccal papilla, and then the suture needle is passed from inside to outside of the diagonally opposite palatal papilla. The suture needle is brought laterally and passed from outside to inside of the other unpierced palatal papilla, needle then passes from inside to outside of the unpierced diagonally opposite buccal papilla creating a crisscross pattern. The suture will be completed with a knot. This allows good securement of the graft and membrane used in ridge preservation

9 Flap Design, Suturing, and Healing

Fig. 9.10 Surgical instruments required for suturing

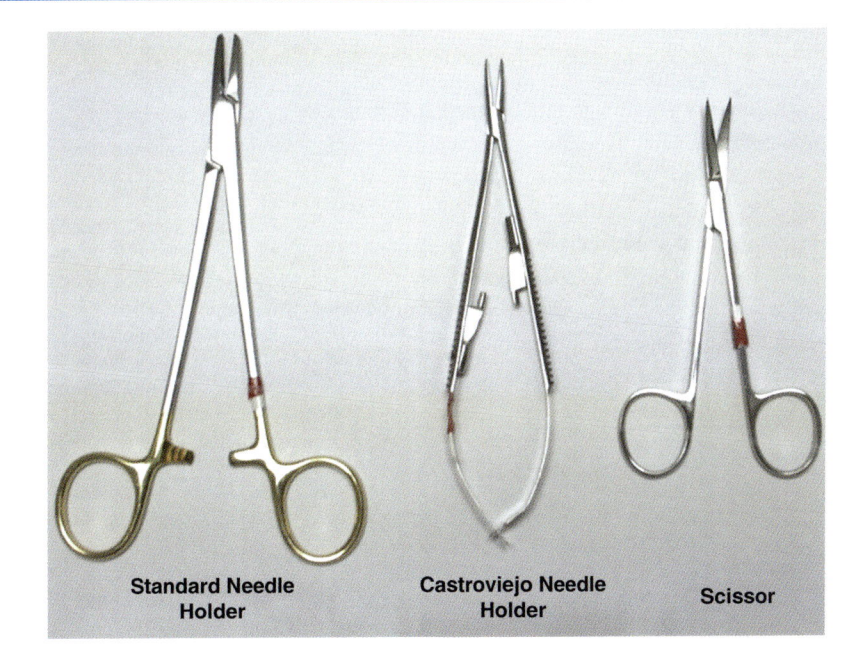

phages that appear within hours followed by lymphocytes. These cells mediate bacterial clearance and phagocytose damaged tissue (DiPietro 1995). Cytokines and growth actors produced in this phase aid fibroblasts, keratinocytes, and endothelial cells in the proliferative phase of healing.

9.3.2 Proliferative Phase

This phase involves rebuilding of damaged structures. The cells involved in this phase include fibroblasts, epithelial cells, and endothelial cells. The epithelial cells proliferate and migrate along the margin of the incision, followed by the fibroblasts in the surrounding mucosa. Granulation tissue is made of fibronectin, deposited by the fibroblasts and by collagen, hyaluronic acid, elastin, and other extracellular matrix components secreted by the fibroblasts. The loss of vascular integrity as a result of the surgical process, in addition to the high oxygen demand for healing, drives endothelial cell migration and proliferation. The demand for oxygen is met by the excess of vasculature formed during healing that recedes to normal levels with the healing of the wound (Risau 1997). The final stages in restoration of barrier function, after the reestablishment of the epithelial barrier, involve the secretion of structural proteins such as involucrin and keratins.

9.3.3 Remodeling Phase

Collagen synthesis, degradation, and reorganization occur during remodeling. The phase follows the proliferative phase and continues for a long period after wound closure. Excess cellularity, a result of the previous phases of healing, is resolved by apoptosis and removal by macrophages. Alternately, cell loss via lysis or necrosis results in inflammation and possibly scarring. The potential for scarring is also increased with a prolonged inflammatory phase or an infection, which in turn leads to an increase in the number of cells (Hunt et al. 2000). Matrix metalloproteinases (MMPs) and tissue inhibitors of metalloproteinases (TIMPs) play a significant role in this phase.

Summary

Careful planning of flap design at every stage of implant surgery is critical to preserve and/or enhance the aesthetics and health of anterior implant restorations. Knowledge of the factors that affect flap design, suturing techniques, and the principles of healing are paramount in obtaining an ideal aesthetic result of an implant restoration that is indistinguishable from adjacent natural dentition.

References

Belser UC, Schmid B, Higginbottom F, Buser D (2004) Outcome analysis of implant restorations located in the anterior maxilla: a review of the recent literature. Int J Oral Maxillofac Implants 19(Suppl):30–42

Bernhart T, Haas R, Mailath G, Watzek G (1998) A minimally invasive second-stage procedure for single-tooth implants. J Prosthet Dent 79(2):217–219

Bichacho N, Landsberg C (1997) Single implant restorations: prosthetically induced soft tissue topography. Pract Periodontics Aesthet Dent PPAD 9(7):745–752

Chen ST, Buser D (2014) Esthetic outcomes following immediate and early implant placement in the anterior maxilla—a systematic review. Int J Oral Maxillofac Implants 29(Suppl):186–215

Cohen BH, Lewis LA, Resnik SS (1975) Would healing: a brief review. Int J Dermatol 14(10):722–726

DiPietro LA (1995) Wound healing: the role of the macrophage and other immune cells. Shock 4(4):233–240

Garg A (2012) Wounds and suturing in dental implant surgery. Dent Implantol Update 23(6):44–48

Gomez-Roman G (2001) Influence of flap design on periimplant interproximal crestal bone loss around single-tooth implants. Int J Oral Maxillofac Implants 16(1):61–67

Happe A, Körner G, Nolte A (2010) The keyhole access expansion technique for flapless implant stage-two surgery: technical note. Int J Periodontics Restorative Dent 30(1):97

Hart J (2002) Inflammation. 1: its role in the healing of acute wounds. J Wound Care 11(6):205–209

Hunt TK, Hopf H, Hussain Z (2000) Physiology of wound healing. Adv Skin Wound Care 13(2 Suppl):6–11

Hertel RC, Blijdorp PA, Kalk W, Baker DL (1994) Stage 2 surgical techniques in endosseous implantation. Int J Oral Maxillofac Implants 9(3):273–278

Hubner G, Brauchle M, Smola H, Madlener M, Fassler R, Werner S (1996) Differential regulation of proinflammatory cytokines during wound healing in normal and glucocorticoid-treated mice. Cytokine 8(7):548–556

Hürzeler M, Weng D (1995) Periimplant tissue management: optimal timing for an aesthetic result. Pract Periodontics Aesthet Dent PPAD 8(9):857–869

Lee E-K, Herr Y, Kwon Y-H, Shin S-I, Lee D-Y, Chung J-H (2010) I-shaped incisions for papilla reconstruction in second stage implant surgery. J Periodontal Implant Sci 40(3):139–143

Luongo R, Bugea C, Baldassarre G, Bianco G, Dimise M, Aliota S (2014) Atraumatic socket preservation with immediate implant placement: a new surgical approach with a non-resorbable membrane intentionally left exposed. Clin Oral Implants Res 25:670

Misch CE, Al-Shammari KF, Wang H-L (2004) Creation of interimplant papillae through a split-finger technique. Implant Dent 13(1):20–27

Nemcovsky CE, Moses O (2002) Rotated palatal flap. A surgical approach to increase keratinized tissue width in maxillary implant uncovering: technique and clinical evaluation. Int J Periodontics Restorative Dent 22(6):607–612

Nemcovsky CE, Moses O, Artzi Z (2000) Interproximal papillae reconstruction in maxillary implants. J Periodontol 71(2):308–314

O'Neal RB, Alleyn CD (1997) Suture materials and techniques. (2008). Curr Opin Periodontol 4:89–95

Palacci P, Nowzari H (2008) Soft tissue enhancement around dental implants. Periodontol 2000 47(1):113–132

Paolantoni G, Cioffi A, Mignogna J, Riccitiello F, Sammartino G (2013) "M" flap design for promoting implant esthetics: technique and cases series. Management 1:2

Park S-H, Wang H-L (2012) Pouch roll technique for implant soft tissue augmentation: a variation of the modified roll technique. Int J Periodontics Restorative Dent 32(3):116–121

Risau W (1997) Mechanisms of angiogenesis. Nature 386(6626):671–674

Sharif MO, Coulthard P (2011) Suturing: an update for the general dental practitioner. Dent Update 38(5):329–330

Silverstein LH, Kurtzman GM (2005) A review of dental suturing for optimal soft-tissue management. Compend Contin Educ Dent 26(3):163–166

Silverstein LH (2005) Essential principles of dental suturing for the implant surgeon. Dent Implantol Update 16(1):1–7

Suchetha A, Phadke P, Sapna N, Rajeshwari H (2014) Optimising esthetics in second stage dental implant surgery: periodontist's ingenuity. J Dental Implants 4(2):170–175. doi:10.4103/0974-6781.140898

Vohra F, Al-Kheraif AA, Almas K, Javed F (2015) Comparison of crestal bone loss around dental implants placed in healed sites using flapped and flapless techniques: a systematic review. J Periodontol 86(2):185–191

Digital Photography and Digital Asset Management

10

Steven H. Goldstein

Abstract

Dental digital photography is commonly used in many of today's dental practices, and high-quality dental images are paramount for laboratory communication, patient communication, and marketing dentistry. This chapter provides an overview of DSLR (digital single-lens reflex) camera settings/parameters required to incorporate clinical and portrait photography into your dental practice and will also discuss postproduction workflow.

10.1 Goals and Objectives

The goal of this chapter is to demonstrate why digital photography is necessary in dentistry and how it is used clinically. Basic professional photographic equipment will be listed as a guide for the armamentarium required. Particular emphasis will be given to the anterior aesthetic group of teeth. A review of fundamental photographic principles and the digital workflow necessary will also be discussed.

10.1.1 Why Digital Photography

Dental digital photography is common in many of today's dental practices, and high-quality dental images are paramount for today's aesthetic dentists and laboratory technicians. Dental photography allows patients to view the quality of your dentistry and to make educated decisions about their treatment, helps the laboratory produce a better product, and makes you a better clinician allowing you to critically evaluate your work over time. Additionally, it also becomes a vital part of the patient's legal record.

Digital photography has revolutionized the world of photography by allowing the user to view the results immediately. Poor images can be deleted easily and replacement images immediately taken. Adjustments to any of the camera settings allow the user to see how the image is affected. Sophisticated auto-controls help the beginner make good images, allowing them to view data of the camera settings (called metadata) afterward to see what parameters the camera chose. This is a great way to learn photography and then compare how various parameters are adjusted to improve the image.

S.H. Goldstein, DDS
10752 N. 89th Place, Suite 217, Scottsdale,
Arizona 85260, USA
e-mail: info@stevenhgoldsteindds.com

10.1.2 High-Quality Images

High-quality images are those that clearly depict the subject, are free from distracting backgrounds, are properly exposed and color-balanced, and are in sharp focus. High-quality images are especially important in the anterior aesthetic zone, as they allow the clinician and laboratory technician to evaluate many important aspects such as papillae shape, display and form, gingival stippling, tooth size, tooth shade, contours and texture, lip position, and smile line (Fig. 10.1). Full-face photos give the technician a "feel" for the patient they are working on and should also be part of the clinician's photo series (Fig. 10.2).

In order to achieve the highest-quality images, professional photographic equipment is required. Without the ideal, the quality of the images will be limited. Below is a list of the required equipment.

- Digital SLR
- Micro lens (105 mm) f-2.8
- Flash
- Cheek retractors
- Mirrors
- Blackout background
- Computer
- Large monitor
- Card reader
- Image software
- Multiple hard disk

Making high-quality images requires the full understanding of the camera settings which will vary for a particular kind of shot. This includes setting up and understanding many of the following parameters: shutter speed, aperture, ISO, white balance, exposure mode, file format (RAW vs JPEG), focus mode, and color mode.

Many books on photography have been written explaining the above terms and how these parameters affect the image. If you are new to photography, a basic course would be beneficial. It is beyond the scope of this chapter to cover all the details, however, a review of many fundamental terms will allow the reader to get an understanding of what they are and why they are important. Optimal learning is by demonstration of the abovementioned principles, with the camera set to the "manual mode" bypassing many of the "automatic" features. This will show the reader exactly how the various settings affect the overall image. All of the images in this chapter were shot using the following camera equipment (Fig. 10.3) – Nikon D200 SLR Digital Camera Body (DX Format Sensor), Micro-Nikkor 105 mm f/2.8G

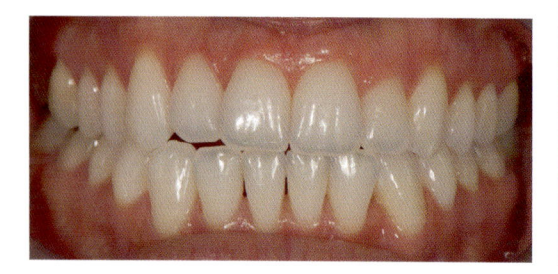

Fig. 10.1 Full smile retracted

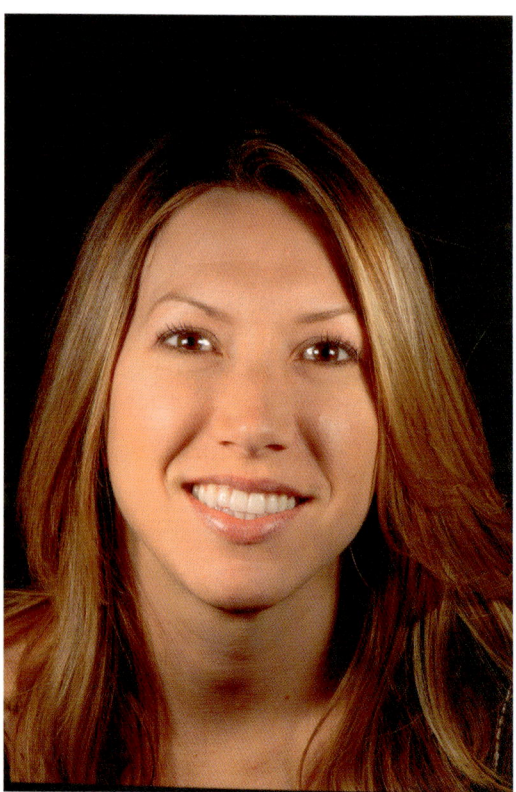

Fig. 10.2 Full-face portrait

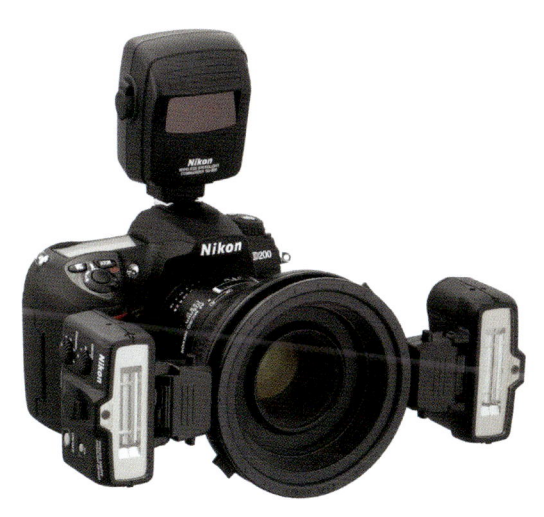

10 Digital Photography and Digital Asset Management

Fig. 10.3 Nikon intraoral DSLR camera setup

IF-ED AF-S VR (Vibration Reduction) Lens, R1C1 Wireless Close-Up Speedlight Flash System with Commander SU-800. Note: the camera body shown in Fig. 10.3 is no longer manufactured; any current Nikon DSLR body will work with this lens and flash setup. Other camera manufactures (Canon and Sony) also make comparable gear.

10.1.3 Dental Photography in the Anterior Dentition

One of the biggest issues a dentist faces in aesthetic dentistry is to meet or exceed patients' expectations. Using simple laboratory procedures in conjunction with dental photography allows the patient and doctor to actually observe a mock-up of the proposed restoration in the mouth prior to starting any definitive treatment (Magne 2002). Portraits and closeup images are taken with and without the mock-up in the mouth, and the images are given to the patient for further evaluation (Figs. 10.4, 10.5, 10.6, and 10.7). The images can be emailed over a HIPAA (Health Insurance Portability and Accountability Act of 1996) compliant network, downloaded to a portable drive, or printed allowing the patient to critique them privately over time and allowing them to decide if they accept

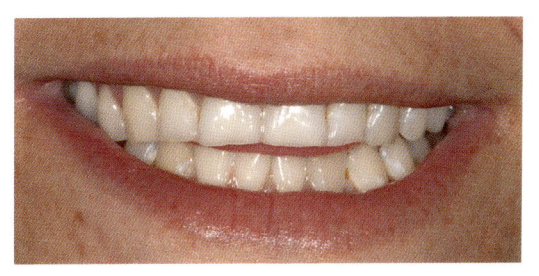

Fig. 10.4 Pre-op full smile close-up

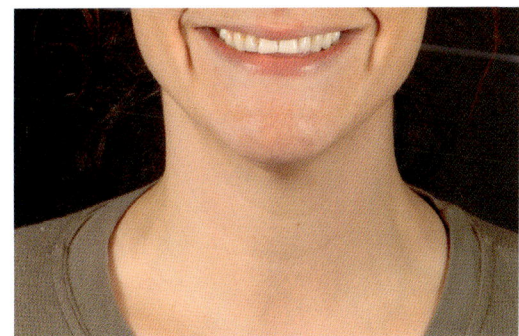

Fig. 10.5 Pre-op full smile

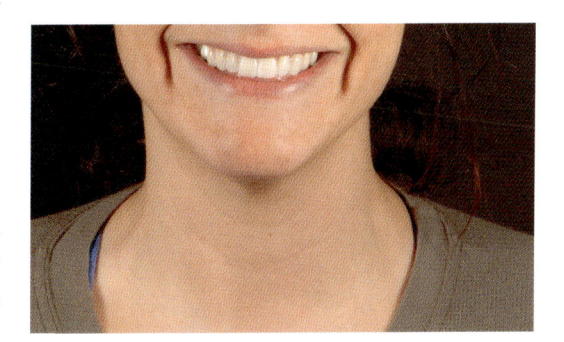

Fig. 10.6 Post-op full smile

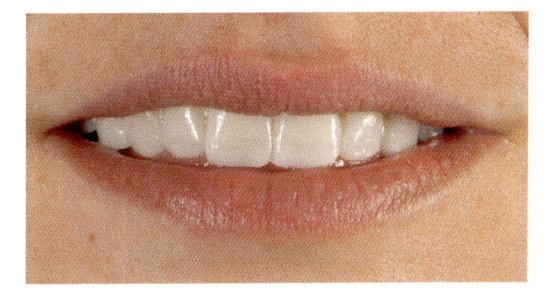

Fig. 10.7 Post-op full smile close-up

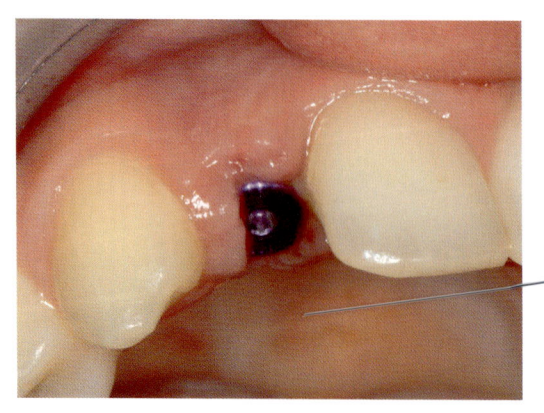

Fig. 10.8 Soft tissue profile

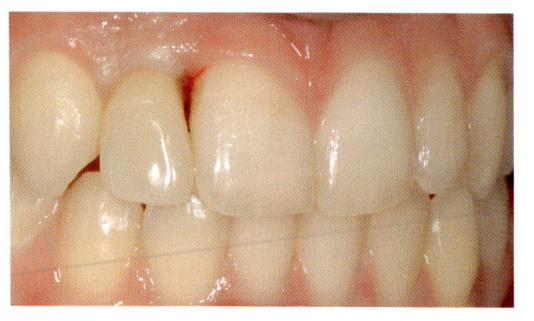

Fig. 10.9 Provisional restoration with soft tissue defect

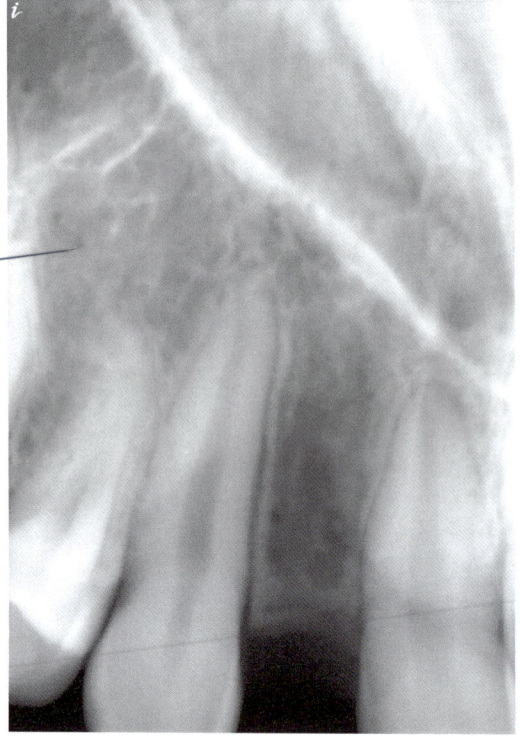

Fig. 10.10 Pre-operative x-ray

the proposed treatment. If the patient does not accept the proposed treatment, the mock-up is modified and the procedure is performed once again. Once the patient approves the proposed digital mock-up, the images are sent to the dental laboratory to aid the technician in the fabrication of the provisional and final restorations. This method allows the patient, doctor, and laboratory technician to have a clear goal for the final restorations.

10.1.4 Implant Restoration

In a case of a congenitally missing lateral incisor, digital photography played a significant role to communicate with the oral surgeon, laboratory technician, and patient during all aspects of the treatment. This image shows the patient shortly after she was released from the surgeon (Fig. 10.8). Note the amorphous gingival tissue. The immediate restorative goal is to fabricate a provisional restoration to aid in the development of a satisfactory soft tissue profile.

The initial provisional was inserted and the lack of the mesial papilla was noted (Fig. 10.9). The radiograph in Fig. 10.10 demonstrates sufficient interproximal bone, and the patient was seen for multiple visits over time to allow for adjustment to the contour of the provisional restoration so that the tissue can fully mature and the mesial papilla to stabilize. Digital images were taken at each visit to monitor the effects of the adjustments. Once the tissue stabilized, a final impression using a custom implant impression coping was made and the case photographed with shade tabs sent to the laboratory (Fig. 10.11).

The final restoration was tried in and photographed again, this time converting the image to black and white to evaluate the "value" of the restoration. The black and white image is an ideal method to evaluate value and is often used by the laboratory for making final shade adjustments (Figs. 10.12, 10.13, and 10.14).

This is a case at the 5-year mark showing good tissue stability and esthetics. This case will be photographed each year in order to monitor its progress (Fig. 10.15).

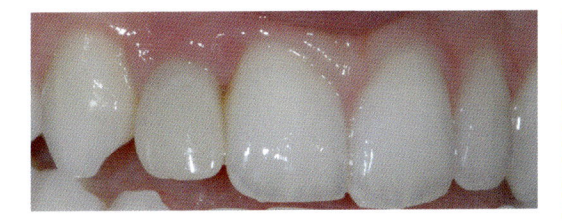

10   Digital Photography and Digital Asset Management

Fig. 10.11 Provisional restoration with final soft tissue contour

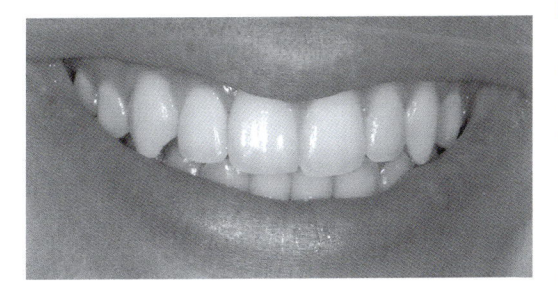

Fig. 10.12 Final restoration B&W

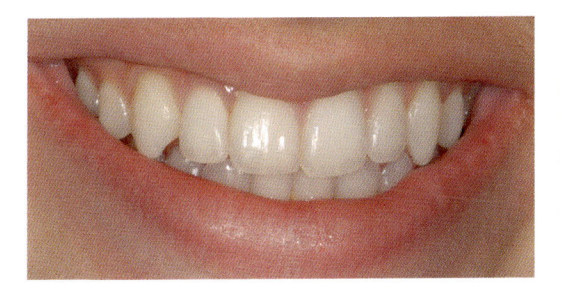

Fig. 10.13 Final restoration color

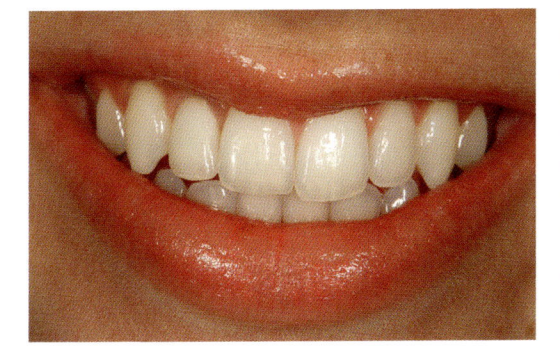

Fig. 10.14 Final restoration. Full smile "glamor shot"

10.1.5 Photography Basics

Below is a review of common photographic terms and their meanings. It is important that the reader fully understand them as well as how they affect the image. The absolute best way to learn photog-

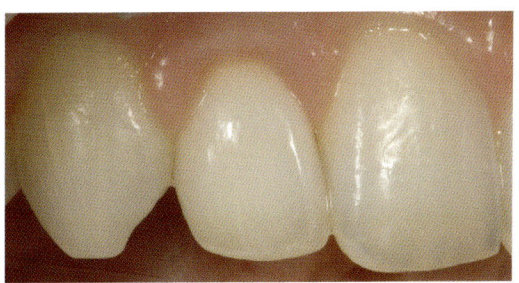

Fig. 10.15 Final restoration at five-years

raphy is to shoot images every day. Experiment and play with the gear, and in a short period of time, it will become second nature.

10.1.6 Exposure

Exposure refers to the brightness values in an image. An overexposed image appears bright and an underexposed image appears dark.

There are three parameters that affect exposure: shutter speed, aperture, and ISO sensitivity. Each parameter can be adjusted individually, however, they are codependent on each other. It is up to the photographer to determine what the "correct" exposure is and to dial in the settings to give them the desired results (Fig. 10.16a–c).

10.1.7 Shutter Speed

The shutter speed controls the amount of time the digital sensor is exposed to light. A fast shutter speed "freezes" motion, while a slow shutter speed will "blur" motion. A convenient rule to follow is to set the minimum shutter speed to 1/focal length of your lens. This will prevent "camera shake" and give you a sharp image. If you are shooting with a 100 mm lens, for example, the slowest shutter speed you would use is 1/100 of a second. In a clinical dental situation, 1/125–1/160 s will yield a very sharp image without the use of a tripod (Fig. 10.17).

10.1.8 Aperture

It is referred to by "f-stop" and corresponds to a specific opening in the lens; the larger the opening, the smaller the f-number (Figs. 10.18 and 10.19).

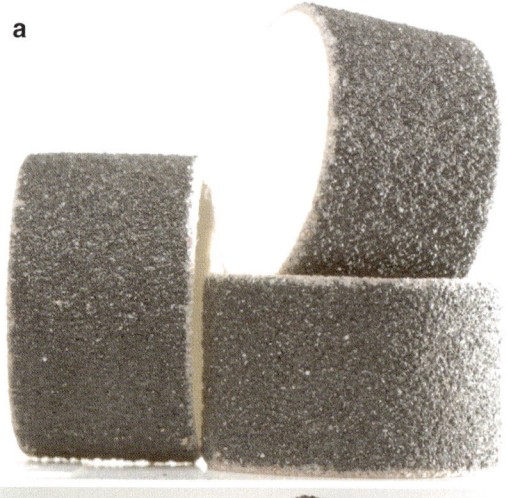

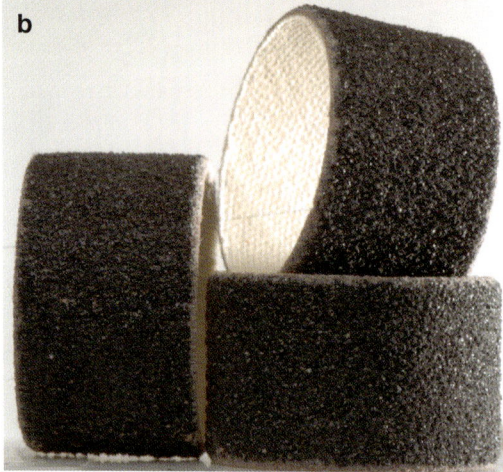

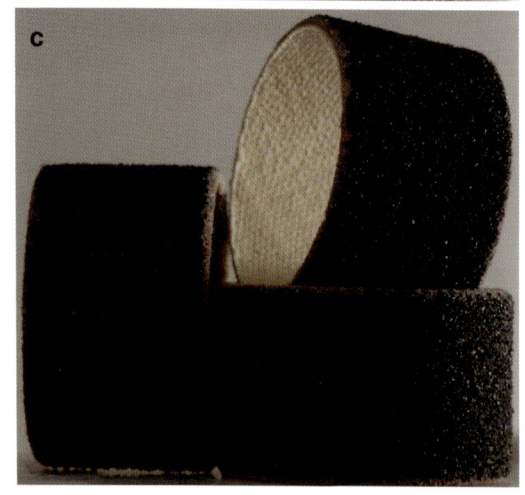

Fig. 10.16 Exposure variations

Fig. 10.17 Shutter speed

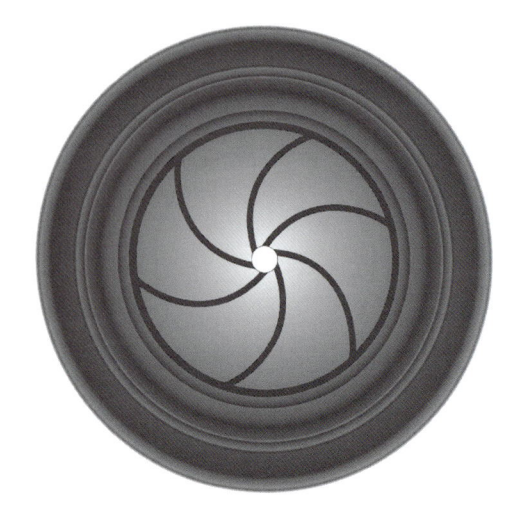

Fig. 10.18 Aperture

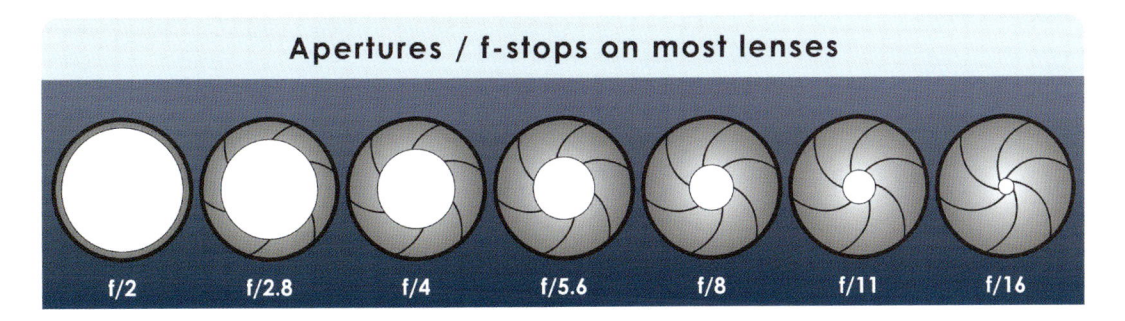

10 Digital Photography and Digital Asset Management

Fig. 10.19 Aperture

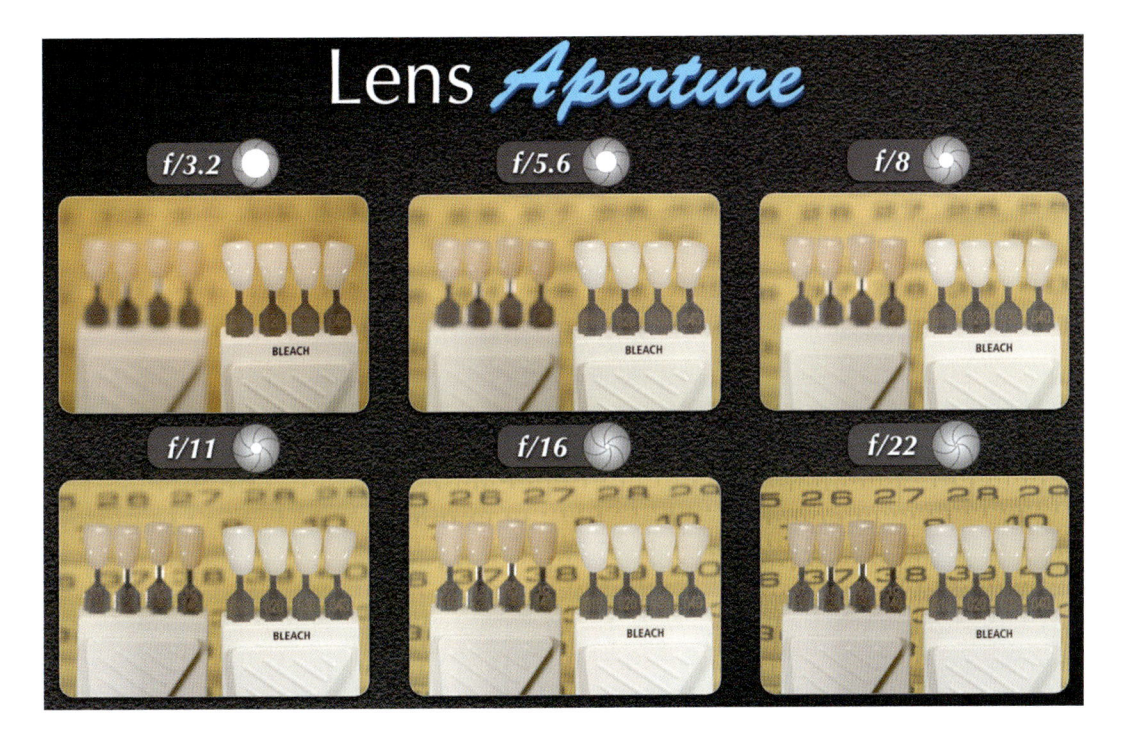

Fig. 10.20 Depth-of-field examples

The lens aperture controls the amount of light exposing the sensor. It also determines "depth of field" which is defined as what is in sharp focus from near to far. This inverse relationship of "f-stop" and the size of the lens opening are often confusing to the beginner photographer. Another way to think of this relationship is the higher the f-stop number, the greater the depth of field.

As shown in the below images of the two shade guides, as the f-stop number is increased so is the depth of field (Fig. 10.20). Note at f-22 both shade guides are in focus as well as the background. This is a good starting point for intraoral photography.

10.1.8.1 Depth of Field
Here's a similar example with a front view of a patient. At f-3.2 the centrals and laterals are the only teeth in focus. At f-22 all the teeth are in focus from the centrals to the molars (Fig. 10.21).

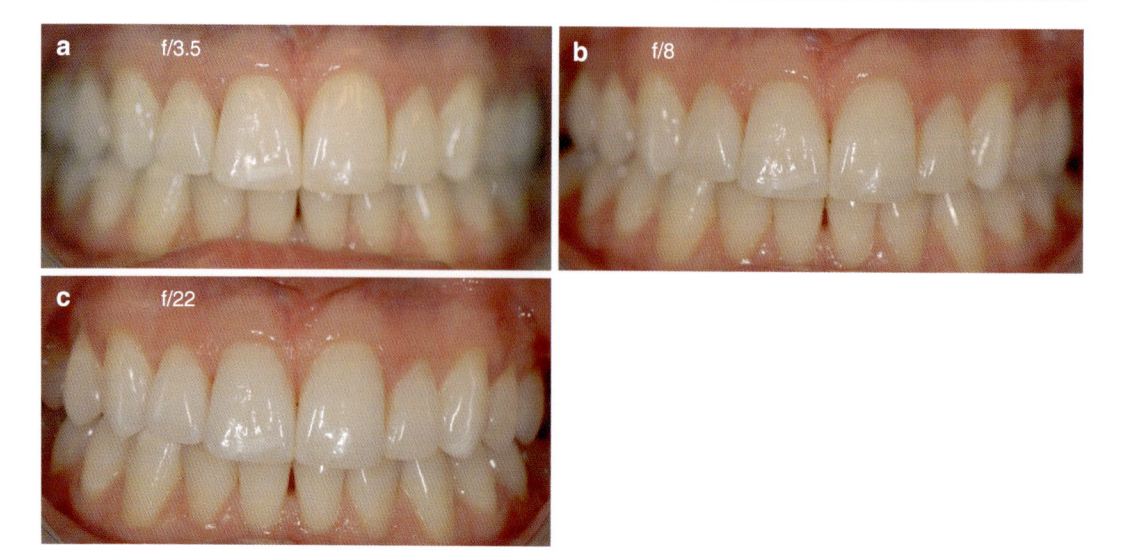

Fig. 10.21 Intraoral depth-of-field examples

Fig. 10.22 High ISO setting resulting in "digital noise"

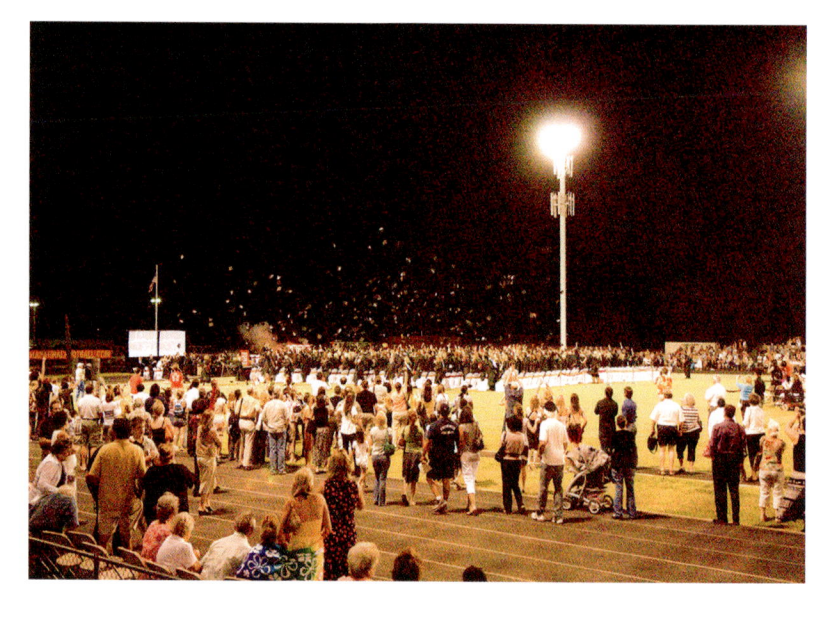

10.1.9 ISO

It is a term coined by the International Organization for Standardization, which determines the sensitivity of the camera's sensor to light. A low ISO number means more light is required to make a good exposure, while a high ISO number means less light is required to make a good exposure. The best quality image will come from a low ISO number since a high ISO number produces more "digital noise" which appears as randomly flecks of unwanted colors. It looks similar to grain found in photographs shot with film. Note the aberrant pixels in surrounding the light, referred to as "digital noise" (Fig. 10.22). Since a powerful flash will be used in clinical dental photography, the lowest ISO setting can be used (which is typically ISO100-200).

10.1.10 Light Meter

How does the camera know what settings to use for a particular image? When set on "auto," the camera's built-in light meter will aid in calculating a good exposure, which is based on a brightness

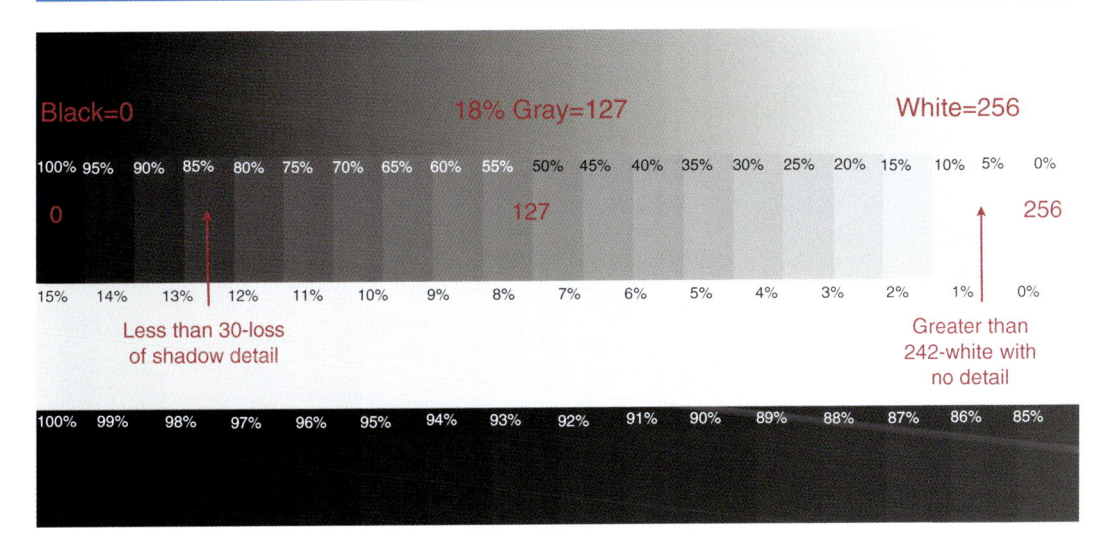

Fig. 10.23 Gray scale

value of 18% gray as shown below (Fig. 10.23). The calculation is done by evaluating the three variable settings (shutter speed, aperture, and ISO) which is commonly referred to as the "exposure triangle." Note that there is really no "correct" exposure since this is based on artistic interpretation and varies among photographers, however, for most images an 18% gray value will appear well exposed.

The abovementioned settings (shutter speed 1/125–1/160 s, aperture f-22, and ISO 200) are ideal for a typical dental intraoral image with a caveat, the use of a sophisticated flash system. Without a flash the exposure would be significantly underexposed (dark).

One of the best methods to learn the "exposure triangle" is to set one parameter to a fixed value (i.e., ISO) and vary the other two using the light meter as a guide to give you an 18% brightness value exposure.

10.1.11 Flash

A flash is used to add light to a subject and is necessary in dental photography. A point flash will give an image shadows and depth, whereas a ring flash will give the image a significantly flatter look. A point source flash is better suited for intraoral photography. A key feature in today's flashes is "through-the-lens" metering (TTL). A TTL flash will evaluate the camera exposure settings (shutter speed, aperture, ISO) and the ambient light and then compute a flash output to make an exposure based on 18% gray. This occurs in a fraction of a second and will keep your images consistently exposed at varying distances from the subject. Of course the flash can be used in the manual mode; however, it requires positioning the camera the same distance from the subject to keep the light output constant.

10.1.12 Focus Area Modes

Most DSLR cameras allow the user to set the focus area mode. This feature communicates with the camera's autofocus system and allows the user to choose and see exactly where the camera will focus through the camera's viewfinder. Typically, there will be a highlighted bracket or dot(s) showing the user where the camera is focusing. There are many different types of modes (e.g., Nikon uses three autofocus (AF) area modes – single-point AF, dynamic area AF, and auto area AF. For intraoral photography we will use the single-point AF mode and adjust it so that it is positioned on what we want in focus. In the example below, the camera was set to focus on the leading edge of the bur and then the trailing edge (Figs. 10.24 and 10.25). With a shallow depth of field, it is easy to see how focusing on different parts of the bur yields two different images. It is up to the photographer to decide what the final image should look like.

In portrait photography, set the camera to focus on the subject's eyes, and in intraoral photography, the focus point is set on the gingival margins or incisal edges of the teeth (Figs. 10.26 and 10.27).

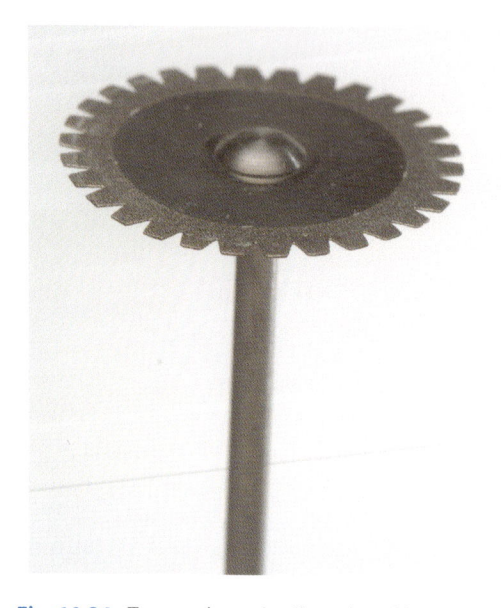

Fig. 10.24 Focus point on leading edge of bur

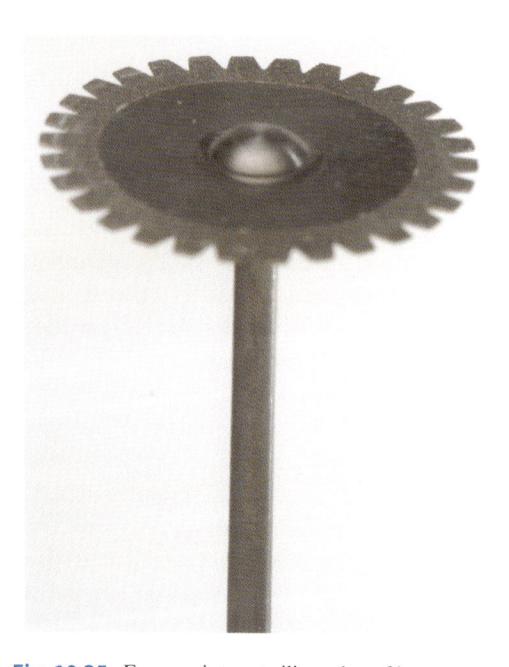

Fig. 10.25 Focus point on trailing edge of bur

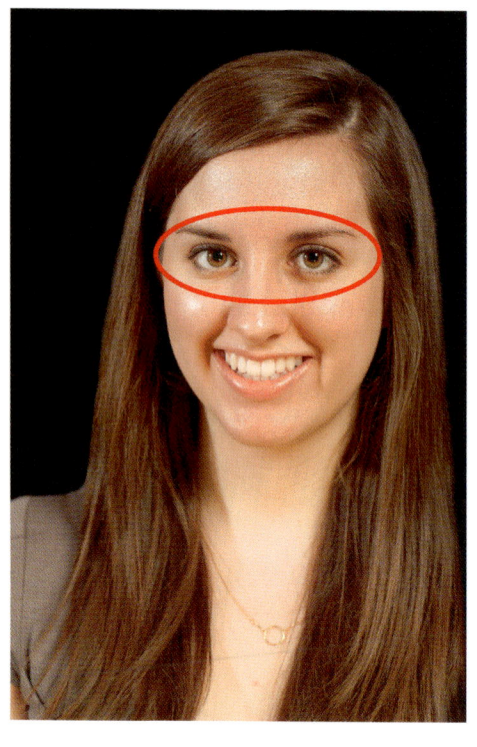

Fig. 10.26 Focus point on eyes

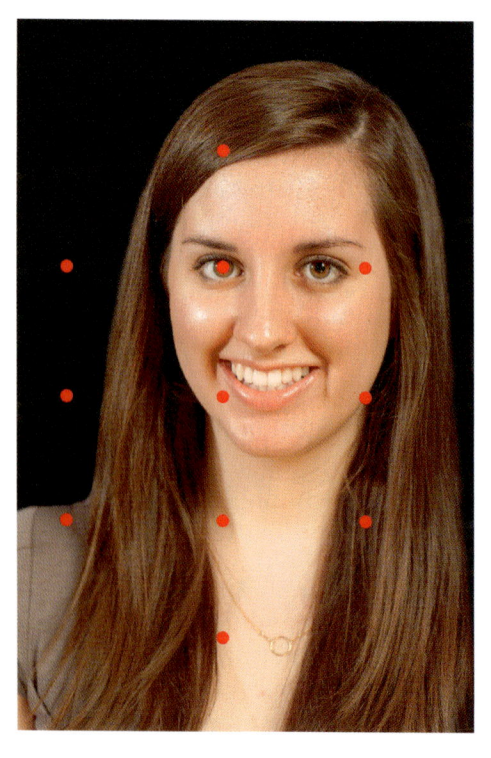

Fig. 10.27 Choice of focus points in camera display

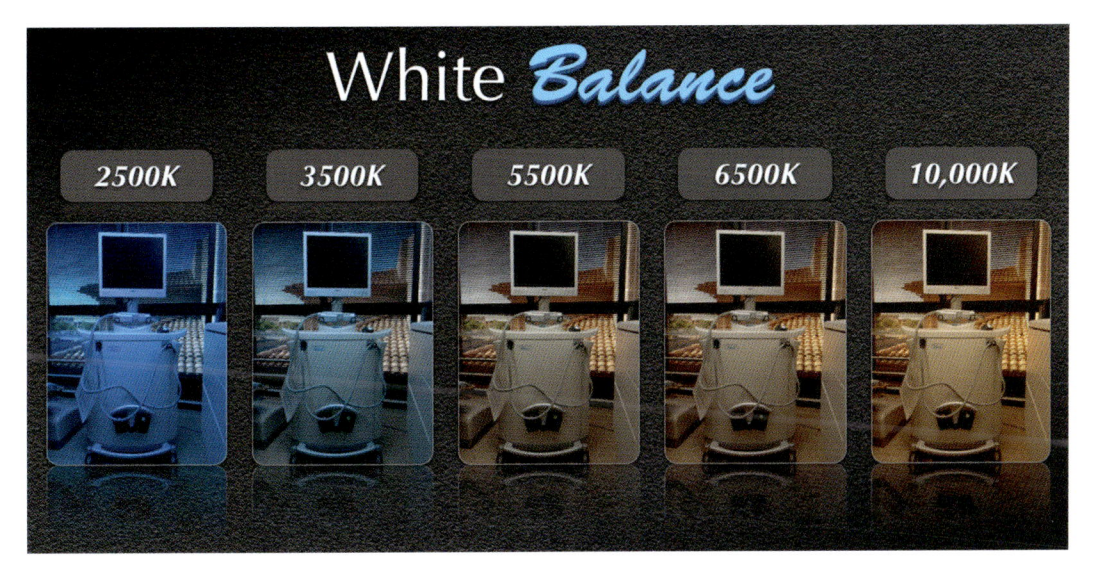

Fig. 10.28 Various white balance settings apply to the same RAW file. Note the shift in colors

10.1.13 White Balance

The human brain is very good at judging what is white under various light sources. Digital cameras cannot emulate the human brain and must be set to adjust color according to the lighting present. White balance (WB) is the process of removing unrealistic color casts, so that objects which appear white in person are rendered white in your photo. In the below example, the same image was assigned a different white balance (Fig. 10.28). Notice the color shift from blue (2,500 K) to yellow (10,000 K). Natural sunlight is around 5,500 K.

Since a flash is being used in the dental office with a known color temperature, the cameras' WB setting should be set to "flash."

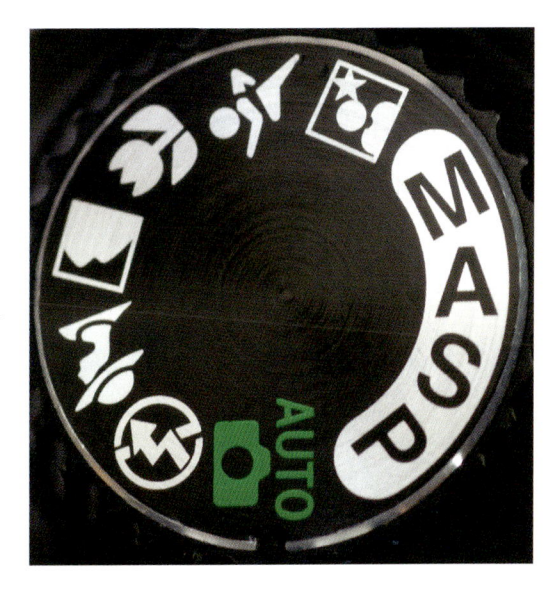

Fig. 10.29 Exposure modes

10.1.13.1 Exposure Modes

Exposure modes allow the user to set the camera up based on user preferences. As stated previously we are using the manual mode giving us full control over shutter speed, aperture, and ISO sensitivity (Fig. 10.29). Here's what the various modes do.

PROGRAM MODE
The camera adjusts both shutter speed and aperture; according to a built-in program.

SHUTTER PRIORITY
The photographer controls the shutter speed and the camera chooses the aperture for a good exposure.

APERTURE PRIORITY
The photographer chooses an f-stop and the camera chooses the shutter speed to achieve a good exposure.

MANUAL MODE

The photographer chooses both an f-stop and the shutter speed to achieve a good exposure. Note that a "good exposure" is based on 18% gray.

10.1.13.2 Image Formats

Various image formats are available for digital images with each one providing certain advantages and disadvantages. Below are the two most commonly used:

JPEG

JPEG Stands for "Joint Photographic Experts Group" and is an international standard for compressing digital photos. JPEG is a "lossy" compression algorithm that will keep the images small for easy file storage and transfer. Lossy compression means that data is actually discarded, decreasing the overall quality of the image. Every time a JPEG file is manipulated and "re-saved," the image will again be slightly degraded. Note that there are typically three types of JPEG compressions: large/fine, medium, and small/normal. The best one to use (having the least amount of compression) is large/fine.

JPEG Advantages: small file sizes and universal format

JPEG Disadvantages: compression (data loss) The solution to this issue is to shoot using the RAW file format. You can easily create a JPEG image from a RAW file without altering the RAW image.

10.1.13.3 RAW

A RAW format file is digital data before it's been processed in-camera.

Advantages

No compression – Highest quality possible

Can change processing afterwards (color tone, sharpening, etc.) without any data loss. Files will get "better" with age with improved postprocessing software algorithms.

Disadvantages

Large file size, more computer manipulation time.

Today, many dental organizations will only accept RAW images for case presentation for entry into their societies. This is due to the fact that a JPEG image can be manipulated without detection, whereas a RAW file cannot.

Why is a RAW file so good? The answer is "bit depth."

10.1.13.4 Bit Depth

Bit depth is the number of available colors present for each pixel, in terms of the number of 0s and 1s, or "bits," which are used to specify each color.

A color image is made up of three channels of color – red, green, and blue (RGB).

A standard JPEG image is an 8-bit image, which for RGB means three channels of 8-bit color. 8-bit information contains a range of 256 tones per channel. With three channels (RGB), we get $256 \times 256 \times 256 = 16.8$ million colors.

A RAW file contains three channels of 16-bit color with a staggering 65,536 tones per channel!

16-bit color offers a possible total of 281.4 trillion colors

$65,536 \times 65,536 \times 65,536 \times 65,536 = 281.4$ trillion colors

As you can see above, a RAW file contains so much data increasing its quality exponentially (Fig. 10.30).

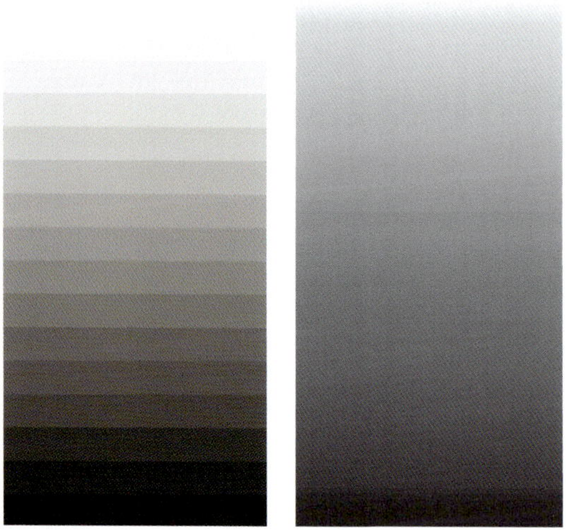

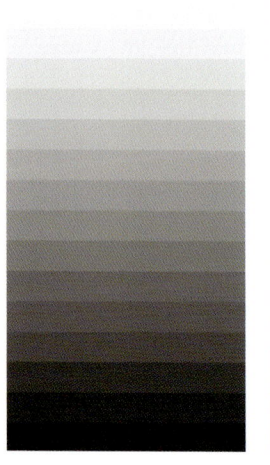

Fig. 10.30 8-bit vs 16-bit gradient scale

10.1.13.5 Intra Oral Camera Setting

Here are the settings for most intraoral images and the reasons why (in parenthesis):

- ISO – 100 or lowest setting (low noise)
- Shutter speed – 1/160 s (will prevent blurring from camera shake)
- Aperture – f-22 minimum (good depth of field for intraoral shots)
- White balance – flash (good color balance)
- Image quality – JPEG/high or RAW (good image quality)
- Flash setup – iTTL or manual (I prefer iTTL allowing the flash to determine the power output keeping my exposures more consistent)
- Exposure modes – manual (allows me to choose the shutter speed, f-stop, and ISO for maximum image quality)
- Focus mode (single focus point)

10.1.13.6 Color Space and Color Management

This is a very complex subject; however, what is necessary for the reader to understand regarding these subjects should be highlighted.

A "color space" describes the color capabilities of a particular device or file. Common color spaces today are Adobe sRGB, Adobe RGB, and ProPhoto RGB (Fig. 10.31). The color spaces shown below indicate what colors are able to be captured or displayed on a digital device. Note that Adobe sRGB is a smaller color space than ProPhoto color space, which means it has less "colors" available to capture or display. Most digital cameras come with the default setting to Adobe sRGB. If possible set the camera to the larger Adobe RGB color space allowing more colors to be captured by the digital sensor. Typically, sRGB is usually used for web designers, and Adobe RGB is most commonly used by professional photographers. Generally, choose the largest color space available for both your capture device (camera) and your software application (the chapter author uses Adobe Lightroom).

A calibrated monitor is crucial in a digital workflow. The colors you see on your monitor should match your digital file precisely. Most monitors brand new out of the box are not properly color calibrated. To calibrate your monitor, a colorimeter is required. This device measures color produced by software from numerically known values to the actual measured screen values. The difference between the screen values and known values is calculated, and a "color profile" is created, a data set that is stored in the computers' operating system and

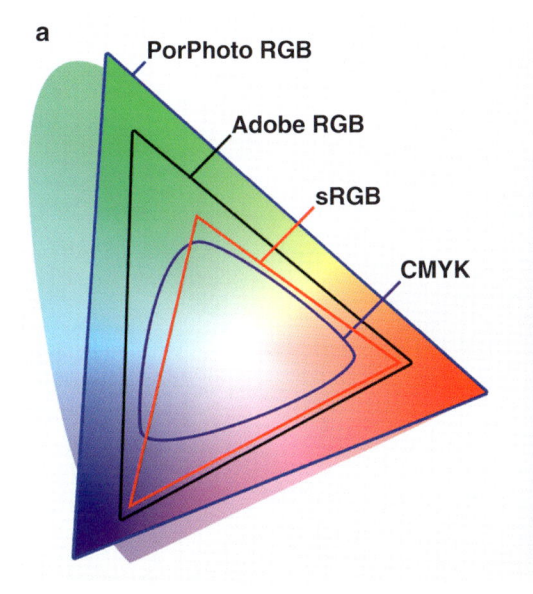

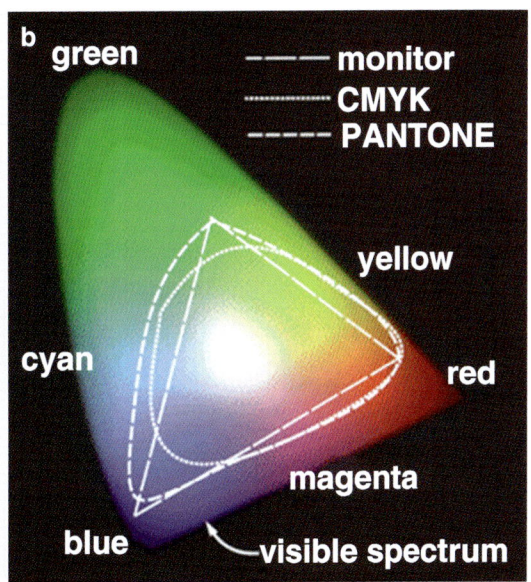

Fig. 10.31 Visible spectrum with various color spaces shown

used to keep the screen and know values the same (the author uses X-Rite's hardware and software). It is easy to do and only takes minutes per month to keep the monitor calibrated.

10.1.13.7 Digital Asset Management

Digital asset management (DAM) refers to the organization and workflow of digital images (called assets). DAM involves importing images into a computer, organizing them so they are easily found, and outputting selected images to various mediums in order to share them with a particular audience. A doctor may elect to email images of anterior veneer restorations captured during a try-in to their dental laboratory, enabling the technician to see how the case appears in the patient's mouth. Conversely, a doctor may want to output images of selected finished cases to an iPad or other electronic devices to show new patients' examples of their work. Other images may be used for marketing on a website or on social media. It is understood that this is only being performed with the patients' written consent and in a HIPAA compliant manner. Dental educators may want to gather and organize hundreds of images to present a particular case or technique to an audience at a dental meeting.

10.1.13.8 The Dilemma

There is a lot of confusion for many dental practitioners regarding how to manage digital images. Since digital photography is a relatively new field (digital SLR cameras became commonplace in 2002 with Nikon's introduction of the D100), most dentists are not trained as professional photographers, nor do they keep up with the most current advances in this area. Hence, many doctors are using dated software technology with limited workflow capabilities. As the demand for dental images increases daily, it is imperative for dental practitioners to be able to perform this task easily and efficiently.

Software bundled with many digital cameras is limited in features offered, and most do not allow for precise image organization and editing. Most are considered "browsers" which allow the user to browse the captured images and have limited output potential as well.

Even worse is trying to use proprietary dental management software (Dentrix, Softdent, MacPractice DDS etc.) with images captured from a digital camera. Dental management software packages do not function as browsers or image editors. They are not designed to store high-quality digital images in various file formats (such as TIFF and RAW), nor will they allow the doctor to find images easily. In addition, adding thousands of images into dental management software will significantly slow up the server. Imagine trying to find completed single tooth implant supported restorations; the doctor would have to recall the names of every patient treated with a single tooth implant! This would be a task not worth performing.

Software packages, such as Adobe Photoshop and Adobe Elements, are specifically designed for image editing and were not designed for browsing, sorting, and sharing images. They are great for creating unique layered images with complete, pixel-level control. They are fairly expensive and have a steep learning curve, which is too time-consuming for most dental practitioners to undertake; plus, the doctor would still require a browser to view the images.

Enter Lightroom (released February 19, 2007) and Apple's Aperture (released in 2005). Both programs are similar in the fact they are both browsers and image-editing software in a single package. The reason many chose Lightroom over Apple's Aperture is that Lightroom works on both Apple and PC platforms, whereas Apple's Aperture only works with Apple computers. In addition, as of 2014 Apple has stopped the future development of Aperture replacing it with the "Photos for OS X" app. When teaching digital photography workshops to dentists, a software that applies to both Apple and PC platforms is preferable.

Lightroom is a professional photography software package with features appealing to the most discerning professional photographer. Lightroom is this author's software of choice for the following reasons:

- Cross platform capabilities
- Designed by photographers for photographers
- Nondestructive editing
- Powerful cataloging and image-editing abilities

10   Digital Photography and Digital Asset Management

- Works with RAW, JPEG, TIFF, and PSD file types
- Output to email, web, slideshow, and print
- Can be used on multiple machines
- Complete digital asset management package; nothing else to buy
- Relatively inexpensive
- Moderate learning curve
- Easily output images to a multitude of devices and books
- Automate backups effortlessly

A key point to understand about Lightroom is that it is cataloging software. It does not physically import (move) images into the software. Images are downloaded from the compact flash card onto the users' hard drive to a predetermined location (e.g., a folder named dental images). Lightroom recognizes where the images are and builds a data catalog. The software never moves or alters the original images. The user can store them physically anywhere (internal or external hard drive). However, if the images are moved from their original location, Lightroom will not be able to find them until the user tells Lightroom the new location. This is a wonderful feature since the images are protected and preserved in their original state.

10.1.13.9   Lightroom Interface

The interface is divided into three main panels: The left panel shows the hard drive (where all the images are stored) and contains all the patient folders. The center panel is the main viewing window. When a particular patient folder in the left panel is selected, the main panel displays all of the images in that folder as thumbnails. The right panel contains data pertaining to an individual image (called metadata). Additional information (such as keywording, ratings, copyright info, etc.) can also be added to the image(s).

10.1.13.10   Lightroom Module Picker

The Lightroom modules are setup to follow a photographer's typical workflow:

Library module: Images are organized, sorted, and key-worded

Develop module: Nondestructive image manipulation

Map module: Images are tagged with GPS coordinates and shown on a map.

The remaining modules are for outputting images to their corresponding titles (Book, Slideshow, Print and Web).

10.1.13.11   Dental Digital Workflow

Importing Images

Images are transferred from the Compact Flash card and sorted into specific patient folders. Images can be stored on the main hard drive or an external drive. Clicking on a folder brings up all the images for that patient. The images can now be browsed and evaluated.

Selecting the "Best" Images

While browsing the images can be enlarged or compared side by side or in a group. Images can also be "flagged" which tags them as "selected" images to be used at a later date. They can also be arranged in any order the user chooses. Once all the best images are selected and flagged, Lightroom allows the user to view only the flagged images, showing only the best images for this particular patient.

Keywording

A huge challenge in managing numerous dental images is finding the exact one you're looking for right when you need it. The solution to this is keywording. Adding user-defined keywords to images makes finding them later on extremely simple. One or more keywords can be assigned to an image, and keywords can be added, removed, or changed in the future. For example, an image depicting a single tooth implant may have the following keywords: implant_single tooth, custom abutment_zirconia, and Straumann. Searching the keyword "implant_single tooth" will bring up every imaged tagged with that keyword. Multiple attributes can also be applied to a search: such as "custom abutment" and "flagged." This search would show the best custom abutment images, filtering out the undesired ones.

Metadata

Metadata means "data about data." It provides information about an image's content. For example, an image's EXIF metadata (exchangeable image file format) contains the file name, file dimensions, date and time information, camera settings, camera make and model, shutter speed, aperture, lens information, ISO settings, and many other parameters. Every digital image taken from every digital camera contains metadata. Lightroom allows the user to edit some of the metadata as well as search for particular items. For example, a doctor may want to view all the images taken on a certain day, or he may want to view every image taken with a particular camera. All of the metadata fields are searchable.

Additionally, the user can add metadata to an image. This may include the user's name, contact information, copyright status, labels, captions, etc. This is useful especially if images are to be given to a third party; they are now tagged with the owner's detailed contact information.

10.1.13.12 Develop

The develop module allows the user to modify the image nondestructively, meaning that any changes made to the image are reversible. With respect to the field of dentistry, the only changes that should be made to an image are global corrections (overall exposure, contrast, and cropping). Specific pixel-based modifications are not accepted for images that are to be used for publication or lecturing.

The main tools used are the crop/straighten and exposure tools. As with any image-editing software, starting with a well-exposed and composed image makes editing simple and quick. This means the doctor should have a good understanding of basic photography principles and know how to set the camera up properly avoid time consuming edits.

10.1.13.13 Output

Now that the best images are organized, selected, keyworded, and cropped, Lightroom allows the user to output the images to a multitude of ways. Collections can be made for a particular case or for a patient presentation or lecture. Think of a collection as a virtual digital scrapbook, containing just the best images you want to show. You may want a collection for a particular patient showing detailed images of the case from start to finish. Or you may want a collection for anterior implant cases. The possibilities are limitless. The collections can be shown as a slideshow, exported for email, printed, or even uploaded to a website, a Facebook page, or a portable tablet. The ability to output images to design and print a book is also possible. All of the above is possible regardless of the file type (RAW, TIFF, JPEG, etc.) due to Lightroom's ability to handle any current file type with ease.

Below is a collection of laboratory items made from selected images (Fig. 10.32).

10.1.13.14 Catalog Backup

Lightroom automatically backs up its catalog and the preview images of your actual images as you exit the program. It does not backup your original images (stored wherever you decide to store them) which should be automated daily using specific software for that purpose. It is recommended to utilize an external drive which is stored off-site from the dental office.

Please note the below advice before using any photo software:

- If your workflow is working for you, do not change it.
- Never experiment with your original data.
- Backup all data BEFORE upgrading or using new software.
- If you want to try a new workflow, do it with sample files and test folders.
- Download the trial version of a particular software and evaluate it before purchasing.
- Research online user comments and opinions.

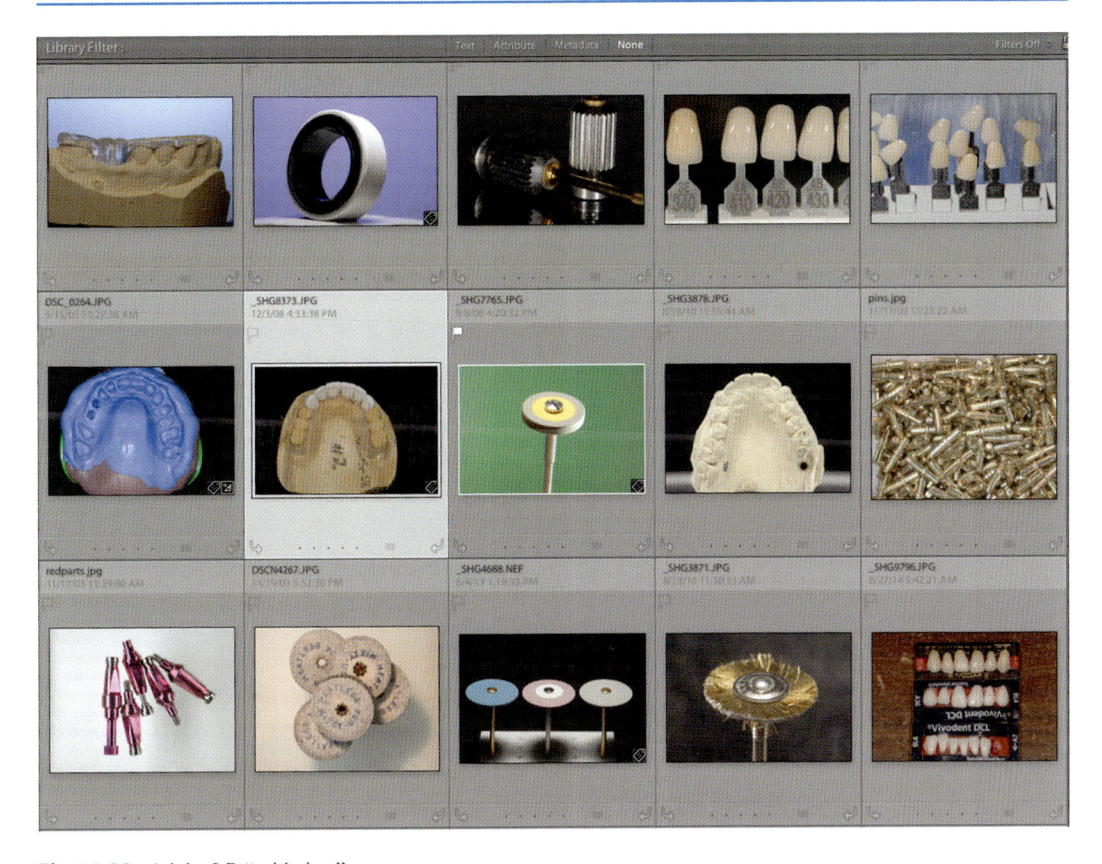

10 Digital Photography and Digital Asset Management

Fig. 10.32 Adobe LR "grid view"

References

Gürel G (2003) The science and art of porcelain laminate veneers. Quintessence

Magne P, Belser U (2002) Bonded porcelain restorations in the anterior dentition: a biomimetic approach. Quintessence, Chicago

Further Reading

McLaren, Edward A. Communicating digitally with the laboratory: design, impressions, shade, and the digital laboratory slip. Dental Ageis Jan/Feb 2011.Vol 7, Issue 1.

McLaren EA, Garber DA, Figueira J (2013) The photoshop smile design technique. (Part 1): digital dental photography. Compendium 34(10):772–779

Part II
Tissue Augmentation Considerations

Preservation of Alveolar Dimensions at the Time of Tooth Extraction

11

Robert A. Horowitz

Abstract

Our patients lose teeth due to advanced periodontal disease, endodontic issues, restorative problems, and trauma. The goal of the dental team that is treating the patient, should be to have the best procedures and materials used to maximize the functional and aesthetic benefits of each and every step of the process. From choosing the appropriate surgical technique to the proper materials will enable the regeneration of an ideal site with vital bone and covered with keratinized tissue. In this way an ideal implant can be placed to support a restoration which is easy to maintain in a clean and healthy state for the rest of the patient's lifetime. This chapter will demonstrate different surgical approaches and biomaterials to help the surgeon make the best educated choice to yield an optimal biologically based, cosmetic outcome. The reader will see clinical cases, histologic validation, and literature source to justify the treatment modalities shown. These are predictable and will assist you in the choices you must make on a daily basis.

The historical record of dental treatment goes back over 9,000 years (Coppa et al. 2006). The beginning of dentistry included drilling through bone to drain abscesses and rudimentary preparations for the use of beeswax and other materials for fillings. There have been mummies found with gold wire prosthetic replacement of missing teeth (Leek 1967). This is a testament to the fact that others have dealt with the issues facing the current dental teams. While our techniques, technologies, and materials have vastly improved, we still have one goal, which is to keep as many teeth for mastication, aesthetics, and lip support and to maintain alveolar stability.

Despite the best efforts of dentists and hygienists at diagnosis, maintenance, and treatment, not all of our patients' teeth are able to be maintained in optimal health and function for the duration of their lives (Hirschfeld and Wasserman 1978). Whether through periodontal disease, caries, or trauma, some or all of their teeth may be lost. The amount of destruction around them is determined by the type of disease process they have undergone, its duration, and the body's

R.A. Horowitz, DDS
2 Overhill Road, Suite 2,
Scarsdale, NY 10583, USA
e-mail: rahdds@gmail.com

response and potential ability to limit the spread of the destruction. The type of insult and exact location has an effect on the prognosis of the tooth. While dental heroics can save all teeth for some time, this may not be advised in all situations. Deep subgingival decay; vertical fractures; severe bone loss; perio-endodontic combined lesions of long-standing, progressive mobility; and other factors may give a questionable or hopeless prognosis to the involved tooth. Medical conditions may leave the patient systemically challenged so that they are not able to heal in the most appropriate manner after certain procedures. Anatomic limitations of proximity to nerves, sinus cavities, or adjacent teeth or implants may also limit the ability to save teeth. Patients need to have their options explained thoroughly so they can make the most informed decision related to the processes in front of them. There are numerous software programs and articles (Anson 2009) that can facilitate the discussions between the dental team members and the patient. Very often, when ideal therapy is proposed to the patient with digital photographs (Horowitz 2003), cone beam tomography, and articulated casts with diagnostic waxups, ideal therapy will be accepted (Fig. 11.1).

For many patients presenting with advanced dental disease, the optimal set of procedures begins with removal of a tooth and its eventual replacement with an implant-supported fixed restoration. There are numerous instruments and techniques that can be utilized to remove the entire tooth from the socket. The size, shape, and location of the roots (Simion et al. 2006a), the amount of root structure retaining the tooth in the socket, and the mobility of the tooth are determining factors in the decision tree the dentist goes through between consultation and completion of the procedure. The surgeon has to determine what the goals of any procedure are, whether it involves saving or removing and eventually replacing the tooth. Depending on the site, there may be a trade-off between hard and soft tissue-directed strategies. If all of the bony walls are intact, volume preservation may be all that is required. However, missing bony walls, high aesthetic demands, and local or systemic factors may tip the balance in favor of augmentation and attempting to increase either bone volume or keratinized tissue or both.

Starting with the end in site has directed human and animal research. The ultimate goals should be maximizing vital bone percentage in the socket (Fig. 11.2) and obtaining a wide

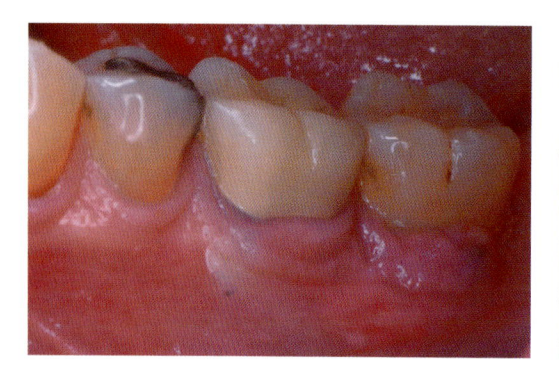

Fig. 11.1 This 82-year-old patient had a large facial infection around a tooth with unsuccessful treatment for a Class III furcation lesion

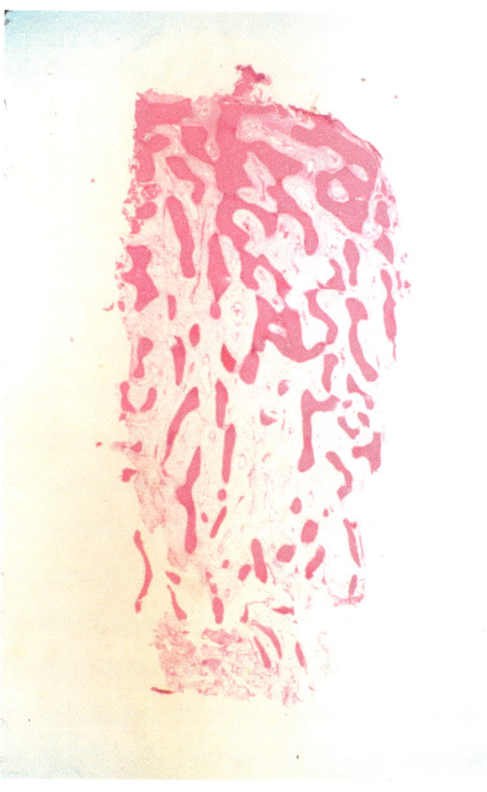

Fig. 11.2 Histologic core of regenerated bone 3 months after a dense PTFE barrier was placed over a blood clot in the extraction socket and removed after 3 weeks

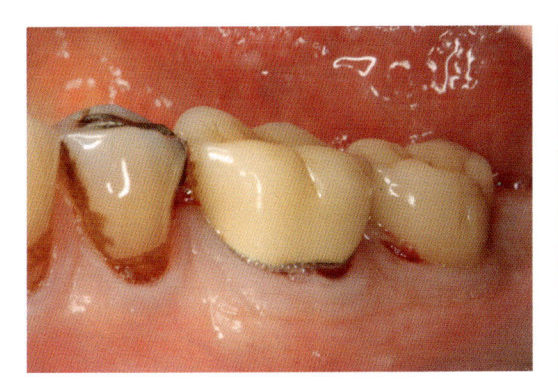

11 Preservation of Alveolar Dimensions at the Time of Tooth Extraction

Fig. 11.3 A clinical view of the same patient 13 years after implant restoration. The tissues are inflamed as at 94 years old, she was undergoing chemotherapy

alveolar ridge covered with sufficient keratinized tissue to enable ideal implant placement and restoration (Fig. 11.3).

11.1 Surgical Approach

Astute dentists have witnessed the results of site collapse. Patients will present with ill-fitting removable prostheses, narrow ridges under fixed prostheses, or where teeth have been lost in the past. Factors leading to this bone loss have been discussed in the dental literature for almost 50 years. The characterization of the location and extent of this bone loss began with researchers looking at patients and dried skull studies. Pietrokovski's group (Pietrokovski and Massler 1967) and others documented the consequences and extent of bone loss following single and multiple tooth extractions. In these publications, bone was predictably lost from the buccal plate primarily. The residual alveolar ridge was located both at a more apical level and further lingually than when the teeth were in place. Histologically, Carlsson et al. (1967) showed that resorption of the buccal plate took place in about 40 days in humans. During that time, new bone filled in most of the extraction socket itself. This left the residual alveolar process further lingual and apical than it would be for ideal support of a removable prosthesis. While these studies looked at the effects of bone resorption on final alveolar shape and position, they did not investigate the specific effects of the type of surgery on tooth removal (Fig. 11.4).

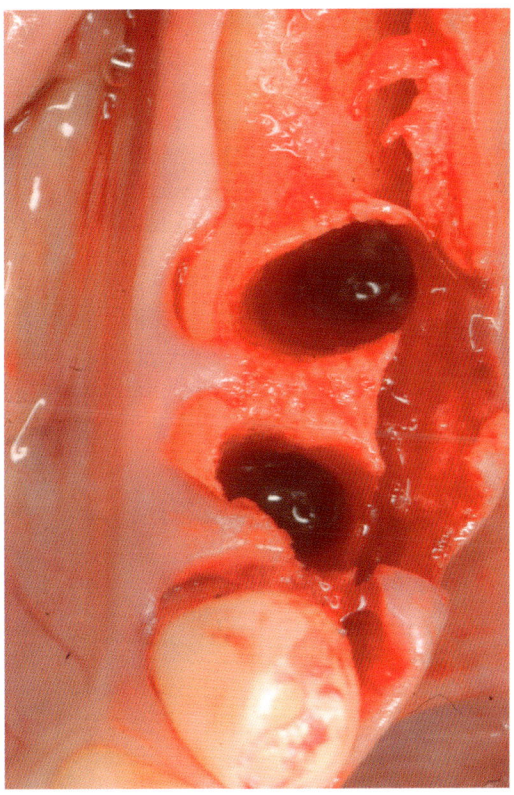

Fig. 11.4 Immediately after extraction, an occlusal view showing thin or absent buccal plates and site collapse in site #19 illustrating the need for bone regeneration

Flap elevation has been documented to result in bone loss when surgical procedures are performed around teeth. Moghaddas and Stahl (1980) showed that approximately 1 mm of bone is lost after raising a full-thickness flap around teeth during periodontal surgery. Fickl et al. (2008) in one of their many papers on the subject looked at the difference between raising full- and partial-thickness flaps around teeth. Notches were made in the facial root surfaces of teeth after one or the other type of flap was elevated. The flaps were repositioned, and the area was investigated by block section retrieval and histologic analysis 4 months later. One result they noticed was that there was significant variability between sites in the same dog. The standard deviation related to the amount of bone loss was less for the partial- than full-thickness flaps. All sites lost bone in both vertical and horizontal dimensions, which is in agreement with other studies done before and after this one. They concluded that around teeth, any flap elevation will result in bone remodeling with more bone loss noticed when a full-thickness flap is elevated.

When a trained surgeon becomes involved in that process, both the alveolar bone and gingival tissues can be preserved. Modified by the skill and experience of the surgeon are the basic procedures called "atraumatic extraction" (Horowitz and Mazor 2010). Proper use of the techniques and materials described later in this chapter will assist healing to obtain ideal physical and biologic results. If these are not employed, more extensive surgical manipulations are required to regain what has been lost. In those instances, alveolar bone and, when possible, keratinized gingiva must be augmented for the patient's return to proper form and function (Fig. 11.5).

Fickl et al. (2008) and their group have looked at numerous aspects of the effects of the type of surgical approach on healing after extraction in dogs. They showed significantly more loss of bone after tooth extraction when surgical flaps were elevated than if a nonsurgical approach was taken. There was approximately 2 mm of bone loss from the coronal portion of the buccal crest when no graft material was placed. With no bone grafting and elevation of a buccal flap, about 2.5 mm of bone was lost coronally. At the same time, for the same two groups, 1.5 and 2 mm of bone, respectively, were lost at the apical portion of the buccal plate. The use of an anorganic bovine bone mineral in a collagen matrix minimally changed the results. The nonsurgical group filled with that graft material and closed with a gingival graft had 1.2–1.4 mm of bone loss along the whole buccal plate. The group grafted in the same manner but where flaps were repositioned exhibited 1.9–2 mm of buccal and 0.4 mm of lingual bone resorption. These results and those of other studies clearly indicate that whenever possible, tooth extraction should be performed without the elevation of mucoperiosteal flaps.

Atraumatic extraction incorporates a set of techniques and instruments to remove the affected tooth or root from the socket with minimal disruption of the cribriform plates and surrounding periodontal tissues (Horowitz and Mazor 2010). The primary goal is to use thin-bladed manual or "powered" instruments to increase the size of the periodontal ligament space. Using periotomes, thin-bladed elevators, and ultrasonic bone surgery instruments or rotary burs helps to increase the mobility of the root(s) to be extracted (Fig. 11.6). Multi-rooted teeth are usually sectioned to facilitate rotation of individual roots. After thorough debridement with hand instruments, appropriate bone replacement graft and/or barrier materials are used to restore

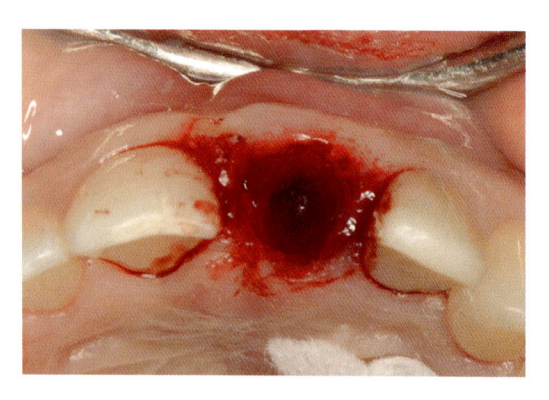

Fig. 11.5 Intact alveolar plates and gingiva after atraumatic extraction

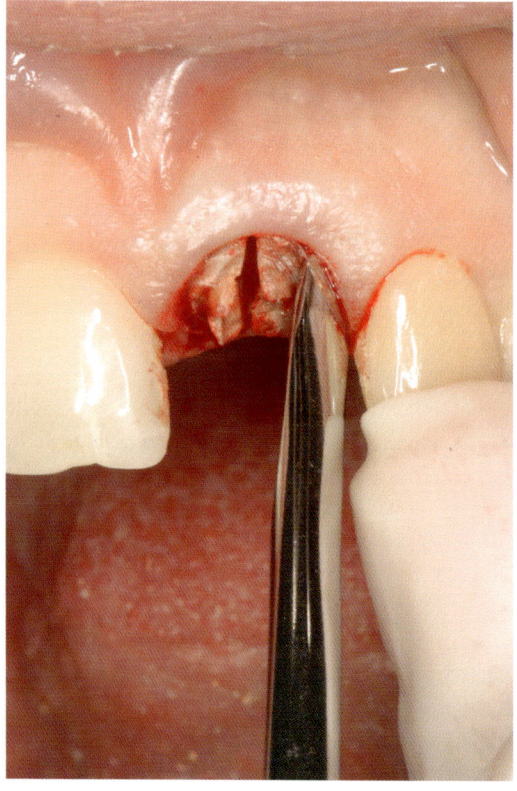

Fig. 11.6 A non-vital maxillary central incisor is sectioned vertically and extracted with periotomes and a straight elevator

both the missing volume of alveolar bone and, when possible, to maximize the amount of vital bone in the treated socket. These techniques were shown in this paper to result in all of the stated goals met using a combination of nanoparticle-sized calcium sulfate (Nanogen, Orthogen, Springfield, NJ, www.orthogencorp.com) and a dense PTFE barrier (Cytoplast TXT, Osteogenics, Lubbock, TX, www.osteogenics.com).

11.2 Socket Filling Materials

Studies in both animals and humans have given greater knowledge to the effects of protective/regenerative techniques and the processes related to the after effects of removal of teeth. Starting with research done by Amler et al. (1960) at NYU, it was shown that an extraction socket that was neither grafted nor barrier protected would fill with vital bone in a few months' time. Knowing that leaving a socket untreated would lead to the patient losing bone in all dimensions gave researchers interesting opportunities. Adding Amler's work to that of Fickl and others led to testing different types of bone replacement graft materials and barriers to see the effect on either the physical loss of bone volume or the biologic regeneration of vital bone inside the socket or both. Iasella et al. (2003) looked at the differences between no therapy and placement of a mineralized allograft in the socket with a collagen barrier over it. Horizontally, the nontreatment group lost 2.7 mm (about 1/3 of the initial width), and the grafted group lost 1.2 mm (1/7th of the original horizontal dimensions). While there was a loss in vertical height of 0.9 mm in the untreated group, there was a gain in vertical height of 1.3 mm in the patients who underwent ridge preservation. The other difference was in the amount of vital bone in the sockets. The grafted sites had only 28% vital bone and 37% residual graft compared to 54% vital bone in the ungrafted sockets. Similar results were obtained by Barone and coworkers (2008) in their research. Their group found significantly less vital bone in the untreated sites (only 26%); they found 35% vital bone and 29% residual graft in all treated sites. These patients also had more resorption in all dimensions than in the Iasella study. There were 2.5 mm horizontal and 0.7 mm vertical bone loss in the grafted sites and 4.3 mm buccolingual and 3.6 mm of vertical loss on the buccal side in the control, non-treated extraction sockets.

Sottosanti (1997) and Anson (2002) showed that a combination of demineralized freeze-dried bone allograft mixed with 20% calcium sulfate formed bone, preserving alveolar ridge dimensions which were suitable for the delayed insertion of endosseous dental implants. More exhaustive analysis on these materials was performed by Vance and his group (2004). This group compared the grafting of extraction sockets with anorganic bovine bone and a collagen barrier to DFDBA/CS in a putty carrier with a calcium sulfate barrier. While both sets of treated sockets lost only 0.5 mm width, there was a 1 mm difference between the moderate height gain of the bovine-grafted sights and a slight loss in the putty- and calcium sulfate barrier-treated ones. The biggest difference between the treated sites was in the histologic comparison. The bovine bone-grafted sockets had 26% vital bone and 16% residual graft compared to 61% vital bone and only 3% residual graft materials in the putty-/CS-treated sockets. This could potentially lead to a decrease in bone to implant contact in the ABBM sites, especially in the early healing period. Surgeons as well as restorative dentists should be aware of these results as it may impact the time between placement and loading of implants in sites treated with different graft materials.

While extractions are frequently done in areas with no active purulent exudate, we surgeons are often called upon to perform similar procedures in the presence of either chronic or acute infection. The presence of this acidic material at a pH of 6.68 (Nekoofer et al. 2009) can affect bone metabolism. When there is a nutritional imbalance in the pH relating to an acidic condition (Bushinsky 2001; Arnett 2003), other sequelae are seen. This leads to an increase in osteoclastic bone resorption and decreased bone formation by osteoblasts. There is little literature describing studies or even case reports where bone regenerative graft materials were inserted at the time of extracting teeth with active infection. In one paper, autologous platelet-rich fibrin was placed in the socket and the shape protected using titanium mesh barriers (Kfir et al. 2007). The most frequent complication in these patients was an almost 50% exposure rate of the barrier. Only 8 of the 15 patients in the study received implants without additional bone grafting procedures.

Wang and coworkers (2004) wrote a technique paper on tooth extraction, detailing the steps for atraumatic extraction and socket grafting. In the abstract, they mentioned (without citing literature) that infected sites should not be grafted but later in the paper described how to stimulate bleeding in the socket after aggressive curettage of the apical and lateral portions of the socket. In contrast to this statement, a paper by Crespi et al. (2010) in which 30 patients had dental implants placed in new extraction sockets and prosthetically loaded. One half of the sites demonstrated initial periapical radiolucencies but no suppuration, fistula, or pain. The success rate of these implants 2 years after placement was 100% as it was in the other sockets with no PAP, showing no affect from the infection. Also of concern is treatment of a site adjacent to a tooth that has a periapical infection. Sussman (2004) reported a case where an implant was lost due to infection from an adjacent tooth. In this case, the infection traveled through the mandible leading to infection and the need to replace the implant and tooth. What these articles demonstrate is the potential for infected material to lead to a deleterious outcome of the surgery. If the tissues are handled properly and all infected tissue is removed, there should be just as high a success rate no matter the clinical presentation of the apical tissue when the tooth is removed.

This patient presented in the middle of chemotherapy treatments. There was a large facial abscess on tooth #10. Upon medical clearance, the tooth was extracted and socket debrided leaving a large facial fenestration (Fig. 11.7). In an attempt to maximize the patient's healing potential, the site was filled with a combination of demineralized freeze-dried bone allograft (Surgical Esthetics, Beverly Hills, CA) hydrated in PRF (IntraSpin, Boca Raton, FL) (Fig. 11.8). A biphasic calcium sulfate (3D Bond, Augma Biomaterials, Israel) was added to improve biologic and physical handling characteristics of the graft (Fig. 11.9). For containment and biologic activity, the graft was covered in its entirety

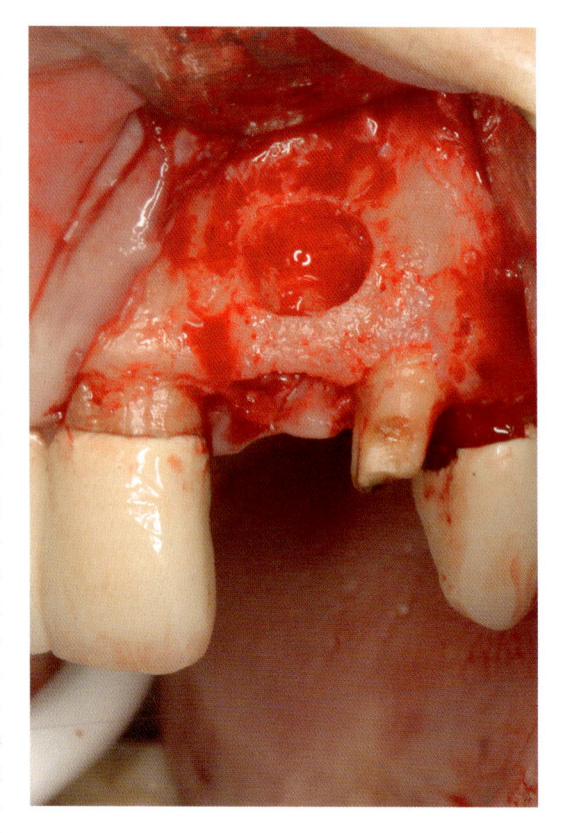

Fig. 11.7 Facial flap elevated to enable debridement after extraction of tooth #10

with an amnion/chorion membrane (BioXclude, Snoasis, Denver, CO, www.snoasismedical.com) (Fig. 11.10) and then PRF membranes and the flaps closed. Three months later, the bone had healed sufficiently to enable the placement of a dental implant in ideal location and orientation (Fig. 11.11). The site was restored with a cementable crown on a custom abutment 4 months later (Fig. 11.12). Histologic evaluation of a retrieved bone core demonstrated significant amounts of vital bone formed (58%) and re-ossification of the demineralized bone graft particles as evidenced by nodules of mineralization (Fig. 11.13). Other studies on this combination of materials have shown a vital bone in extraction socket healing than have been shown with other biomaterials used in similar defects. With the systemic factors and significant amount of total bone loss in this patient, the amount of vital bone regenerated in this site in such a short time period is considered highly successful, especially

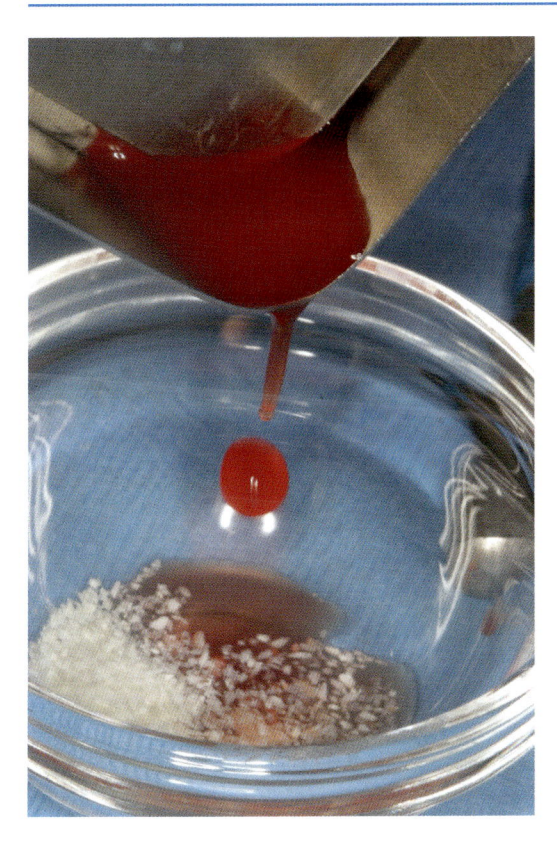

Fig. 11.8 Demineralized freeze-dried bone allograft hydrated in the liquid expressed from fabrication of PRF barrier membranes

compared to other bone replacement graft materials (Iasella et al. 2003; Barone et al. 2008).

An increase in the number and types of bone replacement grafting biomaterials has led to expansion on the bone grafting research performed by Sottosanti, Anson, and others. Multiple sources for xenografts and many types of synthetic grafting materials have been investigated. Their development has been spurred on because there are countries where certain bone replacement graft products, because of their place or species of origin, are not approved by their governing bodies, for sale, and human use. One study recently compared anorganic bovine bone mineral and beta tricalcium phosphate (β TCP) to a blood clot alone in a dog model (Artzi et al. 2004). Healed sites in the alveolus of dogs were prepared with 4 × 5 mm round defects. The sites were either filled with ABBM, β TCP, or a blood clot. Half of the areas were covered with a colla-

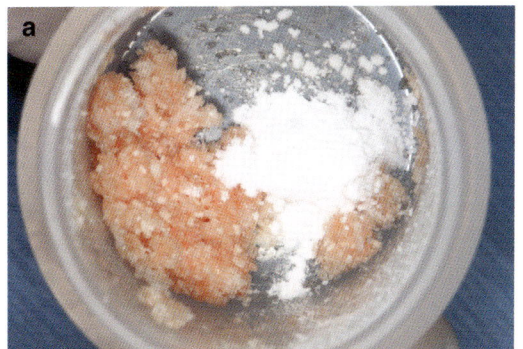

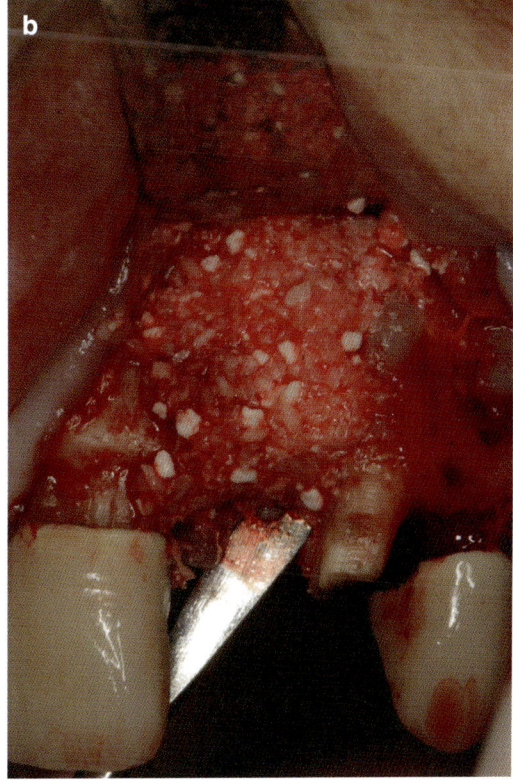

Fig. 11.9 Biphasic calcium sulfate (**a**) mixed with demineralized, freeze-dried allograft used to fill entire defect (**b**)

gen barrier; the others left to heal with the periosteum on top of the treated sites. At 3 months healing time (the equivalent of approximately 9 months in humans), the ABBM sites were filled mostly with bone graft material, vital bone primarily near the edges of the defects. At 6 months, there were minimal numbers of osteoclasts. They were seldom seen near the graft particles, and graft resorption was not typically found. There

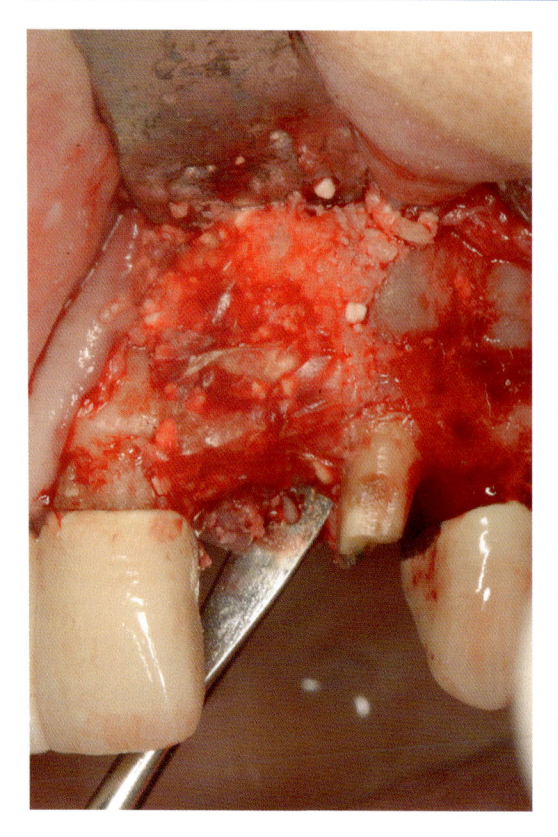

Fig. 11.10 Amnion/chorion barrier membrane placed to enhance bone formation in the regenerating site then covered with two layers of PRF barrier

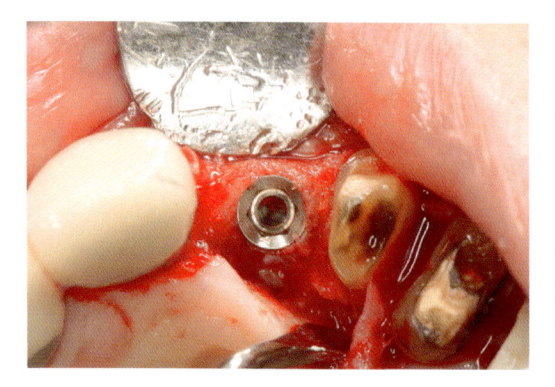

Fig. 11.11 Implant placed 4 months after extraction in dense bone filling the entire site

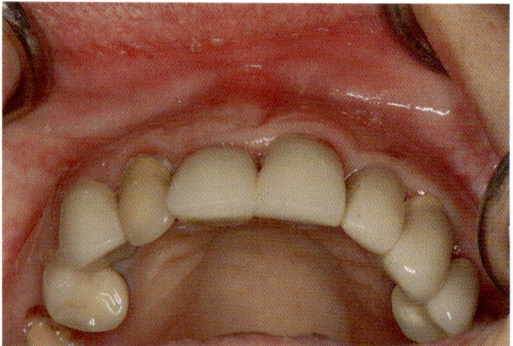

Fig. 11.12 Clinical view of site 2 years after restoration demonstrating healthy, keratinized gingiva

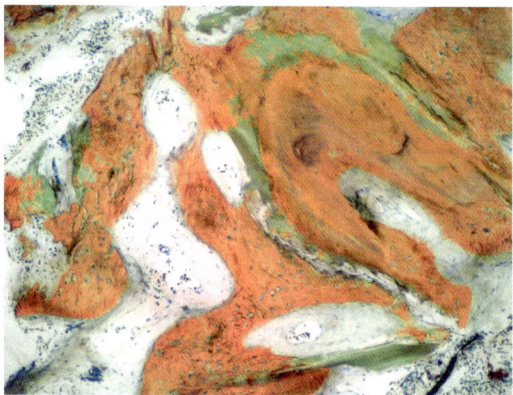

Fig. 11.13 Vital bone formed in socket – 48% bone, 78% vital, 22% residual graft

was new vital bone seen in the β TCP-grafted sites, primarily at the periphery around the graft particles. More vital bone, especially near the surface, was seen in the membrane-protected defects. By 6 months, the β TCP-grafted sites were filled almost completely with new bone. The untreated sites had a significant amount of connective tissue coronally. That amount decreased over time as more vital bone was formed. The results of this and related studies have spurred research into other types of barrier materials to be placed at the time of tooth removal.

Another material placed in extraction sockets is titanium. There are many case reports and longitudinal studies in both humans and animals showing successful restoration of immediate socket dental implants. On the other hand, there are few human histologic studies showing bone-to-implant contact and precise measurements of the alveolar socket changes after immediate socket implantation. The human study by Botticelli et al. (2004) demonstrated some bone fill in the gaps around immediate socket implants. However, their close examination of the data led them to the conclusion that there was "substantial bone resorption from the outside of the ridge" on both the buccal and lingual surfaces. There was vertical loss of bone of 0.3–0.6 mm on average, 30% resorption of the lingual or palatal bone, and 56% width reduction in the alveolar width due to resorption from the buccal.

These results were further validated by a study performed by Vignoletti et al. (2012). After flap elevation and root removal, immediate socket implants were placed in some sockets in dogs, while others were left untreated. There was significant buccal resorption in all sites. The authors concluded that placement of an implant at the time of extraction in the manner studied not only did not preserve the socket dimensions, but there was greater resorption in the immediate socket sites. Ongoing studies of different surgical techniques, graft, and/or barrier combinations have been performed in animals and humans with varying degrees of clinical and histologic success related to ridge preservation, bone-to-implant contact, or bone fill in the "gap." Additionally, many studies look critically at the aesthetic results of these procedures, sometimes combined with restorative therapy (Tarnow et al. 2014).

11.2.1 Barriers

The use of bioexclusive barriers began with correction of areas where the processes of site collapse had occurred. Techniques to regrow the hard and soft tissues around teeth or in place of lost teeth came out of the work of Nyman et al. (1982) and Buser et al. (1990). Nyman and his colleagues treated recession defects in periodontally involved teeth. After surgical flap elevation and debridement of the involved surfaces, a Millipore filter was placed over the defect and then the mucoperiosteal flaps were mobilized to cover it. In this manner, selective nutrient penetration was enabled to the surface of the tooth to be treated. Additionally, cells from the periodontal ligament were able to migrate coronally. This enabled specific cell repopulation of the defect with those cells that would assist in the formation of a new periodontal ligament. This experiment proved that formation of a stable wound, protected by a material that would enable only certain cells to grow underneath it, could be used to improve the health of teeth that had lost bone and gingival support. Buser et al. (1990) removed bone from the mandible of dogs. After healing, that area was covered with an expanded polytetrafluoroethylene (ePTFE) barrier and the space underneath it filled with blood. When the area healed again, it was filled with alveolar bone. Numerous other studies by other teams of researchers have documented different combinations of surgical techniques, graft, and barrier materials all becoming part of guided tissue regeneration.

Studies by Machtei (2001), Simion et al. (1994), and others showed significant complications with healing in periodontal and implant-related defects when ePTFE barriers became exposed during the healing period. Becker showed more threads remaining exposed in an immediate socket implant study when ePTFE barriers were removed earlier than planned due to exposure, infection, or other causes (Becker et al. 1994). One way to avoid these issues is using a different barrier formulation that is completely nonporous. Dense PTFE has been used to assist in both preservation of alveolar ridge width and formation of vital bone in extraction sockets for almost 20 years (Horowitz 2005; Bartee 1995; Hoffman et al. 2008). This material is inserted at the time of extraction over a blood clot alone or a bone replacement graft material in the socket. At approximately 3 weeks postoperatively, with no anesthesia and no surgery, the barrier is removed. At that time the epithelium begins to migrate over the socket adding more keratinized tissue to the biologic processes that are being protected underneath.

Infection and a Class III furcation involvement led to the extraction of tooth #18 in the 81-year-old patient shown earlier (Figs. 11.1 and 11.2). The insertion of a dense PTFE barrier was accomplished without elevating flaps more than the 2 mm needed to tuck this material under the coronal portion of the soft tissue (Fig. 11.14). As shown in Figs. 11.1 and 11.2 from this same patient, the alveolar ridge width and keratinized tissue were preserved quite well enabling the outstanding aesthetic outcome shown in Fig. 11.4. This verifies Buser's research in humans proving that protecting a blood clot in an intra-alveolar lesion with a dense PTFE barrier will enable that defect to completely fill with vital bone. Interestingly, in humans, this process only requires approximately 3 months depending on the buccolingual and mesiodistal widths of the defect. The presence or absence of buccal and lingual plates will also affect the ingrowth of vasculature into the fibrin clot and the proximity of osteoblasts to migrate into the area.

Resorbable barriers have the ability to address some of the concerns related to exposure during early time periods. By being eliminated from the body after recession of the soft tissue over the wound site, there is less of a chance of infection but the ability for graft to wash out and bacteria, food, or quicker migrating connective tissue or epithelial cells to gain access to the site. There is also no need to remove them postoperatively, and there is usually less inflammation due to better tissue compatibility. A study with ePTFE and a glycosylated collagen barrier over deproteinated bone graft particles showed equivalent amounts of vital bone, residual graft, and collagen in humans (Friedmann et al. 2002). Another study with the same membrane showed other interesting characteristics (Zubery et al. 2007). Compared to a conventional porcine collagen membrane, the study membrane ossified adding more volume to the alveolar ridge. Additionally, whereas the standard membrane exhibited variable degradation, the novel membrane consistently remained intact for 18–24 weeks. A longer time of maintained barrier function should enable more predictable volume preservation and vital bone formation either over an extraction or an alveolar ridge defect.

A synthetic resorbable barrier has migrated from the periodontal arena to the extraction/implant side of the surgical armamentarium. Guidor (Guidor®, Sunstar Americas, Inc., www.guidor.com) bioresorbable matrix barrier is made of a polylactic acid with a unique three-dimensional scaffolded design (Rosen and Rosen 2013). With its two perforated layers (Fig. 11.15), many of the criteria for an ideal guided

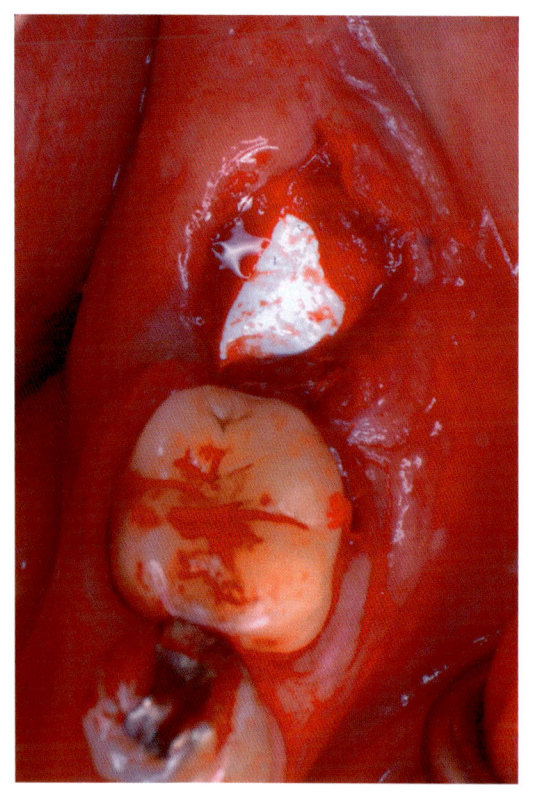

Fig. 11.14 Insertion of dense PTFE barrier over a blood clot in socket 18 from patient shown in Figs. 11.1, 11.2, and 11.3

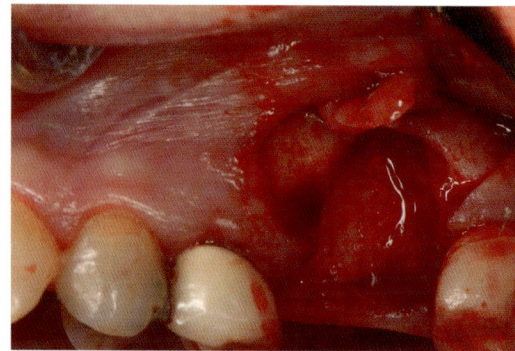

Fig. 11.15 After extraction, site demonstrates no facial plate of bone

tissue membrane have been met. These include the ability for fluids to perfuse from the periosteum to the grafted material, cellular exclusivity to keep connective tissue and epithelial cells from the healing site, and rigidity to maintain the space required for new bone formation. The barrier will stay in place due to integration of the soft tissues at the margins, and the biocompatibility of the material will decrease any postoperative inflammatory response. As shown by Rosen and Rosen, appropriate use of this barrier, with or without bone replacement graft material underneath it, resulted in the preservation of alveolar dimensions without the need for primary closure of the flaps over the barrier. This patient presented with a large facial abscess, leaving no facial plate of bone after extraction (Fig. 11.15). To maximize the volume for implant placement, a putty-like combination of pure phase beta tricalcium phosphate and a biolinker (Easy-graft, Degradable solutions, Schlieren, SW, www.degradable.ch) was inserted in the defect and contoured to ideal form. It was then covered with the semirigid synthetic barrier (Fig. 11.16).

There are also bioactive barriers on the market, some using processed human amnion and chorion tissue as their structure (Koob et al. 2013, 2014a, b; Holtzclaw et al. 2012; Holtzclaw and Toscano 2012, 2013) (Fig. 11.10). One is BioXclude (Snoasis Medical, Denver, CO, www.SnoasisMedical.com) which contains many growth factors and biologic mediators important in bone and keratinized tissue formation (Horowitz 2003, 2005). These include PDGF, VEGF, laminin 5, extracellular matrix proteins, and many types of collagen (Niknejad et al. 2008). It does not require primary closure over it, has been shown to decrease inflammation, and can be used with other barriers. Studies have shown that there is an increase in angiogenic growth factors and human endothelial cells (Koob 2014). Human clinical studies have demonstrated accelerated periodontal healing, quicker flap reattachment, and decreased postoperative recession (Holtzclaw et al. 2012; Holtzclaw and Toscano 2012, 2013).

11.3 Growth Factors/Enhancers

Multiple materials have been advocated for insertion into periodontal or other surgical sites to increase the rate and/or amount of bone formation. Synthesized compounds that are equivalent or similar to cytokines in the human body are called growth factors. This list includes rhPDGF-BB, BMP2, and others that are being developed and tested. One issue with them is their limited "on"-label set of uses and combinations of bone grafts and barriers allowed according to the FDA's guidelines. Research has been conducted on bone morphogenic proteins since the 1960s (Urist 1965). These are a family of compounds that have been shown to induce bone formation and other parts of the healing/regenerative cascade. Being osteoinductive, they can form bone in a part of the body that does not normally do so. Clinical applications of one specific material – Infuse (Medtronic, Minneapolis, MN, www.medtronic.com) – have included repair of extraction sockets, deficient alveolar ridges, and maxillary sinuses (Howell et al. 1997; Nevins et al. 1996; Boyne et al. 2005). There are questions about the legal ability to combine this potent compound with bone replacement grafts or rigid barriers due to restrictions by the US Food and Drug Administration. In some of the studies that have been performed, the resulting bone volume and density have been less than what is seen in native bone despite the potent nature of this

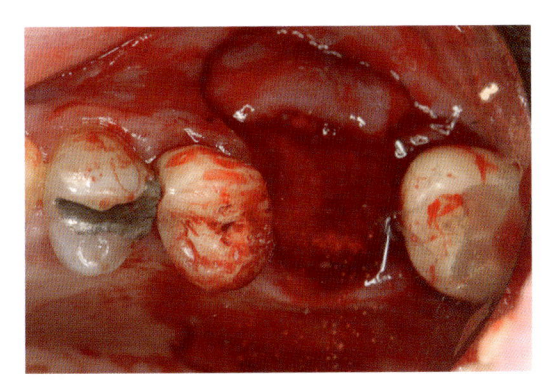

Fig. 11.16 Insertion of semirigid PLLA-PLGA barrier over TCP

growth factor. Another concern with the use of this material is that it may induce root resorption and ankylosis if there are teeth in the segment being treated.

Recombinant human platelet-derived growth factor BB (rhPDGF-BB) has been investigated for over 25 years (Lynch et al. 1989). In periodontal defects (Kaigler et al. 2011; Rosen et al. 2011), alveolar ridge deficiencies (Simion et al. 2006b), and around dental implants (Kaigler et al. 2011), this material has demonstrated the ability to form vital bone around a slowly resorbing bovine bone mineral substrate. Additionally, there have been indications that combined with rhPDGF-BB, there is some resorption of this bovine scaffold not or rarely seen in other histologic studies (Artzi et al. 2000, 2003). Although this material had been released with a beta TCP carrier, many of the studies with this material are combined with anorganic bovine bone mineral. Additionally, there are significant financial costs involved with both of these recombinant compounds that may preclude their widespread incorporation into periodontal, extraction socket, and other regenerative surgical procedures.

More commonly used and less costly for the surgeon are calcium sulfate and L-PRF. Calcium sulfate has been researched by Strocchi et al. (2002) and shown to increase angiogenesis in the grafted site. Multiple forms of calcium sulfate are on the market. One is a self-reinforced biphasic form that sets in both wet and bloody environments (Horowitz et al. 2012). This material is in an easy-to-use syringe and can be inserted alone or mixed with other graft materials (Fig. 11.9). One of the ways that it increases the amount of vital bone in the recipient site is through increasing the amount of vascularity in the grafted site. Additionally, there are sensors on osteoblasts that are stimulated by free calcium in the extracellular matrix (Quarles et al. 1997) as shown by an increase in DNA synthesis when exposed to free calcium in solution in the extracellular matrix.

As has been shown in numerous clinical and scientific papers, adding 20% calcium sulfate to a bone replacement graft material enhances vital bone formation. Al Ruhaimi and coworkers (2000) studied different graft materials in simulated extraction sockets in rabbit femoral condyles. They were inserted alone and mixed with calcium sulfate; the sites were left alone or filled with calcium sulfate alone. At 8 weeks postoperatively, the site where the polymeric graft alone was placed exhibited 13% vital bone in connective tissue with 70% of the site filled with graft particles. Where the resorbable HA was tested, a similar 19% vital bone was observed in the site. However, the residual graft portion was 19% leaving 62% connective tissue. There were only signs of blood vessels and no inflammation in both types of sites. Where calcium sulfate alone was grafted, there were 24% vital bone, blood vessels, and no inflammation in the osteoid matrix. There were large empty spaces but no residual graft material noted. Where calcium sulfate was mixed, the graft healed in a very different manner. The polymer dissolved more and was only responsible for 39% of the site with 29% vital bone. The remaining 32% was filled with empty spaces, connective tissue, and blood vessels. There was 40% vital bone, with a significant amount of lamellar component, in the sites filled with a mixture of HA and calcium sulfate. The 19% remaining graft was dissolving, and there was no inflammation and many blood vessels in the area. In the untreated areas, there were large empty spaces, bone dust, and fat with some borders of bone trabeculae.

Improving on the characteristics of "pure" calcium sulfate is a new, biphasic mixture of hemi- and dihydrate particles (3D Bond or Bond Bone, Augma Biomaterials, Israel, www.augmabio.com). It is self-reinforced and sets in the presence of either blood or saliva. Preliminary clinical and histologic studies demonstrate both volume preservation and significant vital bone formation. In one human clinical case series (Horowitz et al. 2012), three different types of extraction socket defects were treated with this material. A maxillary molar site was grafted and no barrier, no sutures placed. Dense, 32% vital bone was seen with maintenance of the alveolar ridge width. In a mandibular molar site, no buccal plate was present in the coronal 5 mm of the socket so a dense PTFE barrier was placed over the graft for 3 weeks. A bone core was retrieved less than 4 months later at the time of implant placement. The vital bone content of this site was 60%, and the alveolar ridge height was increased by 3 mm on the facial. Where an infected maxillary premolar was extracted, there was no buccal plate. Covering the graft and defect with a resorbable barrier resulted, 4 months later, in an intact ridge with 51% vital bone and no residual graft material.

Leukocyte- and platelet-rich fibrin (L-PRF) is a low-cost, easily processed biomaterial taken from the patient's own venous blood (Dohan et al. 2006). Depending on the size and volume of the defect, an appropriate amount of blood is drawn, usually between 18 and 36 cc. It is spun in a centrifuge at 2,700 RPM for 12 min. The fibrin plug is formed through a slow cicatrization process. This enables the growth factors contained within it to be released over a 7–10 day period (Dohan Ehrenfest et al. 2009a, b) unlike other blood harvested/concentrated products. The leukocytes incorporated into L-PRF play a role in processes involved in healing from being anti-infectious, regulating the immune response, and assisting in remodeling of the matrix to affecting growth factor release. When calcium chloride and thrombin are added to the other products, the growth-stimulating compounds are released over a matter of hours (He et al. 2009). No other steps are required in the processing of L-PRF other than to squeeze the resultant fibrin plug in a perforated metal box. In this manner, barriers or plugs can be formed, and the expressed liquid can be utilized to hydrate bone replacement graft materials. Combining the growth-enhancing properties of the patient's own blood at a minimal cost is very attractive to patients. As numerous researchers have demonstrated, there are biologic bases starting at the cellular level on which to base these therapies. The studies they have published show improved healing in all aspects of surgical therapy from periodontal procedures (Del Corso et al. 2009) to sinus augmentation (Mazor et al. 2009).

When a patient presents with high aesthetic demands, multiple layers of biologically enhanced grafts and barriers are utilized. The maxillary left central incisor in this patient fractured after a new restoration was cemented into place (Fig. 11.17). After atraumatic extraction, a combination allograft with demineralized and mineralized particles in a collagen gelatin matrix tested and shown to be osteoinductive (Optecure with CorticoCancellous chips, Exactech, Gainesville, FL, www.exactech.com) was hydrated in the liquid expressed during the fabrication of L-PRF membranes (Fig. 11.18). After grafting the debrided socket, an amnion/chorion (BioXclude, Snoasis, Denver, CO) barrier was placed over the graft (Fig. 11.19) and then covered with an epithelialized connective tissue graft hydrated in the same liquid. Three months later, the alveolar ridge width is completely preserved, mucogingival level unaltered, and thick, pink, keratinized tissue covers the alveolar crest (Fig. 11.20). A dental implant was inserted and impressions taken for future restoration 4 months after the extraction (Fig. 11.21). One year after the

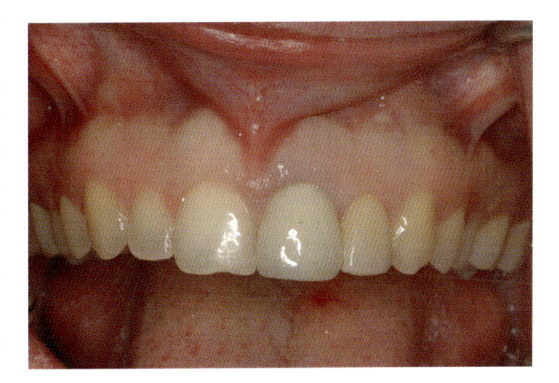

Fig. 11.17 Initial presentation of patient with vertically fractured non-vital root

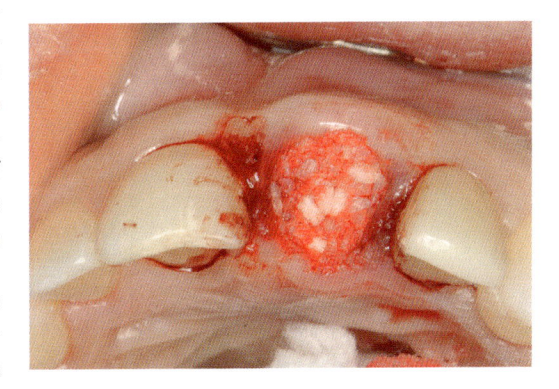

Fig. 11.18 An osteoinductive allograft is hydrated in liquid from L-PRF membranes and used to fill socket

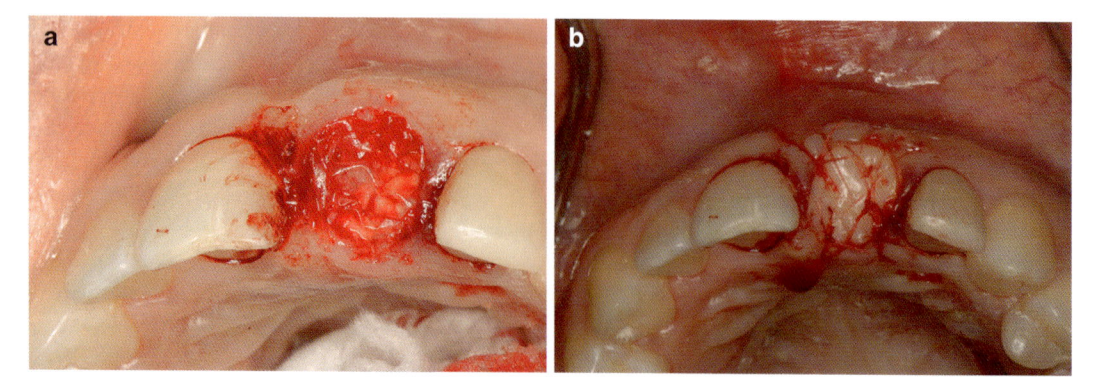

Fig. 11.19 A bioactive amnion/chorion barrier is placed (**a**) then cover with a keratinized graft from the palate hydrated in PRF liquid (**b**)

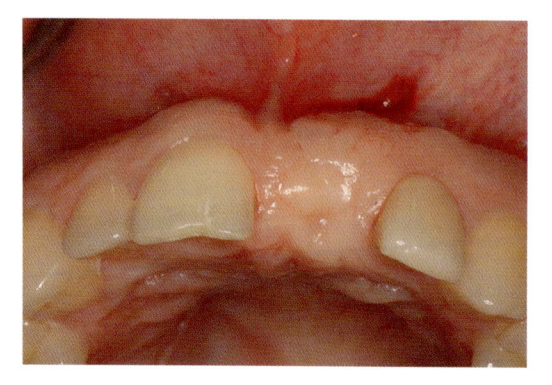

Fig. 11.20 Soft tissues fully healed, ridge width preserved 3 months after growth factor-enhanced extraction

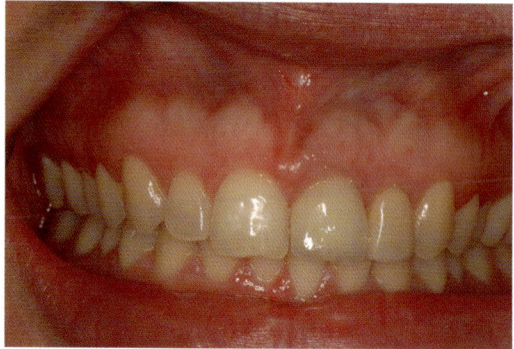

Fig. 11.22 One year post-prosthetic loading of the endosseous implant demonstrated bilateral symmetry and an excellent clinical result

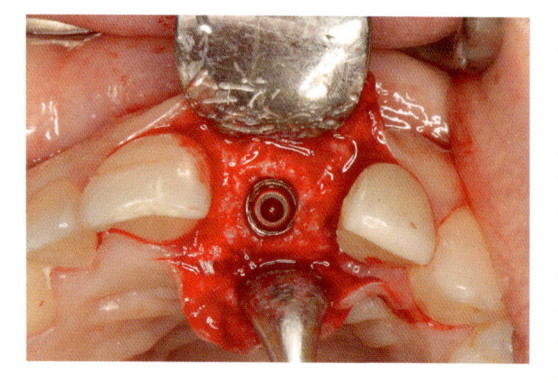

Fig. 11.21 Flap elevation and implant placement into a fully healed ridge with ideal bucco-palatal width

final restoration was placed, the highly aesthetic result is due to the facial margin residing in an ideal location and the papillae which have been maintained (Fig. 11.22).

11.4 Aesthetic Concerns

In the 50 years that dental implants have been placed, the focus has shifted greatly. In the early days, there were a few groups of individuals "pioneering" these exciting technologies including Linkow and Chercheve (1970). There was the group out of Sweden using operating room sterile techniques, vestibular incisions, machined titanium implants of only a single choice of available implant diameter, and those placed solely in the anterior mandible (Branemark et al. 1969). In other parts of the world, there were different diameter and composition, threaded, blade-shaped, and press-fit cylinders, not just screws. We owe a tremendous debt of gratitude to the dentists who pushed the limits of the human body's healing. Additionally, those dental "cripples" who were willing to undergo these "experimental" procedures to restore them to a higher quality of life – occlusal function, phonetics, and aesthetics – deserve our praises as well.

Patients in many areas were not willing to accept the "Scandinavian" restorative options that were often performed in the early 1980s. These screw retained, acrylic over gold restorations did not satisfy the aesthetic demands of many patients. Patients were not just grateful to be able to chew; they wanted to look as they did before they lost the teeth. Implant-supported dental rehabilitation was being required to be functional and aesthetic. A history of the types of implants placed and early superstructures for single and multiple tooth replacements was described in exquisite detail by Albrektsson et al. (1986).

As single and segmental surgically based restorative procedures were being performed, issues arose. Patients expected, and demanded, more ideal restorative outcomes than had been available from sites with collapsed arches. Mecall and Rosenfeld documented how alveolar ridge resorption affected the placement of dental implants in ideal locations (Mecall and Rosenfeld 1991). The increase in prosthetically guided surgery became associated with three-dimensional analysis of the receptor sites. Surgeons and restorative dentists sent patients for CT scan or cone beam CT (CBCT) radiographic studies to determine volume, quality, and quantity of bone in the proposed dental implant sites. Dr. Scott Ganz (2001) and others have published articles describing ways to increase the usefulness of data achieved from these powerful tools. They have also demonstrated the value of specific software analysis for both predictability of the surgical and restorative phases of implant-related therapy and our ability to educate our patients from them.

Utilizing three-dimensional imaging gives a surgeon the ideal view of the area to be treated prior to inception of the surgical procedure. Knowing bone volume, density, and locations of questionable area simplifies the decision-making process at the time of extraction and bone regeneration. Understanding the biology of wound healing in this arena will facilitate ideal choices being made regarding surgical approach and biomaterial selection. Understanding graft resorption and replacement, the need for barrier protection or bioactivity in the site can raise the predictability of each step delivered by the entire dental implant team. All members on the surgical and restorative sides of the equation will have a better understanding of expectations for healing and aesthetics resulting from each part of the multistep procedures.

These combinations of advanced surgical techniques with growth enhancers, barriers, and bone replacement graft materials have been described throughout the dental literature were used to preserve or augment existing alveolar bone and keratinized tissue (Fig. 11.23). Dr. Tarnow and his colleagues (2014) published a recent paper evaluating different methods of preserving alveolar ridge dimensions at the time of immediate socket implant placement. They found the best aesthetic results when placing immediate socket implants, inserting a bone replacement graft in the gap between implant and socket and tunneling a subepithelial connective tissue graft on the facial. These techniques require advanced training of surgeons and restorative dentists to obtain this type of result. Similar results regarding preservation of the alveolar volume can be attained through socket augmentation with implant placement at a later time. Staged procedures may be provided for our patients with lesser training required by the surgical/restorative team and a lower risk of compromise or failure along the way.

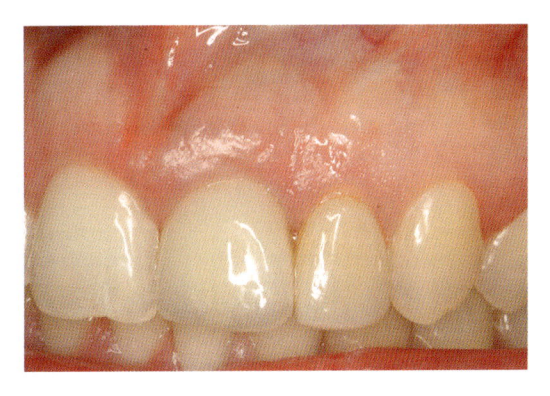

Fig. 11.23 Close-up of restoration 1 year after prosthetic loading

Conclusion

The method by which a tooth is extracted will affect the concomitant loss of the supporting alveolar bone and therefore the position of the marginal gingiva. If surgical flaps are elevated at the time of tooth removal, there is greater loss of bone than would occur from a less invasive approach. Using appropriate bone replacement graft materials and barriers either with or without simultaneous implant placement and restoration can give the patient an acceptable aesthetic result. A three-dimensional analysis of the preoperative condition including the tooth location and surrounding bone volume prior to surgery is critical. It gives the surgeon an indication of the amount of bone present along with locations for potential progenitor cells and vascular supply to populate the grafted site. Merging literature and biology will enable the dental surgeon to choose the ideal combination of surgical approach, bone graft, barrier, and biologic enhancers. In this way the recipient site will be optimized with regard to vital bone, volume, and keratinized tissue. This will lead to a long-term aesthetic success with a fixed prosthetic restoration, in the proper location, framed by an ideal quantity and quality of keratinized gingiva supported by an osseointegrated, endosseous dental implant. Over time, having all of these truly regenerated tissues where there are both proper occlusion and professional maintenance should ensure the longevity of the final result.

References

Albrektsson T, Zarb G, Worthington P, Eriksson AR (1986) The long-term efficacy of currently used dental implants: a review and proposed criteria of success. Int J Oral Maxillofac Implants 1(1):11–25

al Ruhaimi KA (2000) Effect of adding resorbable calcium sulfate to grafting materials on early bone regeneration in osseous defects in rabbits. Int J Oral Maxillofac Implants 15(6):859–864

Amler MH, Johnson PL, Salman I (1960) Histological and histochemical investigation of human alveolar socket healing in undisturbed extraction wounds. J Am Dent Assoc 6:46–48

Anson D (2002) Maxillary anterior esthetic extractions with delayed single-stage implant placement. Compend Contin Educ Dent 23(9):829–830 833–6

Anson D (2009) CE 2-The changing treatment planning paradigm: save the tooth or place an implant. Compend Contin Educ Dent 30(8):506

Arnett T (2003) Regulation of bone cell function by acid–base balance. Proc Nutr Soc 62(02):511–520

Artzi Z, Tal H, Dayan D (2000) Porous bovine bone mineral in healing of human extraction sockets. Part 1: histomorphometric evaluations at 9 months. J Periodontol 71:1015–1023

Artzi Z, Givol N, Rohrer MD et al (2003) Qualitative and quantitative expression of bovine bone mineral in experimental bone defects. Part 2: morphometric analysis. J Periodontol 74(8):1153–1160

Artzi Z, Weinreb M, Givol N, Rohrer MD, Nemcovsky CE, Prasad HS, Tal H (2004) Biomaterial resorption rate and healing site morphology of inorganic bovine bone and beta-tricalcium phosphate in the canine: a 24-month longitudinal histologic study and morphometric analysis. Int J Oral Maxillofac Implants 19(3):357–368

Barone A, Aldini NN, Fini M, Giardino R, Calvo Guirado JL, Covani U (2008) Xenograft versus extraction alone for ridge preservation after tooth removal: a clinical and histomorphometric study. J Periodontol 79:1370–1377

Bartee B (1995) The use of high-density polytetrafluoroethylene membrane to treat osseous defects: clinical reports. Implant Dent 4(1):21–26

Becker W, Dahlin C, Becker B, Lekholm U, van Steenberghe D, Higuchi K, Kultje C (1994) The use of e-PTFE barrier membranes for bone promotion around titanium implants placed into extraction sockets: a prospective multicenter study. Int J O Ral Maxillofac Implants 9:31–40

Botticelli D, Berglundh T, Lindhe J (2004) Hard-tissue alterations following immediate implant placement in extraction sites. J Clin Periodontol 31:820–828

Boyne PJ, Lilly LC, Marx RE et al (2005) De novo bone induction by recombinant human bone morphogenetic protein-2 (rhBMP-2) in maxillary sinus floor augmentation. J Oral Maxillofac Surg 63:1693–1707

Brånemark PI, Adell R, Breine U, Hansson BO, Lindström J, Ohlsson A (1969) Intra-osseous anchorage of dental prostheses. I. Experimental studies. Scand J Plast Reconstr Surg 3(2):81–100

Buser D, Bragger U, Lang NB, Nyman S (1990) Regeneration and enlargement of jaw bone using guided tissue regeneration. Clin Oral Implants Res 1:22–30

Bushinsky DA (2001) Acid-base imbalance and the skeleton. Eur J Nutr 40(5):238–244

Carlsson GE, Thilander H, Hedegard B (1967) Histologic changes in the upper alveolar process after extractions with or without insertion of an immediate full denture. Acta Odontol Scand 25:1

Coppa A, Bondioli L, Cucina A, Frayer DW, Jarrige C, Jarrige JF et al (2006) Palaeontology: early neolithic tradition of dentistry. Nature 440:755–756

Crespi R, Capparè P, Gherlone E (2010) Immediate loading of dental implants placed in periodontally infected and non-infected sites: a 4-year follow-up clinical study. J Periodontol 81(8):1140–1146

Del Corso M, Sammartino G, Dohan Ehrenfest DM (2009) Choukroun's platelet-rich fibrin (PRF) membranes in periodontal surgery: understanding the biomaterial or believing into the magic of growth factors? J Periodontol 80(11):1694–1697

Dohan DM, Choukroun J, Diss A, Dohan SL, Dohan AJ, Mouhyi J, Gogly B (2006) Platelet-rich fibrin (PRF): a second-generation platelet concentrate. Part I: technological concepts and evolution. Oral Surg Oral Med Oral Pathol Oral Radiol Endod 101(3):37–44

Dohan Ehrenfest DM, de Peppo GM, Doglioli P, Sammartino G (2009a) Slow release of growth factors and thrombospondin-1 in Choukroun's platelet-rich fibrin (PRF): a gold standard to achieve for all surgical platelet concentrates technologies. Growth Factors 27:63–69

Dohan Ehrenfest DM, Diss A, Odin G, Doglioli P, Hippolyte MP, Charrier JB (2009b) In vitro effects of Choukroun's PRF (platelet rich fibrin) on human gingival fibroblasts, dermal prekeratinocytes, preadipocytes and maxillofacial osteoblasts in primary cultures. Oral Surg Oral Med Oral Pathol Oral Radiol Endod. 108(3):341–352

Fickl S, Zuhr O, Wachtel H, Bolz W, Hurzeler M (2008) Tissue alterations after tooth extraction with and without surgical trauma: a volumetric study in the beagle dog. J Clin Periodontol 35:356–363

Friedmann A, Strietzel FP, Maretzki B, Pitaru S, Bernimoulin JP (2002) Histological assessment of augmented jaw bone utilizing a new collagen barrier membrane compared to a standard barrier membrane to protect a granular bone substitute material. Clin Oral Implants Res 13(6):587–594

Ganz SD (2001) CT Scan technology—an evolving tool for predictable implant placement and restoration. Int Mag Oral Implantol 1:6–13

He L, Lin Y, Hu X, Zhang Y, Wu HA (2009) Comparative study of platelet-rich fibrin (PRF) and platelet-rich plasma (PRP) on the effect of proliferation and differentiation of rat osteoblasts in vitro. Oral Surg Oral Med Oral Pathol Oral Radiol Endod 108(5):707–713

Hirschfeld L, Wasserman BA (1978) Long-term survey of tooth loss in 600 treated periodontal patients. J Periodontol 49:225–237

Hoffmann O, Bartee BK, Beaumont C, Kasaj A, Deli G, Zafiropoulos GG (2008) Alveolar bone preservation in extraction sockets using non-resorbable dPTFE membranes: a retrospective non-randomized study. J Periodontol 79(8):1355–1369

Holtzclaw D, Toscano N (2012) Amnion chorion allograft barrier: indications and techniques update. J Imp Adv Clin Dent 4(2):25–38

Holtzclaw D, Hinze F, Toscano N (2012) Gingival flap attachment healing with amnion-chorion allograft membrane: a controlled, split mouth case report replication of the classic 1968 Hiatt study. J Imp Adv Clin Dent 4(5):19–25

Holtzclaw D, Toscano N (2013) Amnion–chorion allograft barrier used for guided tissue regeneration treatment of periodontal intrabony defects: a retrospective observational report of 64 patients. Clin Adv Perio 3(3):131–137

Horowitz RA (2003) Case acceptance – increasing profitability through digital photography. Contemp Esthet Restor Pract 2:2–5

Horowitz RA (2005) Extraction environment Enhancement™ – Critical evaluation of early socket healing in long-term barrier protected extraction sockets. Comp Cont Ed Dent 26(10):619–630

Horowitz RA, Mazor Z (2010) Atraumatic extraction: advantages and implementation. Insid Dent 6(7):420–428

Horowitz RA, Rohrer MD, Prasad HS, Tovar N, Mazor Z (2012) Enhancing extraction socket therapy with a biphasic calcium sulfate. Compend Contin Educ Dent 33(6):420–426

Howell TH, Fiorellini J, Jones A et al (1997) A feasibility study evaluating rhBMP-2/absorbable collagen sponge device for local alveolar ridge preservation or augmentation. Int J Periodontics Restorative Dent 17:124–139

Iasella JM, Greenwell H, Miller RL, Hill M, Drisko C, Bohra AA et al (2003) Ridge preservation with freeze-dried bone allograft and a collagen membrane compared to extraction alone for implant site development: a clinical and histologic study in humans. J Periodontol 74(7):990–999

Kaigler D, Avila G, Wisner-Lynch L et al (2011) Platelet-derived growth factor applications in periodontal and peri-implant bone regeneration. Expert Opin Biol Ther 11:375–385

Kfir E, Kfir V, Kaluski E (2007) Immediate bone augmentation after infected tooth extraction using titanium membranes. J Oral Implantol 33(3):133–138

Koob T, Rennert R, Zabek N et al (2013) Biological properties of dehydrated human amnion/chorion composite graft: implications for chronic wound healing. Int Wound J. doi:10.1111/iwj.12140

Koob T, Lim J, Zabek N (2014a) Cytokines in single layer amnion allografts compared to multilayer amnion/chorion allografts for wound healing. J Biomed Mater Res B. doi:10.1002/jbm.b.33265

Koob T, Li W, Gurtner G et al (2014b) Angiogenic properties of dehydrated human amnion/chorion allografts: therapeutic potential for soft tissue repair and regeneration. Vas Cell 4(10):6–10

Leek FE (1967) The practice of dentistry in ancient egypt. J Egypt Archaeol 53:51

Linkow LI, Cherchève R (1970) Theories and techniques of oral implantology. C.V. Mosby Co., St. Louis, pp 1–154

Lynch SE, Williams RC, Polson AM, Howell TH, Reddy MS, Zappa Antoniades HN (1989) A combination of platelet-derived and insulin-like growth factor enhanced periodontal regeneration. J Clin Periodontol 16:545–548

Machtei EE (2001) The effect of membrane exposure on the outcome of regenerative procedures in humans: a meta-analysis. J Periodontol 72:512–516

Mazor Z, Horowitz RA, Del Corso M, Prasad HS, Rohrer MD, Dohan Ehrenfest DM (2009) Sinus floor augmentation with simultaneous implant placement using Choukroun's PRF (platelet-rich fibrin) as sole grafting material: a radiological and histological study at 6 months. J Periodontol 80(12):2056–2064

Mecall RA, Rosenfeld AL (1991) Influence of residual ridge resorption patterns on implant fixture placement and tooth position. Int J Period RestDent 11(1):8–23

Moghaddas H, Stahl SS (1980) Alveolar bone remodeling following osseous surgery. A clinical study. J Periodontol 51(7):376–381

Nekoofar MH, Namazikhah MS, Sheykhrezae MS, Mohammadi MM, Kazemi A, Aseeley Z, Dummer PMH (2009) pH of pus collected from periapical abscesses. Int Endod J 42(6):534–538

Nevins M, Kirker-Head C, Nevins M, Wozney JA, Palmer R, Graham D (1996) Bone formation in the goat maxillary sinus induced by absorbable collagen sponge implants impregnated with recombinant human bone morphogenetic protein-2. Int J Periodontics Restor Dent 16:8–19

Niknejad H, Peirovi H, Jorjani M et al (2008) Properties of the amniotic membrane for potential use in tissue engineering. Euro Cells Mat 15:88–89

Nyman S, Lindhe J, Karring T, Rylander H (1982) New attachment following surgical treatment of human periodontal disease. J Clin Periodontol 9:290–296

Pietrokovski J, Massler M (1967) Alveolar ridge resorption following tooth extraction. J Prosthet Dent 17:21–27

Quarles LD, Hartle JE, Siddhanti SR, Guo R, Hinson TK (1997) A distinct cation-sensing mechanism in MC3T3-E1 osteoblasts functionally related to the calcium receptor. J Bone Miner Res 12(3):393–402

Rosen PS, Toscano N, Holtzclaw D, Reynolds M (2011) A retrospective consecutive case series using mineralized allograft with recombinant human platelet-derived growth factor BB to treat moderate to severe osseous lesions. Int J Periodontics Restor Dent 31:335–341

Rosen PS, Rosen AD (2013) Purposeful exposure of a polylactic acid barrier to achieve socket preservation for placement of dental implants: case series report. Compend Contin Educ Dent 34(1):34–38

Simion M, Baldoni M, Rossi P et al (1994) A comparative study of the effectiveness of e-PTFE membranes with and without early exposure during the healing period. Int J Periodontics Restor Dent 14:166–180

Simion M, Tinti C, Wagenberg B (2006a) A study of the fate of the buccal wall of extraction sockets of teeth with prominent roots. Int J Periodontics Restor Dent 26:19–29

Simion M, Rocchietta I, Kim D, Nevins M, Fiorellini J (2006b) Vertical ridge augmentation by means of deproteinized bovine bone block and recombinant human platelet derived growth factor-BB: a histologic study in a dog model. Int J Periodontics Restor Dent 2:415–423

Sottosanti JS (1997) Calcium sulfate: a valuable addition to the implant/bone regeneration complex. Dent Implantol Updat 8(4):25–29

Strocchi R, Orsini G, Iezzi G, Scarano A, Rubini C, Pecora G, Piattelli A (2002) Bone regeneration with calcium sulfate: evidence for increased angiogenesis in rabbits. J Oral Implantol 28(6):273–278

Sussman HI (2004) Periapical infections adjacent to freshly placed implants. Oral Surg Oral Med Oral Pathol Oral Radiol Endod 98(2):136

Tarnow DP, Chu SJ, Salama MA, Stappert CF, Salama H, Garber DA, Sarnachiaro GO, Sarnachiaro E, Gotta SL, Saito H (2014) Flapless postextraction socket implant placement in the esthetic zone: part 1. The effect of bone grafting and/or provisional restoration on facial-palatal ridge dimensional change-a retrospective cohort study. Int J Periodontics Restor Dent 34(3):323–331

Urist MR (1965) Bone: formation by autoinduction. Science 150:893–899

Vance GS, Greenwell H, Miller RL, Hill M, Johnston H, Scheetz JP (2004) Comparison of an allograft in an experimental putty carrier and a bovine-derived xenograft used in ridge preservation: a clinical and histologic study in human. Int J Oral Maxillofac Implants 19(4):491–497

Vignoletti F, Discepoli N, Muller A, de Sanctis M, Muñoz F, Sanz M (2012) Bone modelling at fresh extraction sockets: immediate implant placement versus spontaneous healing. An experimental study in the beagle dog. J Clin Periodontol 39:91–97

Wang HL, Kiyonobu K, Neiva RF (2004) Socket augmentation: rationale and technique. Implant Dent 13(4):286–296

Zubery Y, Goldlust A, Alves A, Nir E (2007) Ossification of a novel cross-linked porcine collagen barrier in guided bone regeneration in dogs. J Periodontol 78(1):112–121

Development of Hard Tissues with Block Grafting Techniques

12

John Russo

Abstract

Adequate bone and soft tissue volume is necessary for long-term functional and aesthetic success of dental implants. This article discussed how much bone is needed for implant success as well as how to diagnose bone volume with the use of cone beam computed tomography. Options such as ridge split, guided bone regeneration with titanium membranes, and titanium mesh are discussed, but the focus of this chapter is block grafts. A decision tree is given for choosing a donor site for block grafts considering anatomic factors and patient comfort-related factors. For block grafts in the anterior mandible, the mandibular symphysis is the donor site of choice. The posterior mandible lends itself to harvest bone from the external oblique ridge or ramus. For the premaxilla, block allografts are the donor bone of choice. This chapter is dedicated to block allografts in the aesthetic zone of the premaxilla. The technique of incision design; recipient site preparation; releasing buccal flaps; placing fixation screws; shaping the block, particulate bone, and membranes; and suturing is covered. Complications of block grafting are briefly covered.

Implant aesthetics in the premaxilla will always begin with a comprehensive examination and an accurate diagnosis. Cone beam computed tomography (CBCT) has given the profession three-dimensional views of proposed implant sites rather than relying on the traditional two-dimensional radiographs (Figs. 12.1 and 12.2).

J. Russo, DDS, MHS
Division of Periodontics, Medical University of South Carolina, Private Practice 1704 Bay Road, Sarasota, FL 34239, USA
e-mail: russoimplant@comcast.net

Many times a scan appliance can be made by simply placing temporary radiopaque cement on a temporary removable appliance or a temporary bridge (Figs. 12.3, 12.4, and 12.5). When the temporary restoration with radiopaque cement is worn during the scan, it will provide a point of reference of where the restored tooth or teeth need to be. This facilitates using a third-party software to perform a virtual implant placement. If so desired, a surgical guide can be made from the scan and the plan (Figs. 12.6 and 12.7).

When making measurements of bone width and height, it is necessary to know the anatomic

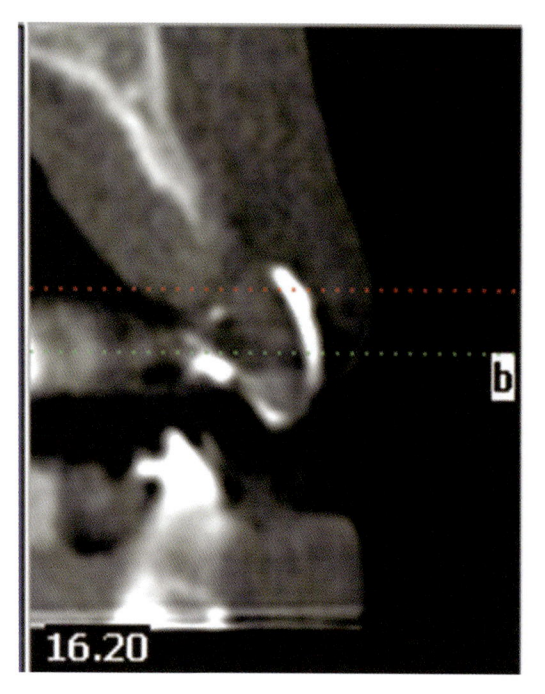

Fig. 12.1 Thin maxillary ridge

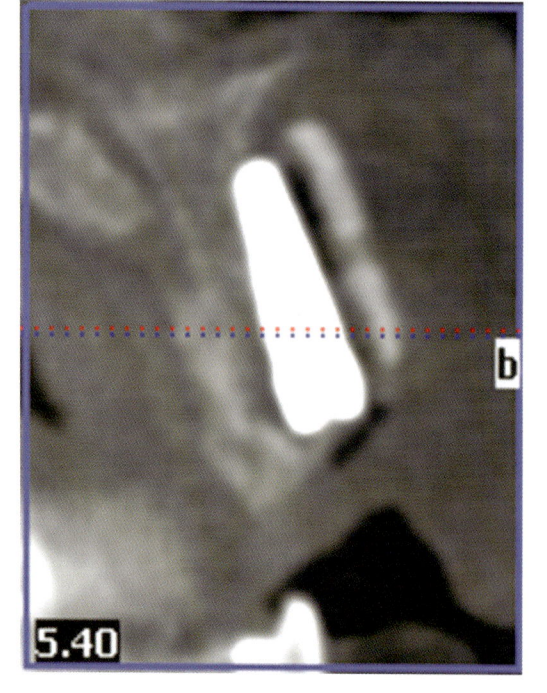

Fig. 12.2 Implant placed in block

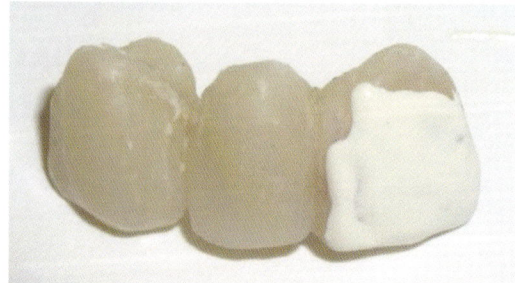

Fig. 12.3 Radiopaque material on temporary bridge

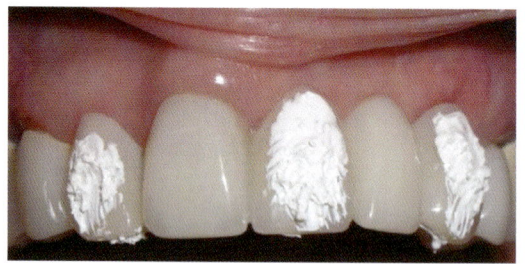

Fig. 12.4 Using temporary bridge as a scan appliance

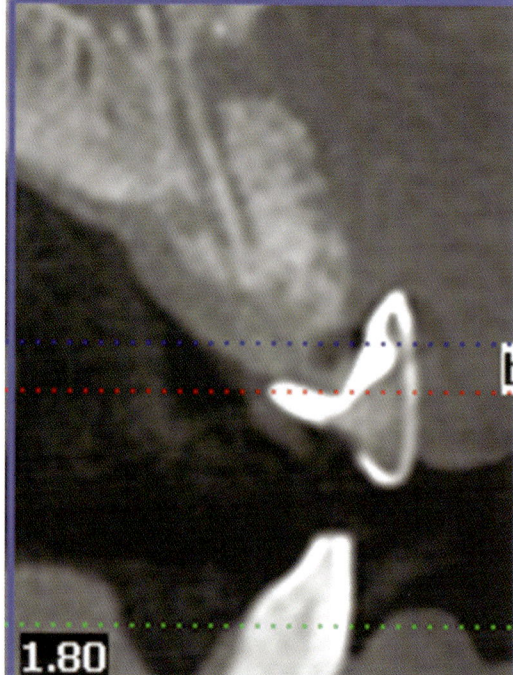

Fig. 12.5 Scan appliance with radiopaque material

structures providing limitations such as the mandibular canal, the maxillary sinus, and floor of the nose. For long-term success of dental implants, 2–3 mm of bone on the buccal of each implant will allow for a blood supply to nourish the buccal bone. To prevent recession of the

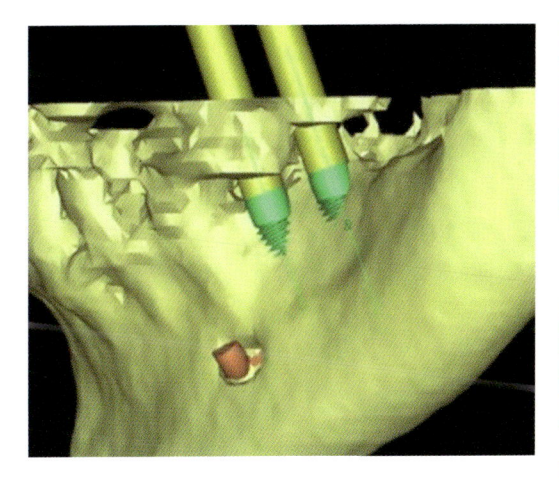

12 Development of Hard Tissues with Block Grafting Techniques

Fig. 12.6 Software helping diagnosis and treatment plan

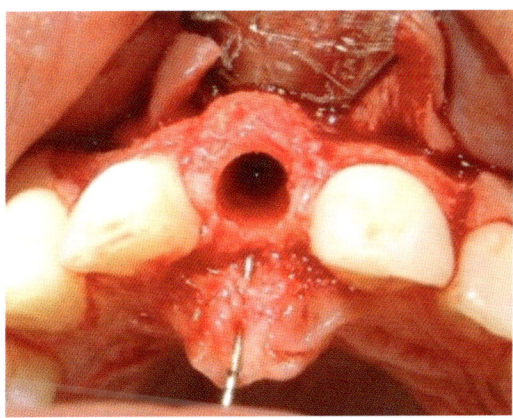

Fig. 12.8 Occlusal view of osteotomy demonstrating 2 mm of bone remaining on the facial of the implant

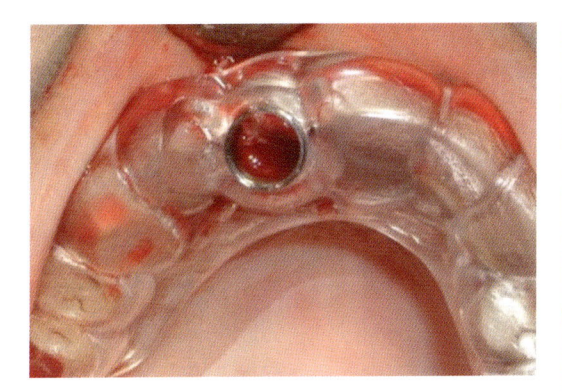

Fig. 12.7 Static surgical guide demonstrating guide tube

peri-implant soft tissue in cases with multiple implants, buccal bone augmentation of more than 2 mm from the implant platform is necessary to overcome the normal pattern of bone remodeling (Fig. 12.8) (Ishikawa et al. 2007).The bone supports the tissue, so that if the buccal bone resorbs due to lack of thickness and lack of blood supply, the tissue will eventually recede (Figs. 12.9 and 12.10). There are biologic limits of the soft tissue dimension around implants; therefore, the limiting factor for the aesthetic result of implant therapy is the bone level at the implant site. Clinicians must focus on the 3-D bone-to-implant relationship to establish the basis for an ideal and harmonic soft tissue situation that is stable over a long period (Grunder et al. 2005). This recession can cause a cosmetic compromise described as an aesthetic failure in the premaxilla. The thicker the soft tissue over this critical buccal plate, the

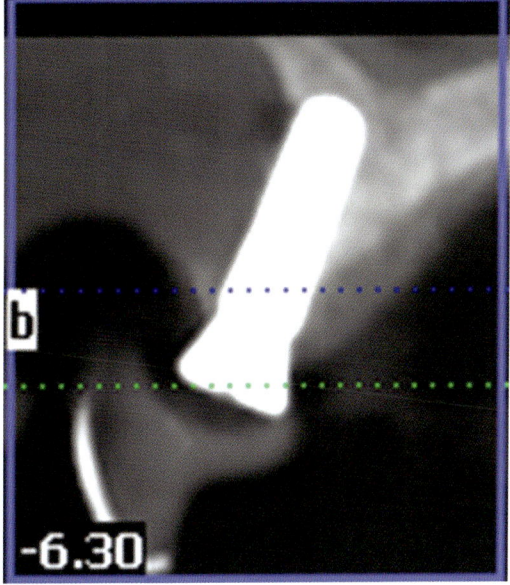

Fig. 12.9 Cross-sectional view from a cone beam computed tomography demonstrating minimal bone on the facial of the implant

less likely recession will occur (Fig. 12.11). Initial gingival tissue thickness at the crest may be considered as a significant influence on marginal bone stability around implants. If the tissue thickness is 2.0 mm or less, crestal bone loss up to 1.45 mm may occur, despite a supracrestal position of the implant–abutment interface (Lincivicius et al. 2009).

The first diagnosis to be made with a CBCT is bone quantity and quality. The second diagnosis

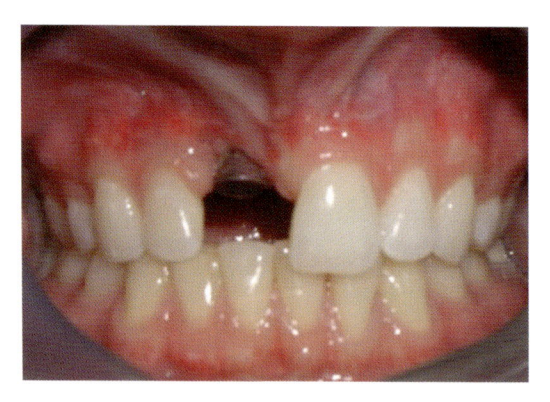

Fig. 12.10 Facial of a dental implant lacking adequate bone and soft tissue thickness necessary for long-term stability

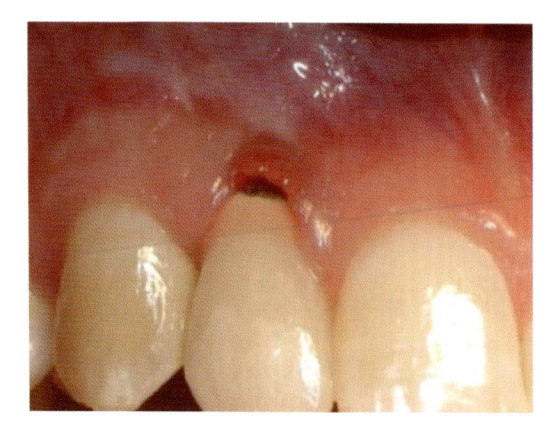

Fig. 12.11 Clinical view demonstrating result of lack of bone on the facial of a dental implant. Bone supports the soft tissue

which is made visually is an assessment of the quantity and quality of the soft tissue. In the maxilla, we have an abundance of thick keratinized on the palate which can be surgically moved to the facial of our implants. It can also be repositioned with releasing flaps. If there have been recent extractions, it may take up to 3 months for the collagen in the soft tissue to mature prior to reentering this site for a block graft. Healed tissue with mature collagen is more resistant to incision line opening over a block graft. After bone augmentation, the mucogingival junction often moves in a coronal direction, and the soft tissue thickness over the barrier membrane is reduced because of the compromised blood supply to the area (Iasella et al. 2003).

For large one-wall bone defects in the premaxilla, our treatment options are ridge split, particulate (Iasella et al. 2003) with space maintainers such as titanium mesh, titanium-reinforced membranes, and/or tenting screws. Intraoral block grafts from the symphysis or ramus and block allografts have also been shown to be very successful in the premaxilla. This chapter will provide a decision tree for donor bone for block grafting in the aesthetic zone of the premaxilla. Although there are other alternatives for grafting of the premaxilla, this chapter will describe block allografts. Autogenous blocks grafts will also be discussed and compared.

12.1 Decision Tree for Donor Site

A decision tree for choosing which technique to use is based on the intraoral location to be grafted (Table 12.1). The goals are to avoid donor site morbidity, increase patient acceptance, and to provide predictable results without limitations of quantity of bone available for grafting. If autogenous bone is the donor of choice, the goal is to keep the donor and recipient site within the same quadrant to decrease morbidity for the patient.

For the *premaxilla*, the literature supports the use of block allografts. With block allografts, a second donor site is avoided that can decrease morbidity and decreased patient acceptance. This allograft provides an unlimited supply to treat multiple sites.

For the *anterior mandible*, the symphysis provides good quality bone (Misch et al. 1992; Misch and Misch 1995; Pikos 1996). This keeps the donor and recipient sites in the same sextant. The buccal lingual dimension needs to be measured with the use of cone beam computed tomography prior to harvesting so as not to harvest a bi-cortical graft. The location of the apices of the remaining tooth roots needs to be identified and avoided.

Table 12.1 Decision tree for donor site

Anterior mandible	Symphysis	Same sextant
Posterior mandible	External oblique ridge	Same sextant
Maxilla	Cortico-cancellous block allograft	Eliminate donor site

12 Development of Hard Tissues with Block Grafting Techniques

For the *posterior mandible*, the external oblique ridge or ramus has been documented as a suitable donor site (Misch 1996; Pikos 1999). This choice of donor site will keep the donor and recipient sites in the same sextant to decrease morbidity for the patient. This is also reported to have less morbidity than the symphysis (Misch 1997) (Fig. 12.12).

The keys to block grafting are the same whether using autogenous bone or a cortico-cancellous block allograft. These keys are space maintenance, recipient site preparation, blood supply/regional acceleratory phenomenon, immobility of the graft, use of a membrane, adequate periosteal release of the flap for passive closure, and primary closure of the flap.

The technique for both autogenous blocks and block allografts in the premaxilla will be the same with regard to recipient site preparation, blood supply, immobility, use of a membrane, periosteal release, and primary closure. Those steps will be reviewed.

A full-thickness mucoperiosteal flap is reflected to allow access to the bone (Fig. 12.13). Typically vertical incisions are made at least one tooth/implant to either side of the graft site. For ease of suturing, the papilla is included in the flap. A small bur can be used to decorticate the recipient site to allow for a blood supply to the graft as well as to initiate the regional acceleratory phenomenon (Fig. 12.14). The buccal flap is released with a shallow incision just through the periosteum from vertical incision to vertical incision. This shallow incision can then be widened with a blunt dissection with the blade turned sideways or by spreading with a blunt hemostat-type instrument. The block will be fixated with at least two lag-type fixation screws that will slide passively through the block but engage the recipient site by undersizing the osteotomy (Fig. 12.15).

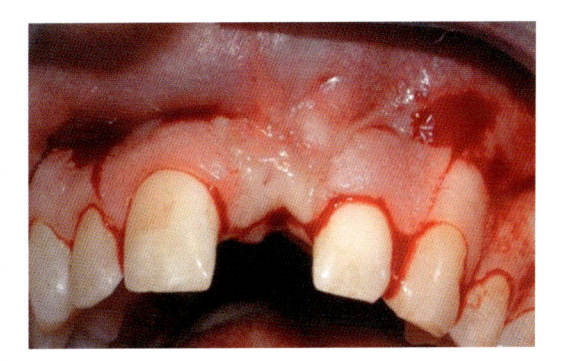

Fig. 12.13 Flap design for a block graft

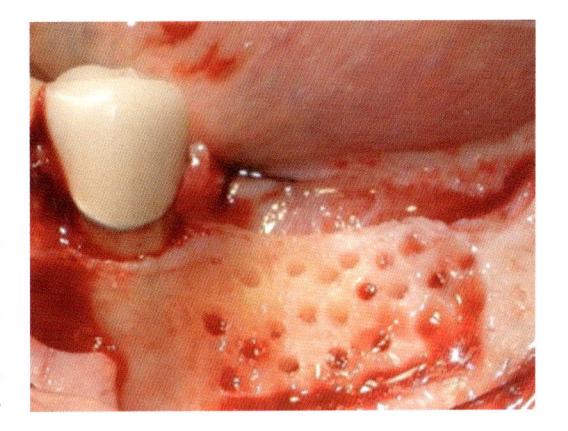

Fig. 12.14 Decortication of recipient site

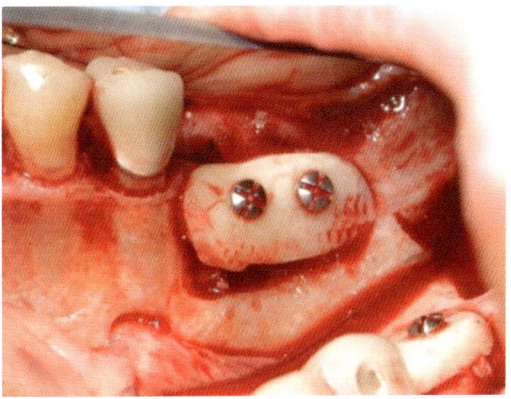

Fig. 12.15 Ramus graft with two fixation screws

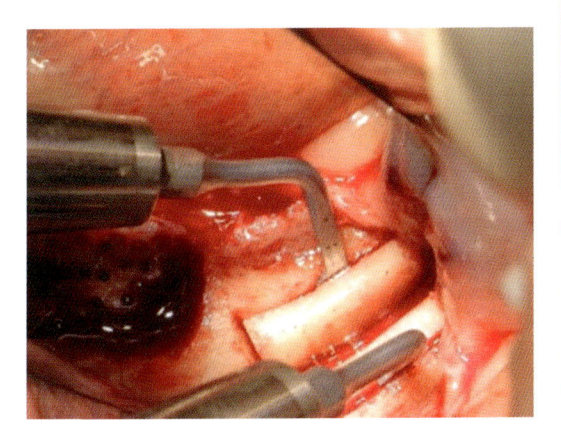

Fig. 12.12 Piezo technology making cut for a ramus graft

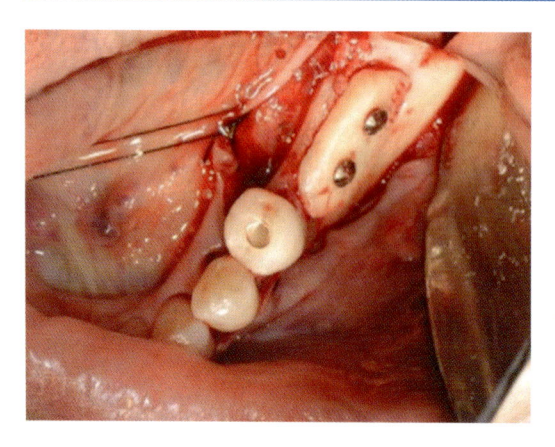

Fig. 12.16 Occlusal view of ramus graft and fixation screws through the opposing cortical plate

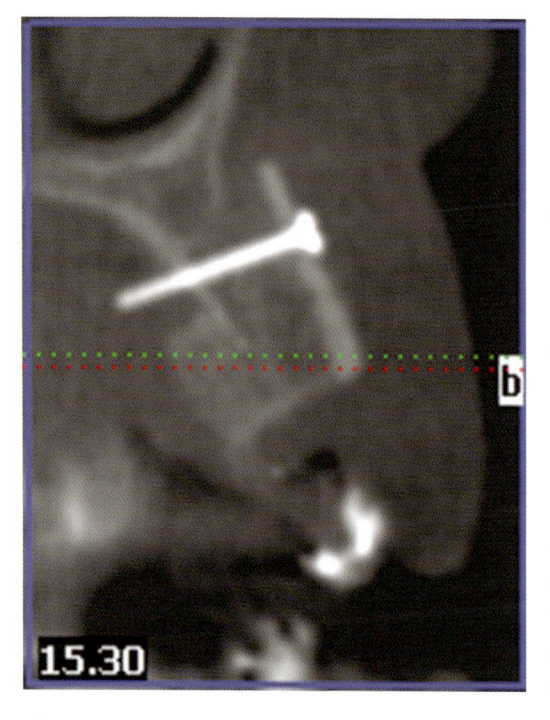

Fig. 12.17 Cross section of CBCT with fixation screw through palatal bone but not through thick keratinized tissue

It is important to place the screw all the way through the opposing cortical plate of the recipient site (Fig. 12.16). In the mandible, it is necessary to reflect the lingual flap and to cut off the excess tip of the screw so as not to irritate the thin lingual mucosa. In most instances in the maxilla, this step is not necessary due to the thickness of the palatal keratinized tissue (Fig. 12.17).

All three choices of donor bone (allograft, ramus, symphysis) can be used for grafting the premaxilla. Based on the decision tree, block allografts are the donor material of choice for the aesthetic zone of the premaxilla.

12.2 Block Allografts

Autogenous grafts have widely been considered the gold standard, primarily because of the growth factors contained in the donor bone (Rubens and West 1989). Block allografts performed in the premaxilla have been reported to have equal success rates compared with autogenous block grafts. Leonetti and Petrungaro provided case reports stating allogenic bone block material use was an effective alternative to harvesting and grafting autogenous bone for implant site development. These cases clinically demonstrate the efficacy of using a block allograft in generating effective new bone fill for dental implant placement. The allograft material was a highly effective modality for restoring the case, and it may significantly reduce the need to obtain autogenous bone from a secondary site (Leonetti and Koup 2003; Petrungaro and Amar 2005; Waasdorp and Reynolds 2010; Chaushu 2010; Keith et al. 2006). One of the theories that block allografts are successful in the premaxilla and not as successful in the posterior mandible is due to the pressure from overlying muscles on very porous cancellous bone. Block allografts are approximately 75% cancellous bone. Although Keith has a very high success rate with block allografts, 71% of his block failures occurred in the posterior mandible. Many of the blocks will be provided from the tissue bank as a bi-cortical piece of bone (Fig. 12.18). These cortico-cancellous block allografts originate from the donor iliac crest. Therefore, the cortical bone is thin (1.5–3.0 mm), and the cancellous zone is much thicker (Fig. 12.19). Due to the lack of consistency of the cortical thickness, a large

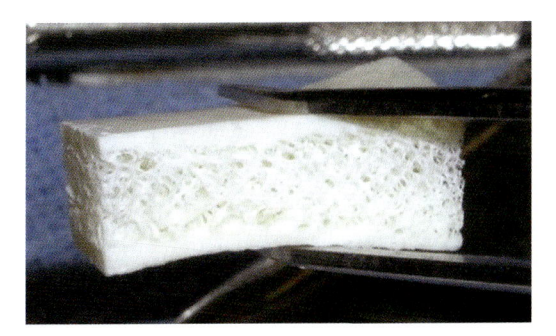

12 Development of Hard Tissues with Block Grafting Techniques

Fig. 12.18 Bi-cortical block allograft

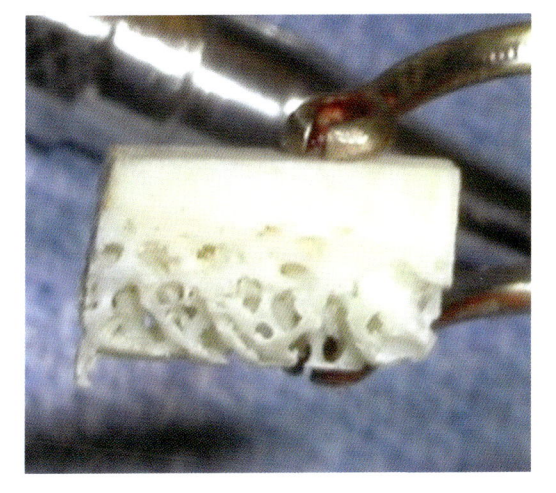

Fig. 12.19 Block allograft demonstrating cortical and cancellous bone

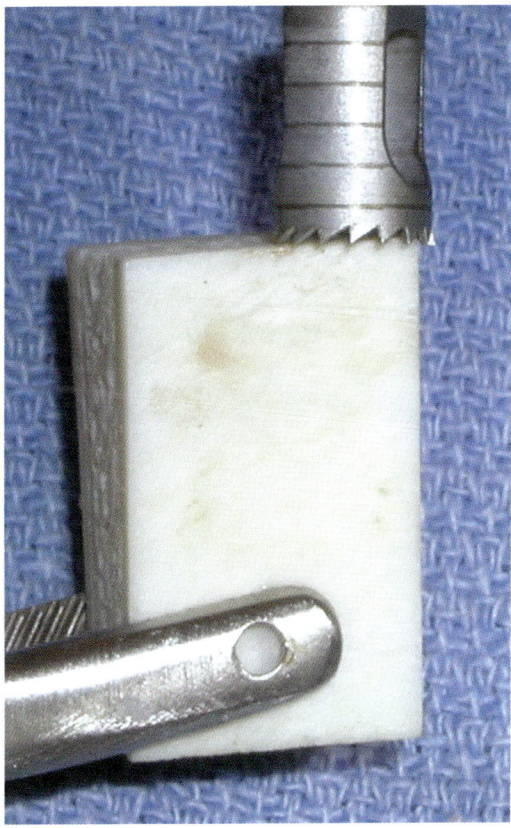

Fig. 12.20 Trephine cutting and shaping block allograft

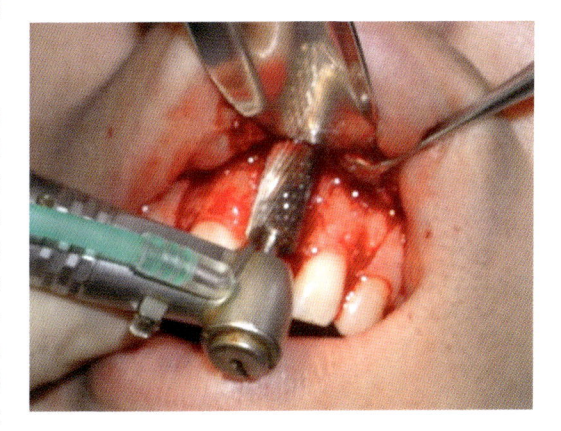

Fig. 12.21 Cylinder bur preparing recipient site for block allograft

piece of bone is provided to allow the surgeon choices for shaping the block to allow the desired thickness of cortical plate (Fig. 12.20). This requires that one of the cortical layers be removed. When the block is fixed, the cancellous portion should be in intimate contact with the recipient site. By using a trephine and corresponding barrel-shaped bur, a very uniform recipient site and donor bone can be created making this a very simple procedure to master with a short learning curve (Figs. 12.21 and 12.22). If more than a single site is necessary, the bone will have to be shaped with a bone saw, piezotome, or a bur. Unlike autogenous bone, this bone is not vital, so it is not necessary to irrigate the block while cutting. Before the block is fixated to the recipient site, it should be hydrated with saline to avoid trapping air into the cancellous portion. A "rapid hydration" technique consists of placing

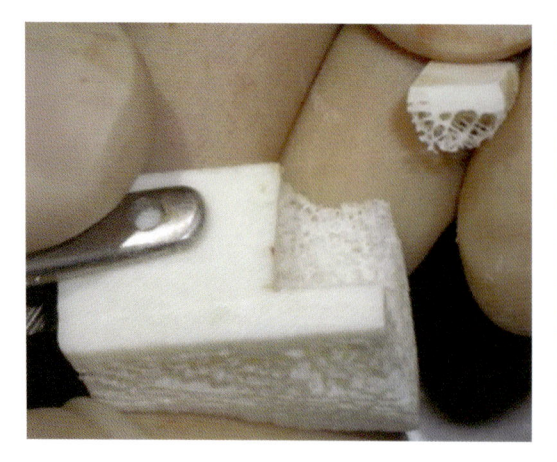

Fig. 12.22 Uniform-shaped block allograft

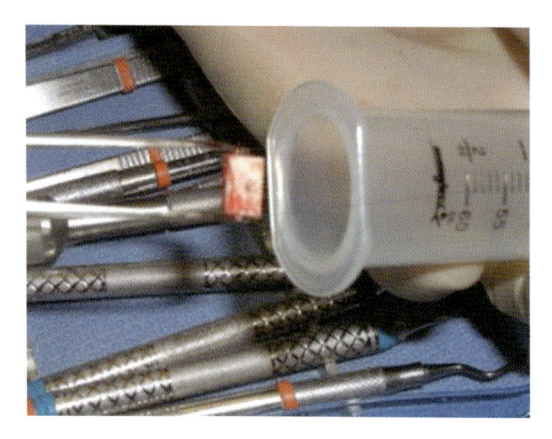

Fig. 12.23 Placing block into syringe for rapid hydration

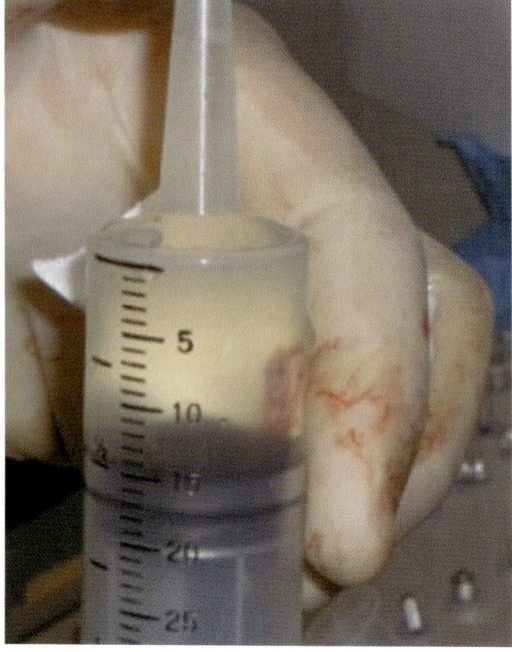

Fig. 12.24 Rapid hydration of block allograft

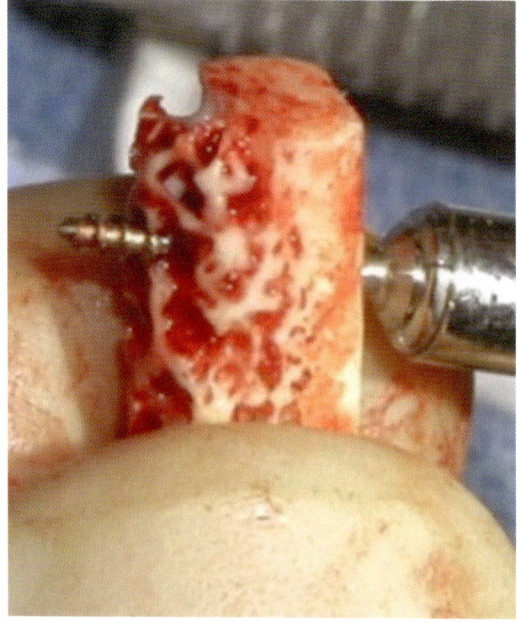

Fig. 12.25 Testing passivity of fixation screw in block allograft

the block in a sterile syringe with sterile saline. The end of the syringe is capped, and the plunger is moved to create a vacuum inside of the syringe. This forces air out of the block while forcing saline into the cancellous portion. When the air bubbles stop coming out of the block, it is hydrated (Figs. 12.23 and 12.24). Once the block has been shaped to fit the recipient site, holes are created to place a passive fixation screw (Fig. 12.25). If the trephine technique is used, only one screw hole is necessary due to the parallel walls providing antirotation of the block. It is not recommended to remove any cortical bone of the allograft. This cortical bone provides the space maintenance. Without this cortical plate, all that

12.3 Ramus Graft

Based on the decision tree, the external oblique ridge is the donor site of choice for block grafting mandibular premolars and molars. This keeps the donor and recipient site in the same sextant reducing morbidity for the patient (Fig. 12.28). Although ramus bone can be used in the premaxilla, block allografts are so predictable that it may not make sense to create an additional surgical site for the patient to harvest ramus bone.

Prior to harvesting bone from the external oblique ridge, a CBCT will provide a three-dimensional view of the donor site. This will help to identify the location of the mandibular canal as well as the thickness of the bone to be harvested. The ramus donor site can be accessed with a midcrestal incision in keratinized tissue, a sulcular incision around any adjacent teeth, and a "hockey stick" releasing incision just distal to the retromolar pad. Special attention is paid to not make the "hockey stick" incision higher than the occlusal plane so as not to expose the buccal fat as well as to avoid the buccal artery. The mesial vertical incision is typically made mesial to the cuspid to avoid damaging the contents of the mental foramen. After a full-thickness mucoperiosteal flap is reflected, the third molar site is identified, and the cuts are made approximately 15 mm long, 4 mm medial, and 8–10 mm apical. Use of a piezotome may minimize bleeding, minimize the potential to damage soft tissue vital structures (contents of the mandibular canal), and provide a thin cut maximizing the volume of bone remaining in the graft (Figs. 12.29 and 12.30). Based on individual anatomy, a much larger block many times can be harvested with respect to the anatomy. The block is approximately 4 mm of cortical bone (Smith and Rajchel 1992; Rajchel et al. 1986). With this density of bone, it is possible to hold the block with a bone block clamp and shape and smooth any sharp corners and round the edges. Due to the location of the incision line directly over the donor bone, particulate bone is not placed in the donor site. It would lead to sequestration of the particulate bone and delayed heal-

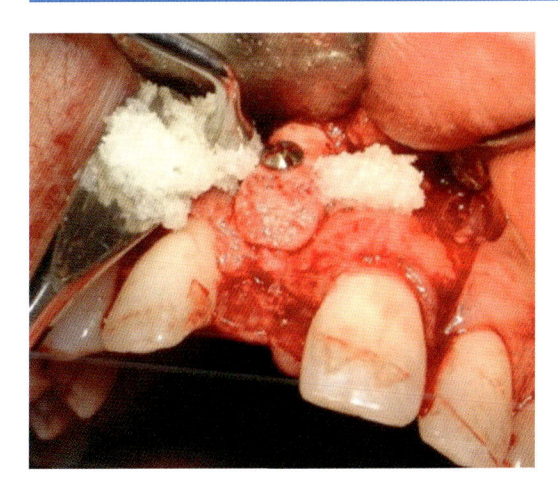

Fig. 12.26 Ramping of bone with mineralized cancellous particulate allograft material

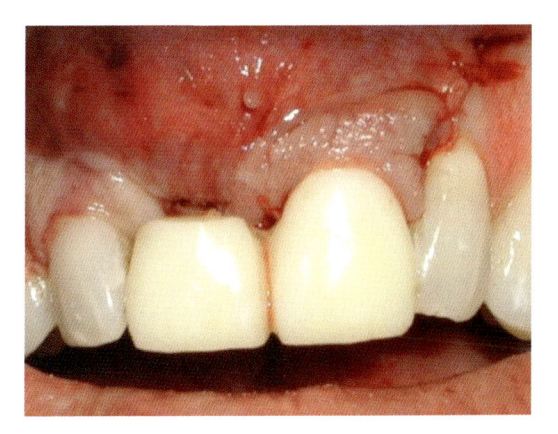

Fig. 12.27 Primary closure with temporary bridge relieved

is left is cancellous bone which is not predictable with regard to volume of resorption. The cortical bone also provides stability for the fixation screw, whereas the cancellous bone may allow mobility around the fixation screw creating a foreign body reaction and ultimate failure of the graft. Once the fixation screws are placed, particulate bone is ramped around the block, including the apex, and a resorbable membrane is used to contain the graft material (Fig. 12.26). Horizontal mattress sutures over the recipient site will be most resistant to incision line opening (Fig. 12.27).

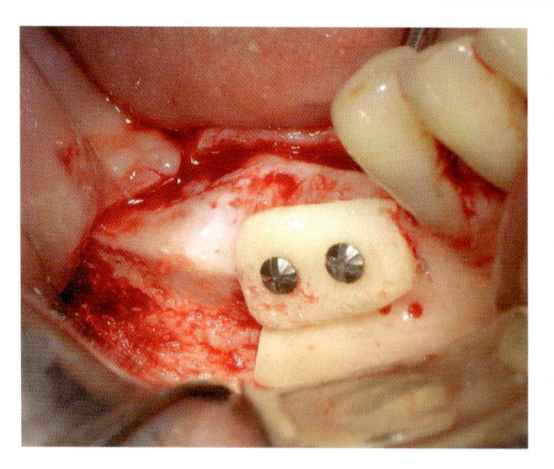

Fig. 12.28 Ramus graft; donor and recipient sites kept in same sextant of mouth

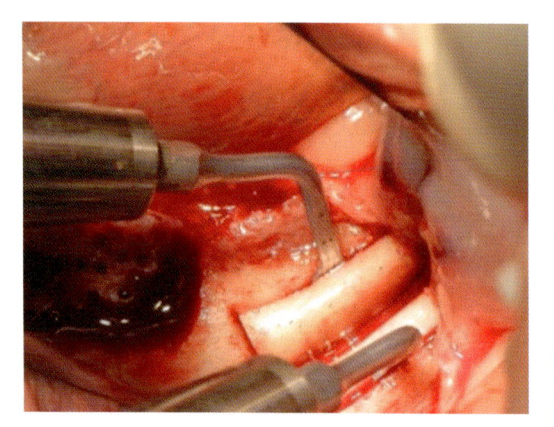

Fig. 12.29 Piezo technology making cut for block graft

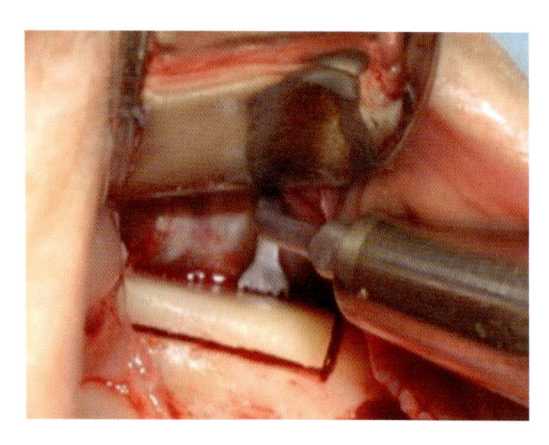

Fig. 12.30 Piezo bone saw making a perpendicular cut in an area lateral to the mandibular canal

ing. An autogenous blood product concentrating the patient's own platelets may be used to facilitate soft tissue healing over the donor site. This site can be sutured with interrupted sutures. There will not be much tension on the donor site. If the donor bone were being used in the posterior mandible, the suture of choice would be a horizontal mattress to evert the flap making it more resistant to incision line opening.

12.4 Chin Graft

Based on the decision tree donor bone from the mandibular symphysis is the donor of choice for block grafting mandibular cuspids and incisors. This keeps the donor and recipient site in the same sextant, reducing morbidity for the patient. Prior to harvesting bone from the symphysis, a CBCT will provide a three-dimensional view of the donor site (Figs. 12.31, 12.32, and 12.33). This will help to identify the location of the mental foramen as well as the thickness of the bone to be harvested and the location of any root apices. A sulcular incision around any remaining

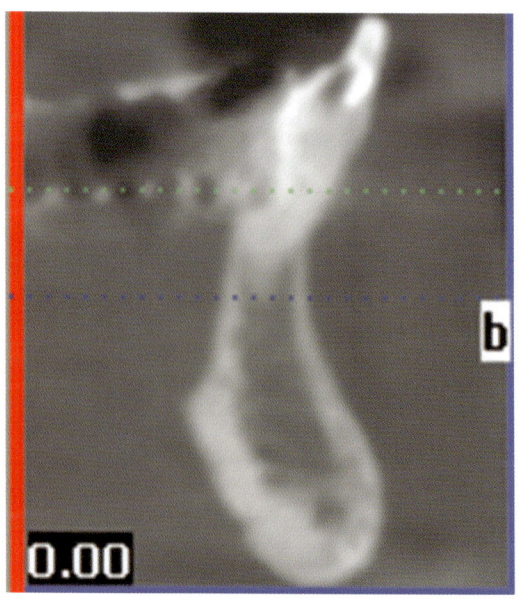

Fig. 12.31 Cross section of CBCT demonstrating location of root apices as well as the thickness of the bone

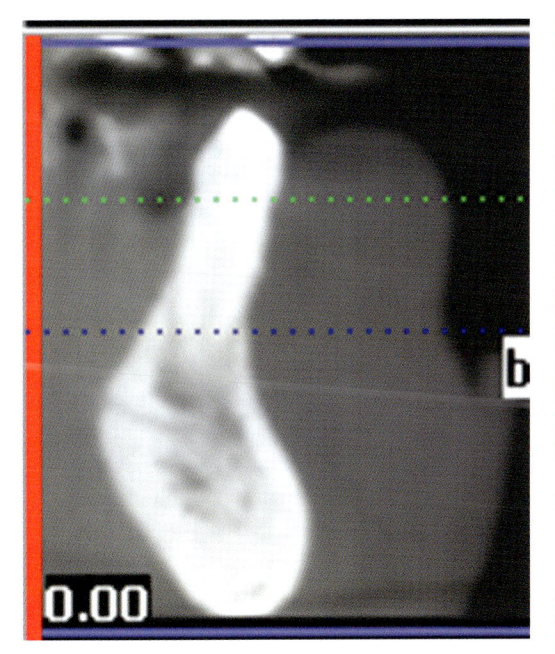

12 Development of Hard Tissues with Block Grafting Techniques   199

Fig. 12.32 Cross section of CBCT demonstrating location of root apices as well as the thickness of the bone

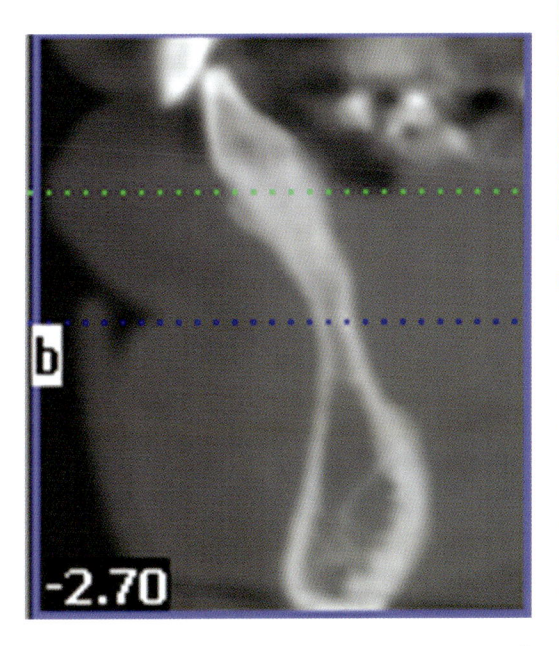

Fig. 12.33 Very thin mandible, block graft contraindication

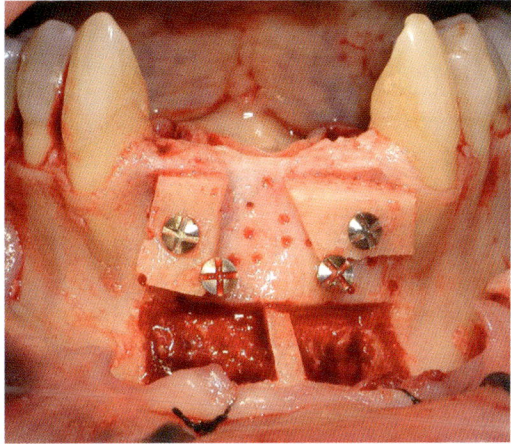

Fig. 12.34 Block graft from chin keeping recipient and donor sites in same quadrant

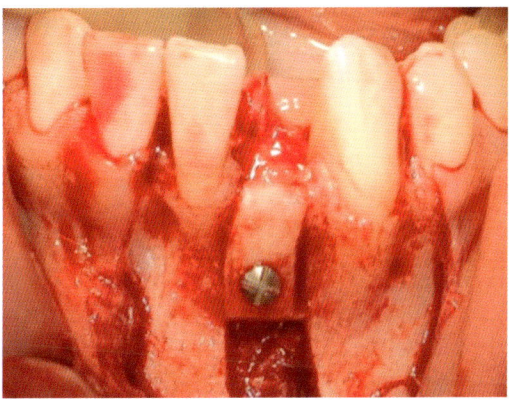

Fig. 12.35 Block graft from chin keeping recipient and donor sites in same sextant

teeth versus a vestibular incision will minimize incision line opening, infection, and scarring (Misch 1997). Vertical releasing incisions need to avoid the area of the mental foramen so as not to damage the contents. After reviewing the CBCT and evaluating the site clinically, a zone of safety is identified. This will start at least 5 mm apical to the apices of any remaining incisors. The bone can be harvested with a bur or a piezotome. The piezotome will be of benefit for the same reasons already mentioned above (Figs. 12.34, 12.35, and 12.36). Care is taken to not take a bi-cortical graft. Once the outline has been made, the block can be harvested with bone spreaders or chisels. Because the flap margin will be far enough away from the borders of the donor site, it is possible to place particulate allograft into the donor site for

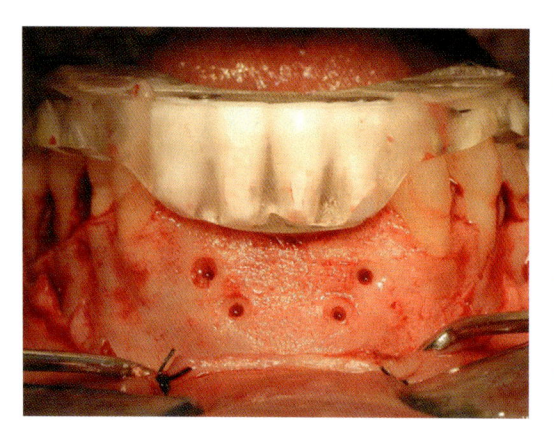

Fig. 12.36 Block graft from chin keeping recipient and donor sites in same sextant

faster healing. The block should be stored in saline and should be irrigated when being shaped and prepared for the lag screw. The block will be mostly cortical bone and needs to be shaped with a rotary instrument and a bone block clamp. The intimate adaptation of the block to the recipient site can be challenging due to the cortical nature of both donor and recipient bone. The more intimate the adaptation, the less concern with micromovement of the graft. Typically, two fixation screws are placed for antirotation, and particulate bone is used to fill in any gaps between the donor and recipient bone. A resorbable membrane is always recommended to contain the particulate bone. At least two fixation screws are used to prevent antirotation of the block.

12.5 Concepts for All Blocks

Temporization of the grafted area may consist of an Essix retainer, a temporary bridge, or a removable partial denture. It is critical that the temporary restoration not touch or load the tissue so as not to cause micromovement of the graft. The surgeon may have to aggressively relieve the temporary restoration to facilitate space for swelling of the tissue and advancement of the flap. As the tissue heals, the temporary restoration can be modified for cosmetics. The patient needs to be compliant with a soft diet so as not to load the graft.

Healing time depends largely on the age of the patient. The literature supports 4–6 months healing prior to placing implants (Misch et al. 1992; Misch and Misch 1995; Pikos 1996). The fixation screw needs to be removed at the time of the implant placement.

12.6 Complications

Complications can occur at the donor as well as the recipient sites. The recipient site complications are typically incision line opening (Figs. 12.37, 12.38, 12.39, and 12.40) (Misch 1997). With incision line opening over a block graft, the treatment is usually removal of the block; wait for 3 months healing and regraft. However, complications from the donor site may have more consequences. Complications from the donor site may include infection, pain, bleeding, and temporary or permanent paresthesia (Hunt and Jovanovic 1999; Nkenke et al. 2001; Raghoebar et al. 2001; Nkenke 2002; Von Arx and Kurt 1998; Cordaro et al. 2002; Cordaro and Rosini 2004). Nkenke reported that at a 1-year follow-up exam of chin grafts, 11.4% of anterior teeth had lost their pulp sensitivity, and permanent changes in lip sensibility were found in 10% of their patients. They considered this procedure to have a high rate of complications (Nkenke et al. 2001). Cordaro described a unique complication after chin bone harvesting. Fracture and posterior dis-

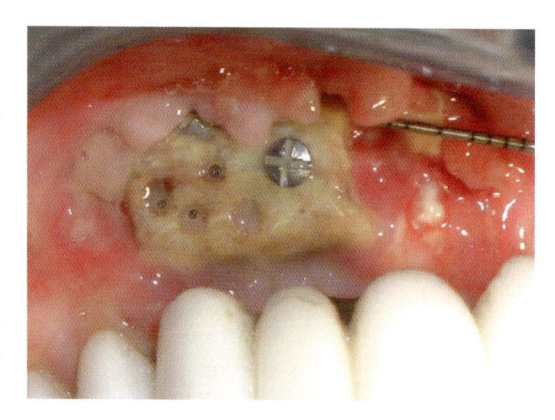

Fig. 12.37 Incision line opening and block allograft exposure

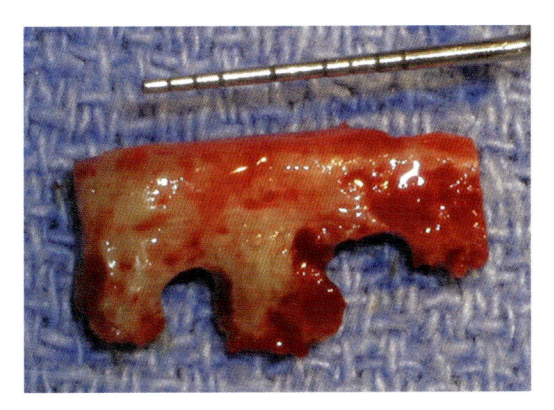

Fig. 12.38 Block allograft after removal demonstration resorption

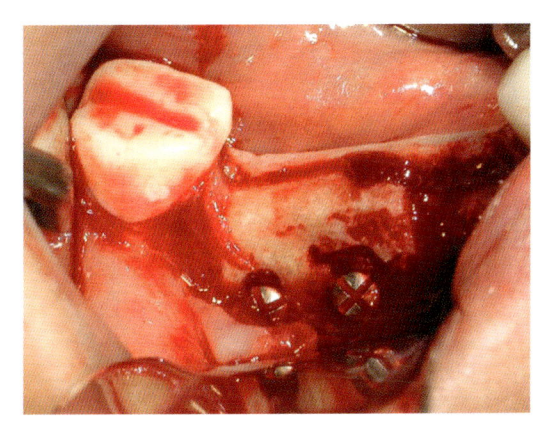

Fig. 12.39 Block allograft in the posterior mandible demonstrating block loose around fixation screws

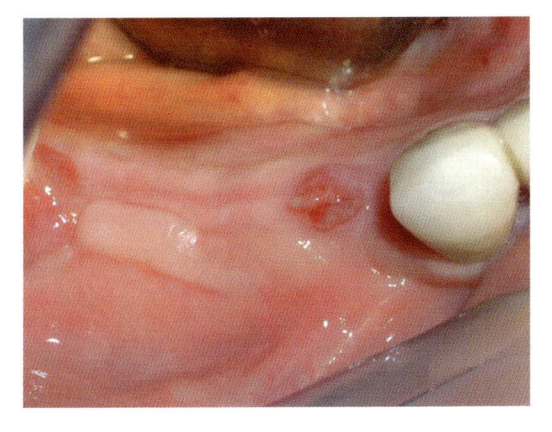

Fig. 12.40 Fistulas due to mobility of block allograft causing inflammatory reaction

placement of the lingual cortical plate did not occur at the time of the operation but during the healing phase. Diagnosis was made by chance with the aid of a postoperative CT scan (Cordaro and Rosini 2004). When considering use of a block allograft or an autogenous graft, these complications from the donor site should be considered.

12.7 Autograft vs. Allograft

The physical/mechanical difference between an autogenous, monocortical block graft and a monocortical block allograft is that the autograft will be approximately 4 mm of dense cortical bone. The allograft will provide approximately 1–2 mm of cortical bone, and remaining bone will be cancellous. The donor source for the allograft is typically the iliac crest. Therefore, it is important to not countersink the screw in the allograft and to keep as much of the cortical bone intact. The cortical bone of the allograft is what creates the space maintenance. To avoid sharp edges, particulate allograft bone is typically placed around the edges of autogenous grafts and block allografts. This ramps the bone, and with the use of a resorbable membrane, the particulate can be contained. Resorption of both grafts is reported to be less than 25% (Misch et al. 1992; Pikos 1999). However, it must be pointed out that a cancellous block allograft without a cortical layer has an unpredictable resorption rate (Wallace and Gellin 2010).

Like many other surgical techniques, bone grafting techniques may be popular for a while, they are replaced with other techniques that appear sexy at the time, and then they come full circle and are in vogue again. When considering which bone grafting technique to use, review the literature, and carefully consider the predictability of the technique and the skill and experience of the surgeon. These factors will definitely provide bias, but most of all choose the treatment plan and option that will provide the most conservative and predictable result for long-term success for your patient.

References

Chaushu (2010) Analysis of complications following augmentation with cancellous block allografts. J Periodontol 81:1759–1764

Cordaro L, Rosini C (2004) Fracture and displacement of lingual cortical plate of mandibular symphysis following bone harvesting: case report. Implant Dent 13:202–206

Cordaro L, Sarzi Amade D, Cordaro M (2002) Clinical results of alveolar ridge augmentation with mandibular block bone grafts in partially edentulous patients prior to implant placement. Clin Oral Impl Res 13:103–111

Hunt DR, Jovanovic SA (1999) Autogenous bone harvesting: a chin graft technique for particulate or monocortical bone blocks. Int J Periodontics Restorative Dent 19:165–173

Grunder U, Gracis S, Capelli M (2005) Influence of the 3-D bone-to-implant relationship on esthetics. Int J Periodontics Restor Dent 25:113–119

Iasella JM, Greenwell H, Miller RL et al (2003) Ridge preservation with freeze-dried bone allograft and a collagen membrane compared to extraction alone for implant site development: a clinical and histologic study in humans. J Periodontol 74:990–999

Ishikawa T, Salama M et al (2007) Three-dimensional bone and soft tissue requirements for optimizing esthetic results in compromised cases with multiple implants. Int J Periodontics Restor Dent 27(3):251–257

Keith et al (2006) Clinical and histologic evaluation of a mineralized block allograft: results from the developmental period (2001–2006). Int J Periodontics Restorative Dent 26:321–327

Leonetti J, Koup R (2003) Localized maxillary ridge augmentation with a block allograft for dental implant placement: case reports. Implant Dent 12:217–226

Linkevicius T et al (2009) The influence of soft tissue thickness on crestal bone changes around implants: a 1-year prospective controlled clinical trial. Int J Oral Maxillofac Implants 24:712–719

Misch CM (1996) Ridge augmentation using mandibular ramus bone grafts for the placement of dental implants: presentation of a technique. Pract Periodontics Aesth Dent 8:127–135

Misch CM (1997) Comparison of intraoral donor sites for onlay grafting prior to implant placement. Int J Oral Maxillofac Implants 12:767–776

Misch CM, Misch CE (1995) The repair of localized severe ridge defects for implant placement using mandibular bone grafts. Implant Dent 4:261–267

Misch DM, Misch CE, Resnik R et al (1992) Reconstruction of maxillary alveolar defects with mandibular symphysis grafts for dental implants: a preliminary procedural report. Int J Oral Maxillofac Implants 7:360–366

Nkenke E (2002) Morbidity of harvesting of retromolar bone grafts: a prospective study. Clin Oral Implants Res 13(5):514–521

Nkenke E, Schultze-Mosgau S, Radespiel-Troger M et al (2001) Morbidity of harvesting of chin grafts: a prospective study. Clin Oral Implants Res 12:495–502

Petrungaro P, Amar S (2005) Localized ridge augmentation with allogenic block grafts prior to implant placement: case reports and histologic evaluations. Implant Dent 14:139–146

Pikos MA (1996) Facilitating implant placement with chin grafts as donor sites for maxillary bone augmentation – Part I. Dent Implantol Update 1995;6:89–92 & Part II. Dent Implantol Update 7:1–4

Pikos MA (1999) Alveolar ridge augmentation with ramus buccal shelf autografts and impacted third molar removal. Dent Implantol Updat 10:27–31

Raghoebar GM, Louwerse C, Kalk WW et al (2001) Morbidity of chin bone harvesting. Clin Oral Implants Res 12:503–507

Rajchel J, Ellis E, Fonseca RJ (1986) The anatomical location of the mandibular canal: its relationship to the sagittal ramus osteotomy. Int J Adult Orthod Orthognath Surg 1:37

Rubens BC, West RA (1989) J Oral Maxillofac Surg 47:359–366

Smith BR, Rajchel JL (1992) Anatomic considerations in mandibular ramus osteotomies. In: Bell WH (ed) Modern practice in orthognathic and reconstructive surgery. WB Saunders, Philadelphia, pp 2347–2360

Von Arx T, Kurt B (1998) endoral donor bone removal for autografts. A comparative clinical study of donor sites in the chin area and the retromolar region. Schweiz Monatsschr Zahnmed 108:446–459

Waasdorp JA, Reynolds MA (2010) Allogeneic block grafts: a systematic review. Int J Oral Maxillofac Implants 25(3):525–531

Wallace SC, Gellin RG (2010) Clinical evaluation of freeze-dried cancellous block allografts for ridge augmentation and implant placement in the maxilla. Implant Dent 19:272–279

Guided Bone Regeneration for Aesthetic Implant Site Development

13

Bach Le

Abstract

Achieving ideal aesthetics with bone augmentation for implant site development is often elusive. Numerous techniques, protocols, and materials in guided bone regeneration (GBR) have been described to manage compromised sites of varying severity. The protocols and techniques employed should be predictable, minimally invasive, aesthetic, and lasting. This evidence-based discussion will describe the latest techniques for GBR for aesthetic site development of the compromised implant site. Topics to be covered include patient evaluation and strategies for dealing with the horizontally and vertically deficient ridge. This chapter will also focus on the most current strategies in minimally invasive bone grafting and tissue management to improve long-term clinical success with dental implants, specifically in the aesthetic zone.

13.1 Introduction

The use of guided bone regeneration (GBR) in implantology is recognized as a method of alveolar ridge augmentation for managing localized defects associated with dental implant placement (Aghaloo and Moy 2007; Chiapasco and Zaniboni 2009; Al-Nawas and Schiegnitz 2014). This concept has been shown clinically to promote osseous regeneration through the creation and maintenance of space under a membrane to allow migration of cells and ingrowth of blood vessels from adjacent osteogenic tissues. The use of GBR has allowed clinicians to provide more predictable restoration of form, function, and aesthetics through more ideal implant placement (Rominger and Triplett 1994; Hammerle et al. 2002). Achieving predictable success in GBR requires proper treatment planning and meticulous execution. The success of GBR is dependent on multiple important variables. These include defect configuration, flap design, space maintenance, graft selection, membrane selection, and implant position. Each of these principles plays a critical role and can influence the success or failure of the procedure.

B. Le, DDS, MD, FICD, FACD
Department of Oral & Maxillofacial Surgery,
The Herman Ostrow School of Dentistry of USC,
USC Medical Center, Los Angeles, CA, USA
e-mail: leb97201@yahoo.com

13.2 Defect Configuration

It is important to realize that certain defects are more challenging than others, and some defects are better managed with alternative techniques. One of the primary goals of augmentation in aesthetic implant site development is the successful placement and long-term maintenance of bone graft in the labial crestal contour of the peri-implant region (Le and Burstein 2008a). This region is largely responsible for the labial soft tissue contour and long-term stability of the gingival margin level. With bone augmentation, graft migration and resorption from this area often result in unaesthetic tissue shrinkage or recession. The challenge in bone depends on a number of critical factors related to defect configuration.

13.2.1 Length of Edentulous Span

Single-tooth defects have a much better aesthetic prognosis than multiple-teeth defects (Belser et al. 2004). This concept is also true for bone augmentation. Particulate grafts in wider edentulous spans are more prone to apical migration.

Wider defects often require the use of containment barrier or space maintenance such as a mesh or a membrane with tacks to contain the bone graft material (Fig. 13.1a, b).

13.2.2 Number of Walls

New bone formation mainly depends on the surface area of exposed bone and bone marrow since the osteogenic and angiogenic cells that form new bone reside in the bone marrow (Schenk et al. 1994). The healing potential of a given defect increases with each bony wall available (Sculean et al. 2008). The number of bony walls available in a defect has a significant influence on the success of the bone augmentation procedure. Three to four wall defects have a better prognosis for containment of graft material within the skeletal borders with minimal migration and space maintenance. Defects with fewer walls are more difficult and often require additional graft procedures to attain the optimal result.

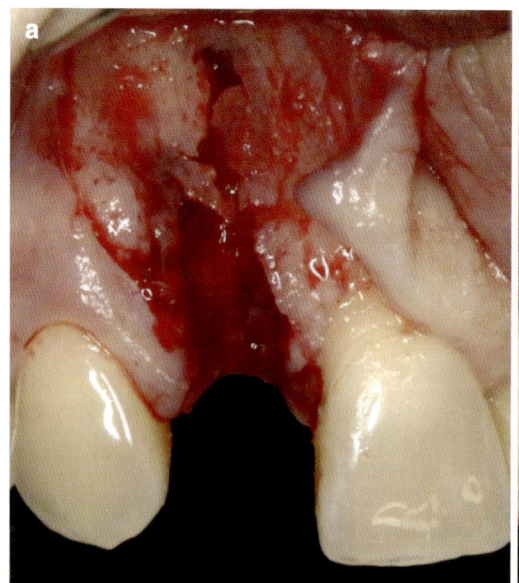

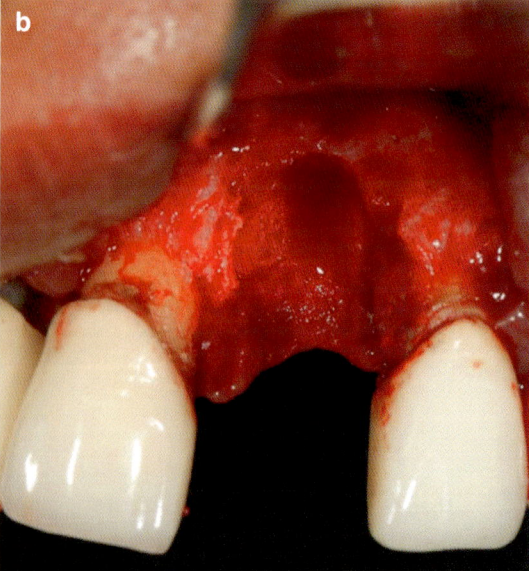

Fig. 13.1 (**a**, **b**) Narrow versus wide defects. Particulate grafts in wider edentulous spans are more prone to migration due to poor graft containment. Wider defects often require the use of containment barrier to contain the bone graft material. (**a**) Narrow buccal wall defect. (**b**) Wide buccal wall defect

13.2.3 Type of Defect

Horizontal defects with bony concavities to contain graft material have better prognosis than those with no walls (Fig. 13.2a, b). Defects with vertical components are the most difficult due to the difficulty in space maintenance. The use of space maintenance devices such as titanium mesh (Roccuzzo et al. 2004) or tenting screws (Le et al. 2010) is recommended in these defects. Distraction osteogenesis and segmental osteotomies have also been described for the management of severe vertical defects (Jensen et al. 2002; Jensen 2014).

13.3 Bone Graft Materials

Various bone graft materials can be used successfully for GBR procedures. An ideal bone graft material would be osteogenic, osteoinductive, osteoconductive, biocompatible, have good handling properties, provide adequate mechanical support to prevent collapse of covering membranes and overlying soft tissues, avoid the need for donor sites and associated morbidity, be of low cost, and resist resorption. Unfortunately, no such graft material exists at present. Autogenous bone has long been considered the gold standard for bone augmentation due to its biocompatibility and osteogenic properties. However, a recent systematic review on bone augmentation concluded there is no evidence that autogenous bone is superior to bone substitute material (Al-Nawas and Schiegnitz 2014). Available biomaterials include allografts (fresh-frozen bone); freeze-dried bone allograft (FDBA); demineralized, freeze-dried bone allograft (DFDBA); xenografts (bovine or equine bone minerals, DBBM); coral minerals, algae minerals, alloplastic materials (e.g., calcium phosphates, polymers, bioactive

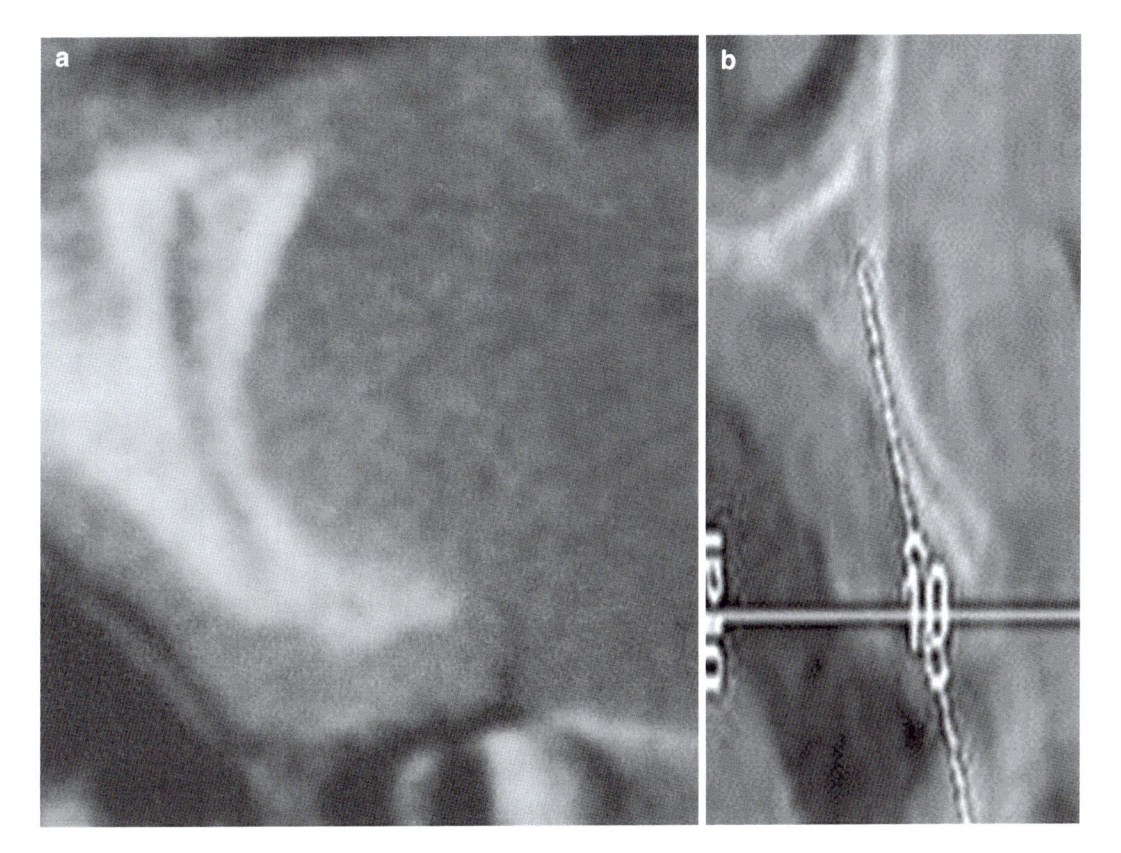

Fig. 13.2 (**a, b**) Defect with walls and defect without walls. (**a**) Horizontal defect with bony concavities to contain graft material. (**b**) Horizontal defect with one wall and no bony concavities are much more challenging to graft with particulate graft material due to apical migration

glass); and genetically engineered bone morphogenic proteins (BMP) and other biologics. Currently, the most widely used materials are autogenous, FDBA, and DBBM.

13.3.1 Autogenous Bone

Autogenous bone has osteogenic, osteoinductive, and osteoconductive properties. It can be harvested from intraoral or extraoral donor sites and, depending on the donor site location, can be primarily cortical, corticocancellous, or cancellous. Intraoral donor sites include the chin, mandibular ramus/body, maxillary tuberosity, anterior nasal spine, and zygomatic body. Extraoral donor sites include the anterior iliac crest, posterior iliac crest, tibia, calvaria, and fibula. Choice of the donor site depends on the size and dimension of the defect being treated as well as the clinicians' preference and consideration of patient morbidity. Particle size of autogenous bone graft is an important consideration since smaller particles have increased surface area allowing more growth factors to be exposed to osteoprogenitor cells (Pallesen et al. 2002).

13.3.2 Allografts

Freeze-dried bone allografts have been utilized with success in GBR procedures (Le et al. 2010; Block and Degen 2004). Studies using histologic analyses of grafted sites have shown adequate bone formation for implant osseointegration (Le et al. 2010; Wang and Tsao 2007; Block et al. 2002). Allografts are available as cortical, corticocancellous, or cancellous bone and can be demineralized or mineralized. The demineralization of allograft material exposes bone-inductive proteins located in the bone matrix (Schwartz et al. 1996), and these crude protein extracts from DFDBA contain immunoreactive BMPs (Shigeyama et al. 1995). However, in a study in mandibles of minipigs, Buser et al. (1998) concluded that DFDBA had only osteoconductive properties. Moreover, DFDBA has decreased mechanical stability compared with FDBA. When compared to DFDBA or bovine xenografts, mineralized allografts (FDBA) have been shown to have higher mean bone density as well as fewer residual particles after site healing (Froum et al. 2006). Our clinical experiences also suggest that FDBA may tolerate wound exposure better than autogenous bone and other biomaterials (Le et al. 2010) (Fig. 13.3a–m).

13.3.3 Xenografts

The most commonly used xenograft in GBR is bovine bone matrix. In its preparation, every effort is made to remove the organic components by chemical treatment with strong alkaline solution, heat treatment to 300–1,000 °C, or a combination of these methods. The resulting mineralized bone matrix is considered to be a safe xenograft with minimal risk of disease transmission (Wenz et al. 2001). In a study by Schwartz et al. (2007), small amounts of protein were found in bovine xenograft material, but these may represent transforming growth factor-beta (TGF-β) and BMP-2 as they were found to be osteoinductive in the nude mouse model when combined with inactive DFDBA.

In an animal model, Araújo et al. demonstrated that bovine bone matrix delayed bone healing in fresh extraction sockets (Araújo et al. 2008, 2009). Only minute amounts of newly formed bone appeared in the grafted sockets after 2 weeks of healing, while large amounts of woven bone had formed in the non-grafted sites. After a 3-month healing period, the newly formed hard tissue in extraction sockets grafted with the bovine material contained a large number of the graft particles that were surrounded by immature woven bone. Indeed, the general consensus is that mineralized bovine bone xenograft is slowly if ever resorbed, and histologic assessment of biopsies from augmented sinuses in humans showed remaining bovine bone particles up to 10 years postoperatively (Piattelli et al. 1999). Although some have found inhibitory effects with bovine bone matrix used in socket preservation, others have found it to be effective in preserving post-extraction alveolar ridge anatomy

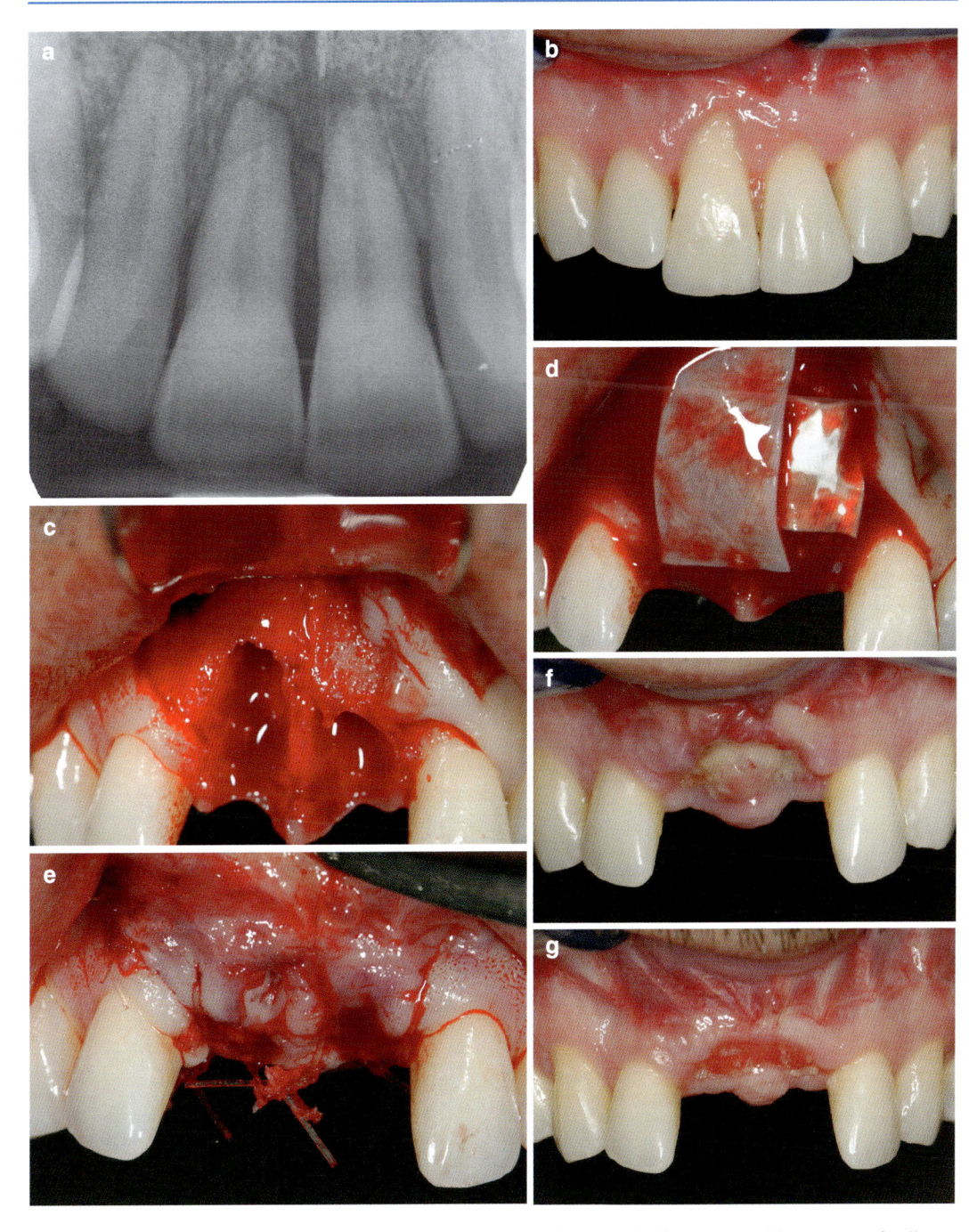

13 Guided Bone Regeneration for Aesthetic Implant Site Development   207

Fig 13.3 (**a–m**) Early wound dehiscence with exposure of mineralized allograft and collagen membrane is better tolerated than with non-resorbable membrane. (**a–e**) Extraction and augmentation of two maxillary central incisor defects with human mineralized allograft and resorbable collagen membrane. (**f**) Early wound dehiscence occurring 1 week after surgery with exposure of collagen membrane and allograft. (**g**) Early granulation of exposed graft. (**h**) Healing at 5 months with flapless implant placement. (**i–k**) Final restorations at 3 years. (**l–m**) CT scan show presence of thick crestal labial bone and soft tissue (Restorative dentist: Baldwin Marchack, DDS, MBA)

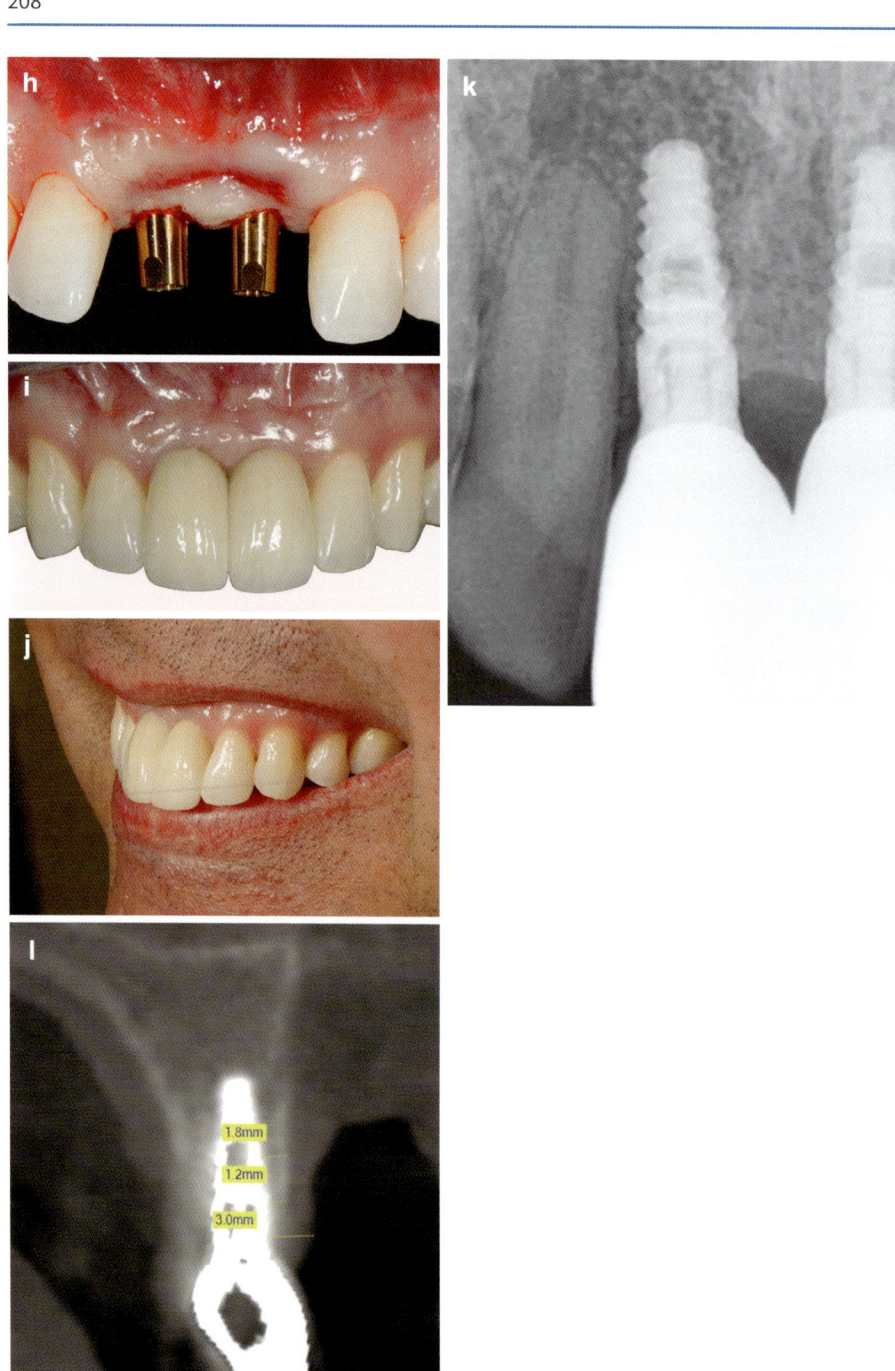

Fig. 13.3 (continued)

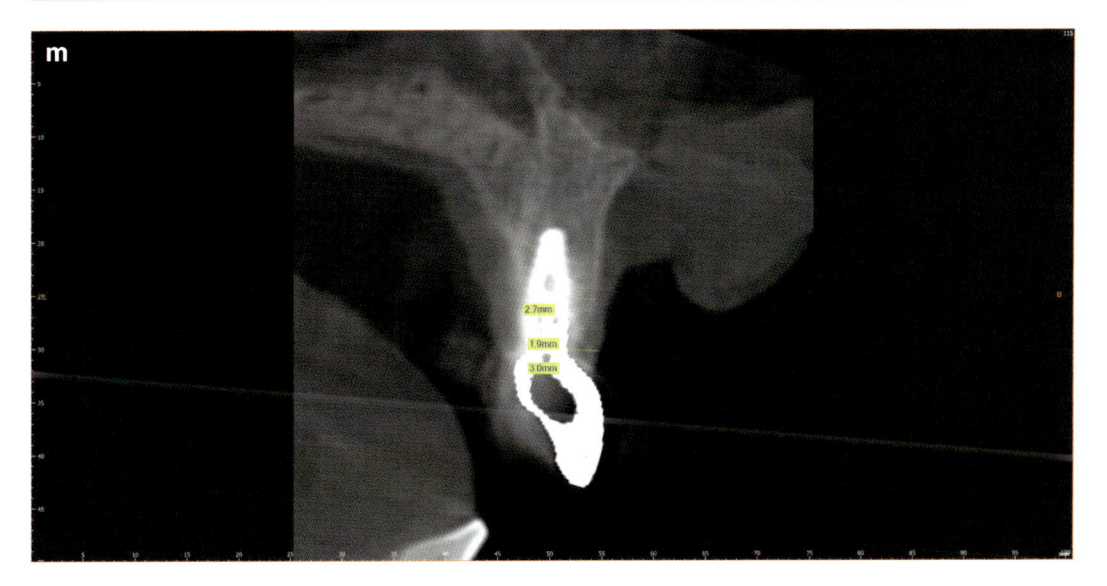

Fig. 13.3 (continued)

with adequate bone formation to allow subsequent successful implant placement (Molly et al. 2008). Given that the material is only osteoconductive, longer time intervals are likely needed between grafting and implant placement to allow for successful osseointegration.

13.4 Barrier Membranes

An ideal barrier membrane should be biocompatible, easy to handle, resorbable to avoid the necessity of an extra procedure for removal, maintain space, have tissue integration, provide cell occlusion, and have minimal susceptibility to complications (Hardwick et al. 1994). The two main categories of barrier membranes are non-resorbable and resorbable membranes. Non-resorbable membranes are generally made from polytetrafluoroethylene (PTFE), while resorbable membranes include polymer membranes and collagen membranes made from a variety of sources.

Bone augmentation can be performed with or without barrier membranes (Louis et al. 2008; Simion et al. 2007; Gielkens et al. 2007). A systemic review of available research to determine if a barrier membrane helped prevent resorption of autogenous onlay grafts concluded that more evidence is needed (Gielkens et al. 2007). Guided tissue regeneration (GTR) and guided bone regeneration (GBR) can be successfully performed using either resorbable or non-resorbable membranes (Laurell et al. 1994; Christgau et al. 1998).

Non-resorbable membranes, particularly those made from expanded PTFE, have significant risk of premature membrane exposure (Machtei 2001; Murphy 1995). They also have higher irritation and infection rates compared to resorbable membranes (Chiapasco and Zaniboni 2009). Collagen membranes are the most widely used resorbable membranes and are derived from modified bovine tendon, bovine dermis, calf skin, or porcine dermis (Bunyaratavej and Wang 2001). It is the author's experience that exposure of crosslinked collagen membranes with use of small particle mineralized allograft is better tolerated and less catastrophic to the graft than exposure with non-resorbable membranes or exposure with autogenous bone (Fig. 13.3a–m).

13.5 Management of Horizontal Defects

Most post-extraction losses of alveolar ridge dimensions occur in the horizontal (width) rather than the vertical (height) plane (Pietrokovski and

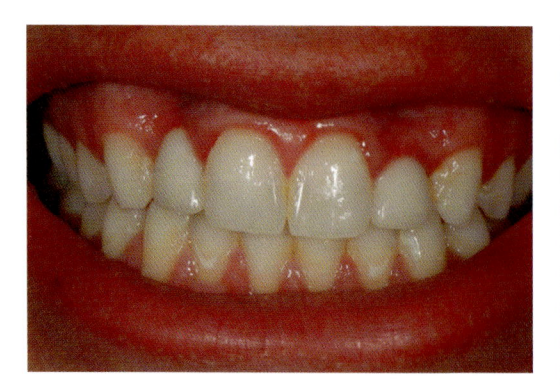

Fig. 13.4 Unnatural appearance of restoration due to collapsed buccal alveolus. Even when there is adequate bone to place implants, irregular ridge anatomy that is not corrected can result in an unnatural appearance of the final restoration

Massler 1967). Even when there is adequate bone to place implants, irregular ridge anatomy that is not corrected can result in an unnatural appearance of the final restoration (Fig. 13.4). Bone augmentation prior to or simultaneously with implant placement may correct ridge contour defects for a more natural-looking restoration and increase facial bone support for long-term peri-implant soft tissue stability (Spray et al. 2000).

Particulate bone has been used for horizontal augmentation with good success for mild to moderately sized defects (Aghaloo and Moy 2007; Chiapasco and Zaniboni 2009; Al-Nawas and Schiegnitz 2014). Utilizing the soft tissue matrix theory, meshes, reinforced membranes, screws, cortical bone, healing abutments, and the graft itself have been used to maintain this expanded space (Le and Burstein 2008a, b; Louis et al. 2008; Frost 1983). A tenting mechanism to prevent collapse of the soft tissue can be advantageous when augmenting vertical or large horizontal defects. Block and Degen (2004) described a minimally invasive tunneling technique using mineralized particulate allograft to horizontally augment partially edentulous defects for successful implant placement. However, a disadvantage of the tunneling technique is that it can be difficult to position and maintain the graft at the labial crest to augment the peri-implant soft tissue. Additional bone grafting is usually necessary at the time of implant placement to address this issue (Le and Burstein 2008a).

Ridge augmentation exclusively using particulate grafts is extremely technique-sensitive and operator dependent. Predictability of lateral ridge augmentation using particulate grafts is largely dependent on the ability to stabilize and maintain the soft tissue matrix. Maintenance of this space becomes more difficult with long edentulous spans or when there is inadequate basal bone support. The analogy of building a sandcastle applies with the use of particulate grafts for ridge augmentation. When building a sandcastle, a wide base is needed first to support the sand at the highest portion (Fig. 13.5a–n). Without adequate basal bone support, the most coronal portion of the graft often migrates apically. If using only particulate graft for larger width correction, basal bone width can be augmented first using a tunneling approach (Block and Degen 2004) or an open approach. The remaining labial crestal defect can be further enhanced at the time of implant placement or during implant uncovering with use of additional particulate graft and a healing abutment in the "aesthetic contour graft" technique" described by Le et al. (Le and Burstein 2008a; Le 2009).

13.5.1 "Aesthetic Contour Graft": Single-Stage Implants with Simultaneous GBR

The traditional GBR procedure is performed as a staged approach with a second surgical procedure to place the implant. If simultaneous bone grafting is performed, it is usually done with the implant submerged underneath the soft tissue. Le et al. described a simultaneous bone grafting with implant placement in a non-submerged single-stage protocol using a healing abutment (Le and Burstein 2008a; Le 2009). This approach offers many advantages. The single-stage protocol minimizes compression and migration of particulate graft material, and it allows the bony and soft tissue architecture to develop around the healing abutment during the healing phase. The placement of a healing abutment, in a single-stage

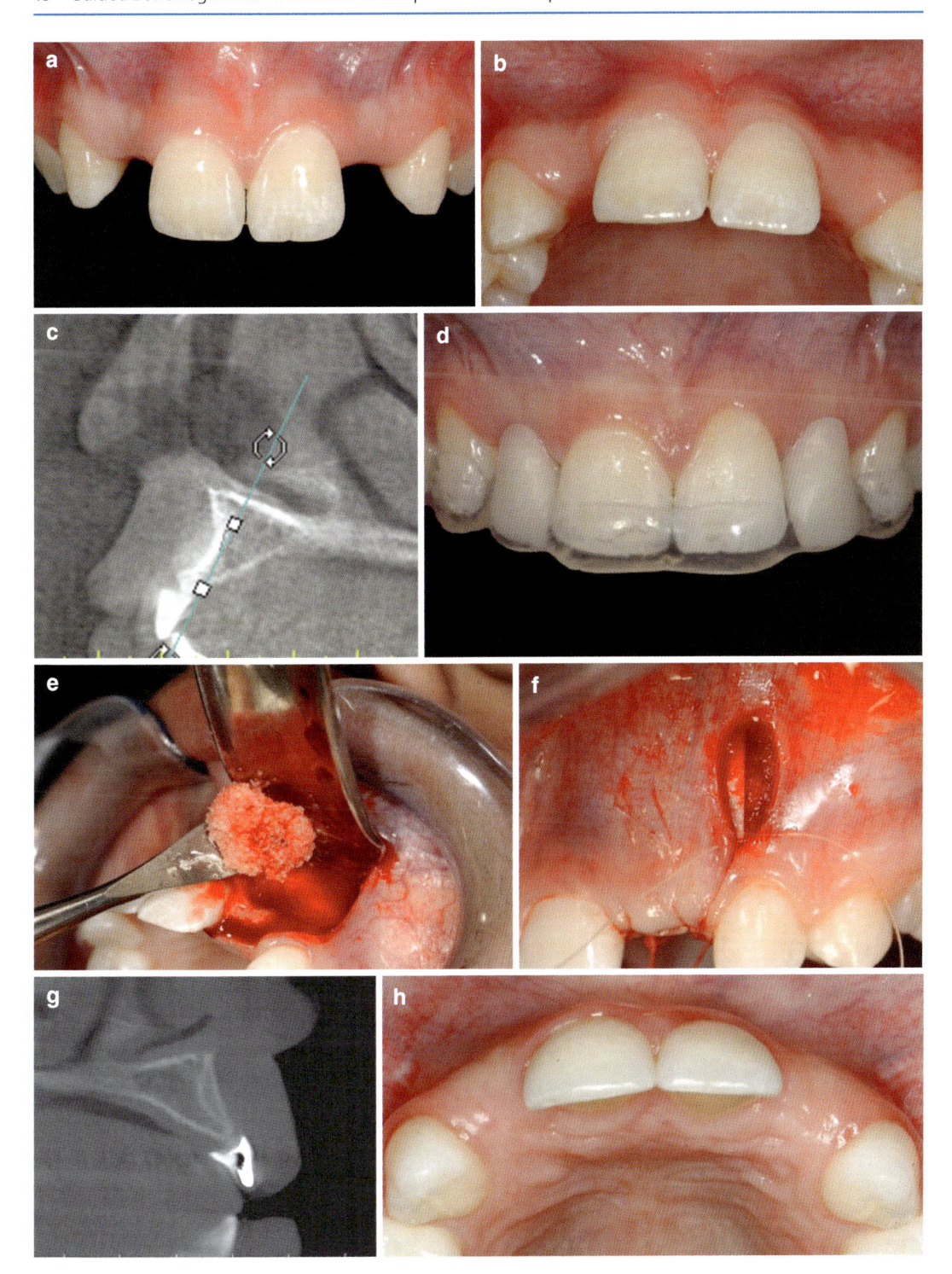

13 Guided Bone Regeneration for Aesthetic Implant Site Development

Fig. 13.5 (**a–n**) Horizontal augmentation with mineralized particulate allograft and resorbable collagen membrane for correction of congenital missing lateral incisor defects. Particulate grafting with GBR principles can be used for horizontal augmentation so long as an adequate bony foundation is already present to support the particulate graft (Restorative dentist, Abdi Sameni, DDS; lab technician, Michel Magne, MDT)

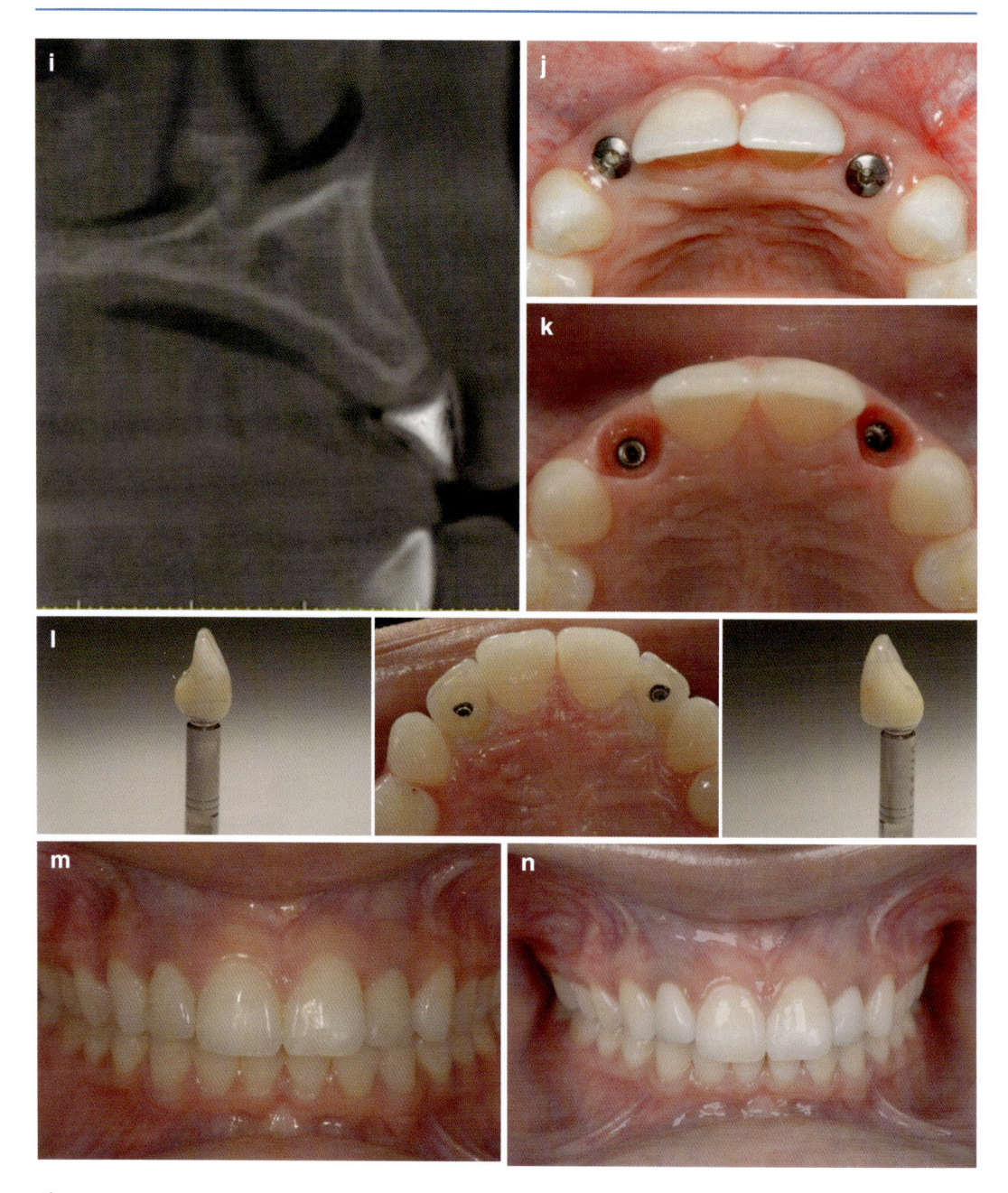

Fig. 13.5 (continued)

placement grafting protocol, provides tenting of the peri-implant soft tissue and results in less apical migration of graft material (Fig. 13.6a–o). This improves the prognosis by safeguarding the width and height of the remaining crestal bone. Grafting at the time of implant placement also takes advantage of the regional acceleratory phenomenon (Frost 1983) that is induced by the trauma of implant placement, leading to a reduced healing time.

Simultaneous bone grafting with two-stage implant placement has shown promising results

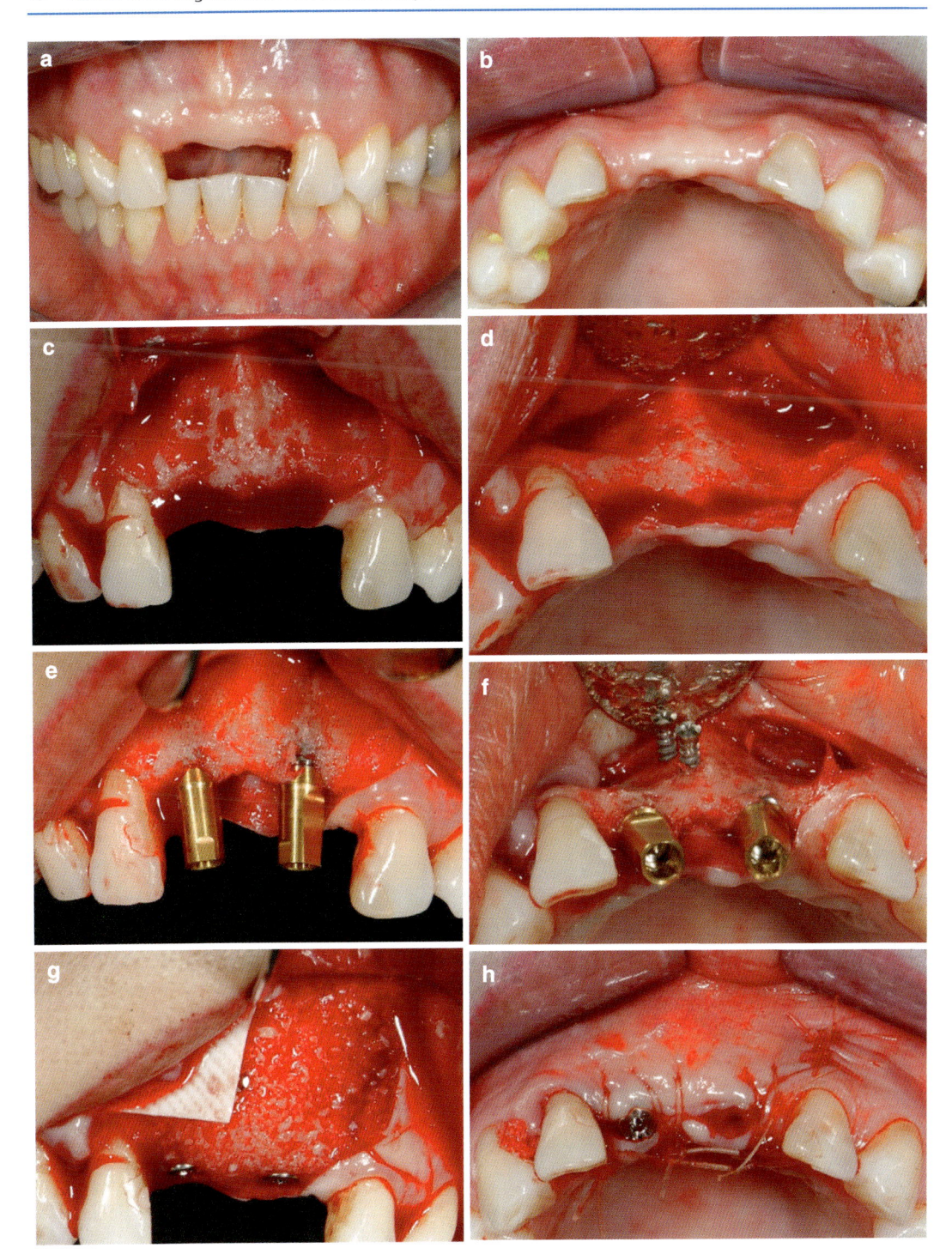

13 Guided Bone Regeneration for Aesthetic Implant Site Development 213

Fig. 13.6 (**a–o**) Aesthetic contour graft – simultaneous non-submerged implant placement and horizontal augmentation. Particulate grafting with GBR principles can be used for horizontal augmentation with simultaneous implant placement to correct small vertical soft tissue defects. In this case, mineralized allograft is placed along with a tenting screw and healing abutments to properly contour the labial peri-implant soft tissue for aesthetic emergence of the restorations (Restorative dentist, Alex Nguyen, DDS; lab, DenTech International)

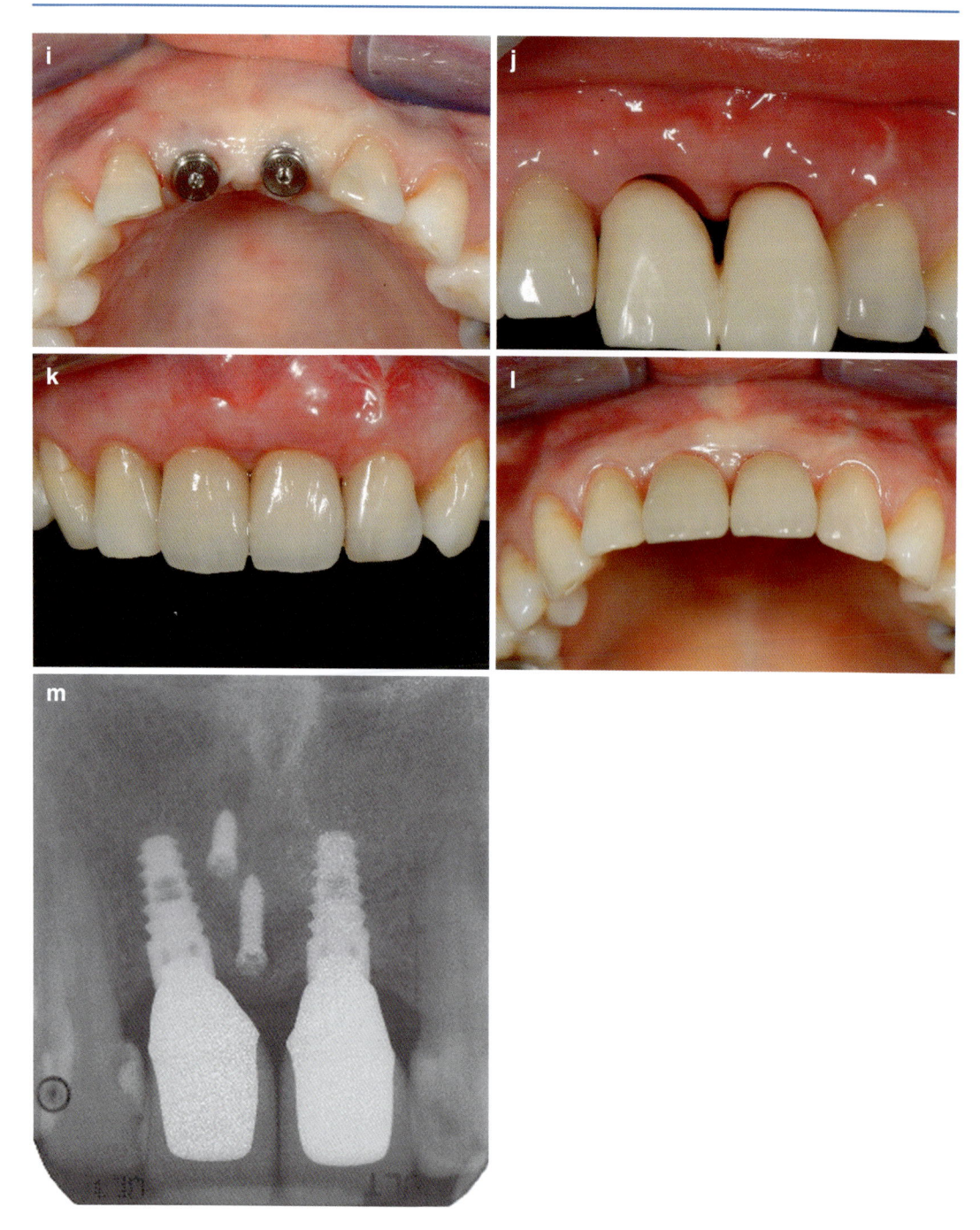

Fig. 13.6 (continued)

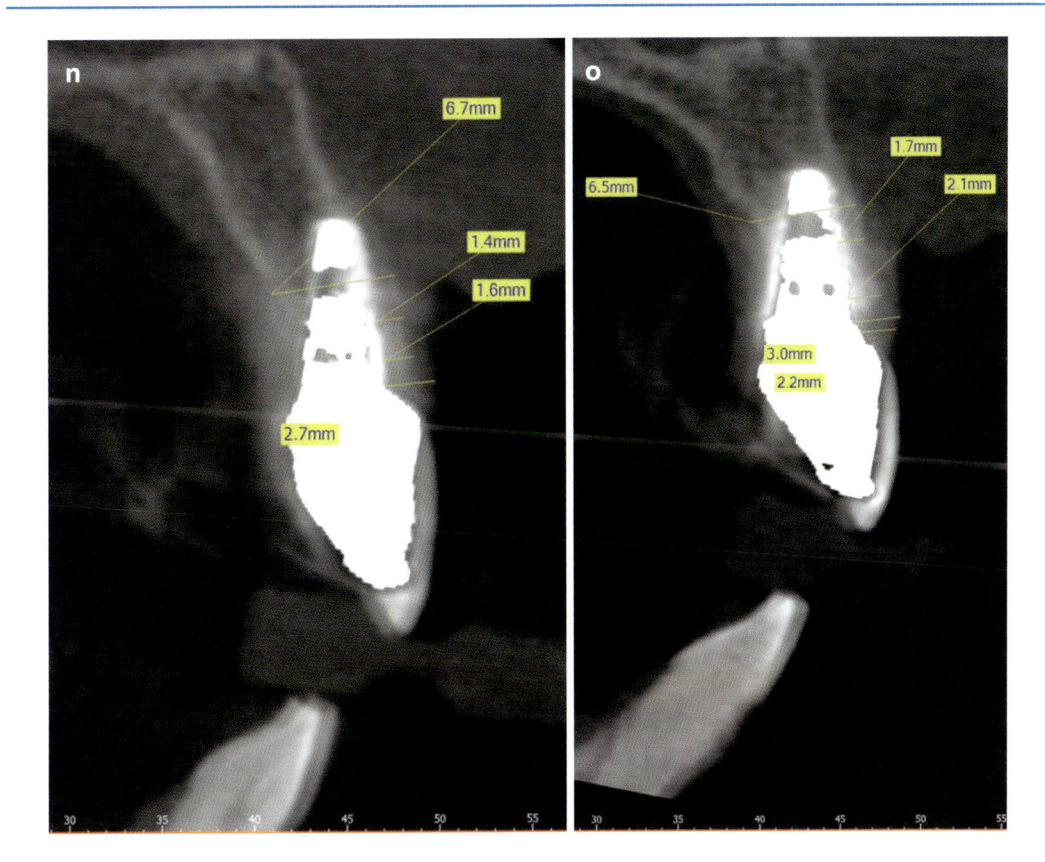

Fig. 13.6 (continued)

(Le 2009). Le et al. assessed the outcome of single-stage (non-submerged) implant placement and simultaneous augmentation of 156 sites with vertical buccal defect using a mineralized particulate allograft covered with collagen membranes (Le and Borzabadi-Farahani 2013). The vertical buccal defects were classified as small (less than 3 mm in depth), medium (3–5 mm in depth), and large (greater than 5 mm in depth). The initial vertical buccal wall defect was recorded by measuring the amount of vertical implant platform's rough surface exposure after implants were placed. Sectional CBCT scans were used at 36 months after graft healing. The site of the original vertical bone defect was evaluated for the presence of any residual vertical bone defect. The results showed the presence of bone in 100% and 79.3% of small and medium size vertical defects, respectively. Large size defects showed only partial improvement without any complete correction. Single-stage implant placement with simultaneous bone grafting to support the soft tissue margin showed promising outcomes in correcting intra-bony sites with vertical buccal wall defects (Le and Borzabadi-Farahani 2013) (Fig. 13.7a–q).

Another recently published article by Jensen et al. (2014) analyzed the long-term stability of contour augmentation during early implant placement (implant placement after 6–8 weeks of healing following tooth extraction) based on human biopsies harvested from the aesthetic zone. The implant placement was performed with simultaneous contour augmentation using deproteinized bovine bone mineral (DBBM) and a collagen barrier membrane. The biopsies were subjected to histologic and histomorphometric analysis. Results showed that the biopsies

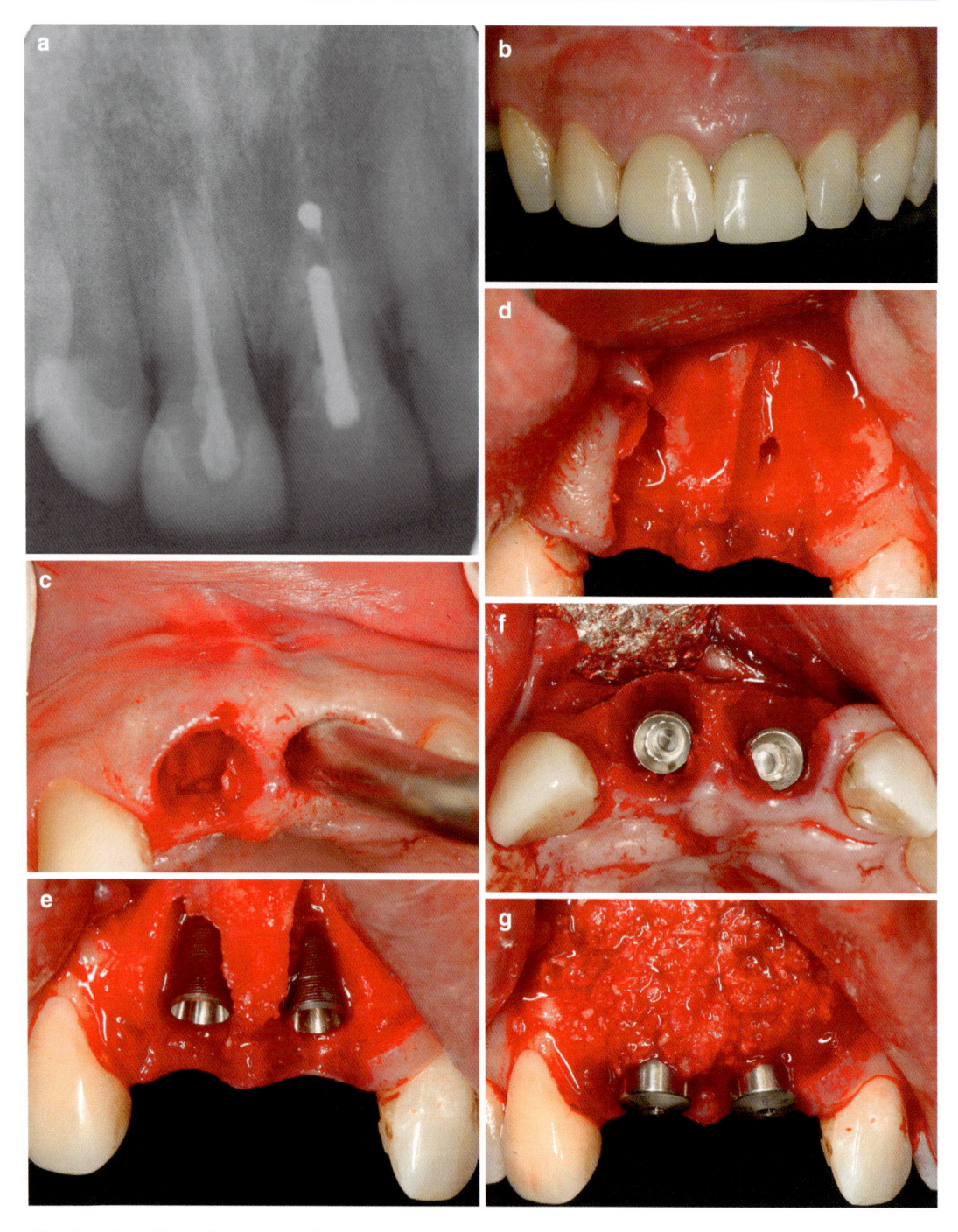

Fig. 13.7 (**a–q**) Immediate implants in extraction sockets with narrow labial wall defect. Sockets with labial wall defects should be managed with an open-flap approach to allow for overcorrection of the defect in anticipation of graft shrinkage from remodeling. Open-book flap design with aesthetic contour graft and non-submerged closure around healing abutment to contour the labial peri-implant soft tissue (Restorative dentist, Kourosh Dianat, DDS; lab, DenTech International)

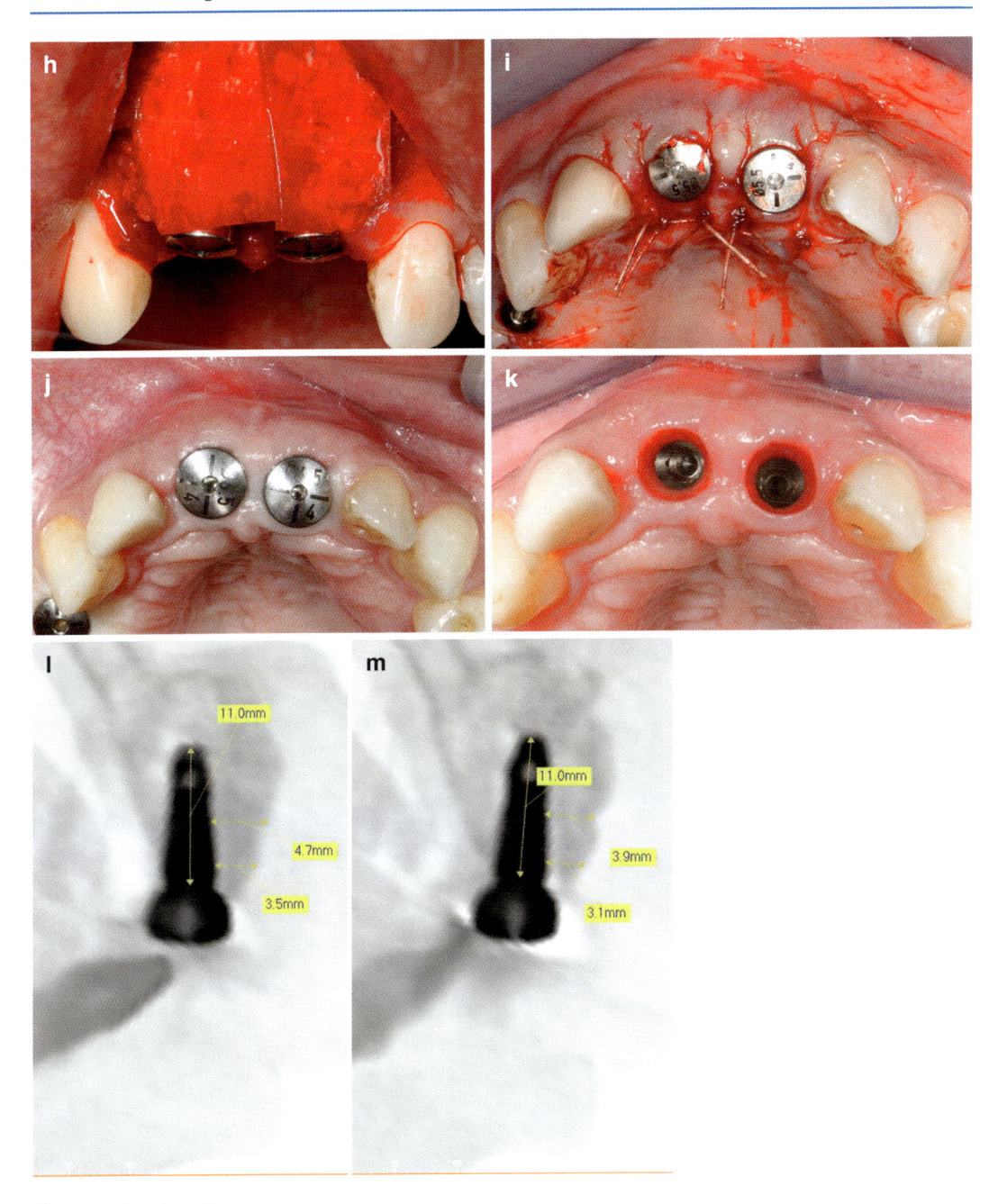

Fig. 13.7 (continued)

consisted of 32.0 ± 9.6% DBBM particles and 40.6 ± 14.6% mature bone. 70.3 ± 14.5% of the DBBM particle surfaces were covered with bone. They concluded that osseointegrated DBBM particles do not tend to undergo substitution over time, confirming previous findings. This low substitution rate supports the clinically and radiographically documented long-term stability of contour augmentation utilizing a combination of autogenous bone chips, DBBM particles, and a collagen membrane (Jensen et al. 2014).

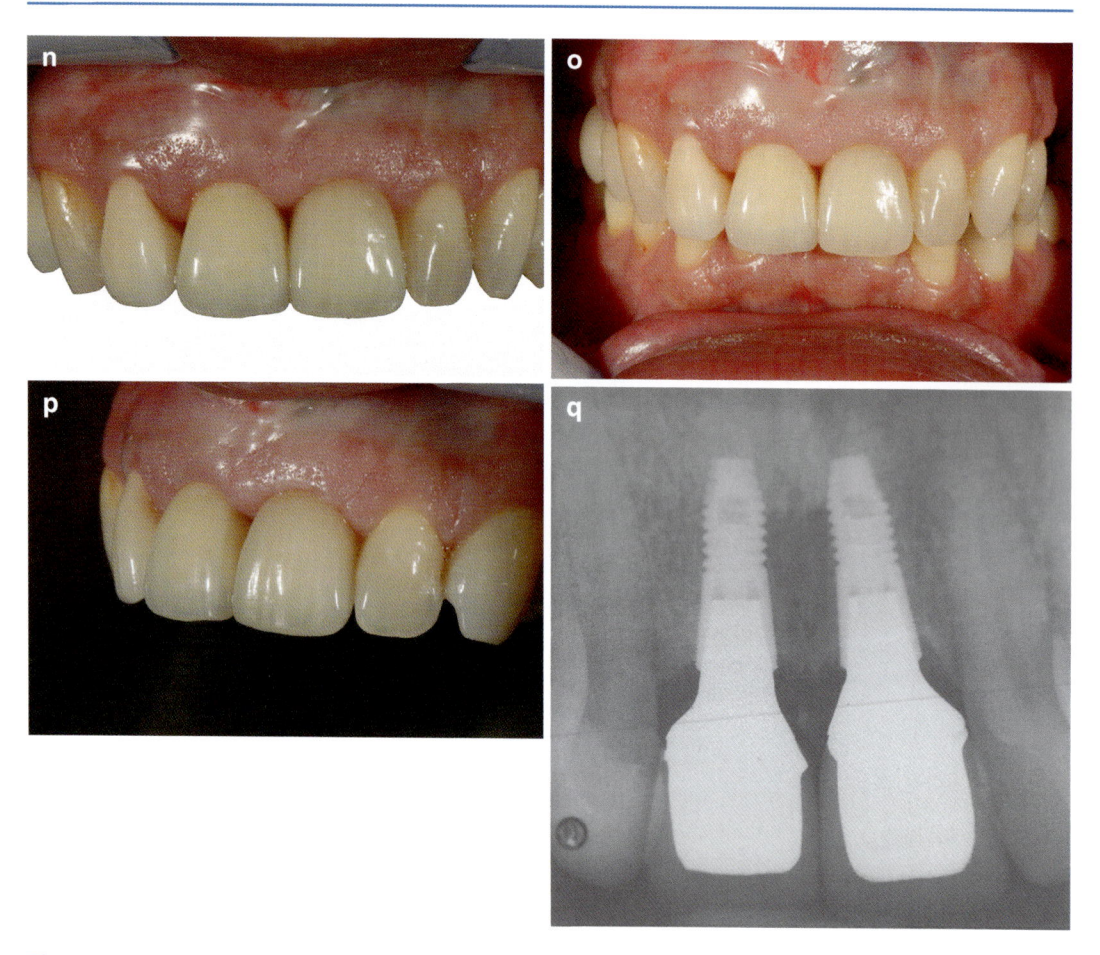

Fig. 13.7 (continued)

13.5.2 Flap Design

Minimizing flap exposure to maximize vascular supply to the surgical site while creating adequate access for graft placement can be delicate. Surgical exposure can be limited to a flapless approach when there is no anticipation for bone augmentation (adequate bone width, height, and keratinized tissue width). A flapless protocol offers many advantages, including faster recovery, less postoperative discomfort, decreased crestal bone loss, and decreased tissue recession. With increasing defect size, surgical exposure will require an incision design using a sulcular flap, envelope flap with extension to adjacent teeth, or vertical releasing incisions. For small ridge defects (<2 mm), a flapless or sulcular incision may be adequate. For larger defects, an open-book flap design may be used to enhance visualization and access to the graft site (Fig. 13.8) (Le and Borzabadi-Farahani 2013). It is important to achieve tension-free adaptation of wound margins during wound closure. Raising a flap for correction of the anatomical defect requires incising or scoring the periosteum for tension-free expansion of the soft tissue matrix. In addition to allowing primary tension-free wound closure, scoring of the periosteum also promotes angiogenesis by creating bleeding into the graft (Wang and Boyapati 2006).

13.5.3 Open-Book Flap Procedure

Grafting of labial wall defects using guided bone regeneration has been described to correct post-

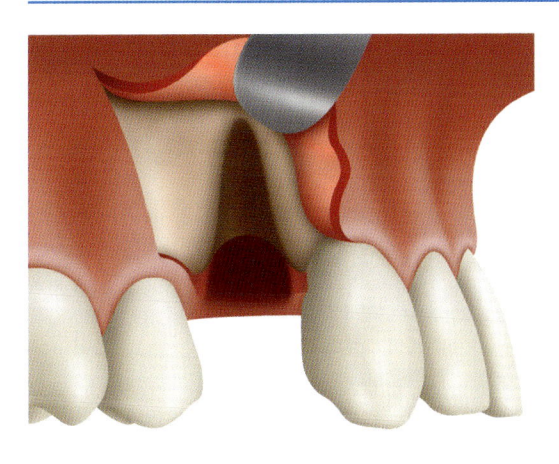

Fig. 13.8 Open-book flap design. The open-book flap design allows for graft containment and coronal advancement of the gingival margin by sliding the flap along the vertical arm of the incision

extraction defects using either a flapless approach, which involves positioning a barrier membrane within the socket and packing mineralized allograft into the socket, or with flap elevation. Although a flapless surgery can be easier to perform, bone regeneration will be limited to the confines of the socket and will likely be subjected to resorption past the confines of the labial wall during the natural resorption and remodeling processes (Kan et al. 2007). As a result, anatomical contours may not be achieved and future bone grafting may still be needed. When labial wall defects are present, grafting with an open-flap approach is recommended and will yield predictable peri-implant tissue and bone stability (Fig. 13.7a–q) (Le and Burstein 2008a; Le and Borzabadi-Farahani 2013; Covani et al. 2008).

The open-book flap is developed with a crestal incision made slightly lingual to the ridge midline to preserve an adequate amount of keratinized tissue in the flap (Fig. 13.6c, d) (Le and Borzabadi-Farahani 2013). This is followed by a distal, curvilinear, vertical incision that follows the gingival margin of the distal tooth, with care to leave approximately 3 mm of gingival cuff. One of the advantages of this incision design is it allows for coronal advancement of the gingival margin in the defect site by sliding the flap along the vertical arm of the incision. This concept is helpful when correcting minor vertical defects in single- or two-teeth defects. A wide subperiosteal reflection is made up to the depth of the vestibule to expose two to three times the treatment area, and then the papilla is reflected on the mesial side of the edentulous site. During implant placement, the implant's restorative platform is positioned to the desired level, and a healing cap is attached to the implant. The peri-implant soft tissue is released and advanced by scoring the periosteum so that a tension-free closure is achieved around the neck of the implant. This is done because moderate graft resorption will occur if there is inadequate tissue seal around the implant neck or if tension-free closure is not achieved. To induce bleeding in the graft site, perform a periosteum release as the last step just prior to graft placement. Pack human mineralized bone allograft into the defect and over-contour by approximately 20–30% to compensate for anticipated apical migration and resorption of the material. Prior to surgery, hydrate the allograft according to the manufacturer's directions and mix with the patient's blood, which serves as a coagulant. It is critical to first place an adequate volume of graft material at the apical depth of the ridge before placing the graft at the crest of the ridge to minimize apical migration of the graft during healing. After grafting, cover the allograft with a resorbable membrane, and attach a wide healing abutment to the implant. Finally, approximate the soft tissues and suture around the healing abutment. This creates a tenting effect over the allograft and, together with the healing abutment, helps to hold the particulate material in place.

Perforating the recipient bone bed is recommended by some surgeons to enhance healing. By perforating the cortical bone with a small round bur, the marrow cavity is opened and bleeding into the defect is induced. Some animal studies have shown that perforations in cortical bone improve healing in a membrane-protected defect (Nishimura et al. 2004; Slotte et al. 2003), while others have shown no effect (Gutta et al. 2009; Lundgren et al. 2000). It was also shown that larger perforations were associated with more rapid new bone formation (Frost 1983). The author of this chapter does not routinely perforate the recipient bone bed and has not seen a difference in the outcome of the graft procedure.

Use of an "aesthetic contour graft" at the time of implant placement may avoid the need for secondary soft tissue augmentation because it augments the underlying bone to restore the natural soft tissue architecture (Fig. 13.6a–o). Clinical observation of labial soft tissue thickening is often noted after successful grafting with particulate allograft and collagen membrane at the time of implant placement. This new concept of "bone-driven tissue transformation" may reduce the need for soft tissue augmentation in some instances and has been reported for the treatment of labial soft tissue recession defects around anterior maxillary implants (Le 2014; Le et al. 2016). Le et al. (Le and Borzabadi-Farahani 2012) showed a high correlation between labial crestal soft tissue thickness and underlying bone thickness, demonstrating that soft tissue thickness can be heavily influenced by the labial bone thickness. In other words, the thicker the bone, the thicker the crestal labial soft tissue around implants and vice versa.

13.5.4 Implant Position

Dental implant therapy should be prosthetically driven and not primarily bone-driven. To this end, the implant must be accurately placed in a 3-D (mesiodistal, labiolingual, and apicocoronal) position with the goal of achieving a proper emergence profile for the final restoration. When the implant position is not accurate, the aesthetic result is often compromised. Implants placed too deep apicocoronally or too labially often result is an unnaturally long restoration. In addition, implant position has been shown to have a direct influence on bone and soft tissue thickness related to the implant (Pluemsakunthai et al. 2015).

Le et al. (2014) studied the relationship between crestal labial soft tissue thickness and implant buccolingual angulation. The buccolingual angulation was recorded as cingulum, incisally, or labially angled based on the position of the screw access hole of the provisional restoration. The implant labial bone thickness was measured at the crestal and mid-implant levels using sectional cone beam computed tomography scans. Of implants with cingulum, incisal, and labial angulations, 3.4%, 20%, and 53.3%, respectively, had crestal labial soft tissue thickness of <2 mm. Implants with cingulum angulation had a mean crestal soft tissue thickness of 2.98 mm, while those with incisal and labial angulation had decreased mean tissue thickness of 2.24 and 1.71 mm, respectively (Fig. 13.9). A significant association between crestal labial soft tissue thickness and implant buccolingual angulation was noted when implant labial bone thickness at crestal level was <2 mm ($P < 0.01$). The investigators concluded that implants with labial angulations carry a higher risk of soft tissue complications when the crestal implant labial bone thickness is <2 mm.

13.6 Management of Vertical Defects

Severe vertical alveolar ridge defects are usually three-dimensional and present a difficult challenge to the implant surgeon. Patients with vertical defects usually have concomitant horizontal defects, and these defects must be fully reconstructed in all dimensions to create an aesthetic and functional result. Furthermore, many vertical defects usually have loss of bone attachment to

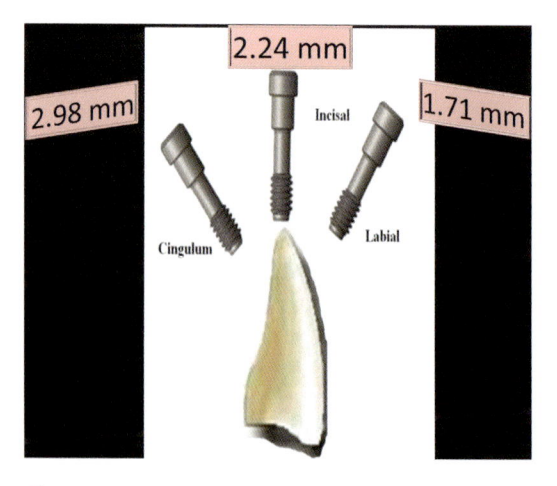

Fig. 13.9 The influence of implant angulation and soft tissue thickness. Implants with cingulum angulation had a mean crestal soft tissue thickness of 2.98 mm, while those with incisal and labial angulation had decreased mean tissue thickness of 2.24 and 1.71 mm, respectively

the teeth adjacent to the defect. In many instances, it is more beneficial to extract these teeth so that a healthy bone attachment level can be attained for bone grafting. If multiple grafting procedures are planned for a severe defect, a consideration should be given to the timing of extraction to minimize the width of the edentulous span and maximize the outcome of any initial grafting procedure.

Autogenous bone graft has long been considered to be the gold standard for grafting severe hard tissue defects. Autogenous block grafts have been described to augment mild to moderate vertical defects, but are prone to significant resorption depending on the type of donor bone (Roccuzzo et al. 2004; Keller et al. 1999). Correction of narrow span vertical defects of 2–4 mm is predictable using autogenous block grafts or particulate graft techniques (Fig. 13.10a–k). Interpositional osteotomies can also be utilized to vertically augment the alveolar ridge, but its use is limited to multiple-teeth moderate size defects ranging from 3 to 6 mm (Block and Haggerty 2009; Jensen 2006). Moderate resorption is also expected using this technique, but with minimal resorption around the implants placed into the augmented bone (Jensen 2006). Distraction osteogenesis has also been described to address the vertically deficient alveolar ridge, but is recommend for severe vertical defects (>6–7 mm) (Klug et al. 2001; Block and Baughman 2005). While all these techniques can be a predictable method for vertical bone augmentation, complications are common and include moderate resorption requiring additional bone augmentation, loss of keratinized tissue, unsatisfactory aesthetic result, and a loss of vestibular depth (Froum et al. 2008). The correction of a severe vertical defect in the aesthetic zone often requires multiple different techniques, strategically staged to achieve ideal hard and soft tissue. Vestibuloplasty with free gingival graft after implant placement is often necessary to

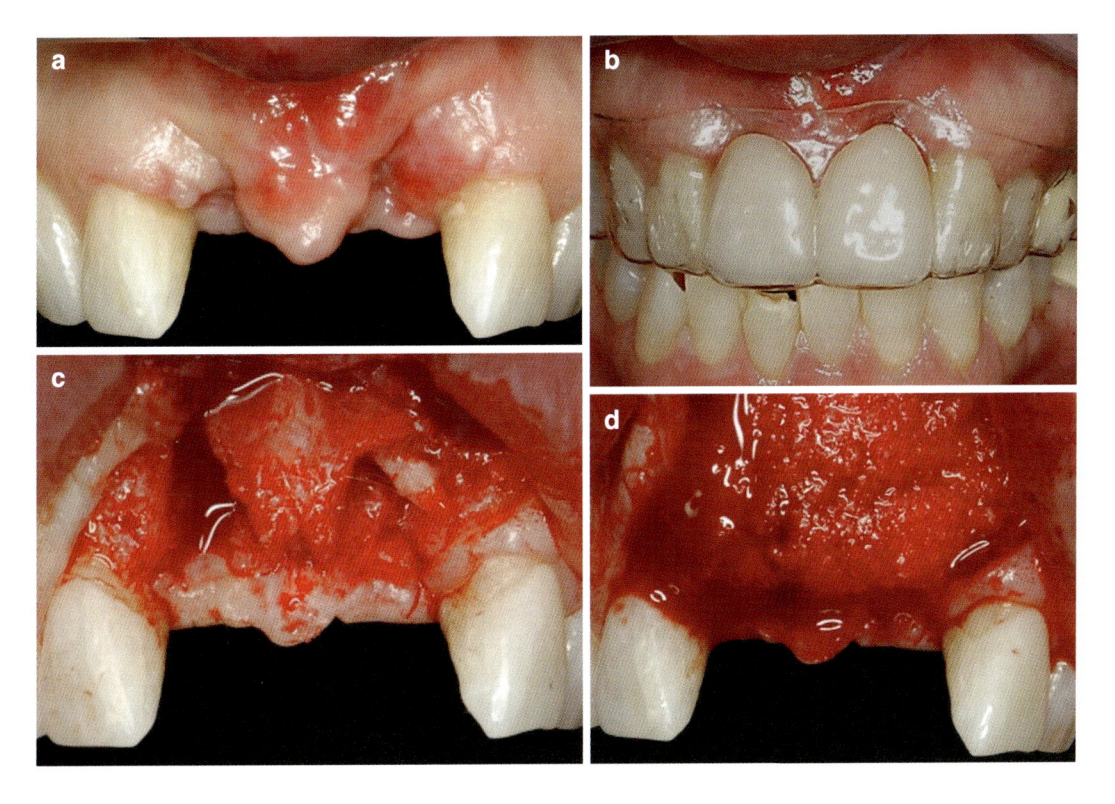

Fig. 13.10 (**a**–**k**) Particulate grafting for minor vertical augmentation. Open-book flap design with particulate grafting to correct a small vertical defect (Restorative dentist, Jon Miller, DDS; lab technician, Tommy Yamashita, DenTech International)

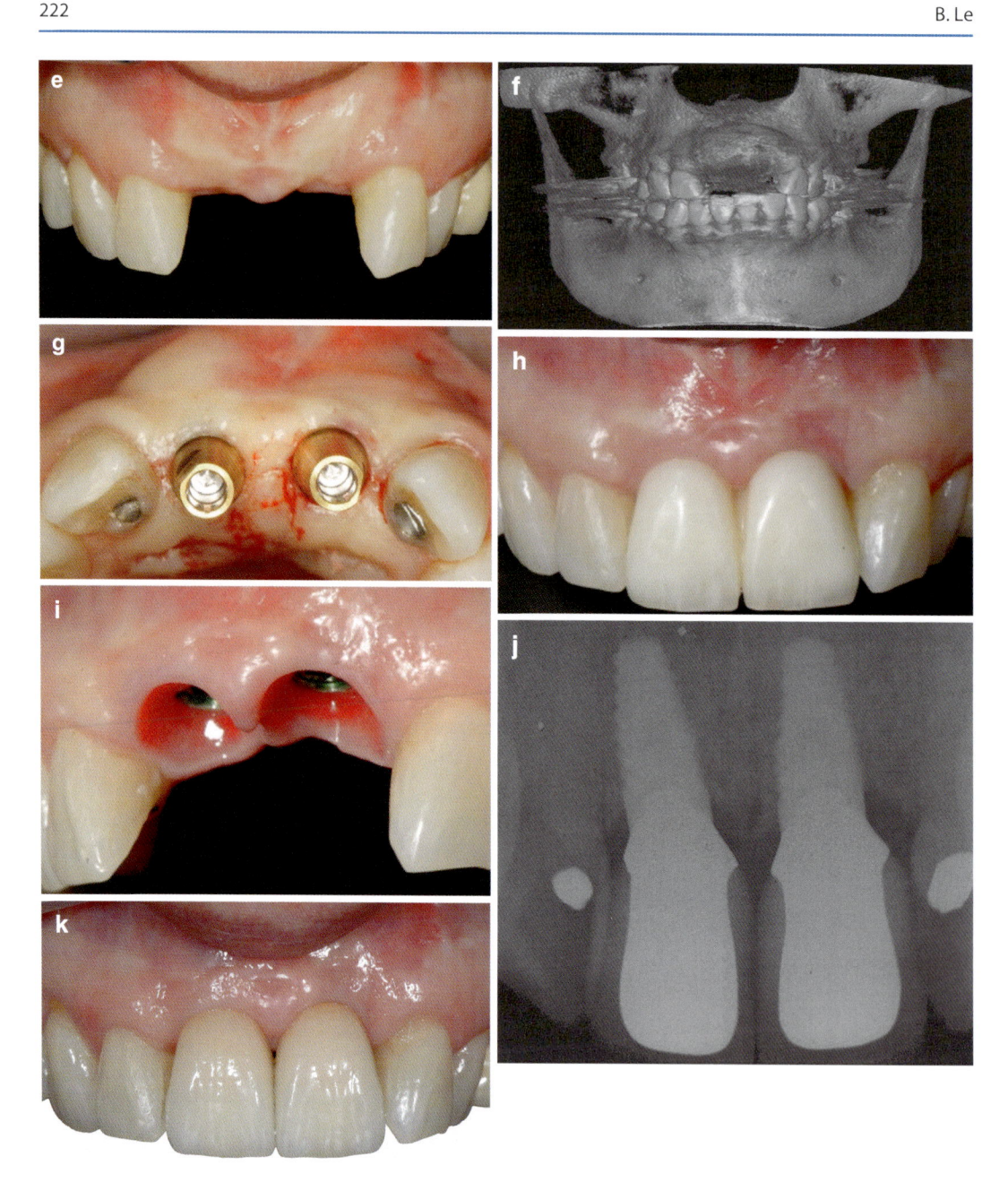

Fig. 13.10 (continued)

increase keratinized tissue attachment and improve aesthetic outcomes (Fig. 13.11a–m).

For management of severe vertical defects, particulate grafts lack the structural rigidity of an only block graft and are subject to graft migration and displacement. Implants can be placed successfully into these grafted sites; however, resorption must be anticipated during treatment planning as further augmentation procedures may be necessary. Screws, implants, meshes, and reinforced membranes have been used as tenting mechanisms to minimize graft migration, displacement, and resorption (Le et al. 2010; Louis et al. 2008; Marx et al. 2002) (Fig. 13.12a–n).

Louis et al. reported on the use of titanium mesh for reconstruction of the severely atrophic maxilla or mandible using iliac crest bone graft with a 97% overall graft success rate, although

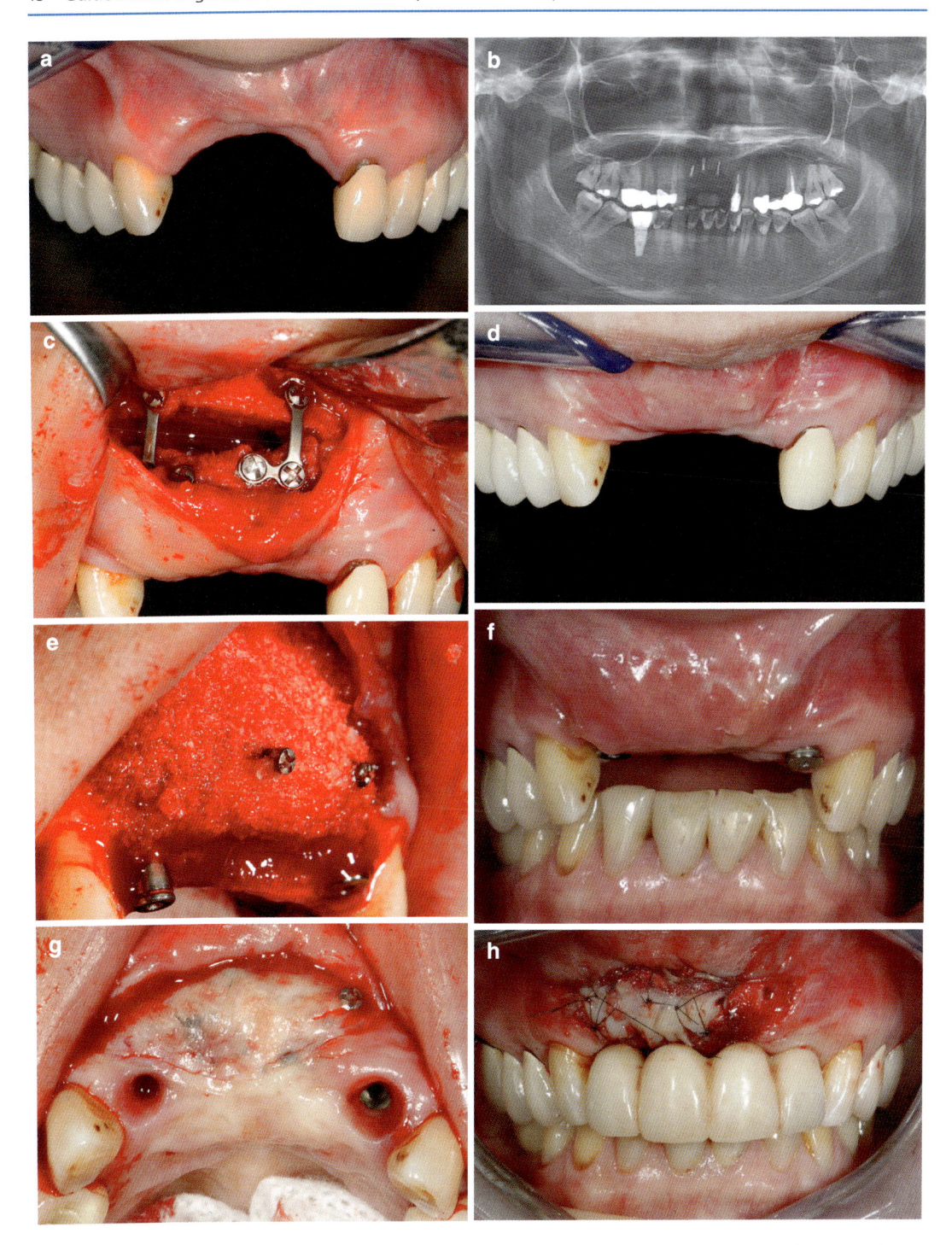

Fig. 13.11 (**a–m**) Severe vertical defect in the anterior maxilla often require multiple different techniques. (**a, b**) Severe vertical defect involving the loss of three failing implants. (**c**) Interpositional osteotomy. (**d**) Healing at 4 months. (**e**) Implant placement using a combination of screw tent-pole and "aesthetic contour grafting" protocol with mineralized allograft and resorbable collagen membrane. (**f**) Healing at 3 months shows correction of bone level, but with a lack of keratinized tissue. (**g, h**) Vestibuloplasty with autogenous free gingival graft. (**i–m**) Final restorations (Restorative dentist: Brian Novak, DDS; Lab technician: Yi-Yuan Chang MDC, USC Oral Design Center)

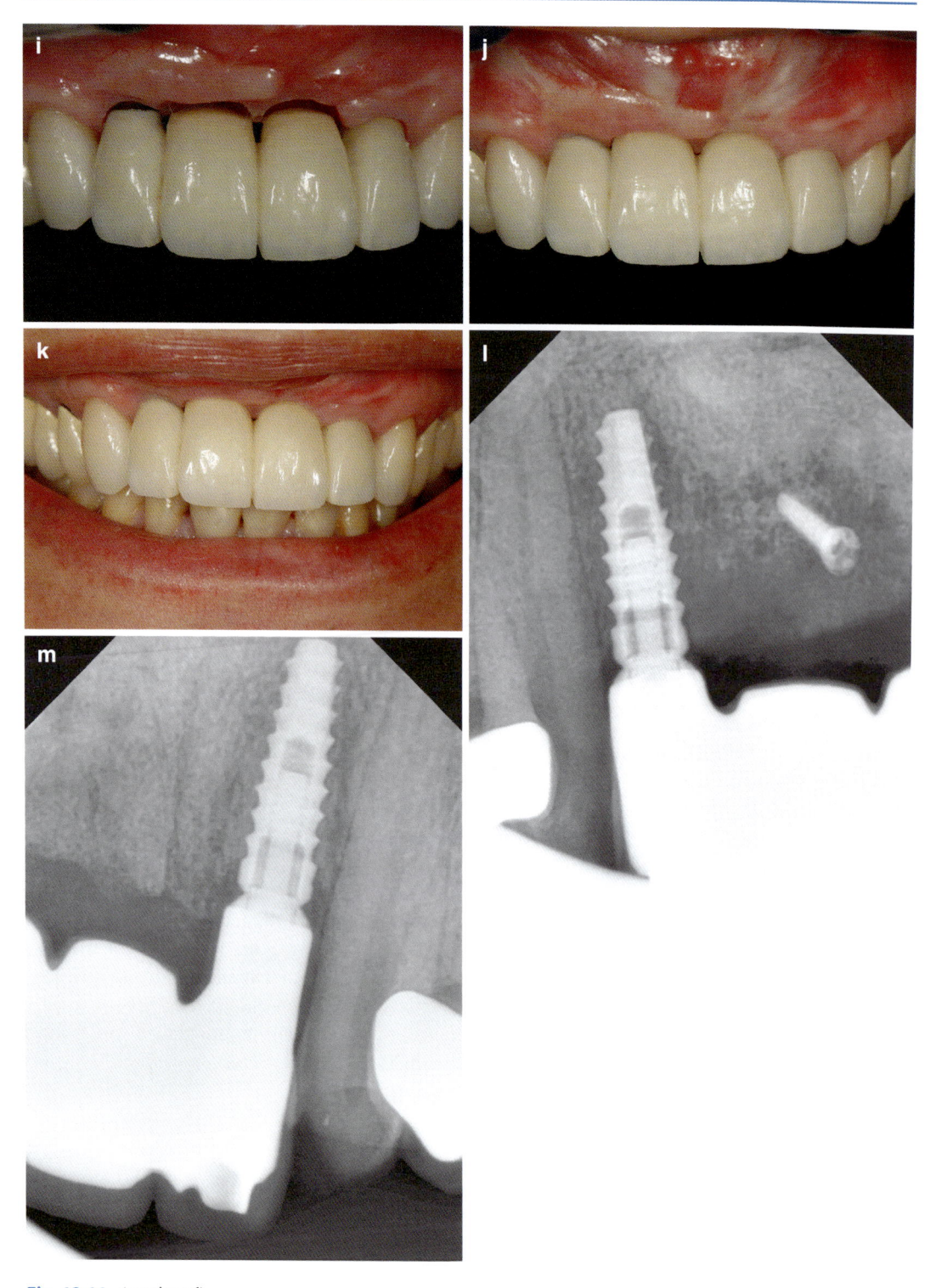

Fig. 13.11 (continued)

exposure of the titanium mesh was reported to be high (52%) (Louis et al. 2008). In addition to the higher resorption rate of iliac crest grafts, other disadvantages include the high costs of hospitalization, risks of general anesthesia, and morbidity of the procedure (Misch 1997).

Mineralized particulate allograft can be used similarly with a tenting mechanism for vertical alveolar ridge augmentation (Le et al. 2010). Using particulate allograft and screws to augment intra-bony defects, an average of 9.2 mm of vertical height was achieved and implants were successfully placed (Le et al. 2010). This "screw tent-pole" technique requires a membrane for optimal results and is technique sensitive (Figs. 13.6f, 13.11e, 13.12c, and 13.13h). Vertical

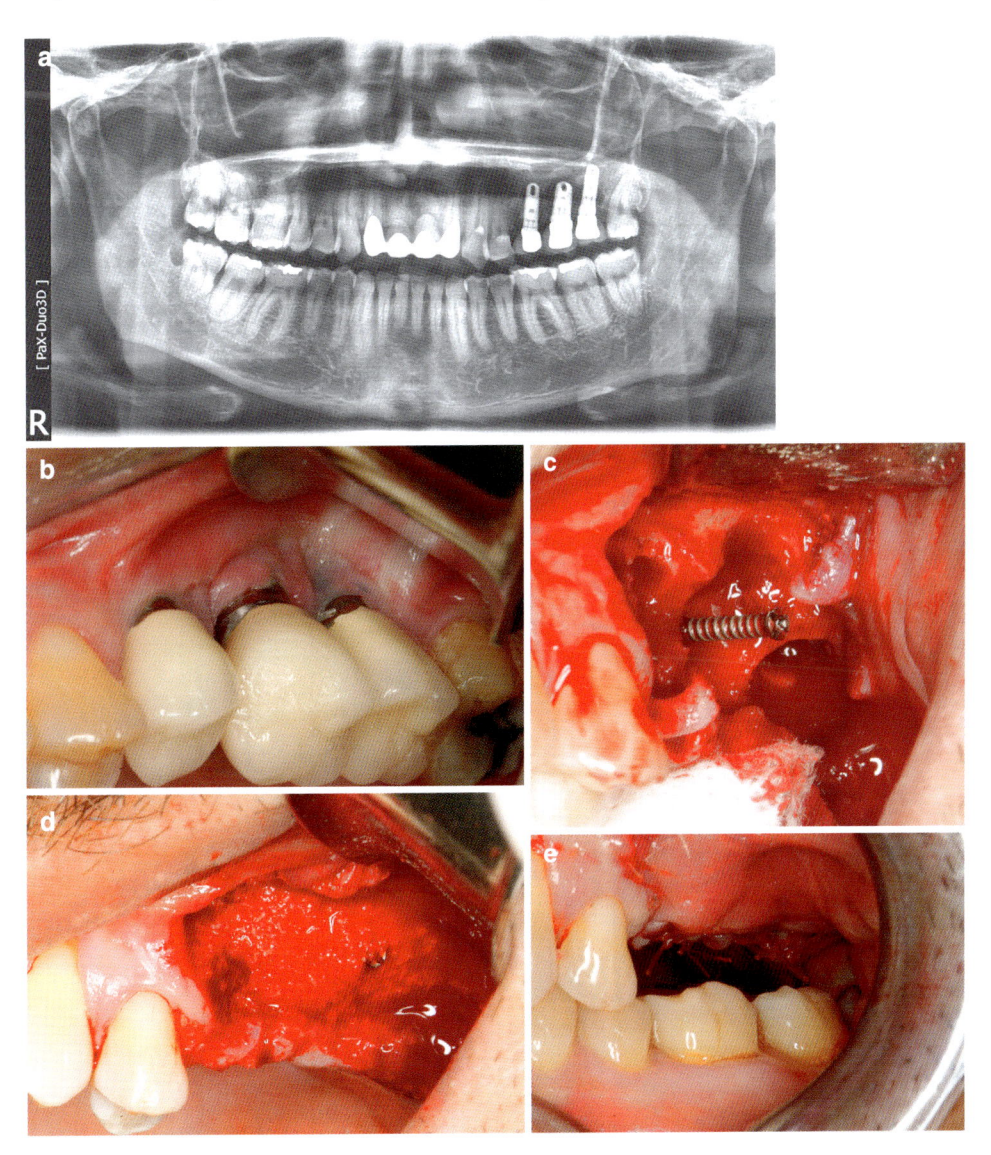

Fig. 13.12 (**a–n**) "Screw Tent-Pole" (STP) grafting technique for vertical augmentation. (**a–e**) Localized vertical alveolar ridge defect after removal of three failing implants. (**d, e**) A tenting screw is placed strategically in combination with human mineralized allograft to tent the soft tissue matrix. (**f**) Healing at 4 months. (**g**) Implant placement with additional grafting using the "aesthetic contour graft" protocol. Bioresorbable membrane is placed over the graft material. (**h**) Healing at 3 months after implant placement shows a lack of keratinized tissue and vestibule depth. (**i–k**) Vestibuloplasty with placement of an autogenous free gingival graft from the palate. (**l**) 3 months after free gingival graft. (**m, n**) Final restorations with maintenance of alveolar bone level (Restorative dentist: Alan Gutierrez, DDS)

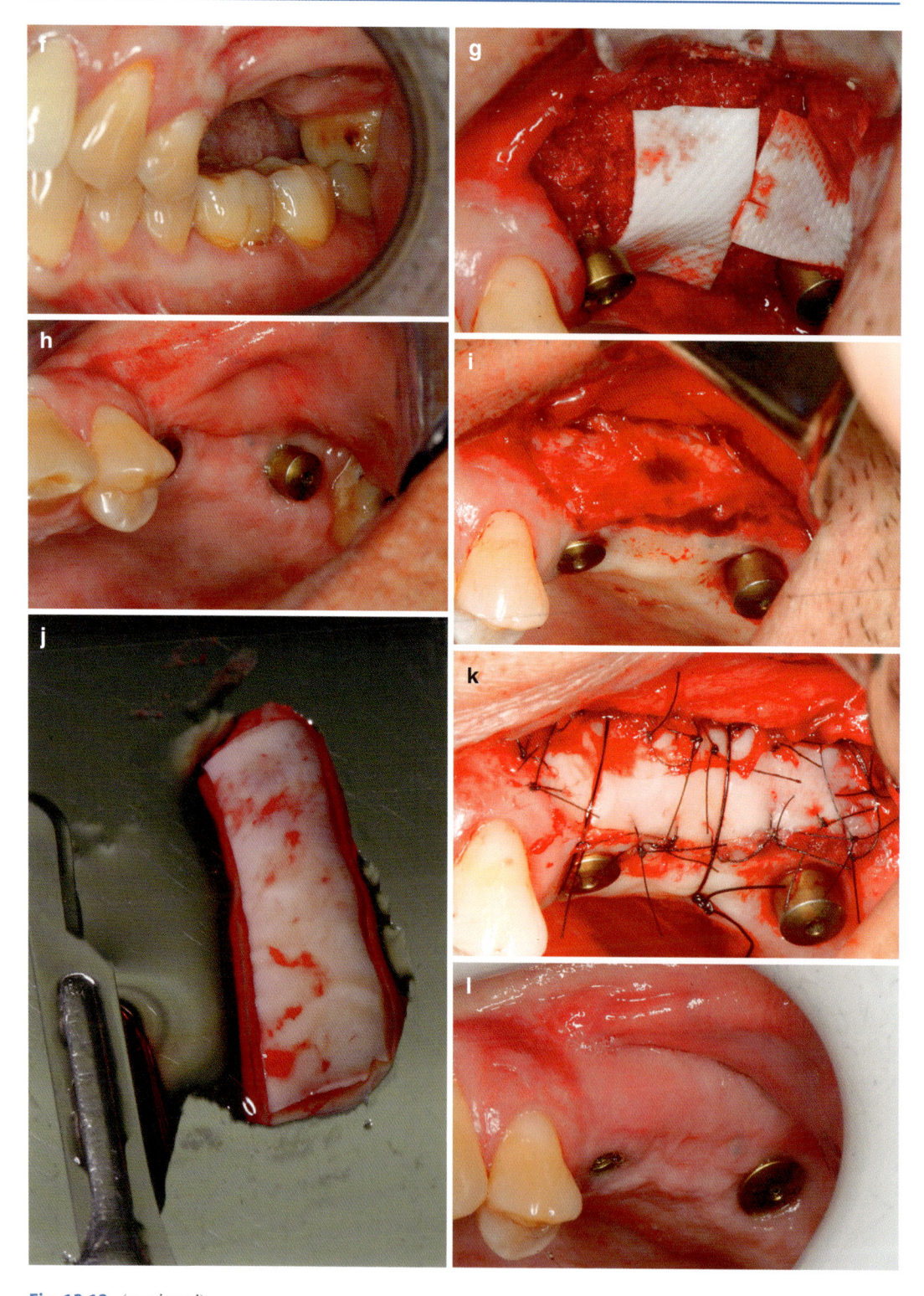

Fig. 13.12 (continued)

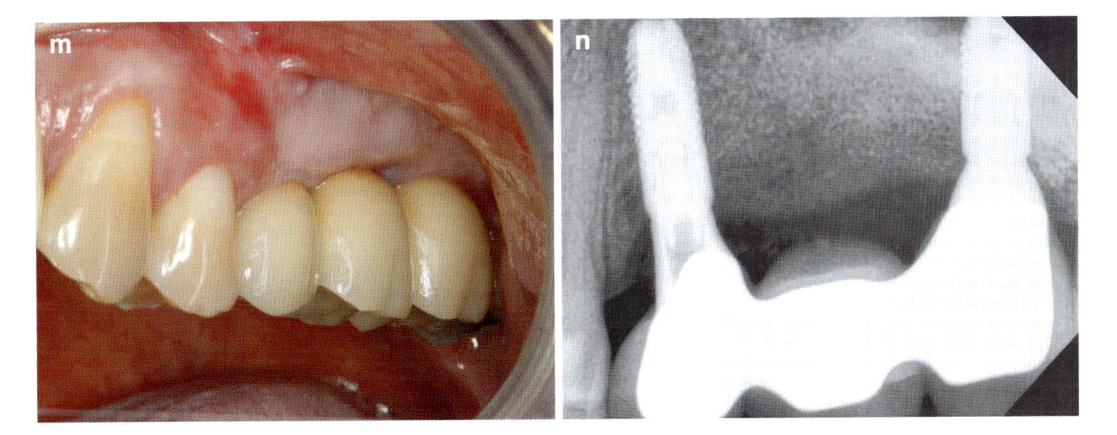

13 Guided Bone Regeneration for Aesthetic Implant Site Development 227

Fig. 13.12 (continued)

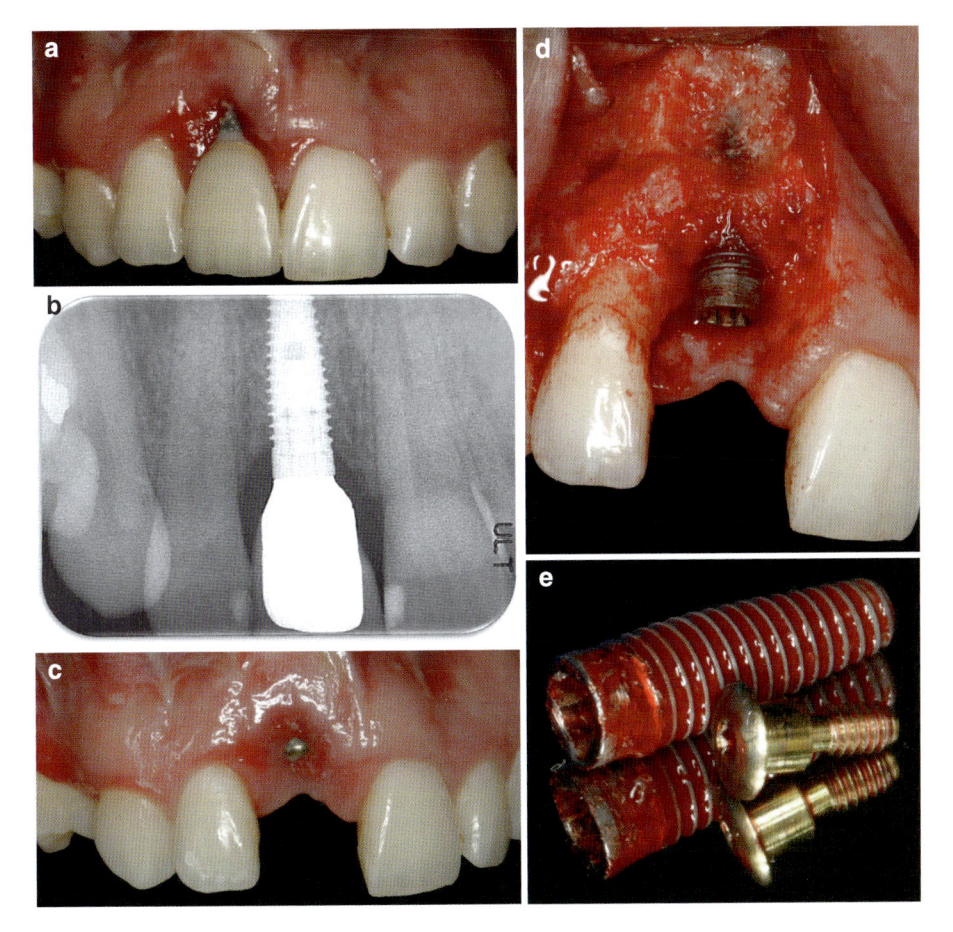

Fig. 13.13 (**a–q**) Vertical defects involving a single missing tooth span may be corrected in a one-staged grafting protocol. (**a–c**) Moderate crestal bone loss around single anterior implant with poor gingival aesthetic requiring removal. (**d–f**) Removing the implant resulted in an intra-bone vertical defect with good interproximal adjacent bone height. (**g**, **h**) Screw tent-pole technique used to tent the soft tissue matrix to support an allograft material. (**i–k**) Radiographic x-ray and CT scan and clinical situation 1 year after graft procedure. (**l**, **m**) Implant placement at 1 year after graft shows good bone height. (**n**, **o**) Screw-retained provisional restoration placed 3 months after implant is integrated. (**p**, **q**) Final restoration at 5 years follow-up (Restorative dentist, Brian Novak, DDS; lab technician, Tommy Yamashita, DenTech International)

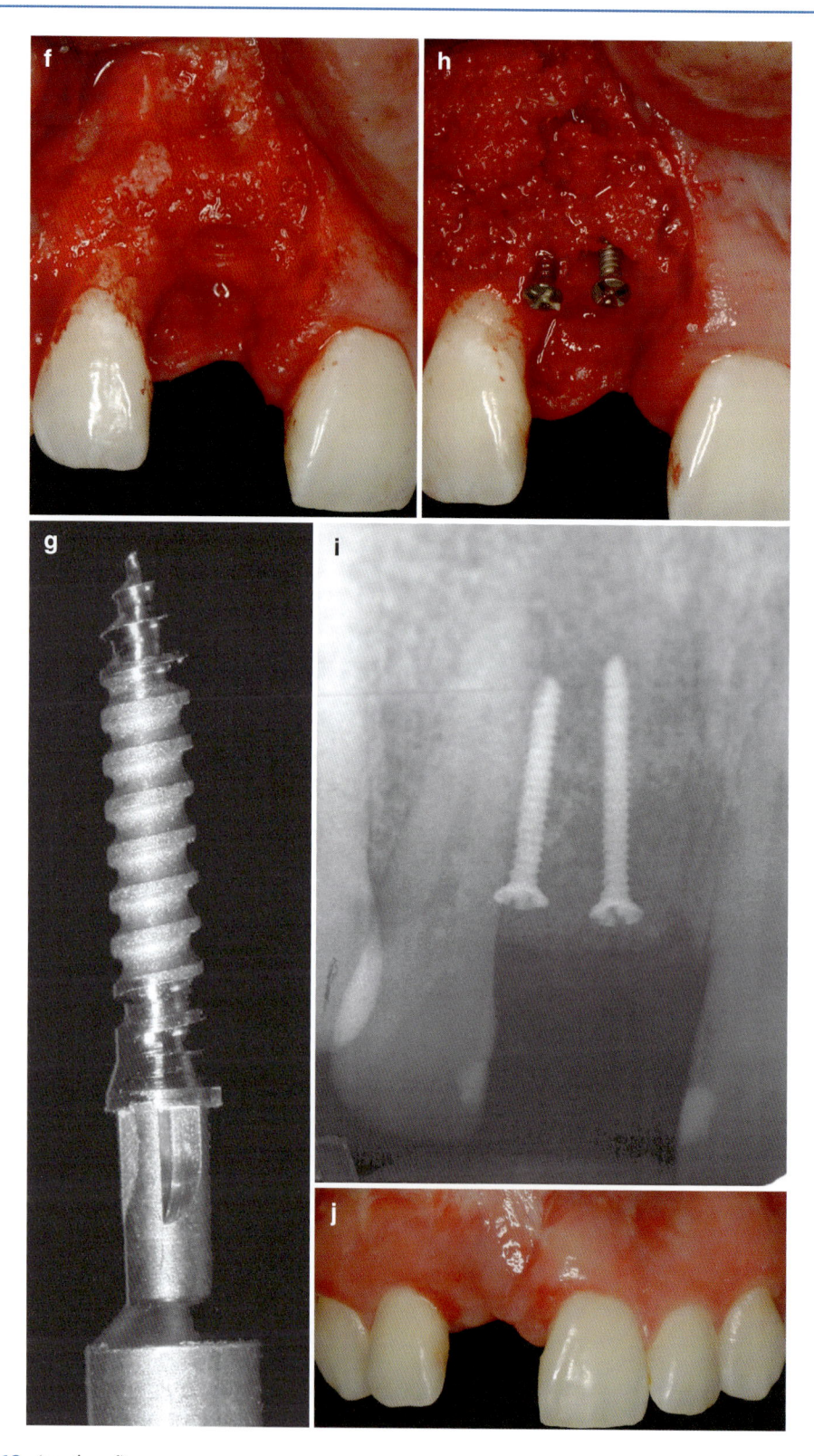

Fig. 13.13 (continued)

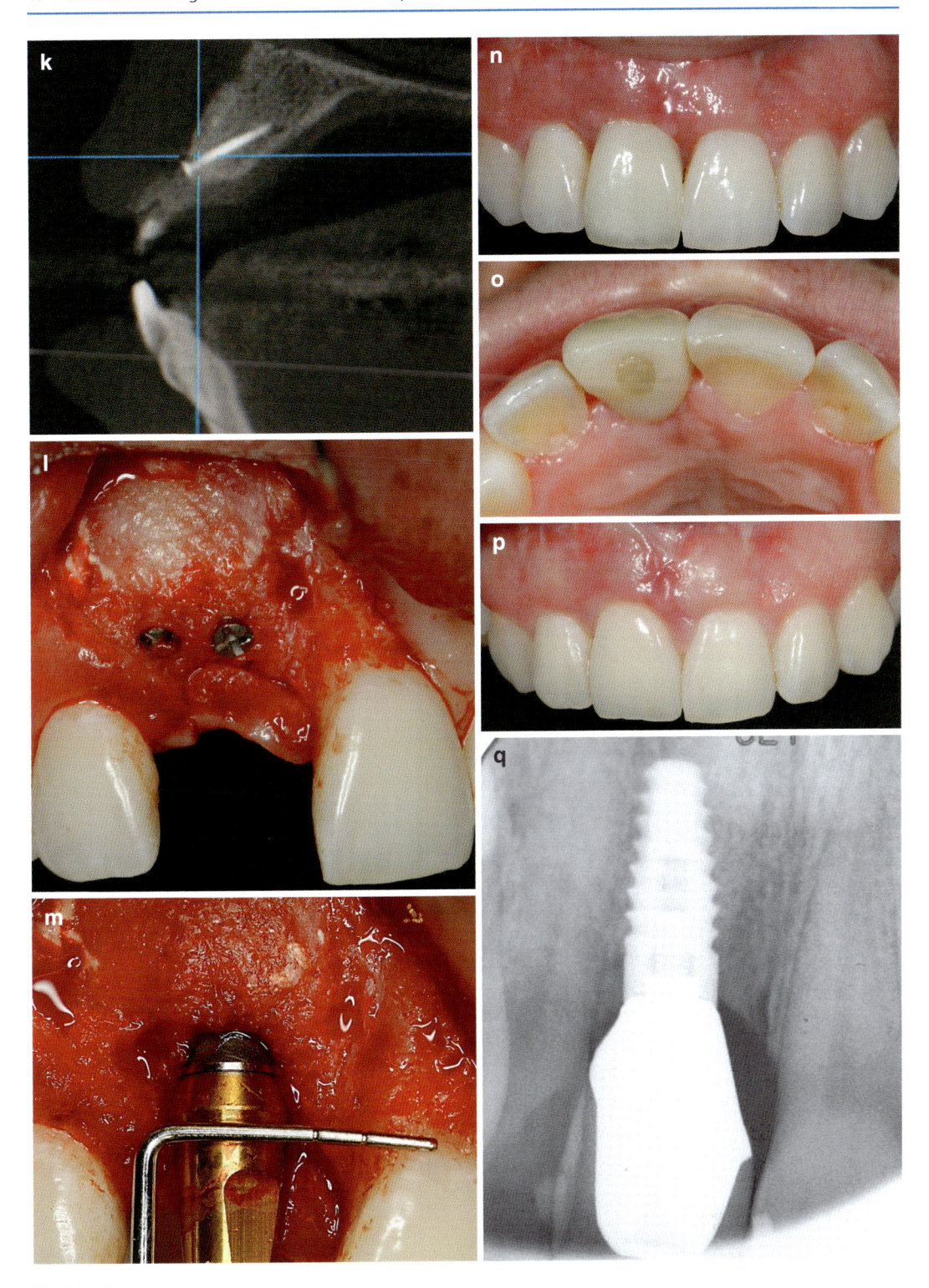

13 Guided Bone Regeneration for Aesthetic Implant Site Development

Fig. 13.13 (continued)

defects with large spans (two missing teeth or more) have a higher risk of wound dehiscence. Correction of these defects in a two-stage grafting protocol restoring smaller increments per graft may reduce the risk of graft dehiscence. Vertical defects involving a single missing tooth span may be corrected in a one-staged surgery protocol (Le et al. 2010) (Fig. 13.13a–q). When there are failures, it is usually the result of inadequate release of the flap leading to bone graft exposure and resorption. Wound dehiscence can lead to more pronounced bone graft resorption. When using particulate bone, maintaining the soft tissue matrix is critical. Proper flap design and manipulation is critical to prevent wound dehiscence when using these techniques.

Multiple surgical procedures are often required to achieve an aesthetic result when bone augmentation is necessary. At times, a combination of the above techniques may be indicated (e.g., only block grafting or GBR and distraction osteogenesis). Sometimes an initial augmentation procedure will still not provide sufficient reconstruction of the missing tissue and an additional procedure may be indicated. No matter how many procedures are required, the implant surgeon and patient must understand that a natural appearing result will be difficult to achieve if the bony structure is insufficient.

Conclusions

The goals of minimally invasive dental implant therapy include minimizing surgical interventions and achieving shorter healing times, while producing predictable and long-term functional and aesthetic results. The decision on which technique to employ should be based on the comfort level of the surgeon, as this will dramatically affect the outcome. Failed guided tissue regeneration done with simultaneous implant placement may lead to exposed implant threads or crown margins. Single-stage implant placement and simultaneous grafting with particulate bone graft and membrane coverage are more predictable on alveolar ridges with small-to-medium-sized horizontal and vertical labial wall defects. The technique becomes more unreliable and more technique-sensitive as the length of the edentulous span increases and if multiple implants are being placed. In wide spans, the tenting screws are needed to prevent collapse of the tissue and graft resorption. The use of a limited flap design to maintain vascular supply and optimize attached tissue and vestibular depth and tension-free closure also are important for the success of this technique.

References

Aghaloo TL, Moy PK (2007) Which hard tissue augmentation techniques are the most successful in furnishing bony support for implant placement? Int J Oral Maxillofac Implants 22(Suppl):49–70

Al-Nawas B, Schiegnitz E (2014) Augmentation procedures using bone substitute materials or autogenous bone – a systematic review and meta-analysis. Eur J Oral Implantol 7(Suppl 2):S219–S234

Araújo M, Linder E, Wennström J, Lindhe J (2008) The influence of Bio-Oss Collagen on healing an extraction socket: an experimental study in the dog. Int J Periodontics Restor Dent 28:123–135

Araújo M, Linder E, Lindhe J (2009) Effect of a xenograft on early bone formation in extraction sockets: an experimental study in dog. Clin Oral Implants Res 20:1–6

Belser UC, Schmid B, Higginbottom F et al (2004) Outcome analysis of implant restorations located in the anterior maxilla: a review of the recent literature. Int J Oral Maxillofac Implants 19:30

Block MS, Baughman DG (2005) Reconstruction of severe maxillary defects using distraction osteogenesis, bone grafts, and implants. J Oral Maxillofac Surg 63:291–297

Block MS, Degen M (2004) Horizontal ridge augmentation using human mineralized particulate bone: preliminary results. Oral Maxillofac Surg 62:67–72

Block M, Haggerty C (2009) Interpositional osteotomy for posterior mandible ridge augmentation. J Oral Maxillofac Surg 67:31–39

Block M, Finger I, Lytle R (2002) Human mineralized bone in extraction sites before implant placement: preliminary results. J Amer Dent Assoc 133:1631–1638

Bunyaratavej P, Wang HL (2001) Collagen membranes: a review. J Periodontol 72:215–229

Buser D, Hoffmann B, Bernard JP, Lussi A, Mettler D, Schenk RK (1998) Evaluation of filling materials in membrane-protected bone defects. a comparative histomorphometric study in the mandible of miniature pigs. Clin Oral Implants Res 9:137–150

Chiapasco MI, Zaniboni M (2009) Clinical outcomes of GBR procedures to correct peri-implant dehiscences and fenestrations: a systematic review. Clin Oral Implants Res 20(Suppl 4):113–123

Christgau M, Bader N, Schmalz G, Hiller KA, Wenzel A (1998) GTR therapy of intrabony defects using 2 different bioabsorbable membranes: 12 month results. J Clin Periodontol 25:499–509

Covani U, Cornelini R, Barone A (2008) Buccal bone augmentation around immediate implants with and without flap elevation: a modified approach. Int J Oral Maxillofac Implants 23:841

Frost HM (1983) The regional acceleratory phenomenon: a review. Henry Ford Hosp Med J 31:3–9

Froum S, Wallace S, Elian N et al (2006) Comparison of mineralized cancellous bone allograft (Puros) and anorganic bovine bone matrix (Bio-Oss) for sinus augmentation histomorphometry at 26 to 32 weeks after grafting. Int J Perio Restor Dent 26:543–551

Froum SJ et al (2008) Distraction osteogenesis for ridge augmentation: prevention and treatment of complications. Thirty case reports. Int J Periodontics Restor Dent 28:337–345

Gielkens P, Bos R, Raghoebar G et al (2007) Is there evidence that barrier membranes prevent bone resorption in autologous bone grafts during the healing period? A systemic review. Int Oral Maxillofac Implants 22:390–398

Gutta R, Baker RA, Bartolucci AA, Louis PJ (2009) Barrier membranes used for ridge augmentation: is there an optimal pore size? JOMS 67(6):1218–1225

Hammerle CH, Jung RE, Feloutzis A (2002) A systematic review of the survival of implants in bone sites augmented with barrier membranes (guided bone regeneration) in partially edentulous patients. J Clin Periodontol 29(Suppl 3):226–231

Hardwick R, Scantlebury TV, Sanchez R et al (1994). Membrane design criteria for guided bone regeneration of the alveolar ridge In: Buser D, Dahlin C, Schenk RK, eds. Guided Bone Regeneration in Implant Dentistry. Chicago, Berlin: Quintessence, pp. 101–136.

Jensen OT (2006) Alveolar segmental sandwich osteotomy for anterior maxillary vertical augmentation prior to implant placement. J Oral Maxillofac Surg 64:290–296

Jensen OT (2014) Segmental alveolar split combined with dental extractions and osteotome sinus floor intrusion in posterior maxilla using BMP-2/ACS allograft for alveolar reconstruction: technical note and report of three cases. J Oral Maxillofac Surg 71:2040–2047

Jensen OT, Cockrell R, Kuhike L et al (2002) Anterior maxillary alveolar distraction osteogenesis: a prospective 5-year clinical study. Int J Oral Maxillofac Implants 17:52

Jensen SS, Bosshardt DD, Gruber R, Buser D (2014) Long-term stability of contour augmentation in the esthetic zone. Histologic and histomorphometric evaluation of 12 human biopsies 14 to 80 months after augmentation. J Periodontol 10:1–15

Kan JY, Rungcharassaeng K, Sclar A, Lozada JL (2007) Effects of the facial osseous defect morphology on gingival dynamics after immediate tooth replacement and guided bone regeneration: 1-year results. J Oral Maxillofac Surg 65:13–19

Keller EE, Tolman DE, Eckert S (1999) Surgical-prosthodontic reconstruction of advanced maxillary bone compromise with autogenous onlay block grafts and osseointegrated implants: a 12 year study of 32 consecutive patients. Int J Oral Maxillofac Implants 14:197–209

Klug CN et al (2001) Preprosthetic vertical distraction osteogenesis of the mandible using an L-shaped osteotomy and titanium membranes for guided bone regeneration. J Oral Maxillofac Surg 59:1302–1308

Laurell L, Falk H, Fornell J, Johard G, Gottlow J (1994) Clinical use of bioabsorbable matrix barrier in guided tissue regeneration therapy. J Periodontol 65:967–975

Le BT (2009) Effectiveness of single-staged implant placement with simultaneous grafting using mineralized allograft. J Oral Maxillofac Surg 67(Suppl 1):57

Le B. Management of the ailing implant: an innovative technique for the treatment of labial gingival recession around dental implants. Abstract. AAOMS Annual Meeting, 2014

Le BT, Borzabadi-Farahani A (2012) Labial bone thickness in area of anterior maxillary implants associated with crestal labial soft tissue thickness. Implant Dent 21:406–410

Le BT, Borzabadi-Farahani A. Simultaneous implant placement and bone grafting with particulate mineralized allograft in sites with buccal wall defects, a 3-year follow-up and review of literature. Journal of Cranio-Maxillofacial Surgery. 2014;42(5):552–9

Le B, Burstein J (2008a) Esthetic grafting for small volume hard and soft tissue contour defects for implant site development. Implant Dent 17:136–141

Le B, Burstein J (2008b) Cortical tenting grafting technique in the severely atrophic alveolar ridge for implant site preparation. Implant Dent 17:40–50

Le BT, Rohrer MD, Prassad HS (2010) Screw "tent-pole" grafting technique for reconstruction of large vertical alveolar ridge defects using human mineralized allograft for implant site preparation. J Oral Maxillofac Surg 68:428–435

Le BT, Borzabadi-Farahani A, Pluemsakunthai W (2014) Is buccolingual angulation of maxillary anterior implants associated with the crestal labial soft tissue thickness? Int J Oral Maxillofac Surg 43:874–878

Le B, Borzabadi-Farahani A, Nielsen B (2016) Treatment of labial soft tissue recession around dental implants in the esthetic zone using guided bone regeneration with mineralized allograft: a retrospective clinical case series. J Oral Maxillofac Surg 74:1552–1561

Louis PJ, Gutta R, Said-Al-Naief N et al (2008) Reconstruction of the maxilla and mandible with particulate bone graft and titanium mesh for implant placement. J Oral Maxillofac Surg 66:235–245

Lundgren AK, Lundgren D, Hämmerle CH, Nyman S, Sennerby L (2000) Influence of decortication of the donor bone on guided bone augmentation. An experimental study in the rabbit skull bone. Clin Oral Implants Res 11(2):99–106

Machtei EE (2001) The effect of membrane exposure on the outcome of regenerative procedures in humans: a meta-analysis. J Periodontol 72:512–516

Marx RE, Shellenberger T, Wimsatt J, Correa P (2002) Severely resorbed mandible: predictable reconstruction with soft tissue matrix expansion (tent pole) grafts. J Oral Maxillofac Surg 60:878–888

Misch CM (1997) Comparison of intraoral donor sites for onlay grafting prior to implant placement. Int J Oral Maxillofac Implants 12:767–776

Molly L, Vandromme H, Quirynen M et al (2008) Bone formation following implantation of bone biomaterials into extraction sites. J Perio 79:1108–1115

Murphy KG (1995) Postoperative healing complications associated with Gore-tex periodontal material. Part II. Effect of complications on regeneration. Int J Perio Restor Dent 15:548–561

Nishimura I, Shimizu Y, Ooya K (2004) Effects of cortical bone perforation on experimental guided bone regeneration. Clin Oral Implants Res 15:293–300

Pallesen L, Schou S, Aaboe M, Hjørting-Hansen E, Nattestad A, Melsen F (2002) Influence of particle size of autogenous bone grafts on the early stages of bone regeneration: a histologic and stereologic study in rabbit calvarium. Int J Oral Maxillofac Implants 17:498–506

Piattelli M, Favero GA, Scarano A, Orsini G, Piattelli A (1999) Bone reactions to anorganic bovine bone (Bio-Oss) used in sinus augmentation procedures: a histologic long-term report of 20 cases in humans. Int J Oral Maxillofac Implants 14:835–840

Pietrokovski J, Massler M (1967) Alveolar ridge resorption following tooth extraction. J Prosthet Dent 17:21–27

Pluemsakunthai W, Le BT, Kasugai S. Alveolar Ridge Alteration Following Immediate Implant Placement in Different Buccal Gap Distance: a microcomputed tomography analysis in dogs. Implant Dent. 2015;24(1):70–6

Roccuzzo M et al (2004) Vertical alveolar ridge augmentation by means of a titanium mesh and autogenous bone grafts. Clin Oral Implants Res 15:73–81

Rominger JW, Triplett RG (1994) The use of guided tissue regeneration to improve implant osseointegration. J Oral Maxillofac Surg 52(2):106–112

Schenk RK, Buser D, Hardwick WR, Dahlin C (1994) Healing pattern of bone regeneration in membrane-protected defects: a histologic study in the canine mandible. Int J Oral Maxillofac Implants 9:13–29

Schwartz Z, Mellonig JT, Carnes DL Jr, de la Fontaine J, Cochran DL, Dean DD, Boyan BD (1996) Ability of commercial demineralized freeze-dried bone allograft to induce new bone formation. J Periodontol 67:918–926

Schwartz Z, Weesner T, van Dijk S et al (2007) Ability of deproteinized cancellous bovine bone to induce new bone formation. J Periodontal 71:1258–1269

Sculean A, Nikolidakis D, Schwarz F (2008) Regeneration of periodontal tissues: combinations of barrier membranes and grafting materials – biological foundation and preclinical evidence: a systematic review. J Clin Periodontol 35(Suppl 8):106–116

Shigeyama Y, D'Errico JA, Stone R, Somerman MJ (1995) Commercially-prepared allograft material has biological activity in vitro. J Periodontol 66:478–487

Simion M, Fontana F, Rasperini G et al (2007) Vertical ridge augmentation by expanded polytetrafluoroethylene membrane and a combination of intraoral autogenous bone graft and deproteinized anorganic bovine bone (Bio Oss). Clin Oral Implants Res 18:620–629

Slotte C, Lundgren D, Sennerby L, Lundgren AK (2003) Surgical intervention in enchondral and membranous bone: intraindividual comparisons in the rabbit. Clin Implant Dent Relat Res 5:263–268

Spray JR et al (2000) The influence of bone thickness on facial marginal bone response: stage 1 placement through stage 2 uncovering. Ann Periodontol 5:119–128

Wang HL, Boyapati L (2006) "PASS" principles for predictable bone regeneration. Implant Dent 15:8

Wang HL, Tsao YP (2007) Mineralized bone allograft-plug socket augmentation: rationale and technique. Implant Dent 16:33–41

Wenz B, Oesch B, Horst M (2001) Analysis of the risk of transmitting bovine spongiform encephalopathy through bone grafts derived from bovine bone. Biomaterials 22:1599–1606

Development of the Soft Tissue with Gingival Grafting

14

David H. Wong

Abstract

The aesthetic success of implant-supported restorations on anterior teeth is largely influenced by the surrounding soft tissue. In considering soft tissue aesthetics, several criteria may be evaluated: gingival volume, contour, color, and consistency. The ideal soft tissue qualities around implants are the same expectations as the soft tissue around natural teeth. As with natural teeth, the gingiva should be dense and firm. The color is often described as "coral pink." The contour is ideally knife edged with a gingival scallop that is consistent with the adjacent teeth. In order to establish these soft tissue goals, several treatment options are available. Commonly, soft tissue grafting is considered. A summary of various grafting sources, surgical design, and timing of procedures is reviewed.

The science of implant dentistry often includes discussions of survival rates and success rates. However, with the predictability of dental implants being established through a vast volume of research, the spotlight of attention is now on dental implant aesthetics.

While aesthetics may be dependent on subjective criteria, there are general objective guidelines that may be used as a reference. Common objective criteria for gingival aesthetics include gingival health, interdental closure, zenith of the gingival contour, and balance of the gingival levels (Magne and Belser 2003).

The aesthetic success of implant-supported restorations is largely influenced by the surrounding soft tissue. However, because aesthetics is the product of both gingival and dental aesthetics working together, it is important to note that defects in the quality of the dental prosthesis and/or the implant placement and position cannot be corrected by periodontal procedures (Magne and Belser 2003). The ideal soft tissue qualities around implants are evaluated by the same criteria as the soft tissue around natural teeth. In regard to tissue quality, the gingiva should be dense and firm. The color is often described as "coral pink." The contour is ideally knife edged with a gingival scallop that is consistent with the adjacent teeth and fills the interdental spaces. In order to establish these soft tissue goals, several treatment options are available. This chapter will

D.H. Wong, DDS
Private Practice, Tulsa, OK, USA
e-mail: david@tulsagums.com

provide an overview of many of the more documented procedures and also provide a discussion as to the timing and sequencing of these surgical options relative to implant therapy.

The aesthetic standard by which any dental implant is measured is often how it compares to the adjacent teeth. While implant aesthetics may be influenced by factors such as implant position and platform, abutment selection, and dental materials, the framing of all of these components is the soft tissue. Perhaps the most important soft tissue topic regarding dental implants is the gingival biotype (Jia-Hui et al. 2011; Linkevicius et al. 2009).

14.1 The Significance of the Gingival Biotype

The gingival biotype is often separated into two categories: thick and thin. Each of these gingival biotypes has observable clinical qualities that can be used to differentiate the two.

Generally, a thin tissue biotype is often associated with a highly scalloped gingival architecture. The surrounding band of keratinized and attached gingiva may be narrow, while the marginal gingiva is often thin and delicate. The underlying bone is also thin and commonly associated with dehiscences or fenestrations in the labial plate. In contrast, a thick gingival biotype is commonly characterized with a wide flat gingival architecture with minimal scalloping. Here, a wider band of keratinized and attached gingiva is often found, while the marginal gingiva is thick and resilient. Thicker underlying bone generally lies beneath a thicker gingival biotype. The clinical significance of these two gingival biotypes is that the thin biotype typically responds to insult or injury with recession of the gingiva, whereas the thicker biotype is much more resistant to gingival recession (Jung et al. 2007; Kao et al. 2008; Kois and Kan 2001).

14.2 The Gingival Biotype and Dental Implants

Much research has been devoted to the significance of the gingival biotype surrounding dental implants. While early studies suggest that the type of tissue surrounding dental implants was unrelated to implant survival and retention, there are a number of papers recognizing the importance of a thick gingival biotype in regenerative procedures as well as preservation of the crestal hard and soft tissues. In dental implant cases where bone grafting is indicated prior to implant placement, a thicker biotype aids in the primary passive closure of the surgical site as well as improved vascularity. Passive primary closure and graft stability are important keys to successful bone grafting. When it comes to dental implant aesthetics, thicker tissue types are important for masking any potential graying areas in the cervical portion of the restoration from either the implant platform or the abutment. Thicker gingival biotypes have also been shown to minimize the amount of crestal bone loss as well as gingival recession once the implant has been restored (Fu et al. 2011).

Tissue thickness is important for the optimal health and aesthetics of a dental implant, but it is important to note that tissue thickness is also affected by implant design, implant position, as well as prosthesis design. Generally, implant-supported crowns and abutments with a more flat or even concave profile allow for thicker tissue than their convex-shaped counterparts (Linkevicius et al. 2009; Rompen et al. 2007). Narrow-diameter implants also afford more gingival tissue than wider-diameter implants (Small et al. 2001). Implant position is important, and more facially positioned implants are associated with thinner tissues and generally more apical crown/abutment margins. The significance of implant position cannot be ignored, as it is a relatively irreversible procedure once the implant has osseointegrated (not absolutely irreversible, implants can be backed out at 300 ncm). Therefore, it is important to understand that grafting procedures are intended to complement and enhance proper implant position; they are not meant to correct deficiencies in implant position (or size) (Lazzara and Porter 2006; Nispakultorn et al. 2010).

14.3 Identifying Gingival Biotype

A number of techniques and methods have been proposed to help identify gingival biotypes (Fu et al. 2011). Unfortunately, many of these methods involve subjective criteria and observations. For example, one common method is simple visual inspection/observation utilizing the common characteristics of a thick or thin biotype: the gingival architecture, the amount of keratinized/attached gingiva, the morphology of the teeth, etc. Another technique is transgingival probing, where the thickness of the tissue can be directly measured by inserting a probe horizontally through the gingiva. While highly accurate, this technique requires the use of local anesthesia which may be considered a somewhat invasive diagnostic procedure. The use of cone beam computed tomography (CBCT) has also been proposed. While not invasive, this adds additional costs to the patient. Perhaps the most reliable method that is both noninvasive and cost-efficient is to simply probe the sulcus around the teeth with a periodontal probe. If the outline of the probe is visible through the tissue, then the gingival biotype is considered thin. If it is not visible, then the biotype is considered thick. Another quantifiable measure relative to edentulous areas (i.e., potential implant sites) is that a thick biotype has tissue thickness equal to or greater than 2.5 mm (Abrahamsson et al. 1996).

14.4 Indications for Gingival Grafting

14.4.1 Correcting Ridge Defects with Gingival Grafting

A common classification system for identifying ridge defects was described by Seibert et al. where three types of ridge deficiencies were identified (Seibert and Salama 1996).

Class I. Horizontal defect exists only. While this may occur on either the facial or lingual aspects of the ridge, Seibert Class I defects typically describe labial/buccal side defects.
Class II. Vertical defect exists only. In Seibert Class II defects, the horizontal dimensions of the edentulous ridge have been preserved, but there is loss of vertical height. These types of defects may also be associated with the loss of the interproximal height of the bone on the adjacent teeth, which is a critical determinant of the final aesthetic outcome.
Class III. Both a horizontal and a vertical defect exist.

A number of soft tissue grafting techniques are particularly useful in the treatment of Seibert Class I, II, and III ridges by restoring lost ridge volume. Additionally, gingival augmentation, bone augmentation, or a combination of both surgeries (performed either simultaneously or performed in sequence) may be used to correct edentulous ridge defects for the purpose of improving aesthetics or to prepare the ridge for implant surgery.

14.5 Converting a Thin Gingival Biotype to a Thick Gingival Biotype

There are several advantages previously mentioned to converting a thin gingival biotype to a thicker gingival biotype (Chung et al. 2006; Kennedy 1974; Kois and Kan 2001; Linkevicius et al. 2009; Warrer et al. 1995).

- Pre-prosthetically, thicker biotypes are better suited to resist gingival recession.
- Thicker biotypes are less prone to inflammation.
- Prior to implant surgery, thicker biotypes aid in primary closure.
- During bone augmentation procedures, a thick biotype offers improved vascularity and graft stability.
- Dental implant-supported fixed prostheses have superior aesthetics when a thicker biotype is present.

There are a number of clinical scenarios where gingival grafting may be indicated.

Gingival grafts are frequently used to convert the existing gingival biotype to aid additional bone grafting or augmenting the size/volume of the tissues for aesthetics (Fu et al. 2011). Gingival grafting may also be used to eliminate unsightly scars such as amalgam tattoos. The "graying" occasionally seen from implant components through thin tissue may also be minimized or removed. Also, inflamed marginal tissue may be restored to health if traditional periodontal procedures aimed at reducing inflammation are unsuccessful. In the event of exposed restoration margins or dental implant threads, gingival grafting is indicated but is limited by several factors. First of all, just as in the case of gingival recession around natural teeth, the amount of root coverage or thread coverage is limited by the height of the interproximal bone (Salama et al. 1998; Seibert and Salama 1996). Secondly, as mentioned earlier, gingival position is influenced by implant position, diameter, and design (Rompen et al. 2007; Small et al. 2001). These are factors that obviously cannot be changed with gingival grafting once the dental implant has been placed.

In reviewing the literature, autografts are the more popular choice for augmenting gingival tissue (Seibert and Salama 1996). Common donor sites include the hard palate, maxillary tuberosity, and edentulous ridges.

Another popular graft material which can be used in a similar manner to autogenous gingival tissue is human acellular dermal graft tissue (Park 2005). This graft material is derived from natural tissue, which is processed to remove the cells that are associated with tissue rejection and graft failure. Its use in dentistry has been thoroughly documented and has been cited several times in both dental and medical literature.

14.6 Gingival Grafting Sources

A brief summary of various graft types/materials along with the basic technique for their use has been included below (Fig. 14.1).

There are several gingival grafting techniques available to correct various soft tissue deficiencies. When discussing gingival grafts, the donor tissue is often classified into two categories: autografts and allografts.

14.7 Common Gingival Grafting Techniques

14.7.1 Free Gingival Graft

The free gingival graft was popularly described by Sullivan and Atkins in 1968. This autogenous graft is typically harvested from the palate (Sullivan and Atkins 1968) but may be harvested at any intraoral location where attached

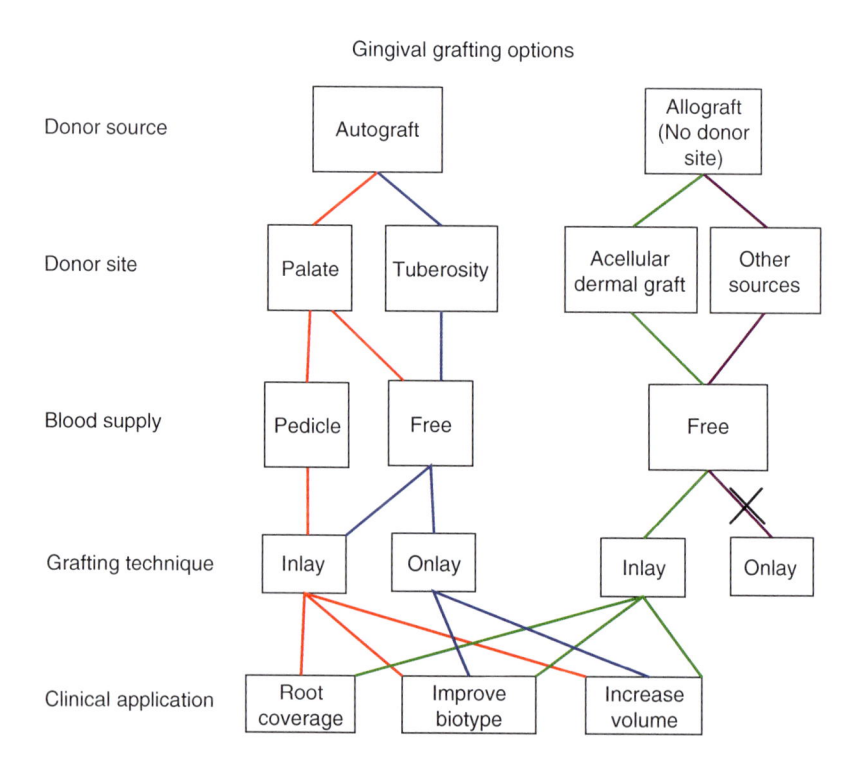

Fig. 14.1 Gingival grafting options

keratinized tissue is present, such as the maxillary tuberosity or an edentulous ridge. When treating the natural dentition or dental implants, free gingival grafts are an effective technique for increasing the band of keratinized and attached gingiva as well as the transgingival thickness of the tissue (Miller 1985). In treating the edentulous ridge, free gingival onlay grafts are effective in treating Seibert Class I, II, or III deficiencies (Seibert and Salama 1996). Once established, the free gingival onlay graft may aid in wound closure, stabilization, and vascularity to future hard tissue ridge augmentations in the area (Fu et al. 2011). Additionally, free gingival grafts may also be used to improve the contours and aesthetics of the final prosthesis (Fig. 14.2a–g).

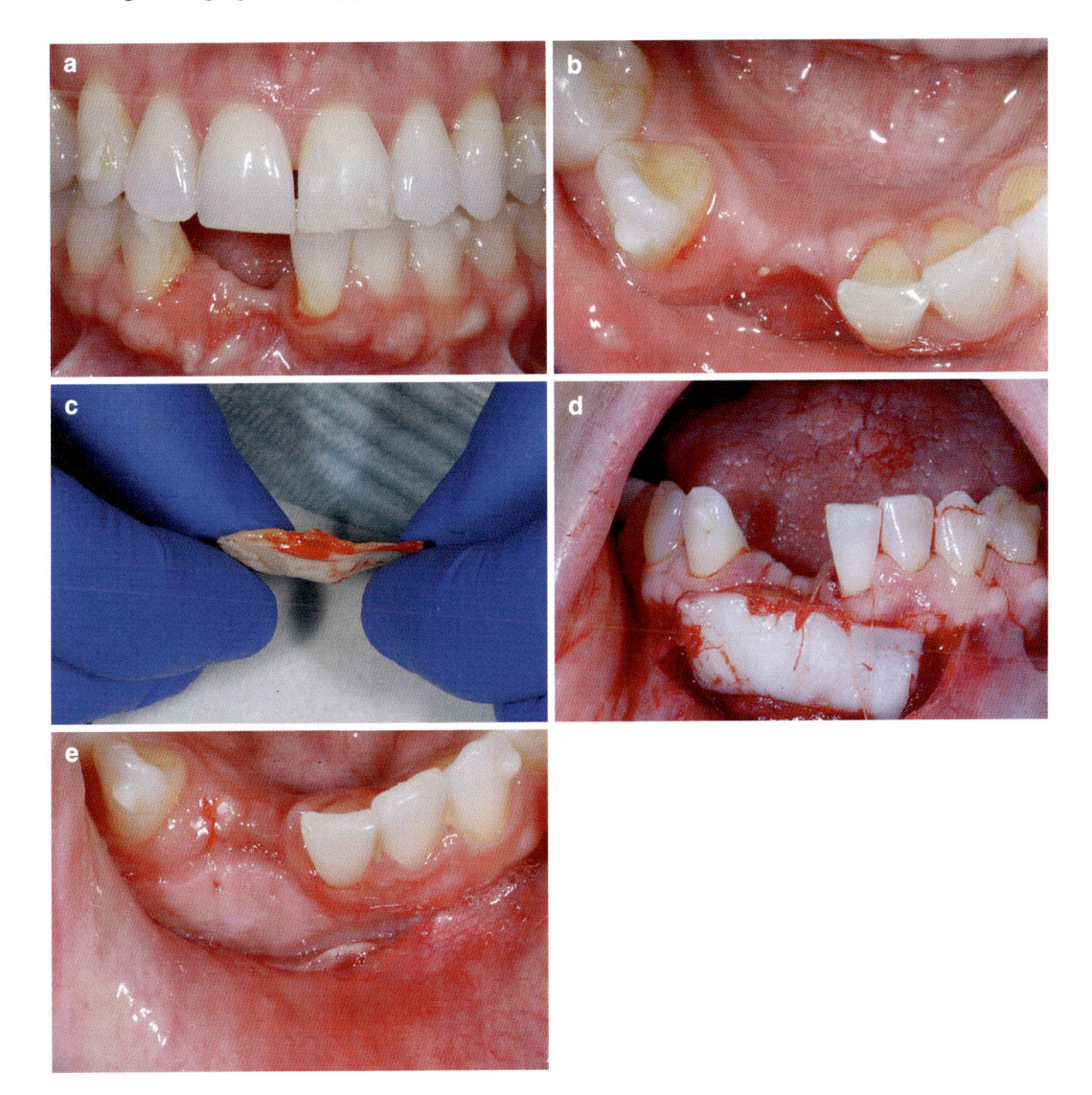

Fig. 14.2 (**a**, **b**) Preoperative view of the vertical and horizontal ridge deficiency related to the edentulous ridge. Soft tissue augmentation with a free gingival graft was prescribed prior to any hard tissue grafting or implant placement. (**c**) The free gingival graft has been harvested from the palate and is approximately 4 mm thick in the center of the graft. (**d**) The graft is sutured to the recipient bed, which is prepared by denuding the existing loose mucosa from the underlying bony ridge. (**e**) Two-week postoperative visit. Sutures will be removed at this visit, but revascularization and maturation of the graft are occurring at this time. (**f**) Radiograph revealing the placement of two dental implants to support a fixed prosthesis. (**g**) Two-year photograph showing the final fixed prosthesis. Note the excellent health and quality of the marginal tissue, the improvement in the gingival biotype, and the architecture of the prosthetic-gingival interface

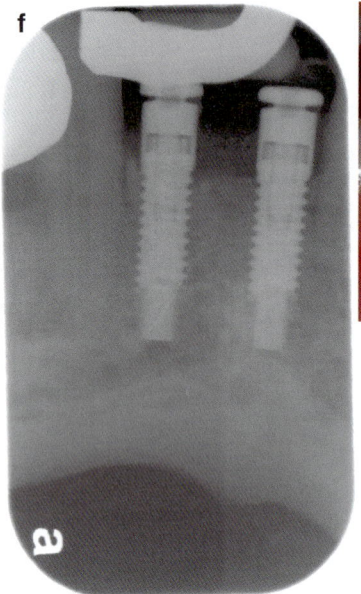

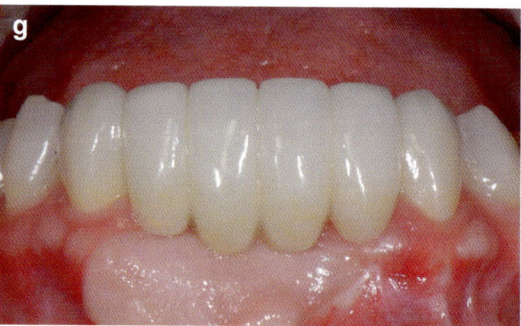

Fig. 14.2 (continued)

One limitation of a free gingival onlay graft is its anatomic variability relative to size and thickness (Reiser et al. 1996). For example, patients may have a limited amount of useful available palatal tissue, which is bound by the height of the palatal vault, the location of vital structures, and the pre-existing thickness of the palatal tissue. Depending on the anatomical limitations as well as the size of the ridge defect, multiple procedures may be required to correct certain edentulous ridge defects. Another limitation is color matching. Free gingival onlay grafts often heal in a way that the margins of the graft are visible and the grafts itself may be a lighter shade than the surrounding gingiva.

14.8 Subepithelial Connective Tissue Graft

The subepithelial connective tissue (SECT) graft is another type of autogenous graft that has several indications for grafting around dental implants. One of its first introductions described its use for correcting gingival recession defects on natural teeth as a predictable method for root coverage (Langer and Langer 1985). The SECT graft is also most commonly harvested from the palate with the same limitations as mentioned for the free gingival graft. The difference between the two graft types, as the name would suggest, is that the SECT does not have a layer of epithelium on its surface (Levine 1991).

Unlike the free gingival graft, a SECT graft can be utilized as either an onlay graft or an inlay graft. Both techniques have an array of clinical applications. As an inlay graft, in which the SECT graft is placed beneath a full- or partial-thickness flap, the gingival biotype may be thickened. Considering how thick and thin biotypes react to local irritants such as bacterial plaque, calculus, retained cement, food impaction, etc. (Kennedy 1974), the SECT graft is an excellent way to treat chronically inflamed gingiva once these local factors are removed (Fig. 14.5a–g). Similarly, the gray shadowing that may transfer through the gingiva from a dental implant may be masked if the SECT graft achieves the necessary thickness of approximately 2 mm (Fu et al. 2011). Please note, however, that this technique does not correct gingival discoloration caused by improper implant positioning and/or size selection. For situations where a modest amount of tissue is desired to augment existing gingiva, the SECT inlay graft may also be a practical, predictable choice of treatment (Fig. 14.3a–f).

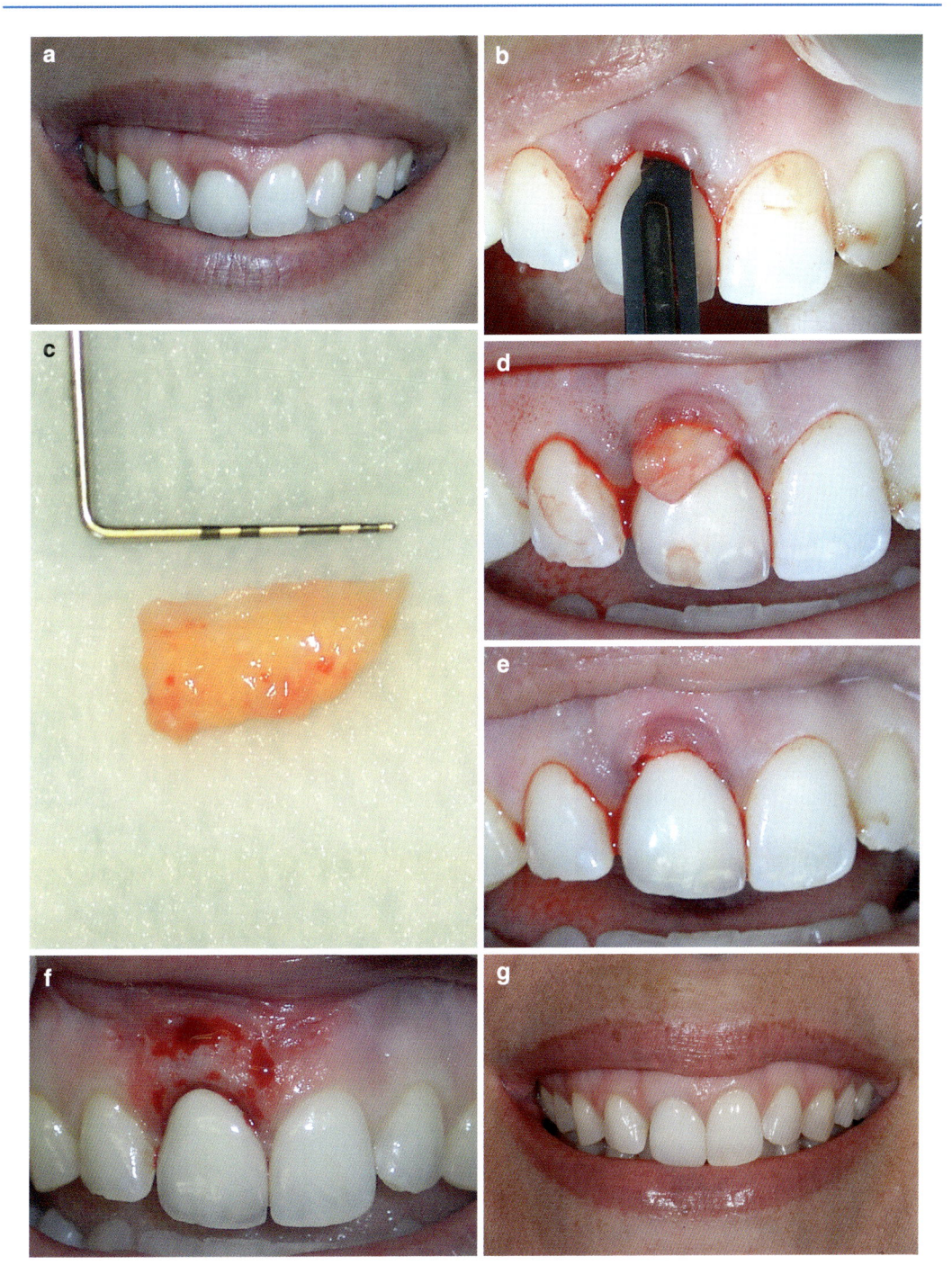

14 Development of the Soft Tissue with Gingival Grafting

Fig. 14.3 (a) Preoperative view of the marginal inflammation that exists around the implant-supported crown #8. The treatment performed was a subepithelial connective tissue (SECT) graft. (b) The initial tunnel flap design is started with sulcular incisions using a #15 scalpel. (c) The SECT graft is removed from the palate with the desired thickness of approximately 1.5–2.0 mm. (d) Once the SECT graft is trimmed to ensure that it covers the entire implant surface and adjacent bony structures, it is inserted underneath the tunnel flap through the facial sulcus. It is recommended that any thread exposure noted be debrided and contaminated as thoroughly as possible. Examples of agents used for implant surface decontamination include a tetracycline slurry, citric acid, or EDTA. (e) The graft is secured beneath the flap with firm pressure with or without the addition of sutures. (f) A gingivoplasty is performed 12 weeks later to remove any undesired contours or scars that may be present. This was performed with a round diamond bur. (g) The final result at 6 years following SECT grafting surgery

When a SECT graft is utilized as an onlay graft, its applications are very similar to those of a free gingival onlay graft. There are a couple of differences that should be pointed out, however. First of all, the SECT graft has a much better color match to the surrounding tissue at the recipient site since the graft does not include the surface epithelium. For aesthetic considerations alone, the SECT graft is often preferred over the free gingival graft, especially in the maxillary arch where gingival display is more prominent (Levine 1991). A SECT onlay graft is effective at both thickening the gingival biotype and correcting small ridge deficiencies and discolorations such as amalgam tattoos (Figs. 14.4a–f and 14.5).

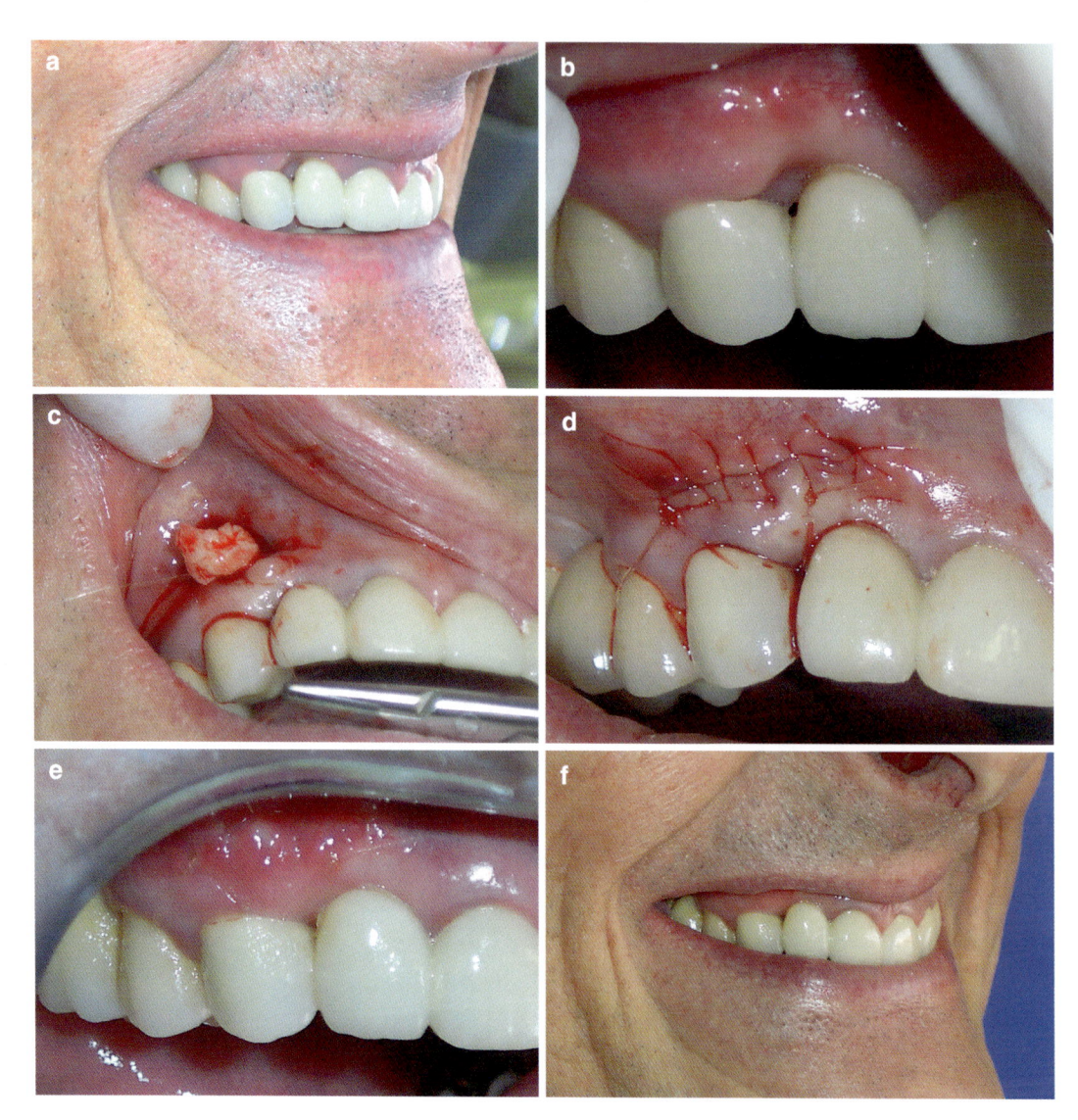

Fig. 14.4 (**a**) For missing teeth #s 6–7, a single dental implant was placed in the #6 position with the final restoration being an implant-supported crown on #6 with a cantilevered pontic to replace #7. (**b**) A close-up view of the gingival deficiency in the papilla between the implant crown #6 and the pontic #7. (**c**) A SECT graft harvested from the maxillary tuberosity was utilized to augment the gingival defect. The recipient bed consists of a straight-line incision apical to the mucogingival junction that extends from #6 to 7. The graft is introduced through the incision and placed in the area of the defect. (**d**) The graft is then secured to the recipient site with resorbable sutures. Primary closure is obtained with non-resorbable sutures. (**e**) Two-week follow-up. Sutures will be removed at this time. Note the significant improvement in the papillary tissue. (**f**) Final photograph 1 year later

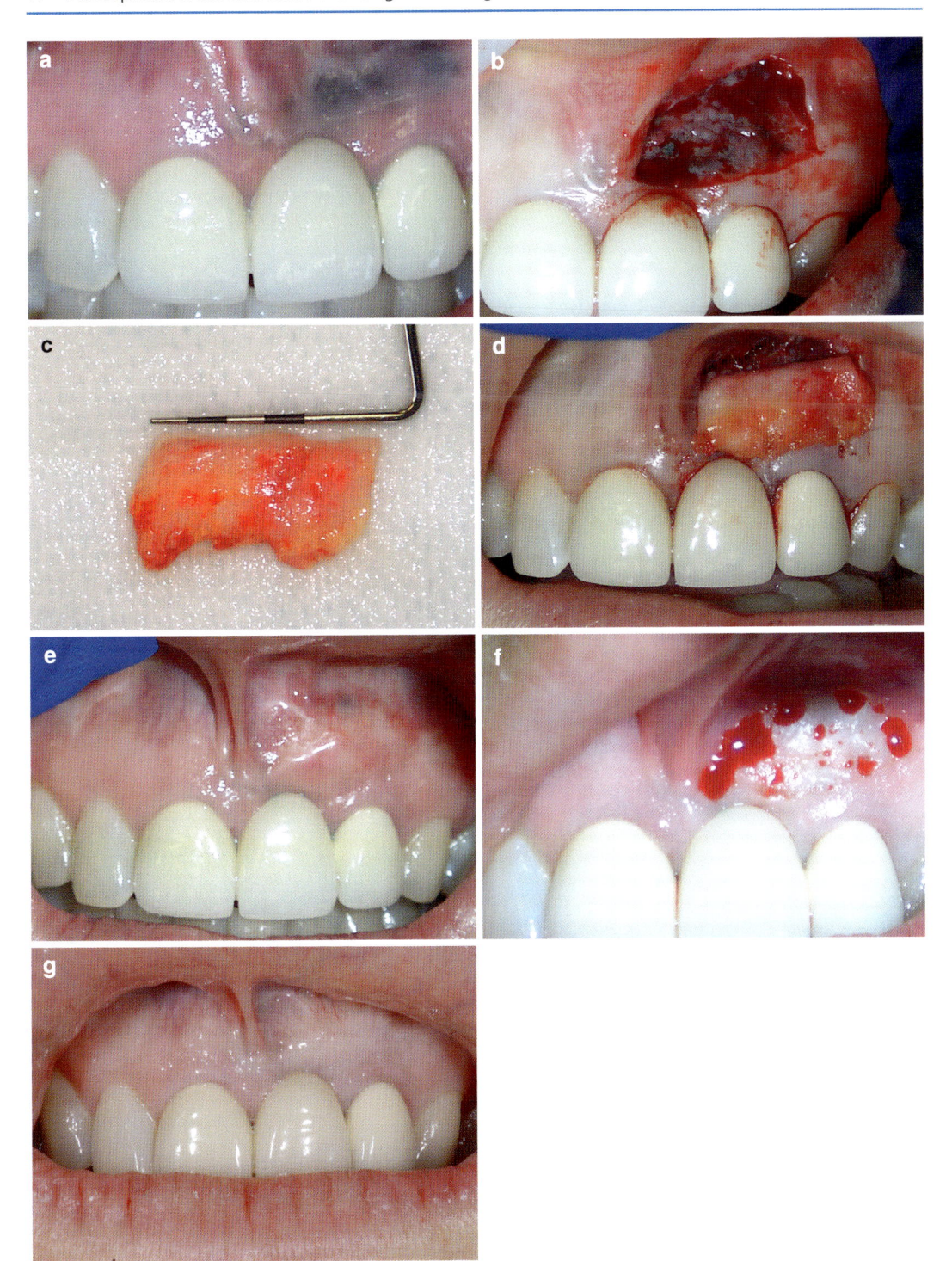

Fig. 14.5 (**a**) Tooth #9 was extracted after a failed root canal treatment as well as a failed attempt at an apicoectomy. A successful implant and crown was eventually placed to satisfactorily restore #9, but the patient is unhappy with the existing amalgam tattoo. (**b**) In preparation for a subepithelial connective tissue (SECT) onlay graft, a recipient bed was prepared over the area of the amalgam tattoo by removing the overlying loose mucosa. (**c**) SECT graft removed from the palate. (**d**) The graft is secured to the bed with non-resorbable sutures. (**e**) At 12 weeks, the SECT onlay graft has healed, eliminating the amalgam tattoo. However, the gingiva is overly thick and unevenly contoured. (**f**) Using a round diamond bur, a gingivoplasty is performed. (**g**) Final result at 5 years. Note the thickness, contour, and quality of the gingiva as well as the stability of the crown/gingiva interface

Another variation of the subepithelial connective tissue graft is the vascularized interpositional periosteal connective tissue (VIP-CT) graft (Sclar 2003). This type of subepithelial connective tissue graft is a pedicle graft, where the base of the graft is left attached as it is simply slid or folded over toward the recipient site (Fig. 14.6a–j). The advantage of this type of graft is that the blood supply to the graft is maintained and never severed. Like the free gingival graft or SECT graft, soft tissue volume may be augmented with this technique. Because this technique involves the connective tissue only, it also provides an excellent tissue color match. This procedure may also be combined with regenerative procedures.

14.9 Acellular Dermal Grafts

One disadvantage of autogenous soft tissue grafts is the need for a second surgical site. This is associated with additional potential complications for the patient including increased bleeding, swelling, pain, and discomfort. In addition, there is a limited amount of tissue available at common intraoral sites such as the palate or maxillary tuberosity.

Acellular dermal grafts are typically allografts derived from human cadavers. They are then processed commonly via proprietary methods to eliminate the cellular component of the graft.

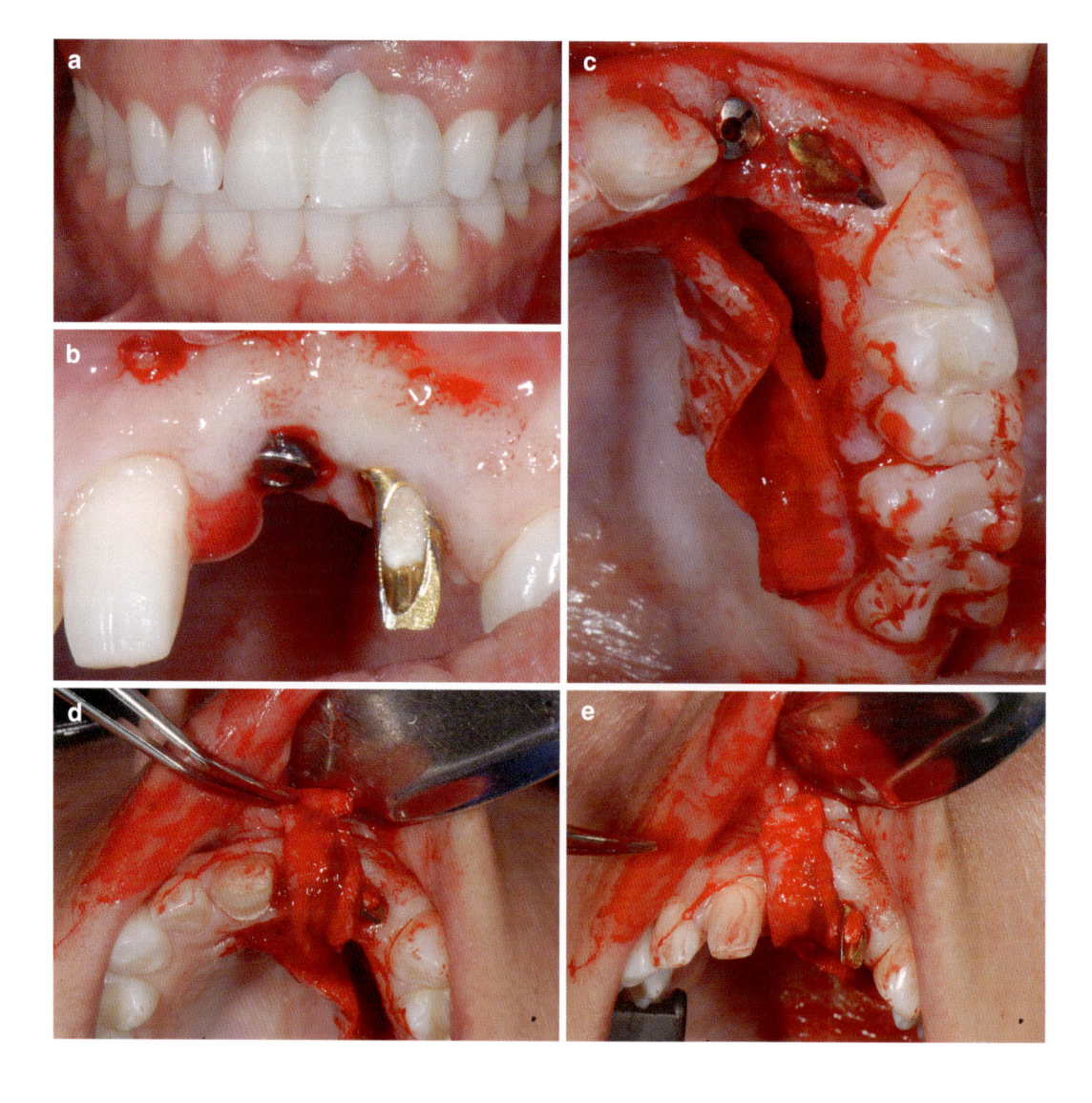

14 Development of the Soft Tissue with Gingival Grafting 243

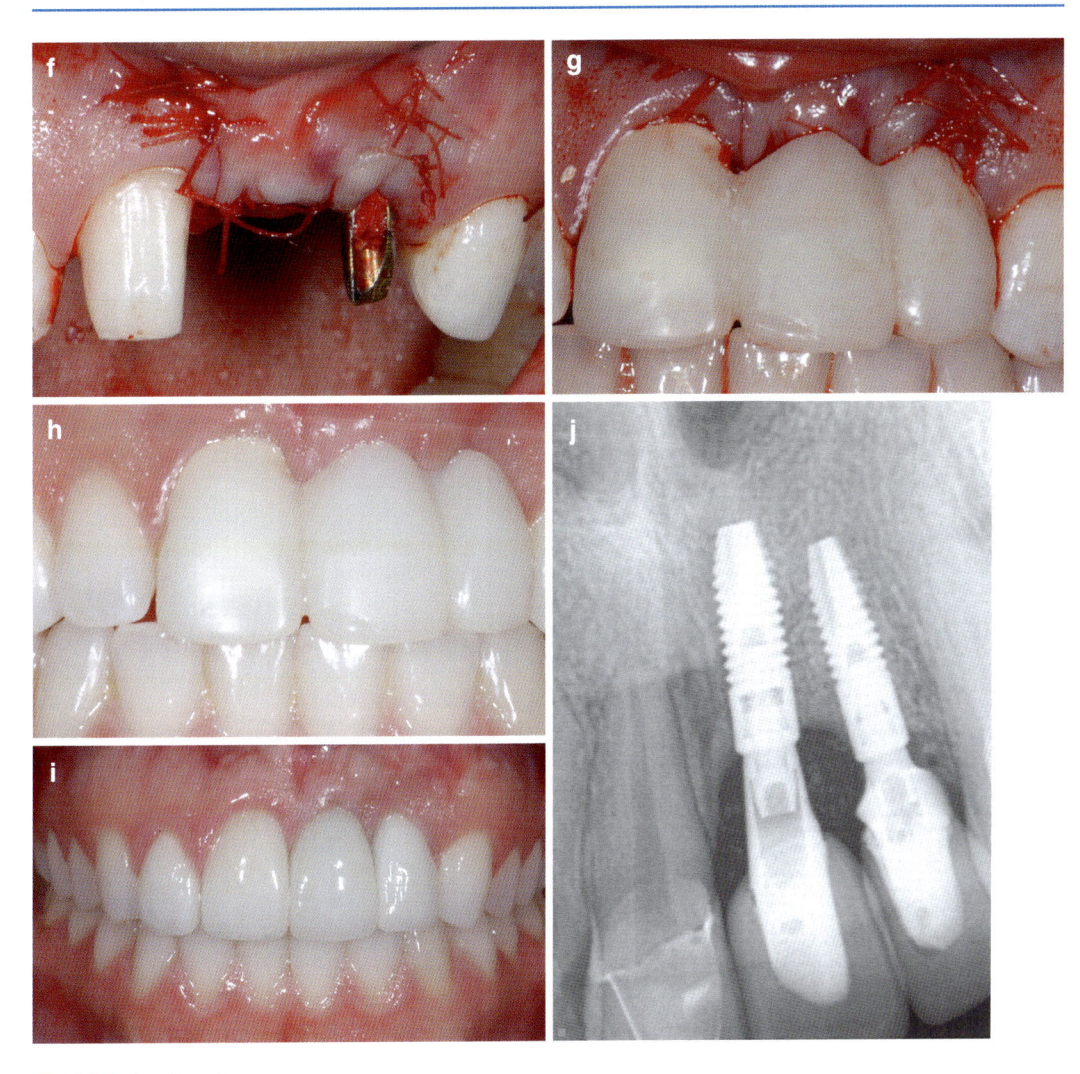

Fig. 14.6 (continued)

Fig. 14.6 (**a**) Following a traumatic accident, this patient lost teeth #s 9 and 10. Following numerous attempts at regeneration, two implants were eventually placed in the #9 and #10 positions. The patient's goal is to establish a more symmetrical gingival height between #8 and 9 as well as the creation of a papilla between the two implants. Prior to surgery, a provisional prosthesis was placed. (**b**) The provisional prosthesis is removed. The recommended treatment in this instance is the vascularized interpositional connective tissue (VIP-CT) graft. (**c**) The connective tissue graft is taken from the left side of the palate, extending from tooth #14 in the posterior to #8 anteriorly. Please note that the VIP-CT graft calls from the graft to maintain fixed to the palate, preserving the blood supply of the graft. (**d**) Once freed from the palate, the VIP-CT graft is then flipped or rotated and placed over the ridge defect. The graft is still secured to the palate near the apex of implant #9. (**e**) Facial view of the VIP-CT graft in place. (**f**) Once the overlying flap is primarily closed over the VIP-CT graft, the increase in anticipated volume can be observed. (**g**) Following final closure of the flaps, the provisional prosthesis is reshaped to ensure light to no contact occurs over the graft, and it is temporarily luted to place. (**h**) Twelve-week follow-up of the patient reveals that excellent healing of the VIP-CT graft has occurred. The majority of the desired volume has been maintained. (**i**) Two-year follow-up. The final prosthesis has been delivered, and the periodontal condition of the crowns is excellent. The gingival zeniths of #8 and #9 are even, and a gingival papilla between #9 and #10 has formed. (**j**) Radiograph at 3 years demonstrates the position of the implants and the relationship of the crestal bone relative to the bone of the adjacent teeth. Note the distance of the crown margins relative to the implant platforms

Clinically, an acellular dermal graft (ADG) is often considered in lieu of the SECT graft (Park 2005). It is recommended that ADGs be completely submerged under passive primary closure. This is in contrast to the SECT graft where the graft may be left partially exposed without compromising the final result. ADGs are not commonly utilized as onlay grafts. These are typically used as inlay grafts and have a number of clinical applications. Like the SECT graft, it is used in the natural dentition to treat and correct gingival recession. It may also be utilized as a membrane during guided tissue regenerations (GTR) and guided bone regeneration (GBR) procedures. In implant-related dentistry, ADGs may be utilized as SECT grafts to establish a thicker biotype and augment ridge defects (Fig. 14.7a–e).

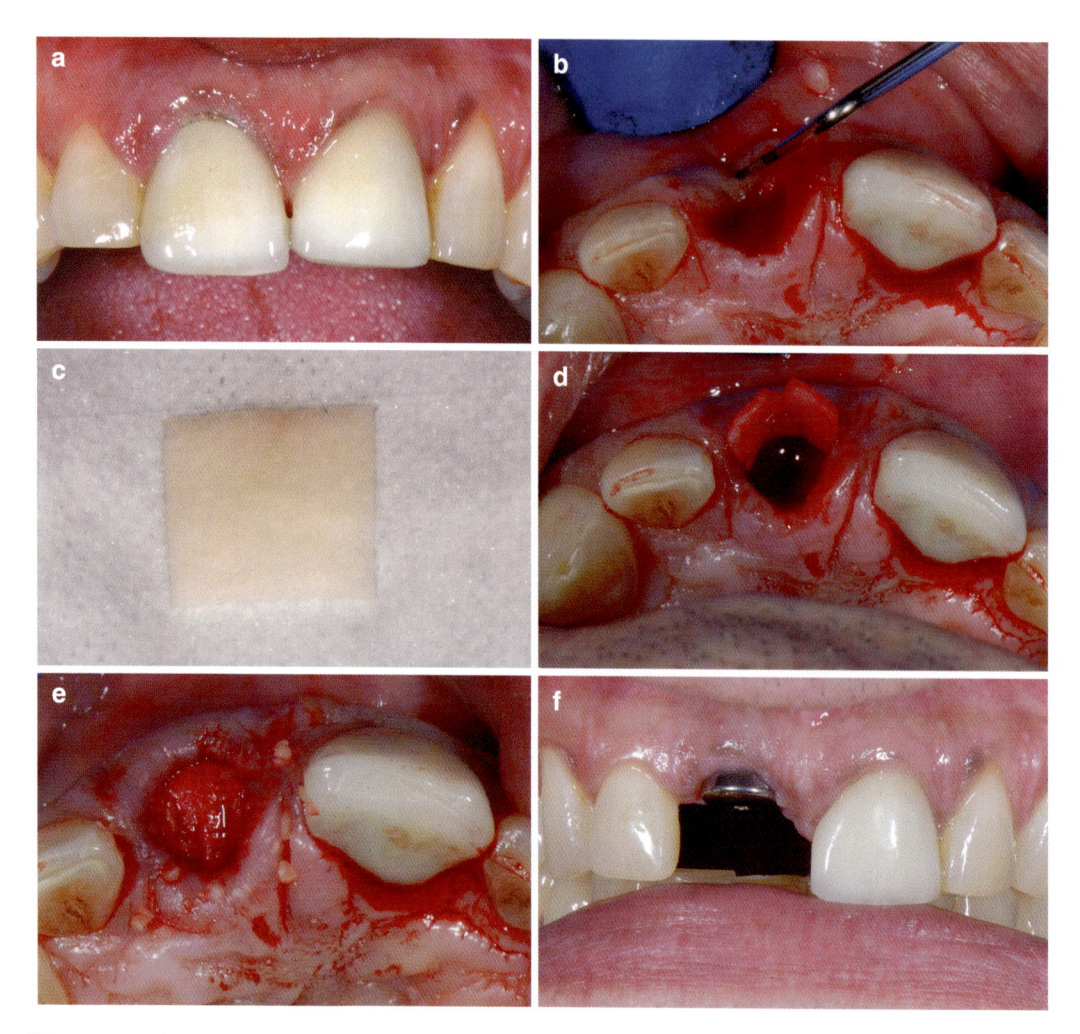

Fig. 14.7 (a) Preoperative photo of tooth #8, which is given a hopeless prognosis due to a horizontal root fracture. An extraction is planned along with simultaneous socket grafting. (b) Once the tooth is extracted, it is apparent that a large dehiscence in the labial plate exists. (c) Prior to placing a socket graft, an acellular dermal graft (ADG) is hydrated in sterile water for 20 min. (d) The ADG is used over the bony dehiscence to serve as a membrane. (e) Following the placement of a bone replacement graft (mineralized cortical bone allograft in this case), the ADG is folded over the coronal portion of the socket and sutured with non-resorbable sutures. (f) This photograph demonstrates the soft tissue contours around the implant healing abutment approximately 4 months after the dental implant has been placed. Please note the gingival symmetry and contour around the healing abutment

Conclusion

During the course of dental implant therapy, the management and development of soft tissues is often vital to the creation of proper gingival architecture for the aesthetics, form, function, and longevity of the final prosthesis. While many techniques and materials are available for purposes such as the transformation of the gingival biotype, the augmentation of soft tissues, or the creation of the desired prosthesis-soft tissue interface, the large majority of procedures involve the use of autografts and allografts. While there are basic indications for each material and technique, the most appropriate decision should be discussed between the surgeon and the patient, taking morbidity, costs, time, practicality, and predictability into consideration.

References

Abrahamsson I, Berglundh T, Wennstrom J, Lindhe J (1996) The periimplant hard and soft tissues at different implant systems. A comparative study in the dog. Clin Oral Implants Res 7(3):212–219

Chung DM, Oh TJ, Shotwell JL, Misch CE, Wang H (2006) Significance of keratinized mucosa in maintenance of dental implants with different surfaces. J Periodontol 77:1410–1420

Fu J, Lee A, Wang HL (2011) Influence of tissue biotype on implant esthetics. Int J Oral Maxillofac Implants 26:499–508

Jia-Hui F, Lee A, Wang HL (2011) Influence of Tissue Biotype on Implant Esthetics. Int J Oral Maxillofac Implants 26:499–508

Jung RE, Sailer I, Hammerle CH, Attin T, Schmidlin P (2007) In vitro color changes of soft tissue caused by restorative materials. Int J Periodont Rest Dent 27:251–257

Kao RT, Fagan MC, Conte GJ (2008) Thick vs thin gingival biotypes: A key determinant in treatment planning for dental implants. J Calif Dent Assoc 36:193–198

Kennedy JE (1974) Effect of inflammation on collateral circulation of the gingiva. J Periodontal Res 9:147–152

Kois JC, Kan JY (2001) Predictable peri-implant gingival aesthetics: surgical and prosthodontics rationales. Pract Proced Aesthet Dent 13:691–698

Langer B, Langer L (1985) Subepithelial connective tissue graft technique for root coverage. J Periodontol 56:715–772

Lazzara RJ, Porter SS (2006) Platform switching: A new concept in implant dentistry for controlling postrestorative crestal bone levels. Int J Perio Rest Dent 26:9–17

Levine RA (1991) Covering denuded root surface with the subepithelial connective tissue graft. Compend Contin Educ Dent 12:568

Linkevicius T, Apse P, Med H, Grybauskas S, Puisys A (2009) The influence of soft tissue thickness on crestal bone changes around implants: a 1-year prospective controlled clinical trial. Int J Oral Maxillofac Implants 24:712–719

Magne P, Belser U (2003) Bonded porcelain restorations in the anterior dentition. A biomimetic approach. Quintessance, Chicago

Miller PD Jr (1985) A classification of marginal tissue recession. Int J Periodont Restor Dent 5:9

Nisapakultorn K, Suphanantachat S, Silkosessak O, Rattanamongkolgul S (2010) Factors affecting soft tissue level around anterior maxillary singe-tooth implants. Clin Oral Implants Res 21:662–670

Park JB (2005) Increasing the width of keratinized mucosa around endosseous implant using acellular dermal matrix allograft. Implant Dent 15:275–281

Reiser G, Bruno J, Mahan P, Larkin L (1996) The subepithelial connective tissue graft palatal donor site: anatomic considerations for surgeons. Intl J Periodontics Restor Dent 6(2):130–137

Rompen E, Raepsaet N, Domken O, Touati B, Van Dooren E (2007) Soft tissue stability at the facial aspect of gingivally converging abutment in the esthetic zone: a pilot clinical study. J Prosthet Dent 97:5119–5125

Salama H, Salama MA, Garber D, Pinhas A (1998) The interproximal height of bone: a guidepost to predictable aesthetic strategies and soft tissue contours in anterior tooth replacement. Pract Periodont Aesthet Dent 10(9):1131–1141

Sclar A (2003) Soft tissue and esthetic considerations in implant therapy. Quintessance, Chicago

Seibert JS, Salama H (1996) Alveolar ridge preservation and reconstruction. Periodontol 2000 11:69–84

Small PN, Tarnow DP, Cho SC (2001) Gingival recession around wide-diameter versus standard-diameter implants: a 3- to 5-year longitudinal prospective study. Pract Proced Aesthet Dent 13:143–146

Sullivan HC, Atkins JC (1968) Free autogenous gingival grafts. III. Utilization of grafts in the treatment of gingival recession. Periodontics 6:152

Warrer K, Buser D, Lang NP, Karring T (1995) Plaque-induced peri-implantitis in the presence or absence of keratinized mucosa. An experimental study in monkeys. Clin Oral Implants Res 6:131–138

Tissue Engineering Approach to Implant Site Development

15

Dan Clark, Igor Roitman, Mark C. Fagan, and Richard T. Kao

Abstract

One of the greatest challenges for the surgical placement of dental implants is the lack of adequate bone volume. Many techniques are available but they are both technique sensitive, and the results are not always predictable. Tissue engineering through the use of biologics provides a strategy for enhancing bone regeneration. Though this is a relatively new strategy, this chapter focuses on technologies that are available for clinicians to utilize at this time.

15.1 What Is Tissue Engineering and Why Use This Approach for Implant Site Development?

Dental implants have enhanced clinicians' ability to provide and promote oral rehabilitation. A common limitation is when the implant site has inadequate bone volume. Tissue engineering is a highly promising field whereby biotechnologies are used to facilitate regeneration of a particular tissue (Fig. 15.1). Tissue engineering constructs may consist of applying biologic signaling molecules (e.g., growth/differentiation factors and plasma preparations), cells (stem cells), and/or scaffolding matrices which are implanted to promote regeneration so that the new tissue is characteristically and functionally indistinguishable from the original (Lynch 1999). The tissue of interest in implant dentistry is the new bone. A recent review discusses the scientific advances of tissue engineering in the oral craniofacial field

D. Clark, DDS
Division of Periodontology, University of California, San Francisco, San Francisco, CA, USA

I. Roitman, DMD, MS
Division of Periodontology, University of California, San Francisco, San Francisco, CA, USA

Private practice, Menlo Park, CA, USA

M.C. Fagan, DDS, MS
Private practice, San Jose, CA, USA

R.T. Kao, DDS, PhD (✉)
Division of Periodontology, University of California, San Francisco, San Francisco, CA, USA

Private practice, Cupertino, CA, USA
e-mail: richkao@sbcglobal.net

Fig. 15.1 Tissue engineering concept is the regeneration of tissues accomplished through the use of signaling molecules, cells, and/or scaffolds. These components can be constructed in the laboratory and directly implanted into a patient to facilitate appropriate tissue regeneration. Clinically available components are highlighted with yellow text (Modified from Lynch 1999)

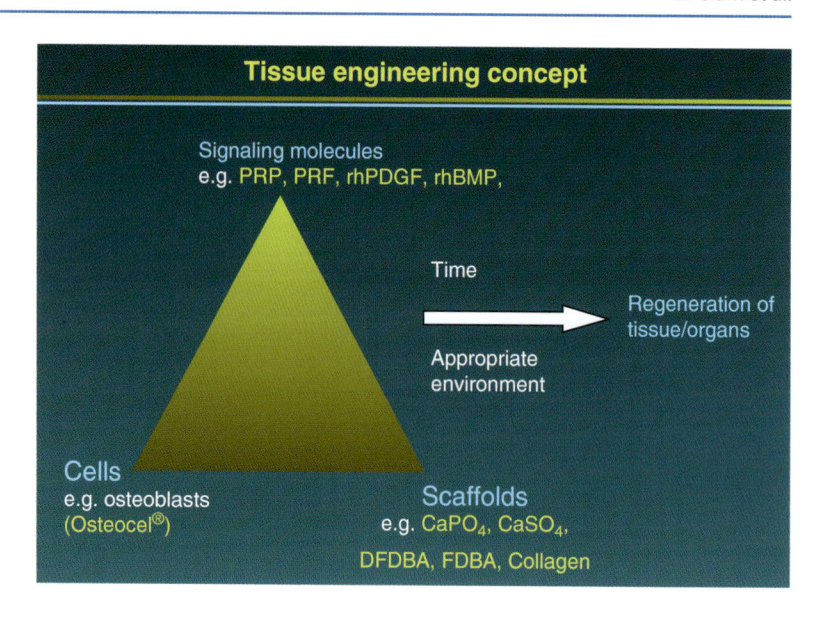

(Pilipchuk et al. 2015). Whereas this review summarizes recent advances in regenerative technologies (scaffolding matrices, cell/gene therapy, and biologic drug delivery), the goal of this chapter is to provide clinicians with an understanding of how certain biotechnologies associated with tissue engineering may be incorporated into implant dentistry. It focuses on clinically available biotechnologies, their scientific merit or potential to improve clinical outcome, and considerations for incorporation into clinical practice.

Clinically, most biologics utilized for implant site preparation are used in conjunction with scaffolding agents (autografts, allografts, and xenografts) with/without guided bone regeneration (GBR) membranes. This chapter will focus on the biologics or signaling molecules currently available for tissue engineering.

15.2 Use of Platelet-Rich Plasma and Platelet-Rich Fibrin for Implant Site Preservation

Platelet-rich plasma (PRP) and platelet-rich fibrin (PRF) are autologous blood concentrate preparations used in dentoalveolar surgery to improve healing and tissue maturation (Choukroun I 2006; Choukroun et al. 2006; Lekovic et al. 2012).

Each product utilizes its own specific preparation protocol; however, both products rely on capturing the natural polypeptide growth factors associated with normal wound healing and delivering them to the surgical site in a highly concentrated form. Proposed applications of PRP and PRF are diverse and include implant site development in combination with bone graft material, applied alone for alveolar ridge preservation, or to increase bone volume via a sinus lift procedure (Anitua 1999; Iasella et al. 2003; Kassolis et al. 2000; Sanchez et al. 2003; Simon et al. 2011; Zhang et al. 2012). Additionally, both preparations have been utilized in surgical application associated with orthopedics, ophthalmology, and plastic surgery (Alio et al. 2015; Del Torto et al. 2014; Sclafani and Azzi 2015).

15.2.1 Platelet-Rich Plasma

Platelet-rich plasma was introduced as an autologous modification of fibrin glue (Hood et al. 1993; Sanchea et al. 2003), a hemostatic and adhesive agent used in various surgical disciplines. Generally, the preparation protocol begins with the initial introduction of anticoagulant to the blood sample, followed by multiple centrifuge and separation cycles that result in a concentrated platelet product. Topical bovine thrombin

(TBT) is then added to activate the platelets and the clotting cascade to obtain an active product with gel-like handling properties.

15.2.2 Platelet-Rich Fibrin

Platelet-rich fibrin is considered a second-generation blood concentrate technique which Choukroun introduced as modification of PRP preparation (Choukroun et al. 2000; Dohan et al. 2006). The production of PRF employs a simpler protocol where collected whole blood is centrifuged at approximately 400 G in a glass tube without the addition of anticoagulants or additives. During the centrifuge process, the fibrin is allowed to slowly polymerize while the blood separates into three distinct layers: an acellular platelet poor plasma on top, a concentrated hematocrit at the base, and the fibrin clot in the middle (Dohan et al. 2006). The fibrin clot is the desired PRF which can be easily isolated and applied surgically (Fig. 15.2).

The production protocol for PRF offers multiple reported advantages over PRP. Notably, there is no addition of anticoagulant, and the clotting cascade occurs naturally with PRF. No TBT is required, eliminating the risk for the development of antibodies to factors V and XI and thrombin (Cmolik et al. 1993; Sanchez et al. 2003). This is of a concern because antibody development can be associated with life-threatening coagulopathies, most notably as a result of factor V deficiency (Cmolik et al. 1993). While complications are rare, there appears to be an increase in susceptibility for their development with increasing exposure to TBT (Cmolik et al. 1993).

15.2.3 In Vitro Characteristics of PRF and PRP

Growth factors released from platelets have been identified and quantified in PRP and PRF. Platelet-associated growth factors include platelet-derived growth factor (PDGF), vascular endothelial growth factor (VEGF), transforming growth factor beta (TGF-β), platelet-derived epidermal growth factor (PDEGF), insulin growth factor 1 (IGF-1), and basic fibroblast growth factor (bFGF) (Dohan et al. 2006; Dohan and de Peppo 2009; He et al. 2009; Sanchez et al. 2003). All of which are involved in hard and soft tissue healing. Multiple studies (Dohan et al. 2006; Dohan and de Peppo 2009; He et al. 2009; Saygin NE, et al. 2000; Sanchez et al. 2003) have compared quantification of these growth factors across PRF, PRP, and whole blood. Schär et al. reported in a 28-day in vitro model in which higher levels of IGF-1 and TGF-β were found in PRF compared to PRP and whole blood (Schär et al. 2015). They also showed PDGF levels did not vary between the three groups, and the VEGF levels were higher in whole blood compared to PRP and PRF. Conversely, He et al. showed higher levels of PDGF and TGF-β in PRF compared to PRP in a similar 28-day in vitro study (He et al. 2009).

Due to the short biologic half-life of these various platelet-associated growth factors, their release kinetics may be critical to sustain biologic changes. A sustained release of growth factors over time may impart better clinical performance than a higher quantity released in a shorter period. Schär et al. showed a difference in the release rates of TGF-β, PDGF, VEGF, and IGF-1 across PRF, PRP, and whole blood (Schär et al. 2015). They reported that PRP released a significantly higher percentage of its total growth factor quantity by day 1, while PRF demonstrated a more sustained release with the highest percentage release at day 3 or 7 (Schär et al. 2015). He et al. confirmed PRP to release more TGF-β and PDGF on day 1 and PRF releasing these two growth factors at a higher concentration on days 14, 21, and 28 (Schär et al. 2015). These release kinetic studies have been confirmed by other investigators (Dohan and de Peppo 2009; Tsay et al. 2005).

The cellular response during in vitro culture analysis also demonstrates the clinical potential of PRF and PRP. The addition of PRP has been shown to increase cell proliferation of adipose-derived stem cells and increase osteogenic gene markers such as alkaline phosphatase, osteopontin, and osteocalcin (Xu et al. 2015). Similarly, rat bone marrow and endothelial cells grown in media

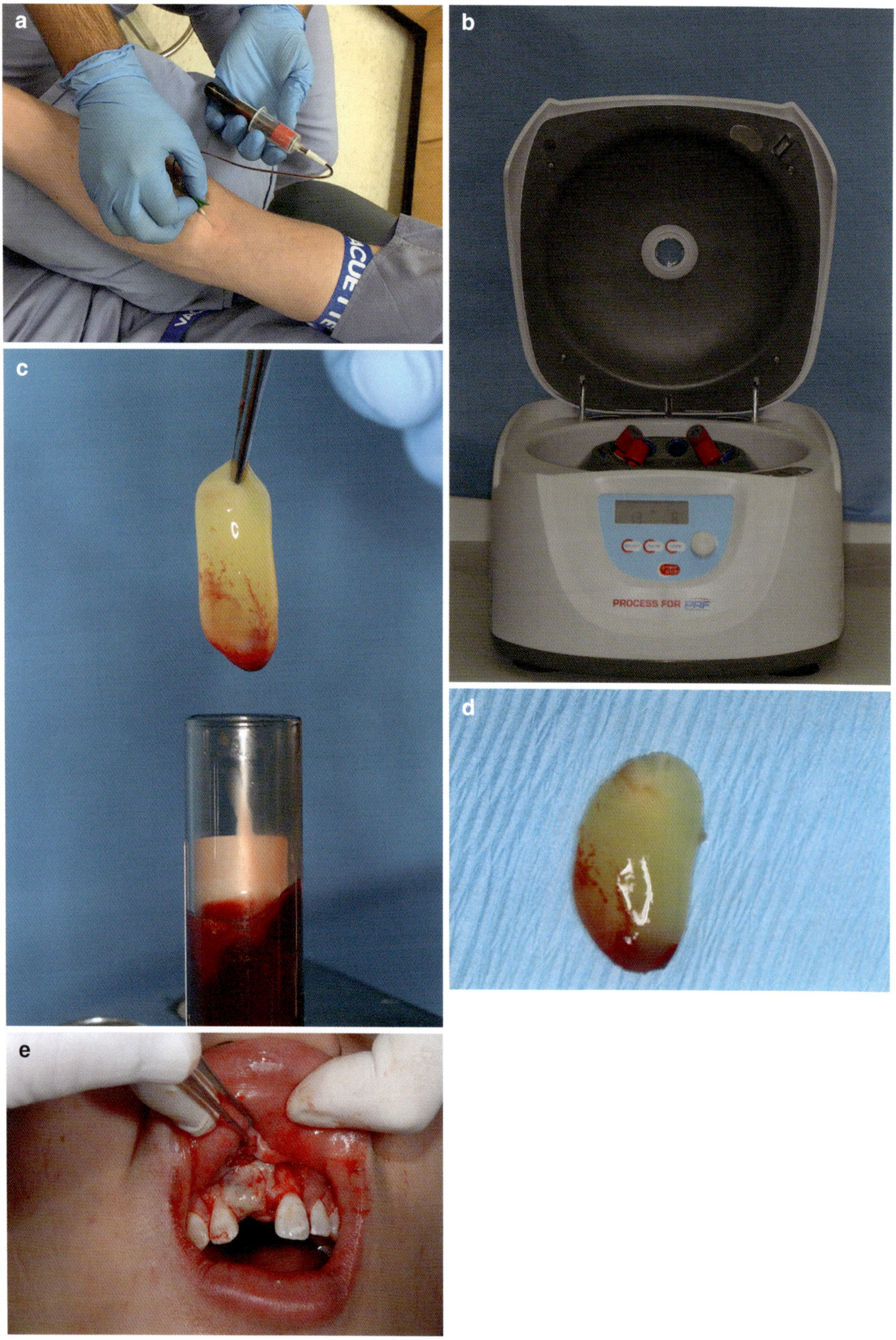
a
b
c
d
e
PROCESS FOR PRF

with PRP demonstrated increased cell proliferation and gene expression for osteocalcin and collagen type I gene expression as compared to cells grown without PRP (Roussy et al. 2007; van den Dolder et al. 2006). Similar in vitro experiments have been performed with PRF. Human osteoblasts have shown increased cellular proliferation in media conditioned with PRF (Clipet et al. 2012; Kang et al. 2011; Tsay et al. 2005; Wu et al. 2012) and gene expression of osteogenic gene markers osteopontin and osteocalcin, as well as osteoblast transcription factor RUNX2 (Clipet et al. 2012; Li et al. 2013). Increased protein expression of lysyl oxidase and heat shock protein 47, two collagen-related proteins involved in forming the extracellular matrices of mineralized tissues, has been shown to be upregulated with PRF-conditioned media (Wu et al. 2012). In comparing the osteogenic potential of PRF to PRP, osteoblast cells grown in PRF-conditioned media showed more robust and faster mineralization formation than the PRP conditioned media group (Kang et al. 2011).

15.2.4 Clinical Applications of PRF and PRP

The purported advantages of PRF and PRP in the surgical field are due to its autogenous nature and low morbidity in harvesting. The application of PRF is further supported due to its simple preparation protocol and low cost. Platelet-rich fibrin production requires only a small tabletop centrifuge and minimal blood collection armamentarium. Training in its production is minimal and can be performed in a matter of minutes by auxiliary staff after the blood is collected by the dentist or staff trained in phlebotomy. The timing between blood collection and PRF preparation is critical; however, once prepared, the PRF is stable for some time until required.

Most clinical reports and studies of PRP utilization describe it for enhancing bone graft material for sinus augmentation or ridge augmentation (Anitua 1999; Froum et al. 2002; Kassolis et al. 2000; Rosenberg and Torosian 2000; Shanaman et al. 2001). Since PRF has been shown to contain similar growth factor concentration as PRP, it has also been used for bone graft enhancement. There are a number of studies and clinical reports showing PRF mixed with graft particulate and demonstrating similar successful treatment as PRP (Simon et al. 2011; Choukroun et al. 2006; Zhang et al. 2012; Li et al. 2013; Suttapreyasri and Leepong 2013). However, the majority of these reports are case studies lacking proper controls and an adequate patient pool for adequate comparisons across different treatment modalities.

In addition to concentrated growth factors and sustained growth factor release, PRF has physical characteristics that make its use advantageous. The fibrin matrix of PRF provides characteristics that can be utilized in two different applications. First, the prepared PRF is a dense fibrin clot which can be applied to the surgical site, where it serves as the stable architecture required in wound healing to promote neovascularization and cell migration and proliferation (Hinsbergh et al. 2001). The PRF clot has been successfully used as a single modality grafting material for sinus augmentation or in extraction sockets for site development for implant placement (Fig. 15.3) (Simon et al. 2011; Simonpieri et al. 2011; Suttapreyasri and Leepong 2013; Tajima et al. 2013). All these studies showed successful healing and successful implant placement at the augmented sites. The second application of PRF is as a membrane. To create the membrane, the PRF clot is compressed, typically between sterile glass slabs or commercially available kits, forcing fluid out and further condensing the dense fibrin matrix. The resulting thin membrane can be applied surgically with good handling

Fig. 15.2 (**a**–**e**) Platelet-rich fibrin preparation. (**a**) Blood collection with butterfly needle and glass vacutainer tube. (**b**) Tubes immediately placed in centrifuge and spun at 400 g. (**c**) After centrifuge, PRF is formed and can be isolated from the remaining hematocrit. (**d**) Isolated PRF clot can be applied directly to the surgical site or pressed into a membrane. (**e**) In this clinical case, the PRF was compressed and placed over a grafted horizontal bony defect prior to soft tissue closure

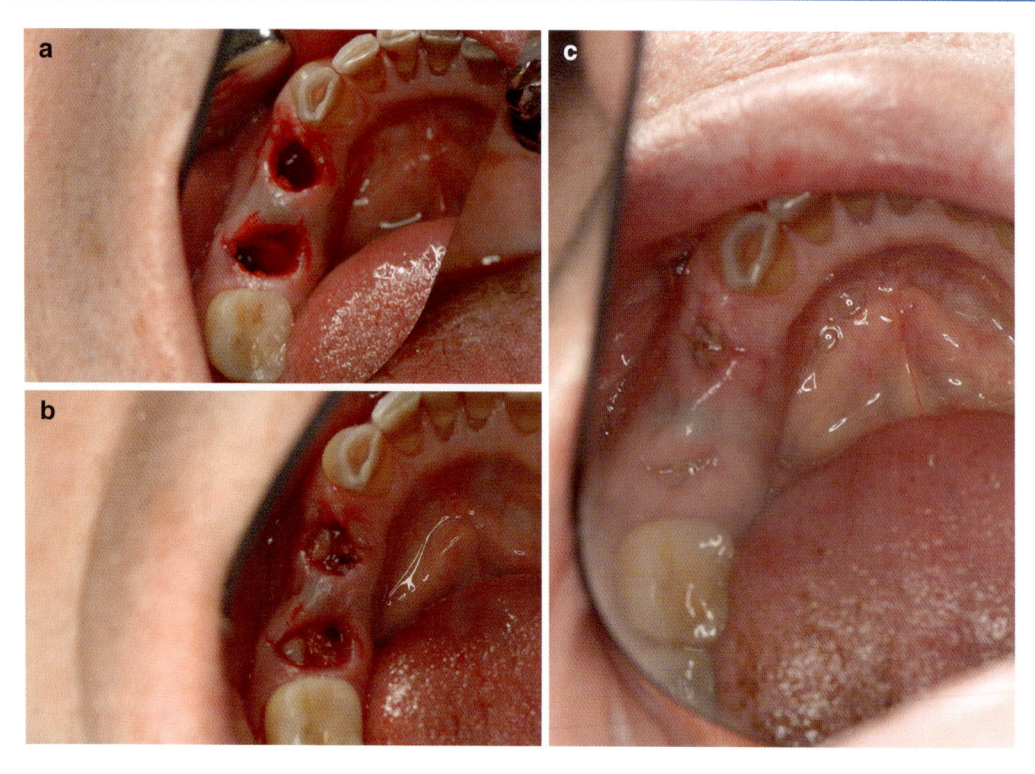

Fig. 15.3 Extraction sockets treated with PRF clot. (**a**) Immediate post-extraction sockets of #28 and 29. (**b**) PRF clot placed directly into socket. (**c**) Healing at 2 weeks postsurgery

characteristics. The dense nature of the membrane allows it to adequately hold a suture and applied as a physical barrier to protect soft tissue from underlying titanium struts or mesh or from tenting or tacking screws. It can also be applied as a traditional membrane material in GTR or GBR applications and to close external sinus windows or repair sinus membrane perforations. However, the true cell occluding properties of the PRF membrane have not been adequately reported in the literature. As the growth factors released by PRF can also promote reepithelialization, it is not surprising that PRF membranes demonstrate rapid and enhanced soft tissue healing over augmented sites.

15.3 Use of Recombinant Bone Morphogenetic Proteins and PDGF for Implant Site Preparation

Bone morphogenetic proteins (BMPs) are a group of differentiation factors that act as morphogenetic signals to orchestrate bone development throughout the body (Reddi and Reddi 2009). Recombinant human BMPs (rhBMPs) are used in orthopedic applications such as spinal fusions and nonunions, and rhBMP-2 has also been FDA approved for sinus augmentation and localized alveolar ridge augmentations (Boyne et al. 2005; Fiorellini et al. 2005; Howell et al. 1997). The product is reconstituted and used in conjunction with an absorbable collagen sponge (ACS). The use of rhBMP-2 and ACS in ridge augmentation and preservation has been shown to be safe (Boyne et al. 2005; Fiorellini et al. 2005; Howell et al. 1997). Clinically, ACS provides minimal structural scaffolding so rhBMP-2 has been used in an off-label fashion with allografts. Additionally, there have been instances where rhBMP caused significant postoperative swelling. Given the poor scaffolding property of rhBMP-ACS, two small case series employed rhBMP-2 and ACS with GBR, such as titanium mesh and inclusion of graft materials, to provide additional three-dimensional support for the graft (Herford and Boyne 2008; Misch and Wang 2011). There is some concern that over-activation of BMP signaling may result in potential development of esophageal adenocarcinoma when used in the proximal portion of the gastrointestinal tract (Bleuming et al. 2007; Milano et al. 2007). A recent meta-analysis has shown rhBMP to be safe (Simmonds et al. 2013). However, the use of rhBMP is not common in implant site development due to its high cost and since comparable end results can be obtained utilizing other techniques.

The second human recombinant signaling molecule available is human recombinant platelet-derived growth factor (rhPDGF). Though well investigated for its ability to correct periodontal intrabony defects (McGuire et al. 2006; Nevins et al. 2005, 2013), the use of rhPDGF for implant site preparation has not been as rigorously examined. PDGF is a protein with the ability to stimulate cell growth, chemotaxis, proliferation, and differentiation (Nevins and Reynolds 2011; Nevins et al. 2011). Growth factors regulate expression of mineral-associated genes that are primarily stored in platelet alpha granules. Secondary producers of these growth factors include osteoblasts, macrophages, and monocytes. Recombinant human PDGF-ββ (rhPDGF-ββ) has been used successfully for implant site preparation in GBR, block graft augmentation, and sinus lifts. rhPDGF-ββ has also been used with autogenous bone, DFDBA, FDBA, xenograft, or mineral collagen bone substitute with and without membranes for successful ridge augmentation (Cardaropoli 2009; Nevins and Reynolds 2011; Nevins et al. 2011; Simion et al. 2007, 2008). Two case reports of sinus lifts where rhPDGF-ββ was used in conjunction with bovine xenograft indicated that significant vital bone is formed as early as 3.5 months postsurgery (Scheyer and McGuire 2011). These studies suggest that rhPDGF added to bone graft may accelerate bone formation, allowing for earlier implant placement; however, more research is needed to confirm this hypothesis.

15.4 Stem Cells

Adequate bone volume, including height, width, and vertical positioning, is required for proper dental implant placement and its subsequent resistance to biomechanical loading. Loss of alveolar bone will compromise implant placement in proper three-dimensional positioning. Alveolar bone can be lost due to odontogenic and non-odontogenic infections, periodontal disease, benign or malignant tumors, trauma, or tooth loss. After tooth loss, bone remodeling continues and further loss of the maxillary or mandibular bone occurs. Ridge or socket preservation and augmentation procedures utilizing bone grafting materials have been developed to successfully maintain or regenerate lost bone volume. Autogenous bone has been the "gold standard" for grafting materials. However, critical limitations for autogenous use include inadequate supply of necessary graft and donor site morbidity. Tissue engineering protocols involving growth factors and stem cell lines have the potential to overcome some of these limitations.

Stem cell protocols have the potential to improve current bone regeneration methods through increased bioactivity of grafting scaffolding, targeted growth factor delivery, and cell recruitment. The concentration of multipotential stromal cells (MSCs) in a cellular bone allograft compared with fresh age-matched iliac crest bone and bone marrow (BM) aspirate was investigated (Baboolal et al. 2014). The authors reported that without cultivation/expansion, the allograft displayed an "osteoinductive" molecular signature and the presence of CD45−CD271+CD73+CD90+CD105+ MSCs with a purity over 100-fold that of iliac crest bone. In comparison with BM, MSC numbers enzymatically released from 1 g of cellular allograft were equivalent to approximately 45 ml of BM aspirate. They concluded that MSC cellular allograft bone represents a unique nonimmune material rich in MSCs and osteocytes. This osteoinductive cellular graft represents an attractive alternative to autograft bone which reduces supply and morbidity issues.

The use of platelet-rich plasma and mononuclear cells from bone marrow aspirate and bone scaffold for maxillary bone augmentation was studied (Filho et al. 2007). They reported an overall 94.7% success rate with adequate ridge dimensions obtained for proper dental implant placement. They noted that grafting failures were due to infection of the maxillary sinus and lack of integration into the host cortical bone. Bone formation with the presence of osteoblasts throughout the trabeculae was noted histologically with minimal marginal bone loss during a 4-year follow-up. Kaigler et al. conducted a randomized controlled feasibility trial to compare the use of tissue repair cells with a conventional GBR technique for alveolar bone regeneration. At implant placement, a second bone grafting procedure was necessary for sockets treated with GBR. The authors also noted that the regenerated bone in the test group exhibited greater density and higher vascularity and acceleration of osteogenesis at 6 weeks (Kaigler 2015).

McAllister described using a cellular allograft for treatment of periodontal defects in both a single-rooted and a multi-rooted tooth (McAllister 2011). In the single-rooted case, a significant reduction in probing was obtained with radiologic evidence of approximately 4 mm of vertical bone fill at 6 months following grafting. In the multi-rooted case, clinical evidence showed decreased probing depths and radiographic bone improvement at 6 months. A cone beam computerized tomography scan taken at 14 months demonstrated three-dimensional bone fill. A similar result was presented in a case report by Koo et al. who described the use of allograft cellular bone matrix containing mesenchymal stem cells in the treatment of a severe periodontal defect (Koo et al. 2012). These case reports indicate a potential resolution of periodontal defects using cellular allograft material.

Successful use of a cellular allograft combined with a titanium mesh to aid in space maintenance for ridge augmentation in both width and vertical dimensions was demonstrated (McAllister and Eshraghi 2013; Rickert et al. 2011). Similar results were obtained using cellular grafting material for ridge augmentation by Sindler et al. (2013). A representative case of a patient presenting with a hopeless maxillary anterior lateral incisor with advanced resorption is shown in Fig. 15.4. In order to aid in soft tissue closure over the anticipated augmentation site, the tooth was extracted, and the soft tissue allowed to heal for 4 weeks. Surgical opening and debridement of the area shows the advanced loss of the facial plate of bone. A tenting pin was inserted to aid in space maintenance, and the site was grafted with a cellular grafting material. A resorbable collagen membrane was placed over the entire site and a primary closure obtained. Following 4 months of healing, the site was reentered for implant placement. The site presented with adequate volume and density for primary implant stability and proper three-dimensional placement. In a histomorphometric analysis of cores obtained during the initial preparation of the implant sites, the presence of 37.0% new bone (range 21.1–57.7%) was found in 12 cores. This compares favorably with a new bone found in the sinus (Gonshor et al. 2011).

Sinus augmentation to increase the necessary bone volume and height for implant placement and stability is common due to the progressive alveolar bone resorption. In a histomorphometric study, bone formation following sinus augmentation procedures using either an allograft cellular bone matrix containing native mesenchymal stem cells or a conventional allograft has been compared (Gonshor et al. 2011). Results over a 3.7-month follow-up healing period of the test group revealed a mean of 32.5% and 4.9% for vital bone and remaining graft content, respectively. In the control group, only 18.3% of the bone content was vital, and 25.8% of residual conventional graft remained. Rickert et al. reported similar results when they compared bovine-derived mineral bone seeded with mononuclear stem cells with bovine-derived mineral bone mixed with autogenous bone (Rickert et al. 2011). Significantly greater bone formation was observed in the test group when compared with the control group at 14 weeks: 17.7% versus 12%, respectively.

Cellular grafting materials and biologics have ushered in an opportunity for clinicians to provide their patients with predictable results that achieve not only quantitative clinical results but also qualitative histologic results demonstrating regeneration of lost periodontium. Clinicians must weigh the benefits versus any risks and cost to determine the best course of treatment for their patients. It should be noted that much of the evidence available is based on limited patient pools. Controlled prospective studies with larger study populations are needed to further determine the clinical promise for stem cell use.

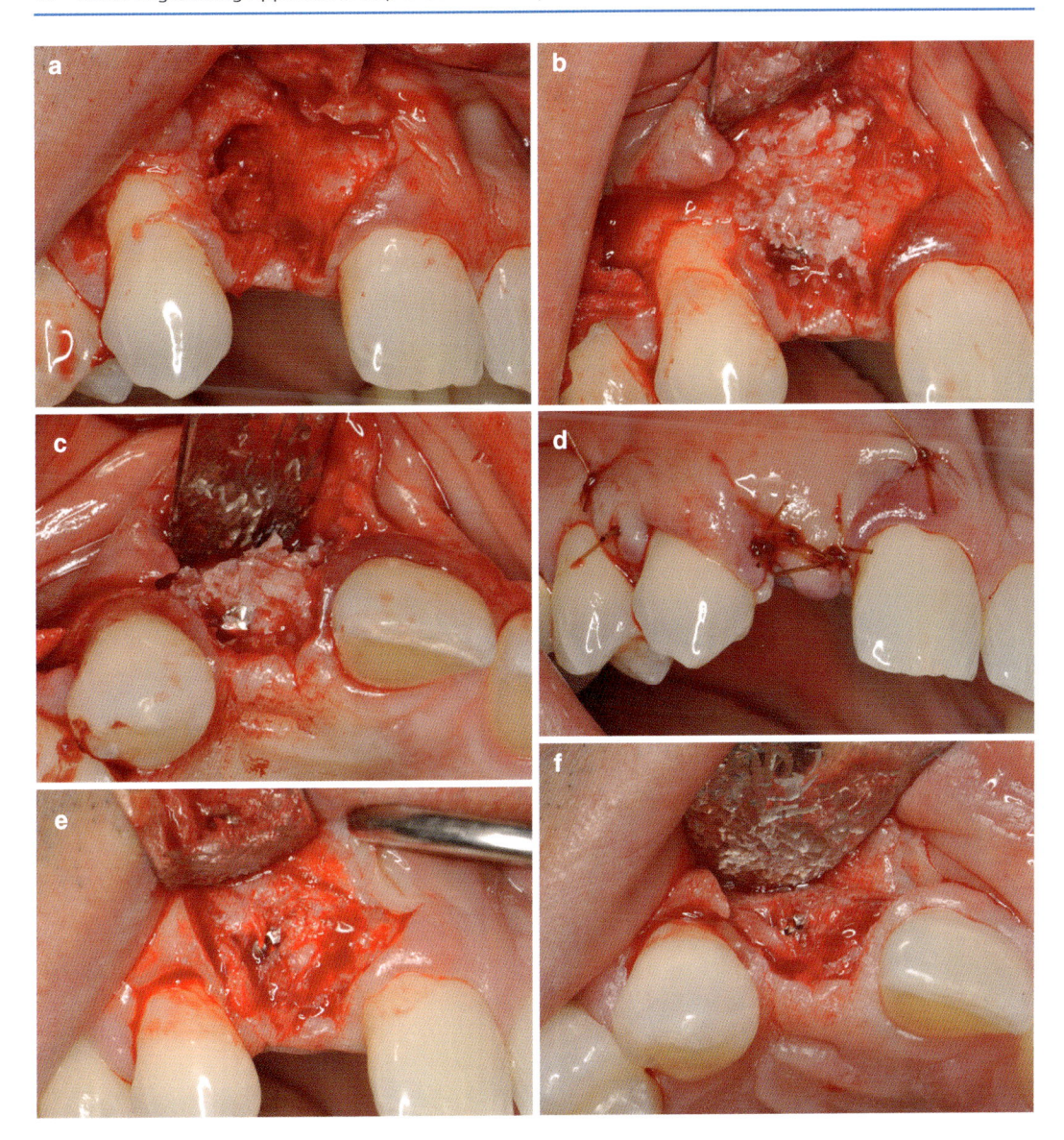

Fig. 15.4 Ridge augmentation with stem cells. (**a**) A previously extracted site was reentered showing almost complete lack of facial bony plate. (**b**) Facial photo of cellular graft material packing after tenting pin placement, noting vertical component needed for proper implant placement. (**c**) Occlusal photo after cellular graft material packed noting the ridge width needed. (**d**) Primary closure after grafting was obtained. (**e**, **f**) Reentry 4 months after grafting indicating both vertical and horizontal ridge augmentation, respectively. (**g**) Implant placement from the occlusal aspects, showing that adequate bone height and width for proper implant placement and stability were obtained. (**h**) Radiograph after implant placement. (**i**) Final restoration on the day of delivery. Root coverage for adjacent teeth obtained and the papilla will blend in over the next 6 months. (**j**) A sample coring of the implant site performed with a 2 mm trephine. The histology (20×) indicates high prevalence of new bone (NB) with minimal residual graft (RG) materials present

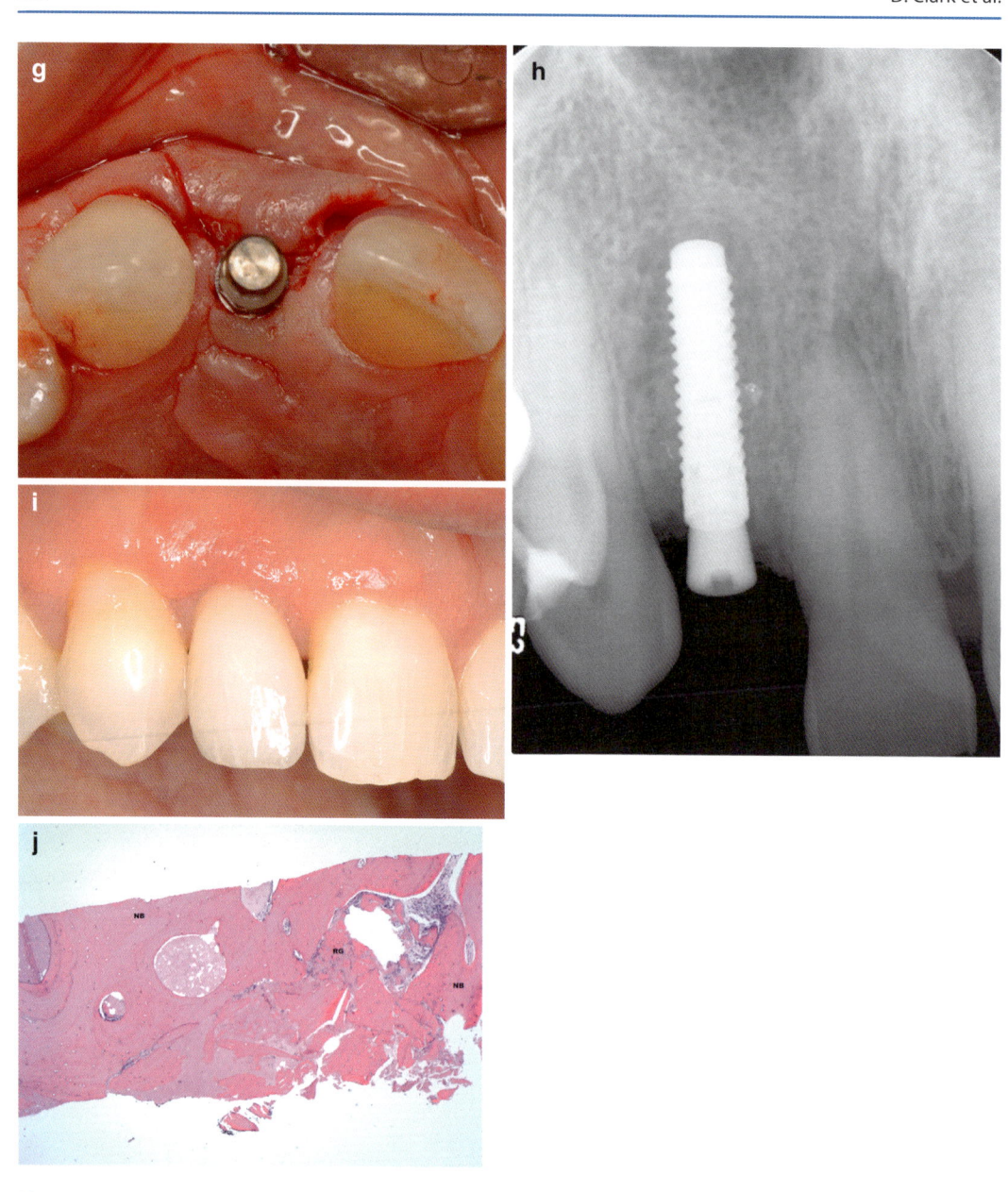

Fig. 15.4 (continued)

Conclusion

Tissue engineering is an emerging technology that may significantly improve our ability for implant site preparation. Through the use of biologics such as PRP, PRF, rhBMP, and rhPDGF-BB along with stem cells, we may be able to increase bone volume without the need for secondary surgical donor site, and surgically these biologics may provide more consistent results. This is a new emerging field that requires additional research, but clinicians should be aware of the potential of tissue engineering and monitor its progress.

References

Alio JL, Rodriguez AE, Wróbel Dudzińska D (2015) Eye platelet-rich plasma in the treatment of ocular surface disorders. Curr Opin Ophthalmol 26:325–326

Anitua E (1999) Plasma rich in growth factors: preliminary results of use in the preparation of future sites for implants. Int J Oral Maxillofac Implants 14:529–535

Baboolal TG, Boxall SA et al (2014) Multipotential stromal cell abundance in cellular bone allograft: comparison with fresh age-matched iliac crest bone and bone marrow aspirate. Regen Med 9:593–607

Bleuming SA, He XC, Kodach LL et al (2007) Bone morphogenetic protein signaling suppress tumorigenesis at gastric epithelial transition zones in mice. Cancer Res 67:8149–8155

Boyne PJ, Lily LC, Marx RE et al (2005) De novo bone induction by recombinant bone morphogenetic protein-2 (rhBMP-2) in maxillary sinus floor augmentation. J Oral Maxillofac Surg 63:1693–1707

Cardaropoli D (2009) Vertical ridge augmentation with the use of recombinant human platelet-derived growth factor-BB and bovine bone mineral: a case report. Int J Periodontics Restor Dent 29:289–295

Choukroun I (2006) Platelet-rich fibrin (PRF): a second-generation platelet concentrate. Part V: histologic evaluations of PRF effects on bone allograft maturation in sinus lift. Oral Surg Oral Med Oral Pathol Oral Radiol Endod 101:299–303

Choukroun J, Adda F, Schoeffler C (2000) Une opportunite´ en paro-implantologie: le PRF. Implantodontie 42:55–62

Choukroun J, Diss A, Simonpieri A et al (2006) Platelet-rich fibrin (PRF): a second-generation platelet concentrate. Part IV: clinical effects on tissue healing. Oral Surg Oral Med Oral Pathol Oral Radiol Endod 101:e56–e60

Clipet F, Tricot S, Alno N, Massot M (2012) In vitro effects of Choukroun's platelet-rich fibrin conditioned medium on 3 different cell lines implicated in dental implantology. Implant Dent 21:51–56

Cmolik BL, Spero JA, Magovern GJ (1993) Redo cardiac surgery: late bleeding complications from topical thrombin-induced factor five deficiency. J Thorac Cardiovasc Surg 105:222–228

Del Torto M, Enea D, Panfoli N et al (2014) Hamstrings anterior cruciate ligament reconstruction with and without platelet rich fibrin matrix. Knee Surg Sports Traumatol Arthrosc 31:1–9

Dohan DM, Choukroun J, Diss A et al (2006) Platelet-rich fibrin (PRF): a second-generation platelet concentrate. Part I: technological concepts and evolution. Oral Surg Oral Med Oral Pathol Oral Radiol Endod 101:e37–e44

Dohan Ehrenfest DM, de Peppo GM (2009) Slow release of growth factors and thrombospondin-1 in Choukroun's platelet-rich fibrin (PRF): a gold standard to achieve for all surgical platelet concentrates technologies. Growth Factors 27:63–69

Filho CH, Kerkis I et al (2007) Allogenous bone grafts improved by bone marrow stem cells and platelet growth factors: clinical case reports. Artif Organs 31:2681 2

Fiorellini JP, Howell TH, Cochran D et al (2005) Randomized study evaluating recombinant human bone morphogenetic protein-2 for extraction socket augmentation. J Periodontol 76:605–613

Froum SJ, Wallace SS, Tarnow DP, Cho SC (2002) Effect of platelet-rich plasma on bone growth and osseointegration in human maxillary sinus grafts: three bilateral case reports. Int J Periodontics Restor Dent 22:45–53

Gonshor A, McAllister BS et al (2011) Histologic and histomorphometric evaluation of an allograft stem cell-based matrix sinus augmentation procedure. Int J Oral Maxillofac Implants 26:123 n a

He L, Lin Y, Hu X et al (2009) A comparative study of platelet-rich fibrin (PRF) and platelet-rich plasma (PRP) on the effect of proliferation and differentiation of rat osteoblasts in vitro. Oral Surg Oral Med Oral Pathol Oral Radiol Endod 108:707–713

Herford AS, Boyne PJ (2008) Reconstruction of mandibular continuity defects with bone morphogenetic protein-2 (rhBMP-2). J Oral Maxillofac Surg 66:616–624

Hinsbergh VW, Collen A, Koolwijk P (2001) Role of fibrin matrix in angiogenesis. Ann N Y Acad Sci 936: 426–437

Hood AG, Hill AG, Reeder GD (1993) Perioperative autologous sequestration. III: a new physiologic glue with wound healing properties. Proc Am Acad Cardiovasc Perfusion 14:126–130

Howell TH, Fiorellini J, Jones A et al (1997) A feasibility study evaluating rhBMP-2/absorbable collage sponge device for local alveolar ridge preservation or augmentation. Int J Periodontics Restor Dent 17:124–139

Iasella JM, Greenwell H, Miller R (2003) Ridge preservation with freeze-dried bone allograft and a collagen membrane compared to extraction alone for implant site development: a clinical and histologic study in humans. J Periodontol 74:990–999

Kaigler A (2015) Bone engineering of maxillary sinus bone deficiencies using enriched CD90+ stem cell therapy: a randomized clinical trial. J Bone Miner Res 30:1206–1216

Kang YH, Jeon SH, Park JY et al (2011) Platelet-rich fibrin is a bioscaffold and reservoir of growth factors for tissue regeneration. Tissue Eng Part A 17:349–359

Kassolis JD, Rosen PS, Reynolds MA (2000) Alveolar ridge and sinus augmentation utilizing platelet-rich plasma in combination with freeze-dried bone allograft: case series. J Periodontol 71:1654–1661

Koo S, Alshihri A et al (2012) Cellular allograft in the treatment of a severe periodontal intrabony defect: a case report. Clin Adv Periodontics 2:35–39

Lekovic V, Milinkovic I, Aleksic Z et al (2012) Platelet-rich fibrin and bovine porous bone mineral vs. platelet-rich fibrin in the treatment of intrabony periodontal defects. J Periodontal Res 47(4):409–417

Li Q, Pan S, Dangaria SJ (2013) Platelet-rich fibrin promotes periodontal regeneration and enhances alveolar bone augmentation. Biomed Res Int 2013:1–13

Lynch SE (1999) Introduction to tissue engineering. In: Lynch SE, Genco RJ, Marx RE (eds) Tissue engineering: applications in maxillofacial and periodontics. Quintessence, Chicago 1999, pp xi–xviii

McAllister B (2011) Stem cell-containing allograft matrix enhances periodontal regeneration: case presentations. Int J Periodontics Restor Dent 31:149–155

McAllister B, Eshraghi T (2013) Alveolar ridge augmentation with allograft stem cell stem cellograft stem cellence; 19. Clin Adv Periodontics 3:1–7

McGuire MK, Kao RT, Nevins M et al (2006) rhPDGF-BB promotes healing of periodontal defects: 24 month clinical and radiographic observations. Int J Periodontics Restor Dent 26:223–231

Milano F, van Baal JW, Buttar NS et al (2007) Bone morphogenetic protein 4 expressed in esophagitis induces a columnar phenotype in esophageal squamous cells. Gastroenterology 132:2412–2421

Misch C, Wang HL (2011) Clinical recombinant human bone morphogenetic protein-2 for bone augmentation before dental implant placement. Clin Adv Periodontics 1:118–131

Nevins ML, Reynolds MA (2011) Tissue engineering with recombinant human platelet-derived growth factor BB for implant site development. Compendium 32:18–28

Nevins M, Giannobile WV, McGuire MK et al (2005) rhPDGF-BB enhances periodontal healing. J Periodontol 76:2205–2215

Nevins ML, Camelo M, Schupbach P et al (2011) Human buccal plate extraction socket regeneration with recombinant platelet-derived growth factor BB or enamel matrix derivative. Int J Periodontics Restor Dent 31:481–492

Nevins M, McGuire MK, Kao RT et al (2013) PDGF promotes periodontal regeneration in localized osseous defects: 36 month extension results from a randomized, controlled, double-masked clinical trial. J Periodontol 84:456–464

Pilipchuk SP, Plonka AB, Monje A et al (2015) Tissue engineering for bone regeneration and osseointegration in the oral cavity. Dent Mater 31:317–338

Reddi AH, Reddi A (2009) Bone morphogenetic proteins (BMPs): from morphogens to metabologens. Cytokine Growth Factor Rev 20:341–342

Rickert D, Sauerbier S et al (2011) Maxillary sinus floor elevation with bovine bone mineral combined with either autogenous bone or autogenous stem cells: a prospective randomized clinical trial. Clin Oral Implants Res 22:251

Rosenberg ES, Torosian J (2000) Sinus grafting using platelet-rich plasma—Initial case presentation. Pract Periodontics Aesthet Dent 12:843–850

Roussy Y, Bertrand Duchesne MP, Gagnon G (2007) Activation of human platelet-rich plasmas: effect on growth factors release, cell division and in vivo bone formation. Clin Oral Implants Res 18:639–648

Sánchez AR, Sheridan PJ, Kupp LI (2003) Is platelet-rich plasma the perfect enhancement factor? A current review. Int J Oral Maxillofac Implants 18(1):93–103

Saygin NE, Tokiyasu Y, Giannobile WV et al (2000) Growth factors regulate expression of mineral associated genes in cementoblasts. J Periodontol 71:1591–1600

Schär MO, Diaz-Romero J, Kohl S et al (2015) Platelet-rich concentrates differentially release growth factors and induce cell migration in vitro. Clin Orthop Relat Res 473:1635–1643

Scheyer ET, McGuire MK (2011) Growth factor-mediated sinus augmentation grafting with recombinant human platelet-derived growth factor-BB (rhPDGF-591-1600-16001-1600n). Clin Adv Periodontics 1:4–15

Sclafani AP, Azzi J (2015) Platelet preparations for use in facial rejuvenation and wound healing: a critical review of current literature. Aesthet Plast Surg 39:495–505

Shanaman R, Filstein MR, Danesh-Meyer MJ (2001) Localized ridge augmentation using GBR and platelet-rich plasma: case reports. Int J Periodontics Restor Dent 21:345–355

Simion M, Rocchietta I, Dellavia C (2007) Three-dimensional ridge augmentation with xenograft and recombinant human platelet-derived growth factor-BB in humans: report of two cases. Int J Periodontics Restor Dent 27:109–115

Simion M, Rocchietta I, Monforte M et al (2008) Three-dimensional alveolar bone reconstruction with a combination of recombinant human platelet-derived growth factor BB and guided bone regeneration. Int J Periodontics Restor Dent 28:239–243

Simmonds MC, Brown JVE, Heirs MK et al (2013) Safety and effectiveness of recombinant human bone morphogenetic protein-2 for spinal fusion: a meta-analysis of individual-participant data. Ann Intern Med 158:877–889

Simon BI, Gupta P, Tajbakhsh S (2011) Quantitative evaluation of extraction socket healing following the use of autologous platelet-rich fibrin matrix in humans. Int J Periodontics Restor Dent 31:285–295

Simonpieri A, Choukroun J, Del Corso M et al (2011) Simultaneous sinus-lift and implantation using micro-threaded implants and leukocyte- and platelet-rich fibrin as sole grafting material: a six-year experience. Implant Dent 20:2–12

Sindler AJ, Behmanesh S, Reynolds MA (2013) Evaluation of allogenic cellular bone graft for ridge augmentation: a case report. Clin Adv Periodontics 3:159–165

Suttapreyasri S, Leepong N (2013) Influence of platelet-rich fibrin on alveolar ridge preservation. J Craniofac Surg 24:1088–1094

Tajima N, Ohba S, Sawase T et al (2013) Evaluation of sinus floor augmentation with simultaneous implant placement using platelet-rich fibrin as sole grafting material. Int J Oral Maxillofac Implants 28:77–83

Tsay RC, Vo J, Burke A et al (2005) Differential growth factor retention by platelet-rich plasma composites. J Oral Maxillofac Surg 63:521–528

van den Dolder J, Mooren R, Vloon AP et al (2006) Platelet-rich plasma: quantification of growth factor levels and the effect on growth and differentiation of rat bone marrow cells. Tissue Eng 12:3067–3073

Wu CL, Lee SS, Tsai CH (2012) Platelet-rich fibrin increases cell attachment, proliferation and collagen-related protein expression of human osteoblasts. Aust Dent J 57:207–212

Xu FT, Li HM, Yin QS et al (2015) Effect of activated autologous platelet-rich plasma on proliferation and osteogenic differentiation of human adipose-derived stem cells in vitro. Am J Transl Res 7:257–270

Zhang Y, Tangl S, Huber CD (2012) Effects of Choukroun's platelet-rich fibrin on bone regeneration in combination with deproteinized bovine bone mineral in maxillary sinus augmentation: a histological and histomorphometric study. J Craniomaxillofac Surg 40:321–328

Part III

Implant Placement and Restoration

Optimal Implant Position in the Aesthetic Zone

16

Jae Seon Kim, Lance Hutchens, Brock Pumphrey, Marko Tadros, Jimmy Londono, and J. Kobi Stern

Abstract

Planning for the optimal implant position in the aesthetic zone requires a thorough communication between the surgeon and the restorative dentist. The implant position is influenced by not only the anatomical morphology but also by the various prosthetic designs of the restoration. The mesial-distal, buccal-lingual, apical-coronal position, and angulation of the implants are all critical factors that will impact the emergence profile and material thickness of the prosthesis. This chapter will outline an interdisciplinary treatment approach to achieve the optimal implant position for the ultimate aesthetic and biologic outcome.

16.1 Introduction

The incorporation of implant dentistry has created a paradigm shift in the way that clinicians approach treatment planning in the aesthetic zone (Misje et al. 2013; Krennmair et al. 2011). There now exist multiple options available for clinicians to restore an edentulous site in the maxilla or mandible. Treatment options require an exponential amount of additional knowledge for the clinician. Implant therapy differs from the natural dentition in a biological, mechanical, and aesthetic perspective. Furthermore, implant prosthetics are comprised of various components, including the implant body, abutment, and the restoration. Often times each component may be fabricated utilizing different materials to achieve a particular aesthetic goal. As a result, there can be at times a complex interplay of components and materials. The biological response to these materials and interfaces may further complicate the environment, in which even the latest research cannot clearly identify. Perhaps this may explain the multiple treatment options that may be suggested for an individual case. Clinicians must be knowledgeable on these variations. Considerable thought should be spent preplanning the treatment from both a restorative and a surgical perspective. In this chapter, the authors will approach the subject of implant position in the aesthetic zone with the most current scientific evidence and an objective review of the evidence in order to provide the clinician with the most predictable and successful outcome.

16.2 Treatment Planning

16.2.1 Wax-Up/Mock-Up

Planning the restorative component of a case is critical in that the position of the definitive prosthesis must be established prior to planning a particular surgical approach (Garber 1995). Although a restoratively driven thought process to implant therapy is ideal, there will always be exceptions. In many instances, the classical restorative position may require a two-stage approach in addition to grafting hard and soft-tissue defects. A compromise should be reached between the restorative and surgical approach to elucidate the optimal aesthetic and functional outcome within the biological environment of the patient (Jivraj and Chee 2006). Prior to any surgical and restorative planning, an aesthetic analysis involving seven specific steps, described by Chiche (2008), should be conducted. The goal of these steps is to establish the proper tooth position and proportion, and this process requires a manual or digital diagnostic wax-up created from accurate impressions or digital scans (Fig. 16.1). Once the ideal shape, proportion, and position of the implant prosthesis are obtained, it can be transferred to the patient's mouth to evaluate how the aesthetics of the diagnostic wax-up integrates into the patient's oral and surrounding environment. This process can be called the "Aesthetic Mock-up," (Fig. 16.2) and can serve as a powerful tool to allow both the patient and the clinician to preview and assess the final outcome (Magne and Belser 2003). One should note that this kind of mock-up is limited to cases of adding tooth or soft-tissue volume and not for reductive cases. When a tooth structure is in the way of the future prosthesis, a digital mock-up can be accomplished using computer illustration software programs (Figs. 16.3 and 16.4). The clinician will be able to visualize and quantify if any soft-tissue/hard-tissue augmentation will be needed. This information can be relayed to the surgeon in order to discuss implant position, site augmentation, or any alterations to the proposed approach (Figs. 16.5 and 16.6).

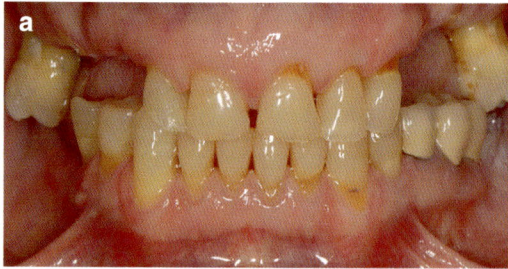

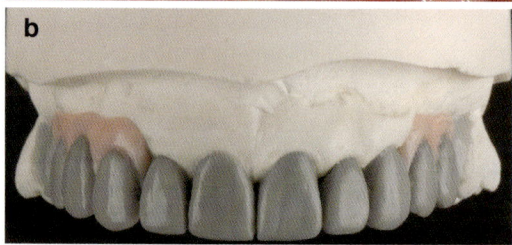

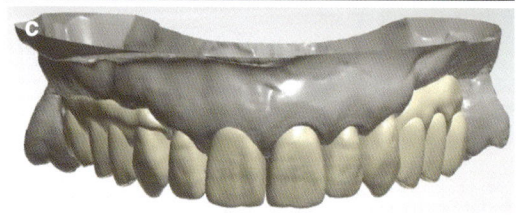

Fig. 16.1 (**a**) Pre-op frontal view in MIP. (**b**) Manual wax-up of anterior dentition. (**c**) Digital wax-up of anterior dentition

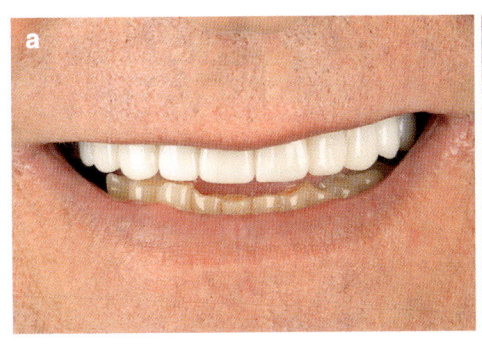

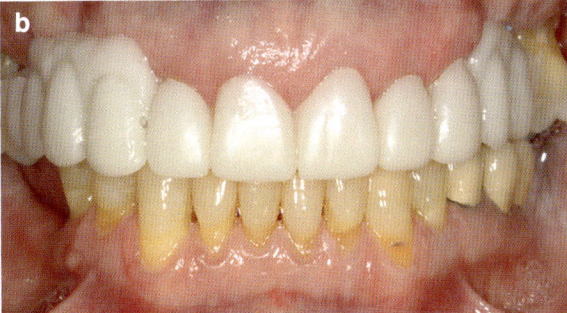

Fig. 16.2 (a) Extraoral evaluation of the aesthetic mock-up is essential to establish the maxillary incisal edge position. (b) Intraoral evaluation of the aesthetic mock-up is mandatory to evaluate the ideal proportion of the teeth and the surrounding soft tissue

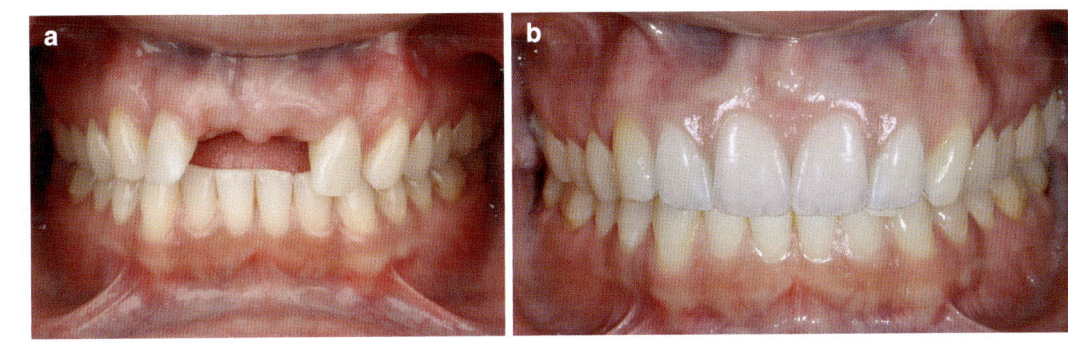

Fig. 16.3 (a) Intraoral view displaying proclination of #7, which will prevent from performing a manual aesthetic mock-up. (b) Digital mock-up of #7–10 using a computer illustration software

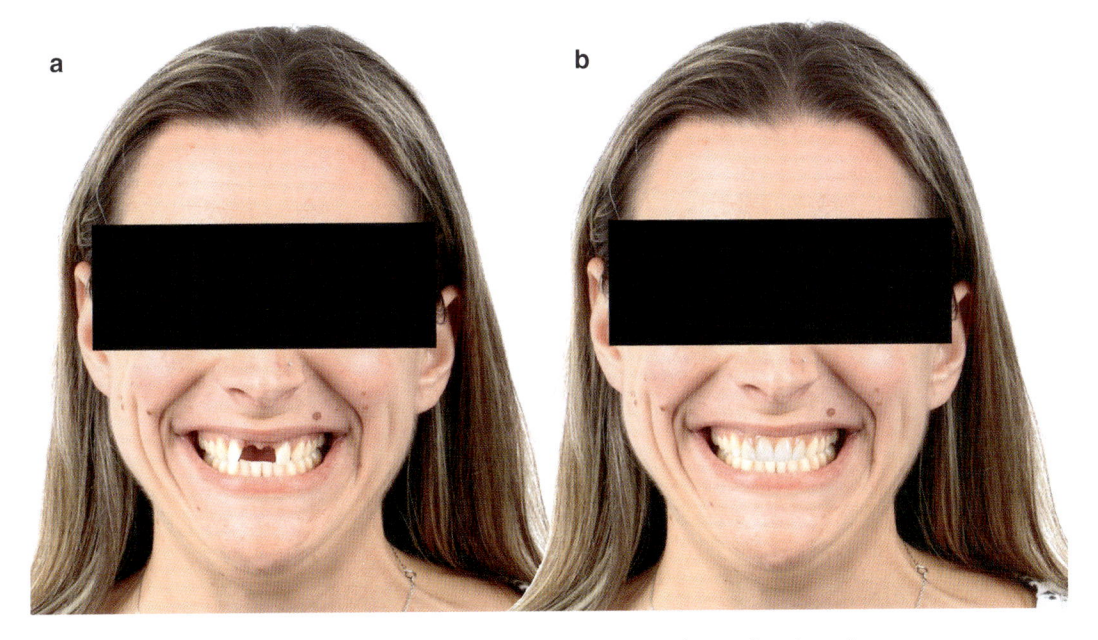

Fig. 16.4 (a) Pre-op smile view of the patient. (b) Digital mock-up superimposed on the patient

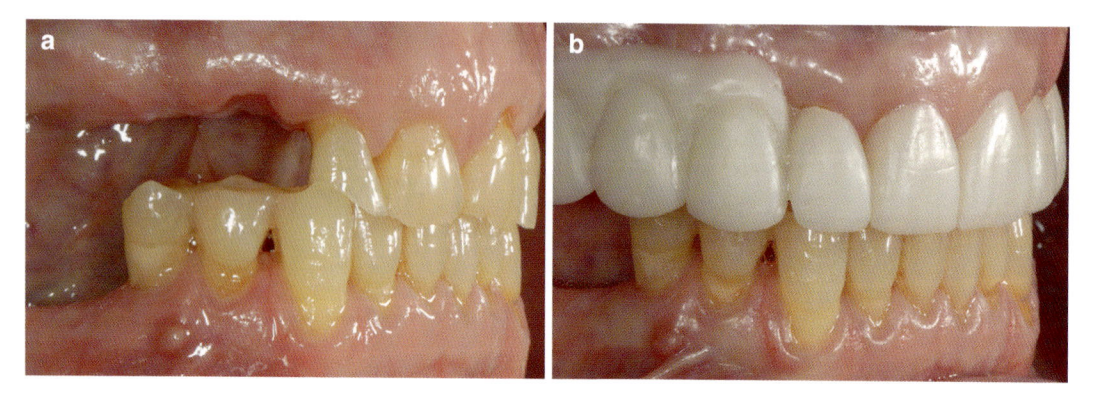

Fig. 16.5 (**a**) Pre-op right lateral view displaying deficient soft and hard tissue in implant sites #4–6. (**b**) Mock-up can show the amount of soft-/hard-tissue augmentation required to overcome the pink deficiency

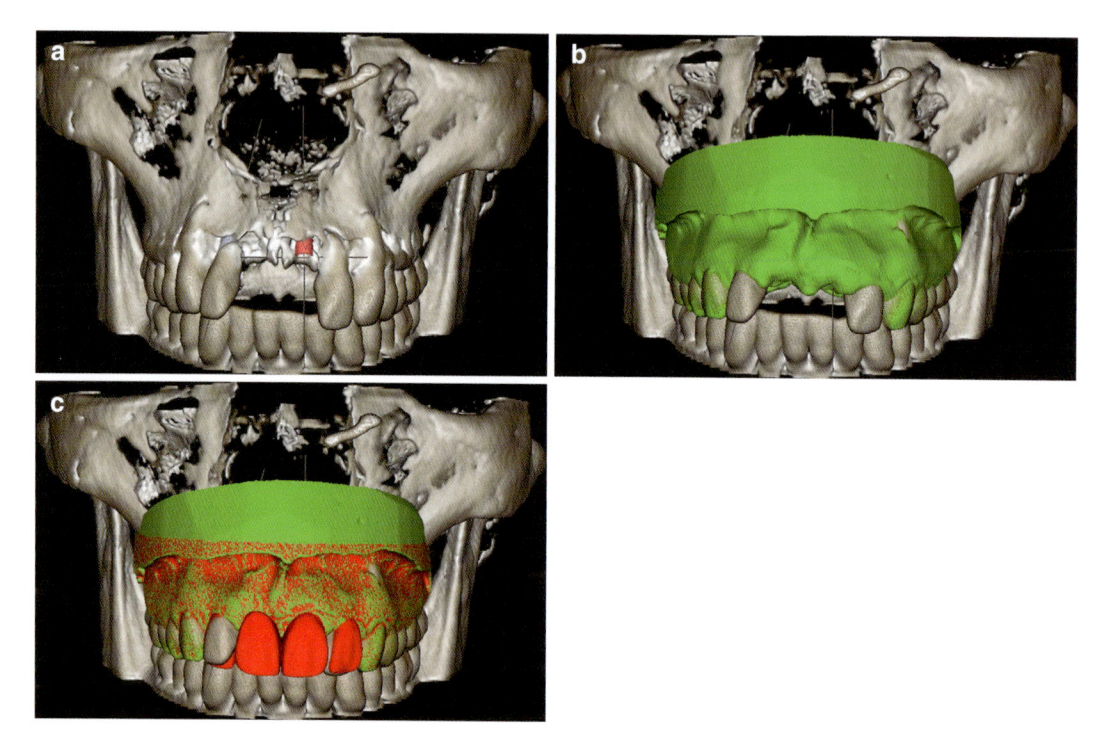

Fig. 16.6 The mock-up of the definitive restoration can be superimposed on the CBCT, and the implant position can be discussed with the surgeon. (**a**) CBCT image of the patient. (**b**) Superimposition of the diagnostic cast with the CBCT Image. (**c**) Virtual simulation on the superimposed images to visualize the final outcome

16.3 Implant Site Evaluation

Prior to surgical placement of implants, the future implant site and the adjacent anatomical structures have to be meticulously evaluated. Alterations in the alveolar ridge have been described as reductions in bone volume following tooth extraction that results in loss of up to 50% of the height and width (Schropp et al. 2003; Araujo and Lindhe 2005). Atraumatic extraction to preserve the remaining bone is essential to minimize future bone loss (Fig. 16.7). Cone beam computed tomography (CBCT) can provide clinicians with accurate three dimensions of the

16 Optimal Implant Position in the Aesthetic Zone

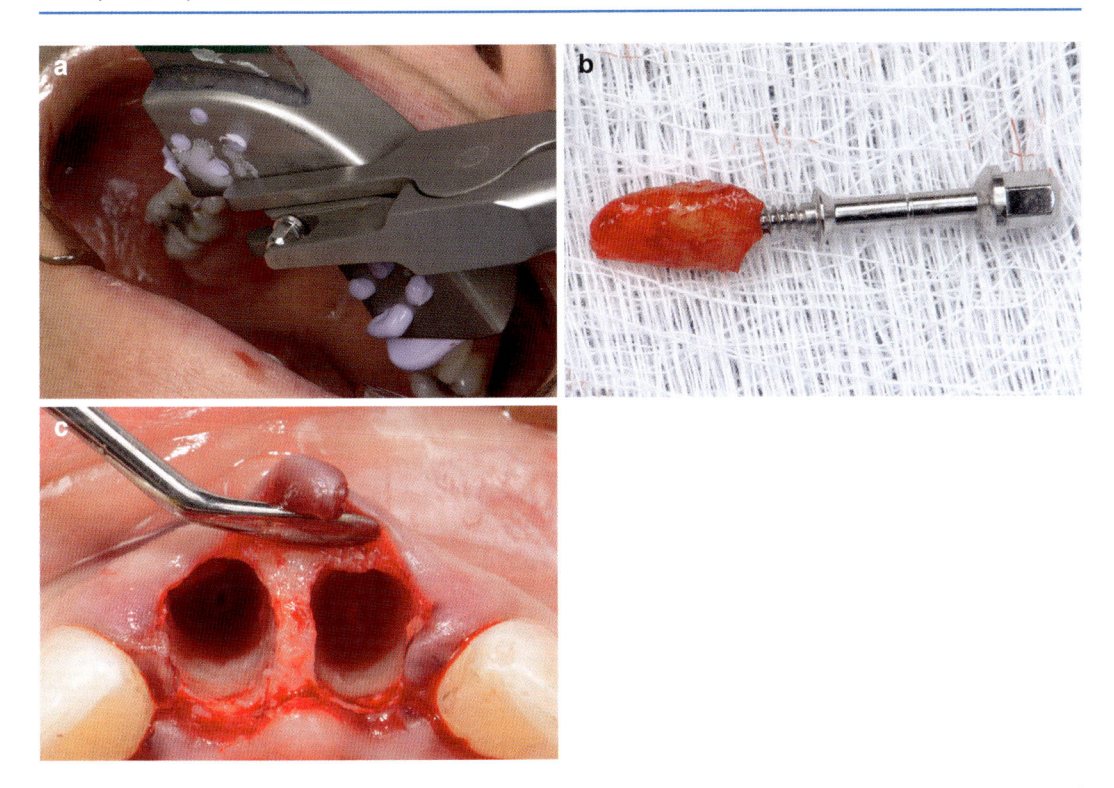

Fig. 16.7 (**a**) Atraumatic extraction being performed by vertically displacing the tooth from the socket. (**b**) Extracted tooth. (**c**) Facial and interproximal bone intact after extraction

existing hard tissue. It is imperative to utilize the CBCT with a radiographic guide whenever possible for the restorative dentist and the surgical team to plan the implant position (Fig. 16.8). The existing bone level has to be evaluated from a height and width perspective. Crestal bone height is regarded as one of the most important factors in the development of satisfactory aesthetic outcomes in implant dentistry (Papalexiou et al. 2006). The existing bone height will be related to the amount of soft-tissue thickness above the bone, which in turn will affect the clinical crown length of the implant restoration. The bone width will impact the emergence of the implant restoration. The lack of width will hinder the restorative dentist from creating a natural emergence of the implant restoration. Instead, there may be a concavity where the apical portion of the restoration meets the gingiva, creating an artificial appearance (Fig. 16.9). The surgeon and the restorative dentist should further discuss alternative treatment options when the hard- and soft-tissue aug-

mentation may not completely fill the bony defect. Utilizing pink restorative material, either of ceramic or composite, can cover the bony defect and create restorations with ideal width to length ratios. However, it is critical that the surgeon discuss with the restorative dentist, the requirement of additional space, which will be requisite for the pink restorative materials. This will necessitate the removal of additional bone to account for this additional spatial need. It is crucial to remove enough bone to hide the junction of the pink restoration and the soft tissue apical to the lip during smile and to allow a convex intaglio surface of the prosthesis to facilitate access for oral hygiene (Fig. 16.10).

The bone level adjacent to the future implant site needs to be evaluated through radiographic findings and bone sounding procedures. Multiple studies have indicated the significance of adjacent bone level on the interproximal soft-tissue aesthetics. The thickness of the buccal plate at the future implant site also needs to be evaluated

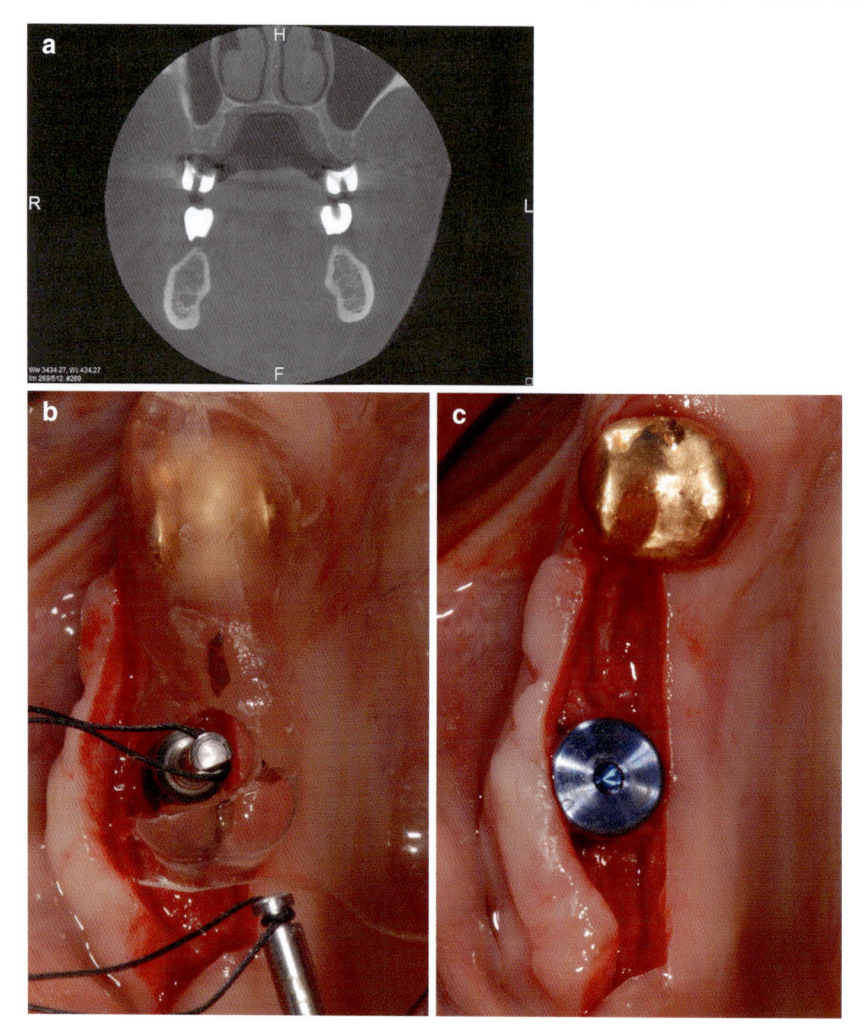

Fig. 16.8 CBCT with a radiographic guide is critical in determining the definitive implant position. (**a**) #3 implant position had to be modified due to a lack of palatal bone and difficulty in grafting the palatal site. (**b**) During the implant surgery, the implant was moved to the buccal to encase the implant within the bony socket. (**c**) Notice the slight buccal position of the implant compared to #5

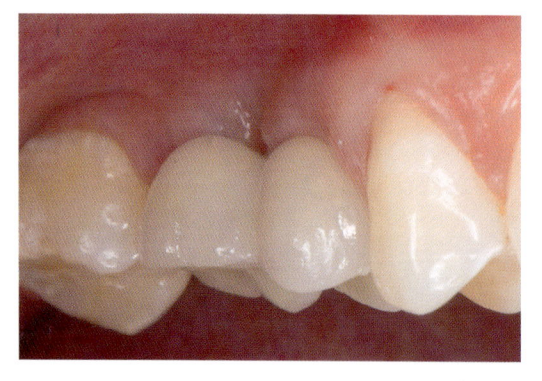

Fig. 16.9 Lack of native bone width may compromise the emergence profile of the restoration

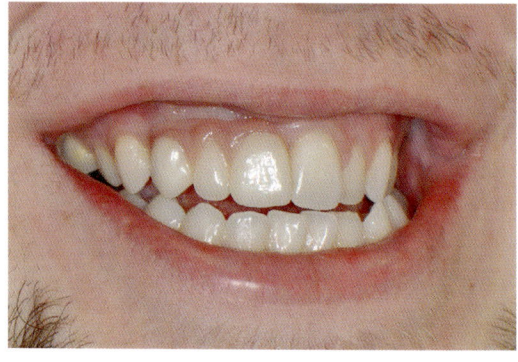

Fig. 16.10 Whenever the gingiva is to be reconstructed with a prosthesis, the restorative-gingival junction has to be apical to the dynamics of the lips to avoid aesthetic compromise

through a cone beam computed tomography (CBCT) scan. Since multiple studies have shown that the average thickness of the buccal plate at the alveolar crest in the maxillary incisor area is less than 1 mm (El Nahass and Naiem 2015; Januário et al. 2011; Braut et al. 2011; Wang et al. 2014), the clinician needs to keep in mind the possible backup plan when this thin plate of bone disappears during surgery or progressively throughout the subsequent postsurgical years (Roe et al. 2012; Kan et al. 2011).

Clinicians should also evaluate the phenotype of the gingival tissue in order to effectively conceal the implant-abutment interface. Multiple studies have shown the thickness of the tissue plays a critical role in masking the abutment substructure (Thoma et al. 2014a, b; Jung et al. 2007). A recent study has also shown that in addition to the tissue thickness, the translucency of the gingiva, which can be affected by the degree of keratinization and the distribution and number of blood vessels, can contribute to the gingival color change by the restorative components (Kim et al. 2015) (Fig. 16.11). The need for soft-tissue grafting can be determined at this diagnostic stage after close observation of the tissue phenotype.

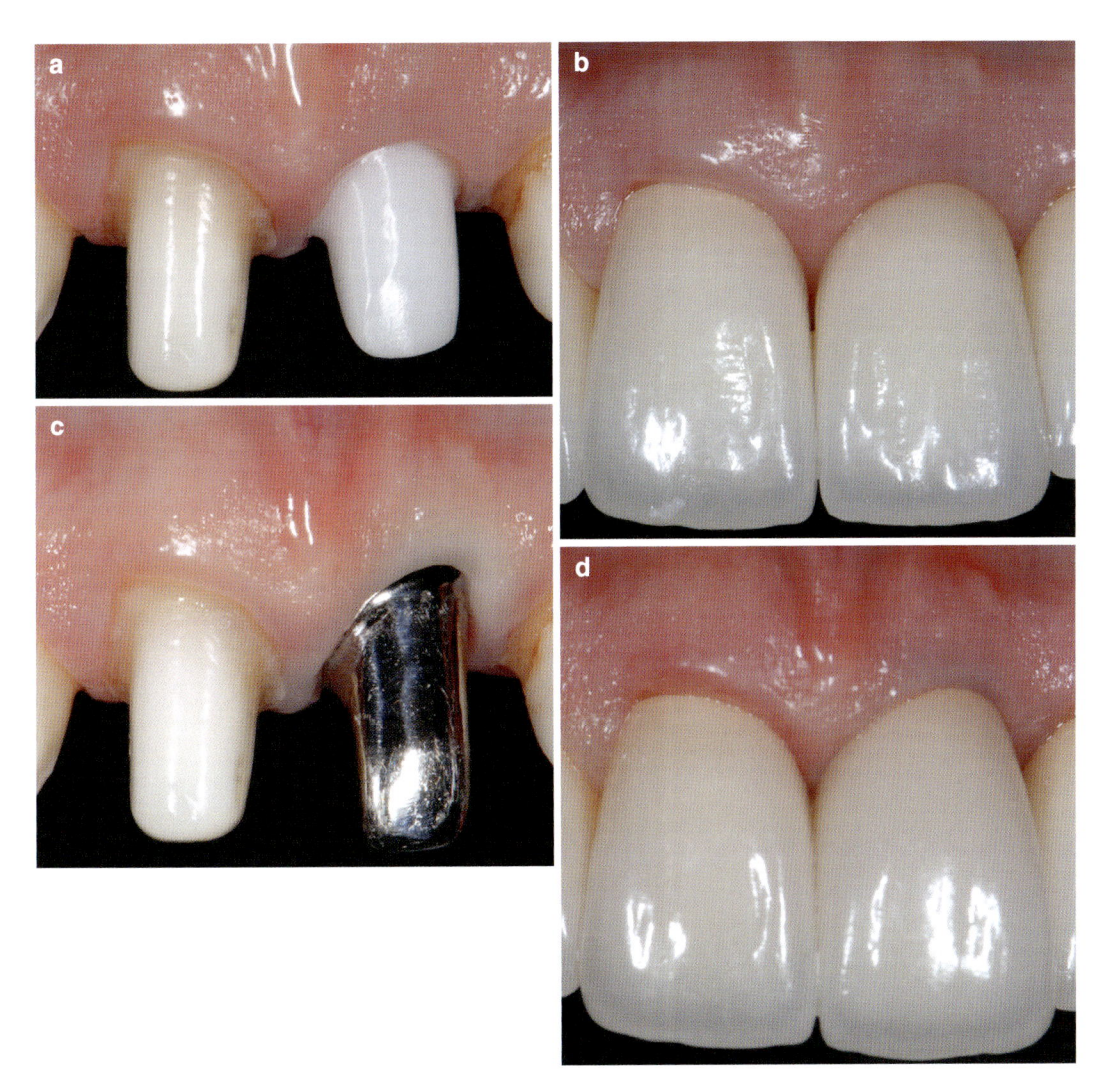

Fig. 16.11 (**a**) Try-in of zirconia abutment on implant #9. (**b**) The color of definitive ceramic restoration with the zirconia abutment blends in well at the abutment/restoration junction. (**c**) Try-in of titanium abutment on implant #9. (**d**) *Gray color* showing at the abutment/restorative junction due to the patient's thin phenotype

16.4 Planning for Optimal Implant Position

Implant position must be discussed between the surgeon and the restorative dentist at length due to its impact on the emergence profile of the implant restoration (Phillips and Kois 1998; Schoenbaum 2015). This in turn will have a direct effect on the overall soft-tissue aesthetic result. The implant position will ultimately play a major role in setting up the stage for the restorative dentist. Guidelines for implant placement were summarized stating that the implant-abutment interface at the alveolar bone crest should be 3 mm apical and 2 mm palatal to the gingival zenith (Cooper and Pin-Harry 2013). These guidelines take into consideration our understanding of the biologic width along the abutment and stability of thicker periosteal tissue and mucosa buccal to a newly placed implant. This section of the chapter will outline the most critical factors to consider when placing implants for screw-retained and cement-retained restorations in the aesthetic zone. The implant position will be discussed in the mesial-distal, buccal-lingual, apical-coronal position, as well as in angulation.

16.4.1 Mesial-Distal

The mesial-distal position of the implant and its impact on the interdental papilla will depend on the adjacent structure of the implant. Inter-implant distance and inter-tooth distance are important when discussing correct positioning of dental implants. Tarnow et al. (1992) showed us that there is greater inter-implant crestal bone loss if the two implants are placed less than 3.0 mm apart. He indicated that the selective utilization of implants with a smaller diameter at the implant-abutment interface may be beneficial when multiple implants are to be placed in the aesthetic zone so that a minimum of 3 mm of bone can be retained between them at the implant-abutment level. Previous investigations have suggested to

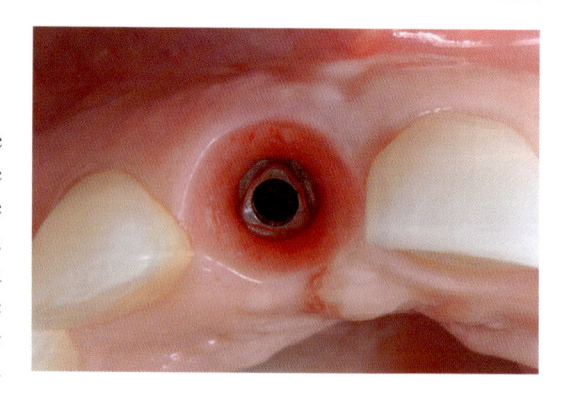

Fig. 16.12 1.5 mm of buffer space is needed around implants in order to prevent interproximal bone loss, which may lead to loss of papilla

leave 1.5 mm between the tooth and an implant to maintain the bone adjacent to the teeth and obtain a good aesthetic outcome (Esposito et al. 1993; Berglundh and Lindhe 1996) (Fig. 16.12). If an implant is placed too close to the adjacent tooth, bone loss, papilla loss, and even root resorption may occur. Animal studies have seen root surface resorption after the placement of mini-implants less than 1 mm from the root surface (Kim and Kim 2011) and that the incidence of root resorption increased when the mini-implants were less than 0.6 mm from the root (Lee et al. 2010). Platform-switched implants have been shown to be successful when placed only 1 mm from the tooth when the surgical guide required it (Vela et al. 2012). Using platform-switching platforms in a limited space between adjacent implants and teeth will allow for a more conservative treatment and may result in a healthier and aesthetically pleasing outcome.

16.4.2 Buccal-Lingual

The buccal-lingual implant position is intricate in that many studies have shown that this position often determines the long-term soft-tissue aesthetics around the implant restoration (Roe et al. 2012; Kan et al. 2011; Chappuis et al. 2013). Recent literature has suggested a lingualized approach to placing immediate implants. Lee et al. (2014) used this approach using the lingual wall of the socket, leaving a gap between surface of the labial socket and the implant surface. In this study he also used a platform switching design to a level 1 mm apical to the buccal alveolar crest and with a lingual orientation, followed by an immediate provisional. At 6 months the alternations in the buccal alveolar plate width were negligible. This lingual approach is essential for both screw- and cement-retained restorations, but screw-retained restorations may require more lingual positioning of the implant so the screw access exits through the palatal aspect. Lingualized position results in a gap between the alveolar wall and the labial implant surface and may also avoid surgical trauma and impingement of the internal aspect of the buccal plate, limiting resorption. In order to ascertain that the implant is not placed too facially, a surgical guide with the palatal surface removed should be utilized during osteotomies and after implant insertion (Fig. 16.13). The buccal-lingual position of the implant will dictate the abutment wall thickness (Fig. 16.14). Therefore, care should be taken to obtain a minimum wall thickness of 0.3 mm for titanium and 0.7 mm for zirconia abutments to prevent abutment fractures (Aboushelib and Salameh 2009; Att et al. 2012).

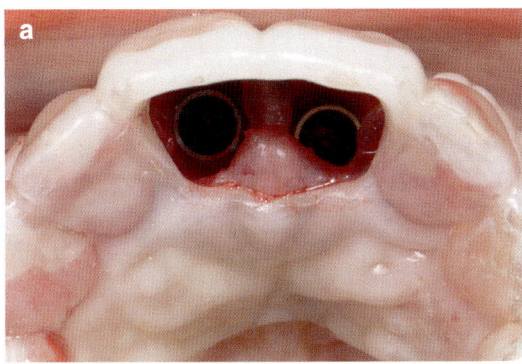

Fig. 16.13 A surgical guide without the palatal surface should be utilized during implant surgery in order to prevent buccal displacement of the implant. (**a**) The implant position on #8, 9 sites are confirmed after placement with a surgical guide. (**b**) The implant position should also be verified with a surgical guide during surgery

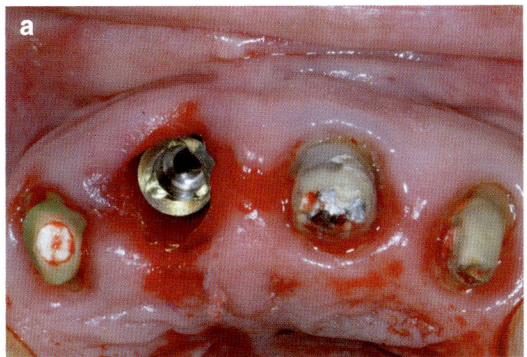

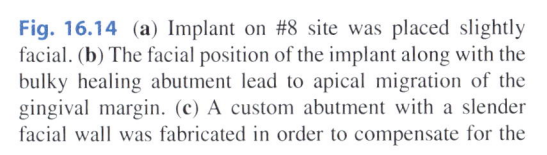

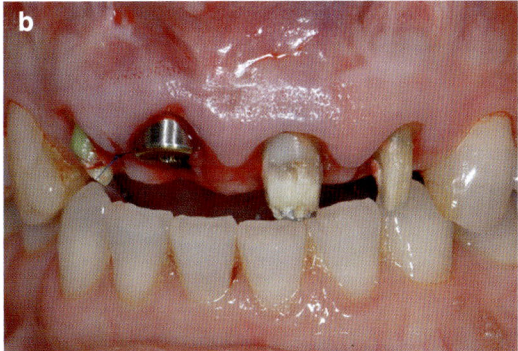

Fig. 16.14 (**a**) Implant on #8 site was placed slightly facial. (**b**) The facial position of the implant along with the bulky healing abutment lead to apical migration of the gingival margin. (**c**) A custom abutment with a slender facial wall was fabricated in order to compensate for the facial implant position. (**d**) Custom abutment in place. Note the symmetrical gingival level between #8 and 9. (**e**) All ceramic definitive restoration bonded to the ceramic abutment for maximum fracture resistance

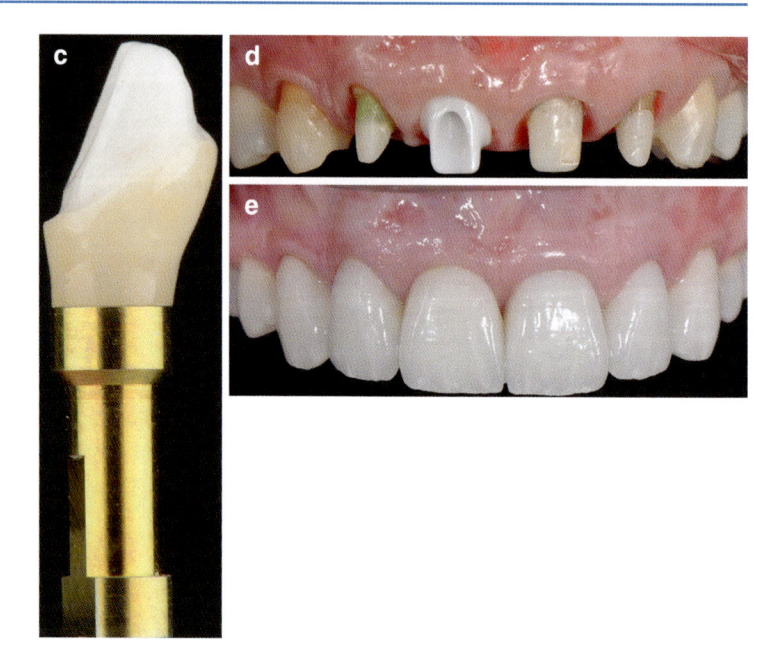

16.4.3 Apical-Coronal

The depth of the implant is critical since the restoration must have sufficient room to create an ideal transition from the implant platform to the prospective gingival margin. Su (Su et al. 2010) has described this area as critical and subcritical contours of the restoration. These contours can be altered to change the gingival levels on the buccal and interproximal surfaces. In order to perform any alteration, an adequate amount of room is required. Many authors have advocated that 3.0–4.0 mm of space is required from the implant platform to the prospective gingival level (Fig. 16.15). This implant depth can be achieved with the help of a surgical guide or an implant depth guide during surgery (Fig. 16.16).

Placing an implant in situations where there is too little, or excess bone surrounding the implant, creates its own subset of problems. When there is too much bone loss and the distance from the crestal bone to the prospective gingival level is more than 4.0 mm, surgeons may be faced with a dilemma. A decision of whether to place the implant supracrestally and graft hard tissue vertically or place the bone at the crest and graft soft tissue vertically must be made. Guided bone regeneration in the vertical direction has shown to be rather unpredictable (Rocchietta et al. 2008; Aghaloo and Moy 2007), and this may result in implant thread exposure and

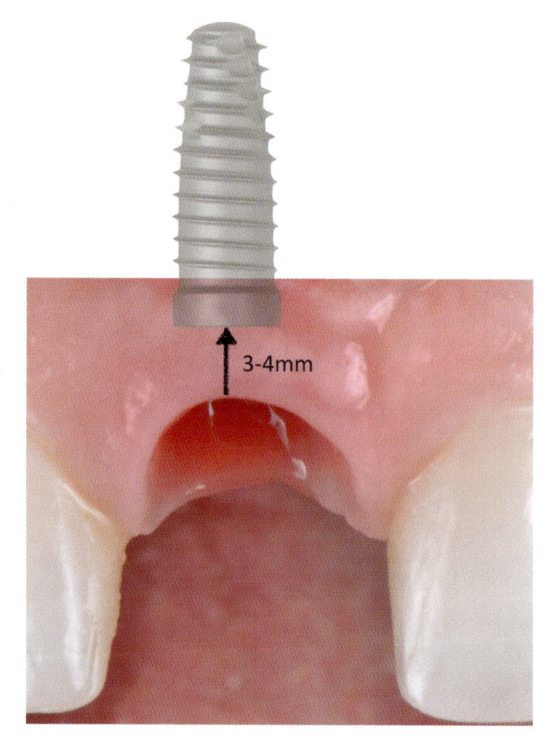

Fig. 16.15 3.0–4.0 mm of space is required from the implant platform to the prospective gingival level to mimic a natural dentition

soft-tissue recession, which may cause tragic aesthetic results. Salama and others (1998) have shown that soft-tissue grafting yields more volume gain and may lead to more predictable soft-tissue aesthetics. In certain situations, hard- and soft-tissue

16 Optimal Implant Position in the Aesthetic Zone

graft must be performed in concert with implant therapy to both maximize the augmentation and satisfy the aesthetic results. This is done in order to reduce the distance between the implant platform and the prospective gingival level. When there is too much bone, such as congenitally missing teeth with retained deciduous teeth or bone created after orthodontic movement, the surgeon may be hesitant to remove the bone (Fig. 16.17). However, when the minimum distance of 3.0 mm is not achieved from the implant platform to the gingival level, it may be impossible to create a smooth transition at the subgingival level and compromise the clinical crown length. When faced with this scenario, the surgeon must verify with the surgical guide the proposed bone level prior to implant placement and remove the bone as needed to ensure 3.0–4.0 mm of space.

The placement depth becomes an important consideration when screw-retained restorations are restoratively planned. Increasing the depth of placement is often required compared to cement-retained restorations due to the fact that the implant must be placed more palatally to compensate for the screw access and exit. The horizontal distance from the implant platform to the facial surface of the restoration becomes greater, therefore, requires more vertical distance to compensate. If the prosthetic component is not placed at the proper depth, the emergence angle will become very abrupt, which may cause apical movement of the soft tissue. This creates an area conducive to plaque formation and inability to maintain hygiene (Fig. 16.18). For these reasons,

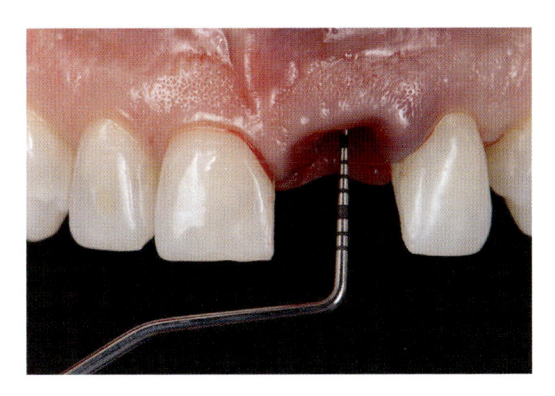

Fig. 16.16 Implant depth should always be verified immediately after implant placement. A periodontal probe is used to measure the distance between the implant platform and the prospective gingival margin

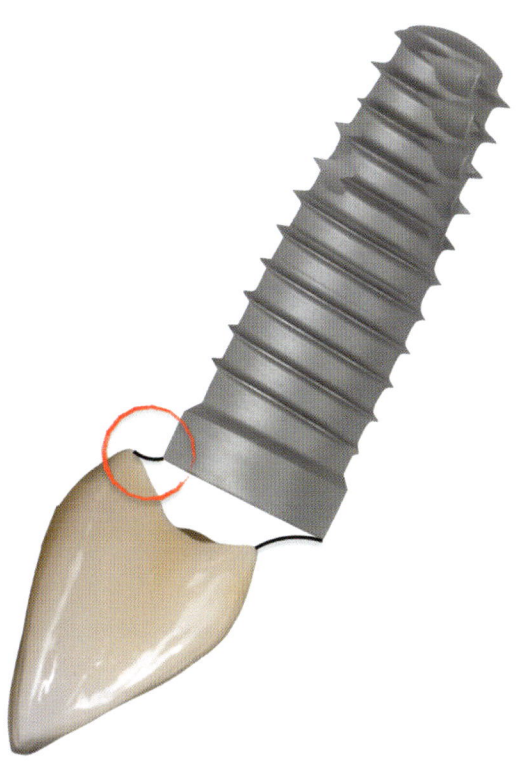

Fig. 16.18 Implants that are placed too shallow will force the facial surface of the restoration to be conducive to gingival recession and plaque accumulation

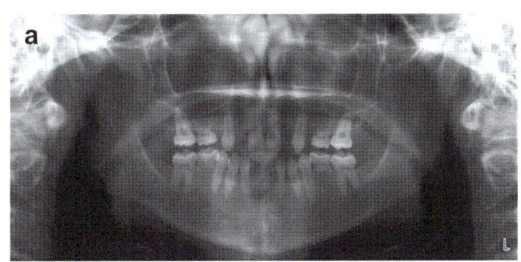

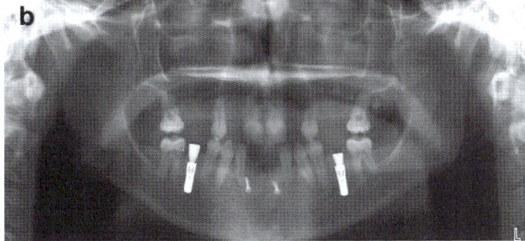

Fig. 16.17 (**a**) Excessive bone present around #K, T. (**b**) Excessive bone was removed prior to implant placement in order to accommodate prosthetic space

a screw-retained restorations should only be considered when the bone level on the adjacent tooth or implant is sufficient. Studies have shown that when implants are placed deeper, more crestal bone loss is present. Proper consideration should be given to this area in the planning phase both surgically and restoratively. Cement-retained restorations, on the other hand, may not require as much distance since the implant may not necessarily have the same palatal placement restrictions. Here, the implant abutment can be customized to simulate a natural dentition with a smooth transition from the implant platform to the gingival margin. It also requires less distance in the vertical and horizontal dimension compared to screw-retained restorations. This can play an important role to protect the bone around the implant and work to preserve the interdental papillae.

16.4.4 Implant Angulation

Improper angulation of implants can lead to root resorption of adjacent teeth, loss of labial plate, apical migration of the gingiva (Fig. 16.19), and prevent the restoration of the implant (Figs. 16.20 and 16.21). The position and morphology of the teeth are a result of the aesthetic and functional determinants. While it is the planned implant prosthesis that dictates the orientation and angulation of implant placement, the anatomy of the jaws and the morphology of the residual ridges can be limitations in any patient. It becomes increasingly more important in the patient for whom tissue augmentation and/or orthodontics/orthognathics is not an option.

It is quite likely that a situation may arise where there is a discrepancy between the

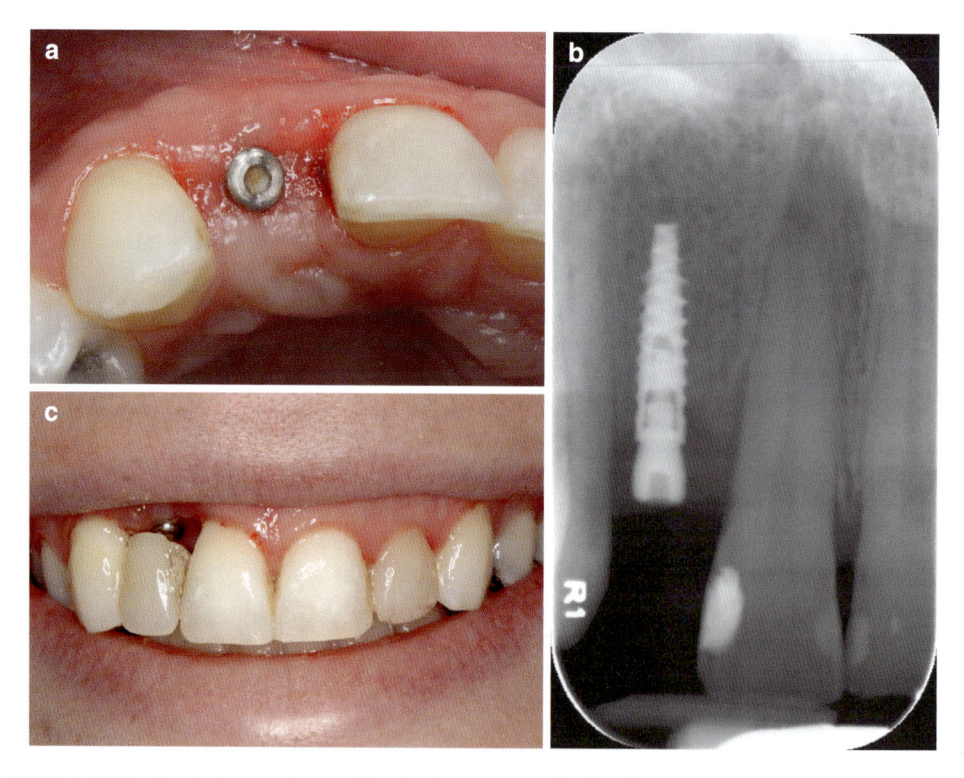

Fig. 16.19 (a) Note the facial angulation of the implant dictating a more apical gingival margin on the future restoration and a compromised facial abutment wall thickness. (b) PA X-ray. Notice the resorbed interproximal height of bone on adjacent teeth. (c) Full-smile view. Notice the *black triangle* and lack of tissue

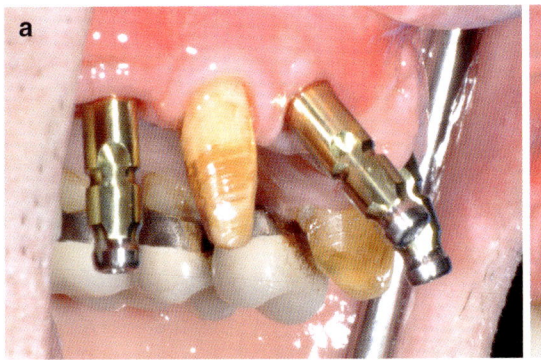

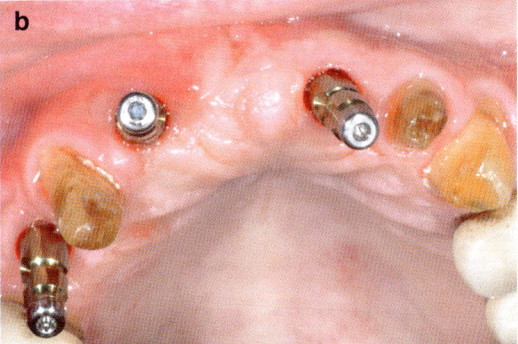

16 Optimal Implant Position in the Aesthetic Zone

Fig. 16.20 (**a**) Implants that are placed too facial can lead to apical migration of the gingiva, and in extreme cases, implants may not be utilized for the definitive restoration. (**b**) Occlusal view showing extreme facial angulation of implant at #7 site

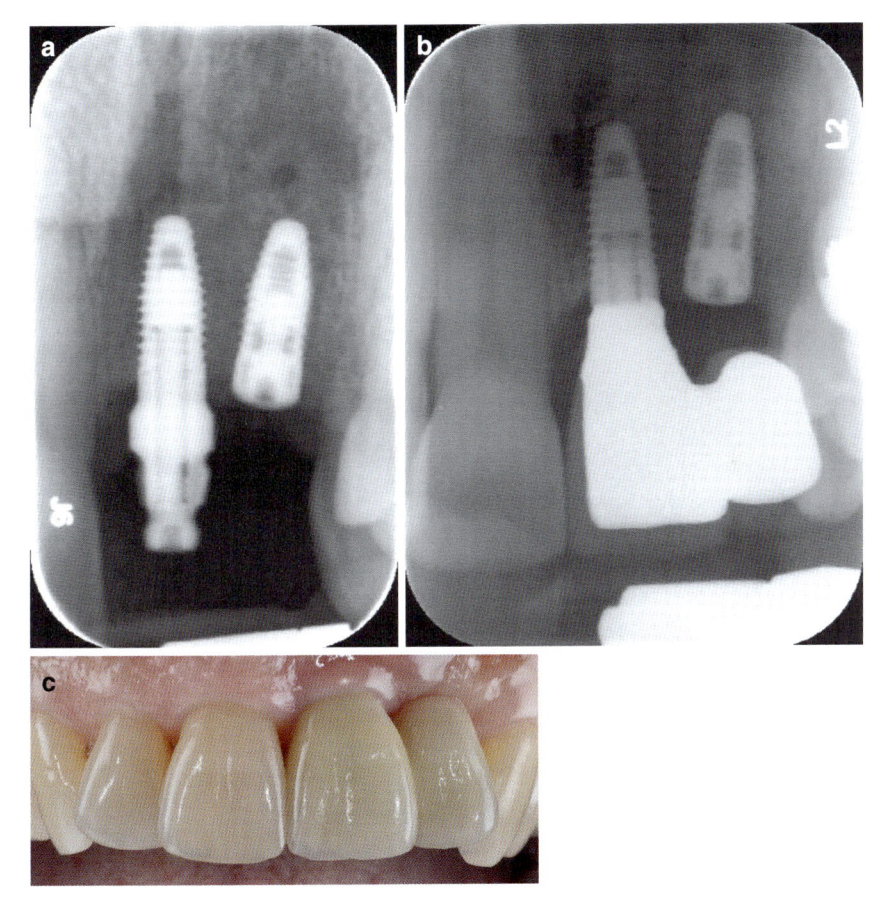

Fig. 16.21 (**a**) Two implants placed in the aesthetic zone. Inclination of implant site #10 did not allow an ideal or correct path of insertion. (**b**) Implant site #10 was not utilized as part of the definitive restoration. (**c**) Intraoral view of the definitive restoration

planned long axis of the implant fixture and the long axis of the implant prosthetics. With planning of dental implant therapy, the clinician must decide between a screw- and cement-retained restoration. For screw-retained restorations, the implant must be angulated to have the screw access exit through the palatal aspect of the restoration. However, care should be taken to examine for any concavities on the facial surfaces. When the implant body is placed in the socket to have the screw access hole exit through the palatal aspect, the apical portion of the implant will be angulated toward the facial (Figs. 16.22 and 16.23). If there is a significant concavity in the patient, the apical portion of the implant can emerge outside of the bony envelope, creating a potential danger for communication of the implant with the intraoral environment and discoloration in the soft tissue. Lately, some implant companies have introduced new prosthetic screws which can compensate the screw channel axis up to 25°. Angulated screw channels have made it possible to alter the access hole angulation so screw-retained restorations can be readily made. Cement-retained restorations can also benefit by having thicker abutment walls for improved strength by changing the screw channel within the abutment. However, more research needs to be conducted on whether torquing the screws at an angle can completely relay all the torque to the implant screws and long-term follow-ups are essential to test the clinical performance of these types of angulated screws. For cement-retained restorations, the implant access hole should still exit along the long axis of the definitive restoration in order to obtain a consistent abutment wall thickness. Even though custom abutments can compensate for the implant angulation, if the angle becomes too excessive, the abutment wall thickness will become too thin and may become the weak link in the implant restoration. The restorative dentist should remember that when the abutment wall becomes thin, a metal abutment, such as titanium or gold, should be utilized, instead of ceramic abutments to prevent abutment fracture (Aboushelib and Salameh 2009; Att et al. 2012) (Fig. 16.24).

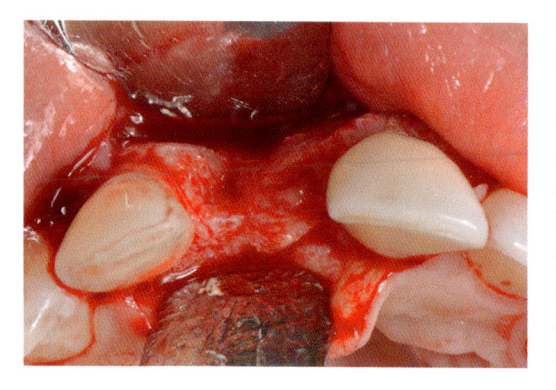

Fig. 16.22 Care should be taken to examine any concavities when planning for screw-retained restorations to prevent the apical portion of the implant from exiting the facial bone

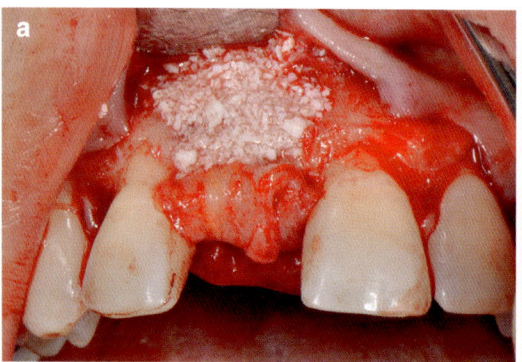

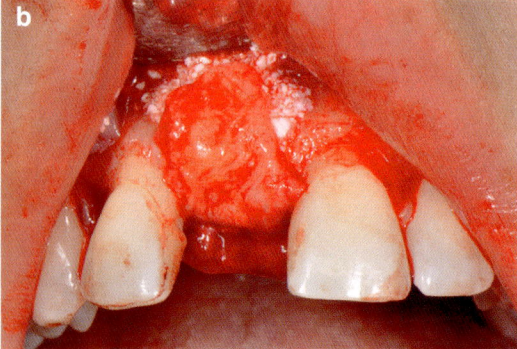

Fig. 16.23 (**a**) Bone graft being placed at #8 site. (**b**) Connective tissue graft being placed over the bone graft to obtain an improved aesthetic profile

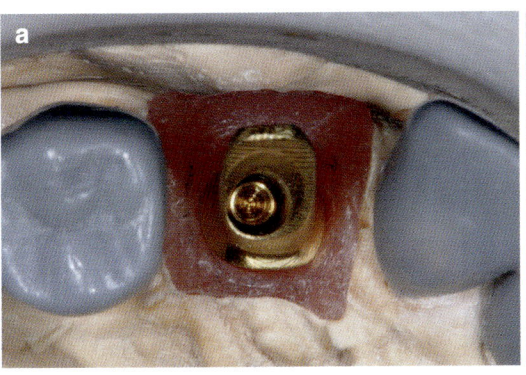

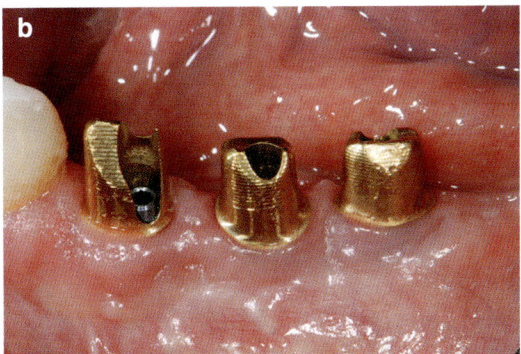

Fig. 16.24 (**a**) A metal abutment was utilized to overcome the thin wall thickness on the distal-lingual of #6. (**b**) Extremely thin axial wall on the distal of #21 due to a distally positioned implant

16.5 Incision and Flap Design in the Aesthetic Zone

In any surgical procedure, incisions are technique sensitive and dependent upon anatomical location and design. The use of a new scalpel blade and sharp dissection is imperative for the survival and healing of the mucosa (Cranin 2002; Mohammed et al. 2012). Flaps can be designed according to which tissues are included (full vs. partial thickness), the number of incisions used to create them (semilunar vs. triangular vs. trapezoidal), or by secondary incisions which dictate the surgical flaps orientation (rotating vs. coronally/apically advancing). In each of these, a portion of the blood supply remains intact to the tissue.

Incision design should begin with consideration of the blood supply to the edentulous midcrestal area, inclusion/avoidance of any adjacent papillae, and if necessary the termination of any releasing incisions (Kleinheinz et al. 2005; Mörmann and Ciancio 1977). Vascularization has been shown to be paramount for any type of healing or regeneration (Mohammed et al. 2012; Kleinheinz et al. 2005; Mörmann and Ciancio 1977; McLean et al. 1995). Blood supply will be most predictable in a posterior to anterior direction, and vessels will typically run parallel to the alveolar ridge, but it cannot be assumed that this is done at regular intervals (Kleinheinz et al. 2005; Mörmann and Ciancio 1977). It has been shown that a wider base is necessary to maintain perfusion to the intact tissues within the surgical flap (Mohammed et al. 2012; McLean et al. 1995), and in the animal model, an interruption in perfusion was shown to last for at least the first 7 days (Mörmann and Ciancio 1977; McLean et al. 1995). Vertical releasing incisions should be located outside the aesthetic zone, avoiding the buccal root prominence, and made short whenever possible (Kleinheinz et al. 2005; Mörmann and Ciancio 1977). It is noteworthy that in the midcrestal region of an edentulous alveolar ridge, there is a 1.0–2.0 mm wide avascular zone with no anastomoses or crossing of the alveolar ridge, making an incision here both safe and predictable (Kleinheinz et al. 2005; Mörmann and Ciancio 1977).

It has been shown that patients with a thin biotype will often show tissue recession around implant sites (Becker and Goldstein 2008). There is a clear relationship between crestal bone height and the stability of soft-tissue determinants of aesthetic success (Papalexiou et al. 2006; Cooper and Pin-Harry 2013). Here, for predictable soft-tissue aesthetics, a crestal bone height of 5.0 mm or less is necessary (Mörmann and Ciancio 1977). When the periosteum is disrupted with the elevation of a full-thickness flap, there will be a 0.5 mm of associated bone loss (Greenstein and Tarnow 2014). There is an abundance of contradictory data as to which technique increases or reduces expected bone loss (Greenstein and Tarnow 2014). However, when a comparison was done between flap elevation with papillae sparing (0–1.0 mm) and flap elevation with papillae elevation (0–3.5 mm), the amount of interproximal bone loss was far less on a papillae-sparing flap/incision (Greenstein and Tarnow 2014). The papillae preservation technique or a flapless surgical technique is associated with a more predictable outcome with respect to the interproximal bone loss (Greenstein and Tarnow 2014).

The decision and length of the vertical releasing incision(s) is always dictated by the need to access, visualize, and accomplish any procedure (Cranin 2002; Greenstein and Tarnow 2014). Previous studies suggested the length to width ratio was shown to be of little consequence, but the revascularization for longer incisions was determined to be poor (Mörmann and Ciancio 1977; Milton 1970). When a vertical release is indicated, it should go all the way to crestal bone and made obliquely to ensure the flap retains a broad base (Cranin 2002; Greenstein and Tarnow 2014). If a site requires hard-tissue augmentation, then the vertical release should be extended into the vestibule with scoring of the periosteum and potentially incising of the submucosa in order to provide release and tension-free coverage of the bone graft material (Greenstein and Tarnow 2014). If soft-tissue grafting is required, then any vertical releasing incisions should extend to the vestibule to be able to either apically position the flap or coronally position it to cover any connective tissue grafting material (Greenstein and Tarnow 2014).

Incomplete coverage of graft material or wound dehiscence is the most common problem associated with grafting procedures (Takei et al. 1984). Providing primary closure in such a way so that the incision is not directly over a defect is important for healing and survivability of any grafted material (Mohammed et al. 2012). Once the extent of the defect is determined clinically via bone sounding and probing, an incision should be designed to be at least 3 mm apical to the margin of the interproximal bony defect to ensure closure that is well separated from the grafted area (Mohammed et al. 2012; Takei et al. 1984). This problem can be exacerbated in the interproximal areas due to surgical technique even if there is apparent tissue approximation at the time of surgical closure (Takei et al. 1984). Beveling the incision allows the connective tissue to be retained on the bone and becomes more important if the mucosal flap cannot be repositioned, and there is a potential for the underlying bone to be exposed (Greenstein and Tarnow 2014).

The surgeon should use extreme caution with very thin and friable tissue, as suturing may be problematic even with slight elevation of the adjacent tissue. Here even with tissues that seem well adapted, there is an increased potential for necrosis along the margins (Greenstein and Tarnow 2014). Healing occurs in predictable stages, but the oral mucosa is less prone to scar formation potentially due to reduced numbers of macrophages in the tissue and the presence of growth factors in saliva (Szpaderska et al. 2003; Gurtner et al. 2008). The buccal mucosa is more prone to scar formation when incised, but the same is not true of attached keratinized gingiva (Larjava et al. 2011). Flap tension and margin adaptation are increasingly important as tissue shrinkage and wound dehiscence increase the likelihood of scar formation (Mohammed et al. 2012; Sclar 2007).

16.6 Types of Incisions and Techniques

If there is an abundance of bone, adequate keratinized tissue, and acceptable osseous contour, a flapless incision can be utilized, but there is inherent risk associated with not being able to visualize the underlying osseous architecture (Kleinheinz et al. 2005). There is no disruption of any of the gingival tissues, and various tissue sculpting techniques can still be implemented post-implant placement. A tissue punch is directed through the mucosa and the gingival tissue removed only in the area where the oste-

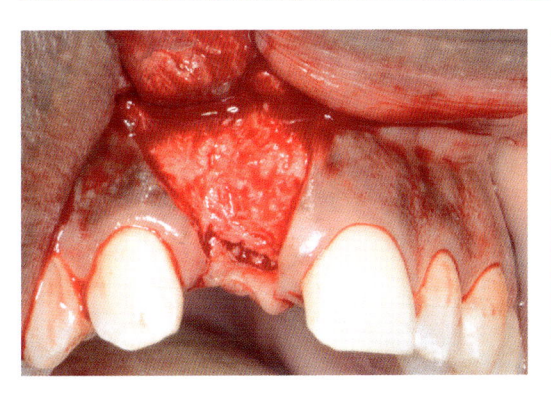

16 Optimal Implant Position in the Aesthetic Zone

Fig. 16.25 Papilla-sparing incision. Reflection of the labial and palatal flap allows for visualization of any defects. Note the width of the interproximal papillae

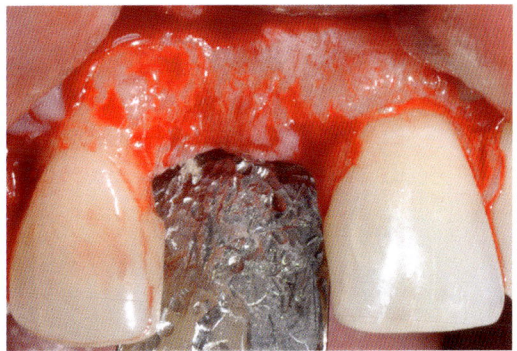

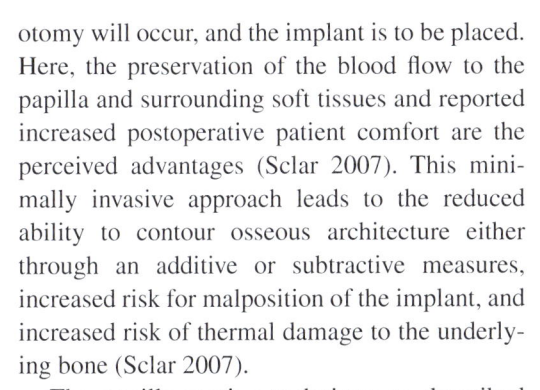

Fig. 16.26 Full-thickness flap is raised when access to underlying bone is indicated either for crown lengthening on adjacent teeth or for augmenting a narrow alveolar ridge. In this case both needs were indicated

otomy will occur, and the implant is to be placed. Here, the preservation of the blood flow to the papilla and surrounding soft tissues and reported increased postoperative patient comfort are the perceived advantages (Sclar 2007). This minimally invasive approach leads to the reduced ability to contour osseous architecture either through an additive or subtractive measures, increased risk for malposition of the implant, and increased risk of thermal damage to the underlying bone (Sclar 2007).

The papilla-sparing technique as described by Greenstein and Tarnow (2014) avoids papillae elevation, which may help to prevent its loss and is highly desirable in the aesthetic zone (Fig. 16.25). This incision begins with a horizontal incision along the midcrestal or palatal ridge and terminates 1.0 mm from the adjacent teeth. Next, bilateral buccal vertical releasing incisions that extend obliquely at an angle should connect to the horizontal incision. The length of the vertical incision should be extended if any grafting is required. In addition, if more access is needed, vertical incisions may also extend bilaterally on the palate (Greenstein and Tarnow 2014).

A full-thickness flap is indicated when the surgeon's access must accommodate grafting of any existing defects (Fig. 16.26). Originally described by Palacci (Palacci and Nowzari 2008), the papilla regeneration technique is a full-thickness flap utilized when there is at least 4.0–5.0 mm of keratinized gingiva on the buccal (Sclar 2007; Palacci and Nowzari 2008). This technique is used to gain circumferential closure around the implant abutment (Sclar 2007). The flap is outlined and elevated along the buccal mucosa. The pedicles are created from the buccal flap designed to correspond to passively fit the interdental space (Sclar 2007). These pedicles are next rotated into the interdental space and secured with a figure eight suture to avoid tension or necrosis (Sclar 2007). There are many slight variations to this technique based on different factors such as the width of keratinized gingiva present on the buccal flap margin, the vestibular depth, the extent/type of the defect, and the number of implants placed.

16.7 Surgical Guide

A surgical guide is critical in assisting the surgeon in implant placement in the aesthetic zone. The radiographic guide can be converted into a surgical guide, or a CBCT-based guide can also be fabricated from the laboratory (Fig. 16.27). The most critical part of the surgical guide is to relay the optimal implant position to the surgeon while making it user friendly. There are times when a surgical guide is not used, and the implant is placed in the most biologically

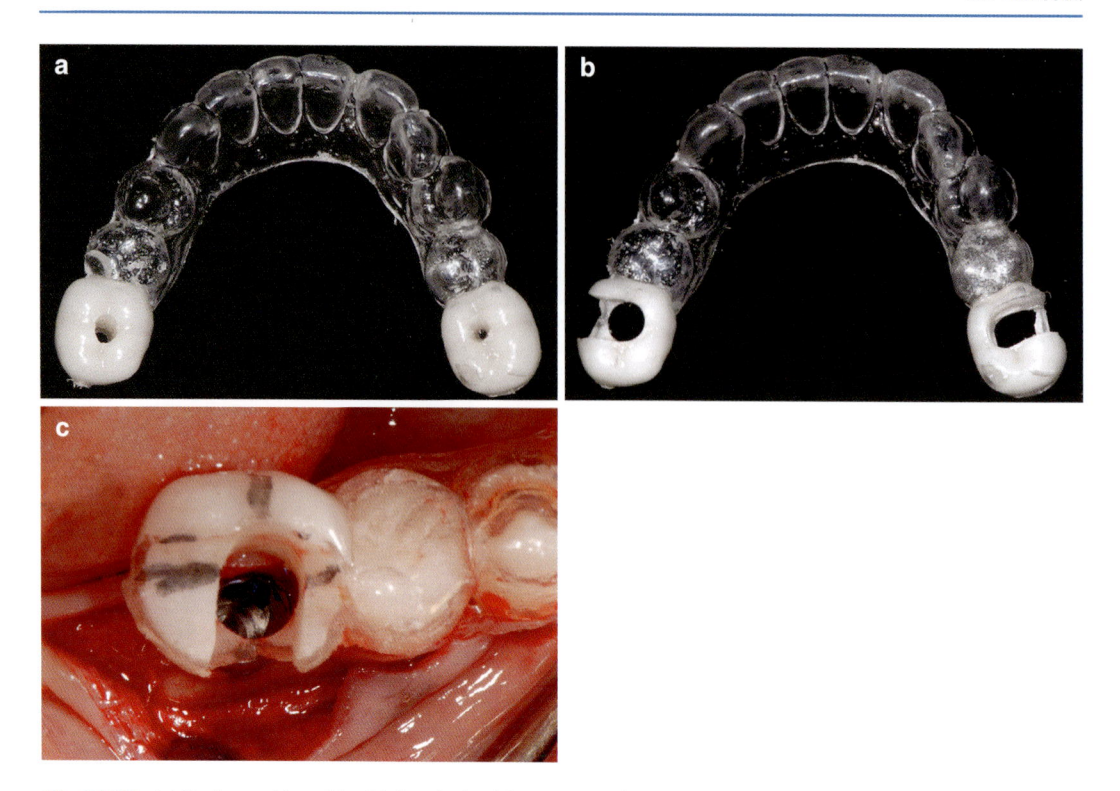

Fig. 16.27 (**a**) Radiographic guide. (**b**) Surgical guide converted from the radiographic guide. (**c**) Surgical guide in use during implant placement

optimal positions. This can be beneficial for the survival of the implant, but the restorative dentist may not be able to deliver the most aesthetically pleasing restorations. Different implant manufacturers advocate using their computer guided surgical guide, which often merges a CBCT scan and the patient's intraoral scan (STL file) and produces a very accurate guide for the surgeon (Fig. 16.28). However, depending on the type of implant, even these types of guides are not fully "guided," in that the guides often have to be removed during the actual placement of the implant. This style of guide provides an increased level of precision for the osteotomy, but not for the actual implant placement. Some implants, such as those with an aggressive thread design, may change the drilling path and angulation, and this three-dimensional change commonly occurs as the implant is being torqued in place; the implant is following the path of least resistance within the alveolus. The surgeon will always benefit from a guide even if only used to verify the implant position. These guides are fabricated from an accurate impression and the subsequent diagnostic wax-up. Two different types of guides may be utilized, one with a facial opening and another with a palatal opening, which are necessary for visualization of the implant position, notably related to the angulation and depth. If the definitive implant position is not confined within the openings of these two styles, the implant should be removed and repositioned at the time of surgery, with the caveat that primary stability is still achievable. If the positioning is unacceptable and creation of a secondary osteotomy will preclude the stability of the replacement fixture, then the procedure should be abandoned, the surgically created defect grafted, and implant placement be tried again after sufficient healing of associated hard and soft tissues.

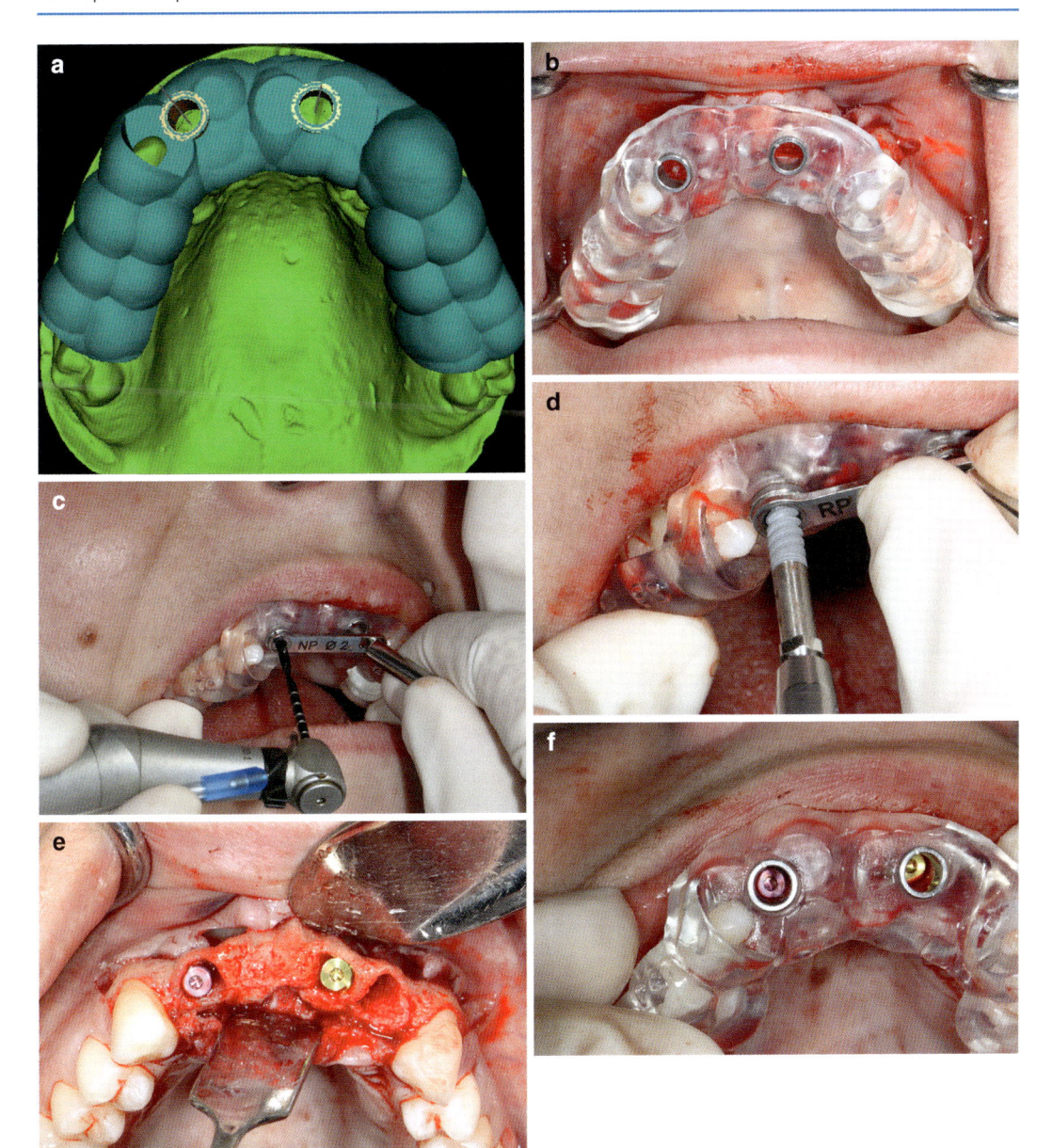

Fig. 16.28 (**a**) CAD-CAM surgical guide fabricated from the laboratory. (**b**) Surgical guide in place. Note the cutback on #6 and 11 to confirm complete seating of the guide. (**c**) Osteotomy through the surgical guide. (**d**) Implant being placed with the surgical guide in place. (**e**) Occlusal view of the implant position. (**f**) Verification of the implant position with the surgical guide in place

16.8 Implant Selection

The criteria for implant selection in the aesthetic zone may be slightly different from that in the posterior region. Often times, patients may be more critical of the soft-tissue aesthetics surrounding an implant in the aesthetic zone. Implant selection in terms of diameter, length, cervical anatomy, and prosthetic options should be discussed with the surgeon, and the restorative dentist, in that biological and restorative options can alter the aesthetic outcome.

16.8.1 Diameter

Multiple implant diameters are available for clinicians to choose from. The surgeon and the restorative dentist must agree on the implant diameter prior to the surgery due to its impact on the soft-tissue aesthetics and biomechanics of the restoration and the implant body. The implant diameter can be directly related to the fracture resistance of the implant platform and the prosthetic abutment, but it is equally critical to house the implant in native bone as much as possible. The collaborating clinicians should find a balance between these two contributing factors to achieve long-term success of the implant restoration. Studies have shown that narrow diameter implants are more prone to fracture than wider ones (Hirata et al. 2014; Shemtov-Yona et al. 2014). Manufacturers have made progressive improvements to the narrow diameter implants to prevent implant fractures, but clinicians should also remember that the abutment width is reduced with narrow diameter implants. With high-function patients, narrow implants and abutments may be prone to failure. Wider diameter implants can have superior mechanical strength over narrow ones, but the implant should only be wide enough to be housed within the bony socket of the implant site. If excessive soft- and hard-tissue grafting is necessary to envelop a wide diameter implant, the long-term soft-tissue aesthetics may be unpredictable. Therefore, it is critical to choose an implant diameter that minimizes potential need for grafting yet provides sufficient abutment thickness for strength. The restorative dentist should choose the abutment material according to the implant diameter for optimal soft-tissue aesthetics and strength.

16.8.2 Length

The criteria for implant length have shifted slightly over the years from studies that have shown that the implant survival rate is not different between long and short implants (Al-Hashedi et al. 2014; Anitua et al. 2014; Annibali et al. 2012). Multiple studies have shown that the implant to bone contact surface area a significant role in osseointegration, rather than just the implant length itself. It is unnecessary to place extremely long implants because occlusal load will only be relayed to the cervical portion of the implant. However, there may be situations where the native bone quality is poor, and in order to gain primary stability, a long implant has to be placed to engage cortical bone (Fig. 16.29). The clinicians have to understand that even though the length of the implant may not always be directly related to the implant survival rate, longer implants may have been utilized to engage the implant in high-quality bone, thereby maximizing the stability of the implant.

16.8.3 Cervical Anatomy

16.8.3.1 Traditional Platform-Matched Fixtures

Once an implant has been placed, peri-implant crestal bone-level alterations occur. These crestal bone changes are typically immediate and occur during exposure to the oral environment. If a procedure is one stage, or after the second-stage surgical approach, the micro-gap between the abutment and the implant could be a source of these alterations. Authors have suggested that the postoperative remodeling is from localized inflammation within the soft tissue located at the implant-abutment interface and is a consequence of the soft tissue's attempt to establish a mucosal barrier, i.e., the bodies effort to establish a biologic width around the top of the implant (Abrahamsson et al. 1998; Ericsson et al. 1995). This remodeling may be more extreme in implants than in natural teeth due to the connective tissue adhesion that is parallel to the implant surface and perpendicular in a natural tooth. These fibers act as a barrier or a seal against bacterial invasion and ingress of food debris into the implant-tissue interface (McKinney et al. 1984). It has been shown that 2.0 mm of vertical bone loss around the implant-abutment junction (IAJ) may be expected regardless of the original level of the bony crest (Cochran et al. 1997). Horizontal

Fig. 16.29 (**a**) PA of #11 implant at initial placement. The implant subsequently failed. (**b**) #11 implant was replaced with a longer implant to engage the apical portion of the implant in the cortical bone. (**c**) Intraoral view of definitive restoration on implant #11

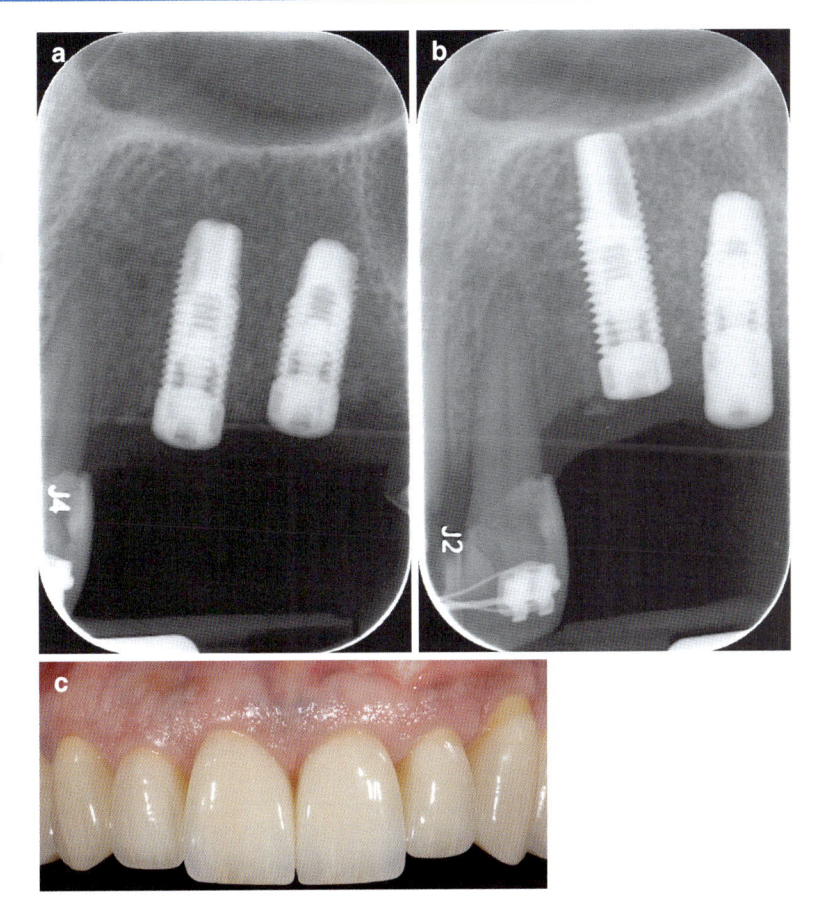

distance is usually around 1.34 mm based on Boticelli et al. (2004). This bone loss usually takes place within the first year of loading. The placement of the IAJ above the crest may result in less bone loss than placing it below the crest because bone resorption increases to establish the biologic width (Hermann et al. 1997, 2000). In a study measuring bone loss around implants placed at different vertical positions at 1 year, it was shown that implants coronal to the facial bone had bone loss of 0.89 mm. This was compared to implants placed more apically which showed a loss of 2.25 mm and level with the bone showing a 1.47 mm of bone loss (Yi et al. 2010).

16.8.3.2 Platform-Switched Fixtures

Lazarra et al. (Lazzara and Porter 2006) first introduced the idea of platform switching due to continued evidence that the IAJ is one of the primary controllers of post-restoration crestal bone position. He concluded after 13 years of observation that greater crestal bone loss was observed with the two-piece matching diameter implant abutment connection when compared to a platform-switched implant and abutment connection.

Platform switching is a prosthetic concept to use an abutment of a narrower diameter than the implant shoulder, so that the micro-gap is located at a greater combined horizontal and vertical distance to the first bone-implant contact. A systematic review in 2010 on platform switching showed that an implant-abutment diameter difference of ≥0.4 was associated with a more favorable bone response compared to platform-matched prostheses (Atieh et al. 2010). It can be concluded from this study that platform switching can be considered a desirable morphologic feature that may prevent the horizontal saucerization and preserve the vertical crestal bone level. Mean bone loss around platform-switched implants has been documented to be 0.65 mm in both the vertical and horizontal directions (Rodríguez-Ciurana et al. 2009), which is approximately half the bone loss documented around non-platform-switched implants. However, there are limitations to the published studies in that it is impossible to accurately measure the amount of bone loss or bone retention from two-dimensional radiographs. It is still controversial whether the discrepancy in the implant diameter and the prosthetic abutment is the sole factor in superior aesthetics or the reduced amount of gap between implant and the abutment through an internal connection design along with the additional soft tissue created with a narrower abutment contributed to the improved aesthetics (Bishti et al. 2014; Caram et al. 2014; Schwarz et al. 2014). Regardless of which implant system or platforms used, the most important driver in the placement of any implant in the aesthetic zone is the thorough evaluation of the overall patient's aesthetics and risks.

16.8.4 Prosthetic Option

Various prosthetic options offered by the implant company can play a major role in implant selection. The restorative component, especially the abutment selection in terms of accuracy of fit, various materials, and shade can have a significant impact on the aesthetic outcome of the implant restorations. In addition to the aesthetic outcome of the implant restoration, the abutment material can cause mechanical wear on the implant platform after extensive period of function in the intraoral environment (Kim et al. 2013; Klotz et al. 2011; Stimmelmayr et al. 2012). This potentially irreversible damage on the implant platform can be detrimental, leading to a dysfunction of the implant due to the loss of intimate fit of the abutment to the implant fixture. Further clinical research is needed to clarify the effect of various abutment materials and fit of the components on the damage to the implant platform. Clinicians should carefully select an implant that is paired with the best fitting components and provide aesthetic features that will ensure the implant restoration mimics the natural dentition.

> **Summary**
> - Diagnostic evaluation utilizing a wax-up and a mock-up is necessary for accurate treatment planning.
> - For optimal aesthetic and biologic integration, a three-dimensional safety zone around the implant is needed (Fig. 16.30). The surgeon should take precautions not to violate this zone and should not hesitate from switching to narrow implants to preserve this zone.
> - Careful evaluation of the surgical site and the need for flap elevation prior to any implant surgery is critical. Whenever possible flapless or minimally invasive surgery should be carried out.

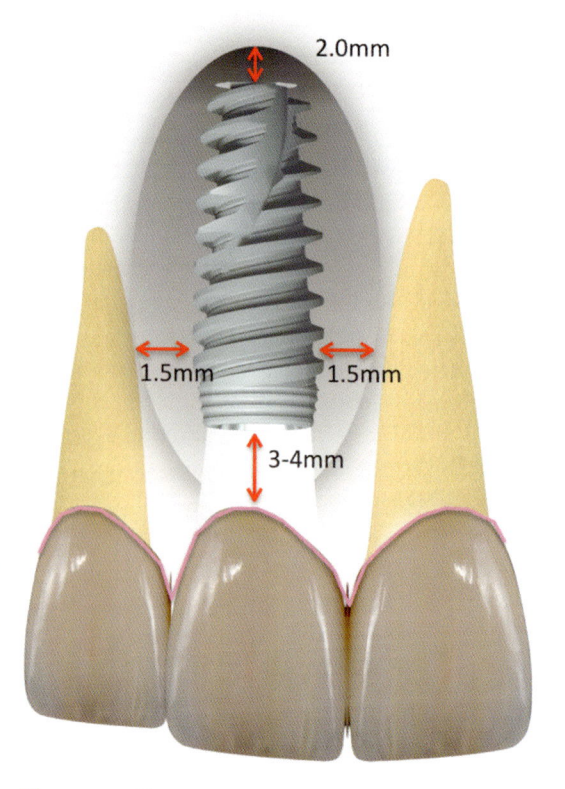

Fig. 16.30 Illustration of the "Implant-Halo"

- Surgical guides should be utilized during implant surgery to help the surgeon in placing the implant in the target zone.
- If the implants are not placed in the ideal position, repositioning of the implant at the time of surgery should be done in order to minimize the prosthetic challenge.
- Implant size and design selection with their restorative options are critical to consider in the aesthetic zone. Platform-switched implants may yield improved soft-tissue aesthetics, although evidence is not clear on whether the reduction of implant-abutment gap in platform switched implants or the additional soft tissue created due to the narrow cervical portion of the abutment is the main factor for this improvement.

References

Aboushelib MN, Salameh Z (2009) Zirconia implant abutment fracture: clinical case reports and precautions for use. Int J Prosthodont 22:616–619

Abrahamsson I, Berglundh T, Lindhe J (1998) Soft tissue response to plaque formation at different implant systems. A comparative study in the dog. Clin Oral Implants Res 9:73–79

Aghaloo TL, Moy PK (2007) Which hard tissue augmentation techniques are the most successful in furnishing bony support for implant placement? Int J Oral Maxillofac Implants 22:49–70

Al-Hashedi AA, Taiyeb Ali TB, Yunus N (2014) Short dental implants: an emerging concept in implant treatment. Quintessence Int 45:499–514

Anitua E, Piñas L, Begoña L, Orive G (2014) Long-term retrospective evaluation of short implants in the posterior areas: clinical results after 10–12 years. J Clin Periodontol 41:404–411

Annibali S, Cristalli MP, Dell'Aquila D, Bignozzi I, La Monaca G, Pilloni A (2012) Short dental implants: a systematic review. J Dent Res 91:25–32

Araujo MG, Lindhe J (2005) Dimensional ridge alterations following tooth extraction. An experimental study in the dog. J Clin Periodontol 32:212–218

Atieh MA, Ibrahim HM, Atieh AH (2010) Platform switching for marginal bone preservation around dental implants: a systematic review and meta-analysis. J Periodontol 81:1350–1366

Att W, Yajima ND, Wolkewitz M, Witkowski S, Strub JR (2012) Influence of preparation and wall thickness on the resistance to fracture of zirconia implant abutments. Clin Implant Dent Relat Res 14:e196–e203

Becker M, Goldstein M (2008) Immediate implant placement: treatment planning and surgical steps for successful outcome. Periodontol 47:79–89

Berglundh T, Lindhe J (1996) Dimension of the peri-implant mucosa. Biological width revisited. J Clin Periodontol 23:971–973

Bishti S, Strub JR, Att W (2014) Effect of the implant-abutment interface on peri-implant tissues: a systematic review. Acta Odontol Scand 72:13–25

Botticelli D, Berglundh T, Lindhe J (2004) Hard-tissue alterations following immediate implant placement in extraction sites. J Clin Periodontol 31:820–828

Braut V, Bornstein MM, Belser U, Buser D (2011) Thickness of the anterior maxillary facial bone wall- a retrospective radiographic study using cone beam computed tomography. Int J Periodontics Restor Dent 31:125–131

Caram SJ, Huynh-Ba G, Schoolfield JD, Jones AA, Cochran DL, Belser UC (2014) Biologic width around different implant-abutment interface configurations. A radiographic evaluation of the effect of horizontal offset and concave abutment profile in the canine mandible. Int J Oral Maxillofac Implants 29:1114–1122

Chappuis V, Engel O, Reyes M, Shahim K, Nolte LP, Buser D (2013) Ridge alterations post-extraction in the esthetic zone: a 3D analysis with CBCT. J Dent Res 92:195S–201S

Chiche GJ (2008) Proportion, display, and length for successful esthetic planning. Interdisciplinary treatment planning: principles, design, implementation. Quintessence Publishing Co, Chicago

Cochran DL, Hermann JS, Schenk RK, Higginbottom FL, Buser D (1997) Biologic width around titanium implants. A histometric analysis of the implanto-gingival junction around unloaded and loaded nonsubmerged implants in the canine mandible. J Periodontol 68:186–198

Cooper LF, Pin-Harry OC (2013) "Rules of Six" – diagnostic and therapeutic guidelines for single-tooth implant success. Compend Contin Educ Dent 34:2–8

Cranin AN (2002) Implant surgery: the management of soft tissues. J Oral Implantol 28:230–237

El Nahass H, Naiem SN (2015) Analysis of the dimensions of the labial bone wall in the anterior maxilla: a cone-beam computed tomography study. Clin Oral Implants Res 26:57–61

Ericsson I, Persson LG, Berglundh T, Marinello CP, Lindhe J, Klinge B (1995) Different types of inflammatory reactions in peri-implant soft tissues. J Clin Periodontol 22:255–261

Esposito M, Ekestubbe A, Grondahl K (1993) Radiological evaluation of marginal bone loss at tooth surfaces facing single Branemark implants. Clin Oral Implants Res 4:151–157

Garber DA (1995) The esthetic dental implant: letting restoration be the guide. J Am Dent Assoc 126:319–325

Greenstein G, Tarnow D (2014) Using the papillae-sparing incisions in the esthetic zone to restore form and function. Compend Contin Educ Dent 35:315–322

Gurtner GC, Werner S, Barrandon Y, Longaker MT (2008) Wound repair and regeneration. Nature 453:314–321

Hermann JS, Cochran DL, Nummikoski PV, Buser D (1997) Crestal bone changes around titanium implants. A radiographic evaluation of unloaded nonsubmerged and submerged implants in the canine mandible. J Periodontol 68:1117–1130

Hermann JS, Schoolfield JD, Nummikoski PV, Buser D, Schenk RK, Cochran DL (2000) Crestal bone changes around titanium implants. A histometric evaluation of unloaded non-submerged and submerged implants in the canine mandible. J Periodontol 71:1412–1424

Hirata R, Bonfante EA, Machado LS, Tovar N, Coelho PG (2014) Mechanical evaluation of four narrow-diameter implant systems. Int J Prosthodont 27:359–362

Januário AL, Duarte WR, Barriviera M, Mesti JC, Araújo MG, Lindhe J (2011) Dimension of the facial bone wall in the anterior maxilla: a cone-beam computed tomography study. Clin Oral Implants Res 22:1168–1171

Jivraj S, Chee W (2006) Treatment planning of implants in the aesthetic zone. Br Dent J 201:77–89

Jung RE, Sailer I, Hämmerle CH, Attin T, Schmidlin P (2007) In vitro color changes of soft tissues caused by restorative materials. Int J Periodontics Restor Dent 27:251–257

Kan JYK, Rungcharassaeng K, Lozada JL, Zimmerman G (2011) Facial gingival tissue stability following immediate placement and provisionalization of maxillary anterior single implants: a 2- to 8-year follow-up. Int J Oral Maxillofac Implants 26:179–187

Kim H, Kim TW (2011) Histologic evaluation of root-surface healing after root contact or approximation during placement of mini-implants. Am J Orthod Dentofac Orthop 139:752–760

Kim JS, Raigrodski AJ, Flinn BD, Rubenstein JE, Chung KH, Mancl LA (2013) In vitro assessment of three types of zirconia implant abutments under static load. J Prosthet Dent 109:255–263

Kim A, Campbell SD, Viana MA, Knoernschild KL (2015) Abutment material effect on peri-implant soft tissue color and perceived esthetics. J Prosthodont 25:634–640

Kleinheinz J, Büchter A, Kruse-Lösler B, Weingart D, Joos U (2005) Incision design in implant dentistry based on vascularization of the mucosa. Clin Oral Implants Res 16:518–523

Klotz MW, Taylor TD, Goldberg AJ (2011) Wear at the titanium-zirconia implant-abutment interface: a pilot study. Int J Oral Maxillofac Implants 26:970–975

Krennmair G, Seemann R, Weinländer M, Wegscheider W, Piehslinger E (2011) Implant-prosthodontic rehabilitation of anterior partial edentulism: a clinical review. Int J Oral Maxillofac Implants 26:1043–1050

Larjava H, Wiebe C, Gallant-Behm C, Hart DA, Heino J, Häkkinen L (2011) Exploring scarless healing of oral soft tissues. J Can Dent Assoc 77:b18

Lazzara RJ, Porter SS (2006) Platform switching: a new concept in implant dentistry for controlling postrestorative crestal bone levels. Int J Periodontics Restor Dent 26:9–17

Lee YK, Kim JW, Baek SH, Kim TW, Chang YI (2010) Root and bone response to the proximity of a mini-implant under orthodontic loading. Angle Orthod 80:452–458

Lee EA, Gonzalez-Martin O, Fiorellini J (2014) Lingualized flapless implant placement into fresh extraction sockets preserves buccal alveolar bone: a cone beam computed tomography study. Int J Periodontics Restor Dent 34:61–68

Magne P, Belser U (2003) Bonded porcelain restorations in the anterior dentition: a biomimetic approach. Quintessence Publishing Co, Carol Stream, IL pp 200–225

McKinney RV Jr, Steflik DE, Koth DL (1984) The biologic response to the single-crystal sapphire endosteal dental implant: scanning electron microscopic observations. J Prosthet Dent 51:372–379

McLean TN, Smith BA, Morrison EC, Nasjleti CE, Caffesse RG (1995) Vascular changes following mucoperiosteal flap surgery: a fluorescein angiography study in dogs. J Periodontol 66:205–210

Milton SH (1970) Pedicle skin flaps: the fallacy of the length: width ratio. Br J Surg 57:501–506

Misje K, Bjørnland T, Saxegaard E, Jensen JL (2013) Treatment outcome of dental implants in the esthetic zone: a 12- to 15-year retrospective study. Int J Prosthodont 26:365–369

Mohammed JA, Shaifulizan ABR, Hasan FD (2012) Principles of flap design in dental implantology. Dent Implantol Updat 23:41–44

Mörmann W, Ciancio SG (1977) Blood supply of human gingiva following periodontal surgery. A fluorescein angiographic study. J Periodontol 48:681–692

Palacci P, Nowzari H (2008) Soft tissue enhancement around dental implants. Periodontol 47:113–132

Papalexiou V, Novaes AB Jr, Ribeiro RF, Muglia V, Oliveira RR (2006) Influence of the interimplant distance on crestal bone resorption and bone density: a histomorphometric study in dogs. J Periodontol 77:614–621

Phillips K, Kois JC (1998) Aesthetic peri-implant site development. The restorative connection. Dent Clin N Am 42:57–70

Rocchietta I, Fontana F, Simion M (2008) Clinical outcomes of vertical bone augmentation to enable dental implant placement: a systematic review. J Clin Periodontol 35:203–215

Rodríguez-Ciurana X, Vela-Nebot X, Segalà-Torres M, Calvo-Guirado JL, Cambra J, Méndez-Blanco V, Tarnow DP (2009) The effect of interimplant distance on the height of the interimplant bone crest when using platform-switched implants. Int J Periodontics Restor Dent 29:141–151

Roe P, Kan JY, Rungcharassaeng K et al (2012) Horizontal and vertical dimensional changes of peri-implant facial bone following immediate placement and provisionalization of maxillary anterior single implants: a 1-year cone beam computed tomography study. Int J Oral Maxillofac Implants 27:393–400

Salama H, Salama MA, Garber D, Adar P (1998) The interproximal height of bone: a guidepost to predictable aesthetic strategies and soft tissue contours in anterior tooth replacement. Pract Periodontics Aesthet Dent 10:1131–1141

Schoenbaum TR (2015) Abutment emergence profile and its effect on peri-implant tissues. Compend Contin Educ Dent 36:474–479

Schropp L et al (2003) Bone healing and soft tissue contour changes following single-tooth extraction: a clinical and radiographic 12-month prospective study. Int J Periodontics Restor Dent 23:313–323

Schwarz F, Hegewald A, Becker J (2014) Impact of implant-abutment connection and positioning of the machined collar/microgap on crestal bone level changes: a systematic review. Clin Oral Implants Res 25:417–425

Sclar AG (2007) Guidelines for flapless surgery. JOMS 65:20–32

Shemtov-Yona K, Rittel D, Levin L, Machtei EE (2014) Effect of dental implant diameter on fatigue performance. Part I: mechanical behavior. Clin Implant Dent Relat Res 16:172–177

Stimmelmayr M, Edelhoff D, Güth JF, Erdelt K, Happe A, Beuer F (2012) Wear at the titanium-titanium and the titanium-zirconia implant-abutment interface: a comparative in vitro study. Dent Mater 28:1215–1220

Su H, Gonzalez-Martin O, Weisgold A, Lee E (2010) Considerations of implant abutment and crown contour: critical contour and subcritical contour. Int J Periodontics Restor Dent 30:335–343

Szpaderska AM, Zukerman JD, DiPietro LA (2003) Differential injury response in oral mucosal and cutaneous wounds. J Dent Res 82:621–626

Takei HH, Han TJ, Carranza FA, Kenney EB, Lekovic V (1984) Flap technique for periodontal bone implants – papilla preservation technique. J Periodontol 56:204–210

Tarnow D, Magner AW, Fletcher P (1992) The effect of the distance from the contact point to the crest of bone on the presence or absence of the interproximal dental papilla. J Periodontol 63:995–996

Thoma DS, Mühlemann S, Jung RE (2014a) Critical soft-tissue dimensions with dental implants and treatment concepts. Periodontol 66:106–118

Thoma DS, Buranawat B, Hämmerle CH, Held U, Jung RE (2014b) Efficacy of soft tissue augmentation around dental implants and in partially edentulous areas: a systematic review. J Clin Periodontol 41:S77–S91

Vela X, Méndez V, Rodríguez X, Segalá M, Tarnow DP (2012) Crestal bone changes on platform-switched implants and adjacent teeth when the tooth-implant distance is less than 1.5 mm. Int J Periodontics Restor Dent 32:149–155

Wang HM, Shen JW, Yu MF, Chen XY, Jiang QH, He FM (2014) Analysis of facial bone wall dimensions and sagittal root position in the maxillary esthetic zone: a retrospective study using cone beam computed tomography. Int J Oral Maxillofac Implants 29:1123–1129

Yi JM, Lee JK, Um HS, Chang BS, Lee MK (2010) Marginal bony changes in relation to different vertical positions of dental implants. J Periodontal Implant Sci 40:244–248

Parameters of Peri-Implant Aesthetics

17

Henriette Lerner

Abstract

Aim: The goal of the following is intended to provide a comprehensive overview of state-of-the-art peri-implant tissue management. This should empower the clinician to choose the most suitable method of implant therapy for a particular patient depending on the clinical findings, the tissue type, and his/her own surgical experience.

Summary: Over the past 50 years, implantology has evolved from an experimental treatment modality into a safe and effective method in dentistry. Today, in addition to osseointegration, aesthetics play a more and more important role including both white and pink aesthetics. The latter is controlled by an elaborate soft tissue management. This starts at the stage of tooth extraction and is perpetuated to the point of recall in the maintenance treatment. However, preserving marginal peri-implant tissues is more than adding improved aesthetics to successful osseointegration; vice versa, a state-of-the-art soft tissue management contributes to maintaining overall functional health and stability in the long term.

Key learning points: It is understood that bone thickness is a major factor in dental implantology. In addition, the periodontal soft tissue biotype should be given attention, as it is decisive for peri-implant soft tissue *and* bone stability. For example, an implant requires around itself 3 mm of tissue height/thickness and 3 mm of attached gingiva to allow for the buildup of a sufficient biological width; an initially thin biotype tissue will even compromise the buccal plate thickness. As a rule, minimally invasive surgical methods should be employed as well as abutment/crown designs for maximally tender soft tissue manipulation.

H. Lerner
HL-Dentclinic, Ludwig-Wilhelm-Str. 17,
Baden-Baden 76530, Germany
e-mail: h-lerner@web.de

17.1 Introduction

Implant dentistry is a symbiosis between art and science.

The art is to visualize the end result of the patient's face, on the other hand, to enable to restore on implants in detail the same precise architecture of the bony structures, soft tissues, and teeth. The structures and aesthetics created in this way should also stay stable and perfectly functional in time.

This means that today, we do not talk about osseointegration success, we talk about aesthetic success.

The art of the tissue reconstruction is to be able to implement the information from the biology, literature, and technologies and constantly implement them into our daily workflow. The philosophy of the treatment should be as follows: Choose the most minimally invasive and effective procedures and techniques, which lead to the maximal aesthetic success.

The evaluation and classification of the aesthetic success of the treatment will be made today by the white aesthetic score (WES) and pink aesthetic score (PES) (Belser 2009) (Fig.17.1). The criteria of the pink aesthetic score were developed by Fürhauser et al. (2005), while the white aesthetic score was defined by Belser et al. (2009).

17.2 Tooth Extraction

Tooth extraction is a traumatic procedure often resulting in immediate destruction and loss of alveolar bone and surrounding soft tissues (Caplanis et al. 2005). The amount of the resorption and residual volume is depending on the general health situation, while the factors which influence the

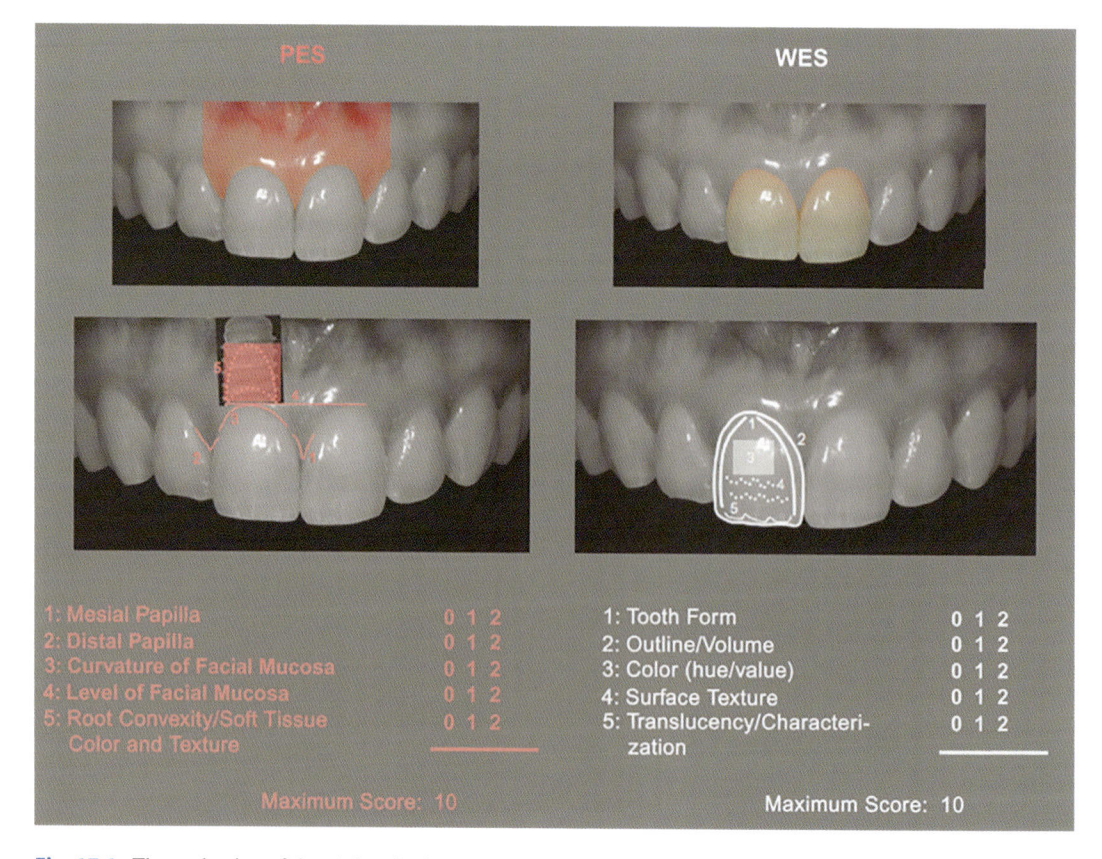

Fig. 17.1 The evaluation of the *pink* and *white* aesthetic score according to Fürhauser and Belser. The authors are showing that, under certain conditions, the volume and structure of the oral tissues stay stable in 95% of the cases in a range of 5–9 years (Buser et al. 2013)

Fig. 17.2 Defect grafting philosophy

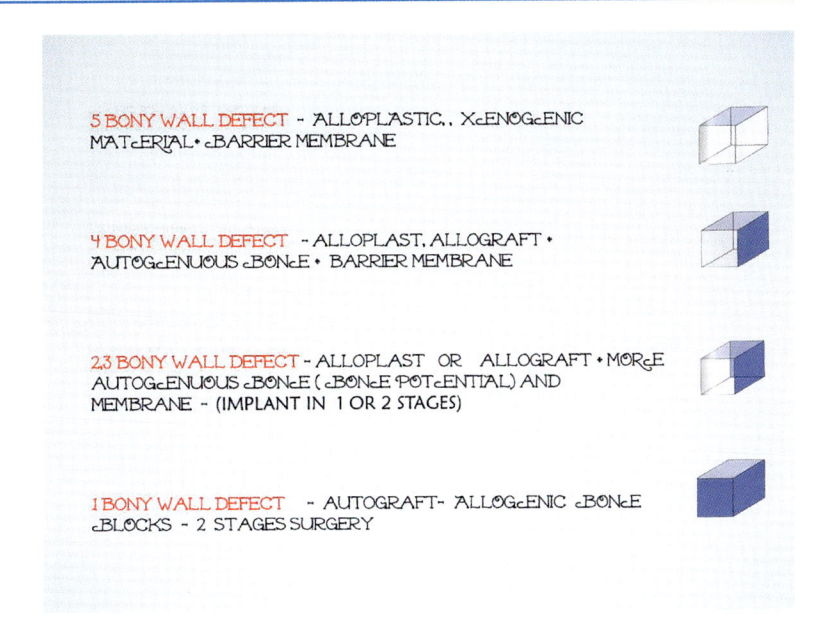

5 BONY WALL DEFECT - ALLOPLASTIC, XENOGENIC MATERIAL + BARRIER MEMBRANE

4 BONY WALL DEFECT - ALLOPLAST, ALLOGRAFT + AUTOGENOUS BONE + BARRIER MEMBRANE

2,3 BONY WALL DEFECT - ALLOPLAST OR ALLOGRAFT + MORE AUTOGENOUS BONE (BONE POTENTIAL) AND MEMBRANE - (IMPLANT IN 1 OR 2 STAGES)

1 BONY WALL DEFECT - AUTOGRAFT - ALLOGENIC BONE BLOCKS - 2 STAGES SURGERY

wound healing should be considered. A detailed dental history and thorough understanding of the pathology leading to the extraction are vital to the assessment and management of the extraction defect.

A detailed aesthetic analysis of the previous tooth should be performed, including photo and video documentations. This should reveal a variety of anomalies of the anatomical structure which are present.

The periodontal assessment should document the periodontal biotype; probing depths; amount of attached gingiva; recession; mobility; furcation involvement, as well as the presence of plaque, including the extent of inflammation; and bleeding on probing.

A subject of particular concern during the periodontal evaluation is the periodontal biotype.

Protective techniques are necessary to extract the tooth using microsurgical instruments (periotomes and other special extraction tools) and minimally invasive procedures, in order to save and protect all 8 of the major gingival fibers, which are needed for predictable healing.

Careful assessment of the extraction defect is therefore paramount to the success of aesthetic implant procedures. Extraction defect assessments can be made with or without flap reflection.

Following tooth extraction, a visual inspection of the socket bony walls is initially performed, whereas the buccal wall has the main importance for the aesthetic outcome.

The grafting of the socket/bone defect for a volume as well as for form maintenance should follow these rules.

The more bone that is initially missing:

- The more volume of bone graft has to be added.
- The more vascularization you have to promote into the graft.
- The more form maintenance has to be achieved through an appropriate membrane technique (Fig. 17.2).

17.3 Peri-Implant Tissue Histology and Modifications After Extraction

Clinical guidelines suggest that a minimal buccal alveolar bone thickness of 1–2 mm is required to maintain the tissue architecture following tooth extraction and implant placement (Vera et al. 2012). The buccal plate is a bundle bone which is connected to the tooth and therefore is prone to resorption after the extraction, and implant placement alone is able to maintain this bone.

It is generally accepted that the placement of an implant immediately after tooth extraction fails to prevent the bone remodeling process that occurs mainly at the buccal bone plate after losing one tooth.

The studies which evaluate the impact of immediate implant placement on the bone healing dynamics have reported heterogeneous results, with a mean resorption (mm) of the buccal bone plate ranging from 0.5mm to 3.14mm. This high variability may be explained by the use of different preclinical models, different healing times, different implant diameters and their respective geometries, as well as varying surgical protocols. The aim is to have a minimum of resorption and volume loss of the tissues. Therefore, certain protocols are established.

17.3.1 Immediate Implant Placement and the Added Grafting Philosophy

Immediate implant placement is a well-documented procedure, with a high aesthetic success rate under certain conditions and parameters.

The skills and knowledge of the clinician are decisive for using these principles and techniques. If the skills and experience are not complete, the clinician should take one step back and choose a more conservative method (two-stage surgery, grafting, implant placement instead of immediate placement and loading).

17.3.2 Immediate Loading/ Immediate Restoration

Immediate loading/immediate restoration is a very predictable procedure, also well documented in the literature (Capelli et al. 2013; Misch et al. 2004; Schnitman et al. 1997; Tarnow et al. 1997; Misch 1998a, b; Wohrle 1998; Schwartz-Arad and Chaushu 1999).

According to the well-accepted immediate loading definition and to consensus conference results (Wang et al. 2006), immediate loading is defined on one/more implants in a single tooth restoration/partially edentulous situation as a provisional crown/bridge which is placed on an implant, in infra-occlusion. The immediate full-arch restoration is a provisional splinted bridge and the requisite diet limited to only soft food for the duration of osseointegration (8–10 weeks).

The conditions for an implant immediately placed in an extraction socket to be immediately loaded are:

- Primary stability (35 Ncm resistant to insertional torque).
- Ideal ISQ value.
- Three-fourths of the surface of the implant should be covered by bone.
- Grafting of the gap.

In clinical cases in which the distance between implant surface and the buccal plate is <4 mm, the combination of internal and external grafting (IEG) is recommended to maintain the volume and the contour of the ridge and achieve a successful aesthetic outcome.

The second-stage surgery is a predictable procedure.

On the path of a minimally invasive surgery, based on less surgical sessions, but aiming for a best aesthetic outcome, we can perform the following grafting and implant placement.

Today, the bone-grafting procedure, additionally to the implant, is tissue thickness typology oriented (Fig. 17.3).

17.3.3 Ideal Socket Situation

In thick tissue types, a flapless approach may be considered. Without raising the flap, this procedure is considered to be minimally invasive. Immediate implant placement and immediate loading can give a predictable aesthetic result. In thin tissue biotype (tissue thickness <2 mm), a connective tissue graft will be added in an envelope or tunneling technique (Fig. 17.4).

IMMEDIATE IMPLANT PLACEMENT	THICK TISSUE BIOTYPE	THIN TISSUE BIOTYPE	
IDEAL	NO FLAP, GAP GRAFTING IIP, IL	GAP GRAFTING, SOFT TISSUE MI GRAFTING, IIP NO IL	
LESS BUCAL PLATE (max 3 mm missing)	HARD AND SOFT TISSUE GRAFTING, IIP	HARD AND SOFT TISSUE GRAFTING, IIP NO IL	
NO BUCCAL PLATE	SANDWICH TECHNIC IIP, NO IL	SANDWICH TECHNIC NO IL	
NO INTERDENTAL BONE	HARD AND SOFT TISSUE GRAFTING, STAGED SURGERY	HARD AND SOFT TISSUE GRAFTING, STAGED SURGERY	

Fig. 17.3 *IP* immediate placement, *IL* immediate loading, *MI* minimally invasive. That is why the measurement of the thickness of the tissue prior to the surgery is an important step for the soft tissue grafting technique, long-term aesthetic, and tissue stability success of the implant treatment

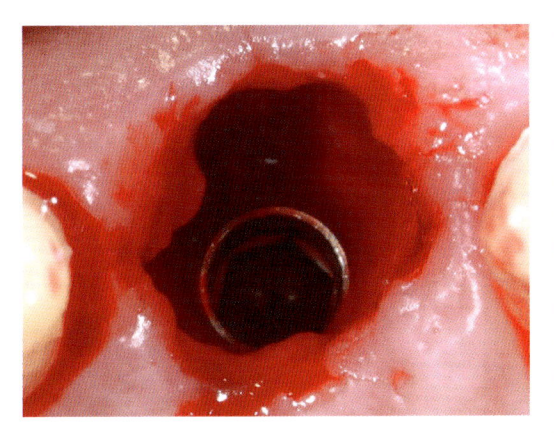

Fig. 17.4 Immediate implant placement in extraction socket. The position of the implant and thick tissue biotype gives the predictability to an aesthetic result

17.3.4 When 3–4 mm Buccal Bone Is Missing

Immediate implant placement is possible; however, immediate loading will not produce as predictable an aesthetic result, even in thick tissue phenology (Cabello et al. 2013).

Grafting both the gap between the implant fixture and the buccal plat of bone and the covering soft tissue are mandatory. The soft tissue grafting is recommended to be done with membranes which can at the same time protect the graft and keep it in form. A connective tissue won't be able to protect the graft; it will rather integrate partly with the grafting, partly with the flap (Fig. 17.5).

Fig. 17.5 Buccal defect of 3.4 mm will be grafted and covered by membrane, immediate implant placement is possible, and a closed healing will be a better solution for a more predictable aesthetic outcome. The inlay socket seal graft gives one of the best solutions to close the implant site, if more than 3 mm buccal plate is missing

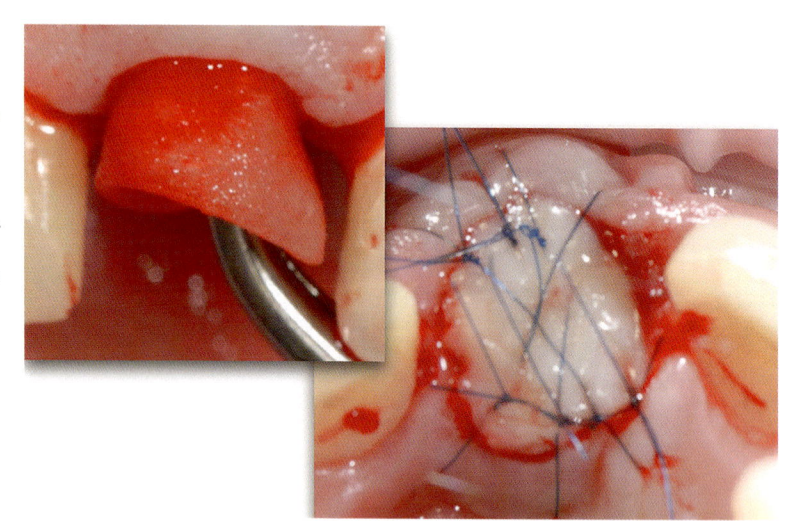

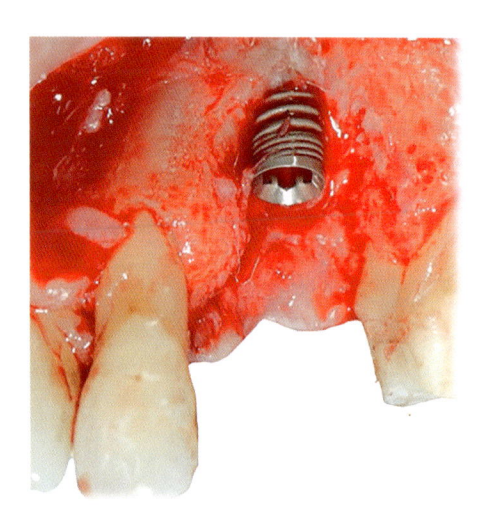

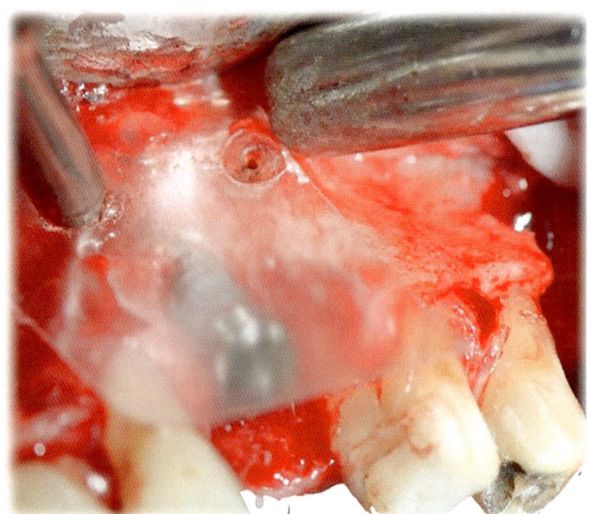

Fig. 17.6 Sandwich technique and a formed long-term stable membrane

When more than 3.4 mm of the buccal plate is missing, a simultaneous implant placement and bone grafting is performed which follows the sandwich technique. A stable membrane is required to maintain the space required for angiogenesis. This technique was first described by Hom-Lay Wang (Fu and Wang 2011) (Fig. 17.6).

17.3.5 Vertical Interdental Bone Loss

Currently, the literature shows that on average, until there is a maximum of 4 mm of bone loss, particulate material (synthetic, bovine, human) can be used for the vertical grafting, sometimes even simultaneously positioned with implant placement. This decision depends on the:

17.4 Peri-implant Tissue Reconstruction Techniques and Principles for Achieving Ideal Aesthetics

The structures to be maintained/rebuilt around implants are:

1. *Buccal plate thickness* and level of the interdental bone
   The buccal plate is a bundle bone connected to the tooth and will resorb horizontally and vertically with the extraction of the tooth (Araújo and Lindhe 2005). That is we try to maintain this bone by means of grafting of the gap with a non-resorbable material. The additional grafting of the soft tissues is performed in order to protect the bone resorption, by the formation of the biological width (Cochran et al. 1997).
2. *Soft tissue biotype*
   Linkevicius (Linkevicius et al. 2013) shows in contemporary studies what also Cochran pointed out in 1997. The tissues and dimension of these structures around teeth are very different than those around implants. The implant has a structure around it, specifically a peri-implant biological width. This is the composition of epithelial attachment, sulcus and connective tissue. And it extends to 3 mm, in average. When the tissues have a height/thickness of 3 mm, this soft tissue structure will be maintained, and the buccal plate will stay at the same level. If the initial tissues are with thin biotype (<2 mm), the biological width will be built on the cost of the bone loss. In conclusion, the tissue biotype is decisive for a peri-implant bone and soft tissue stability. Studies give evidence that the soft tissue biotype is essential for conserving aesthetic and functional stability of the peri-implant tissues. Any loss of more than 1 mm of tissue height/thickness causes a visual discolouration of the tissues (Linkevicius 2013).

In average, based on studies and literature, we can resume that an implant needs:

Three millimeters of tissue height
Three millimeters of tissue thickness

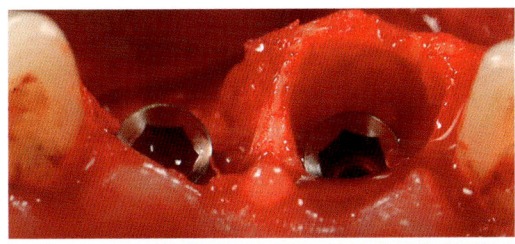

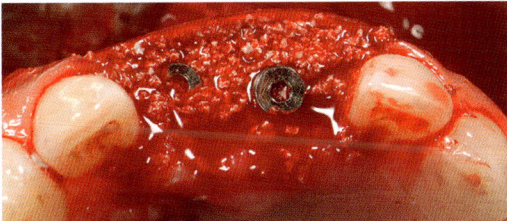

Fig. 17.7 Vertical and horizontal bone grafting with particulate material

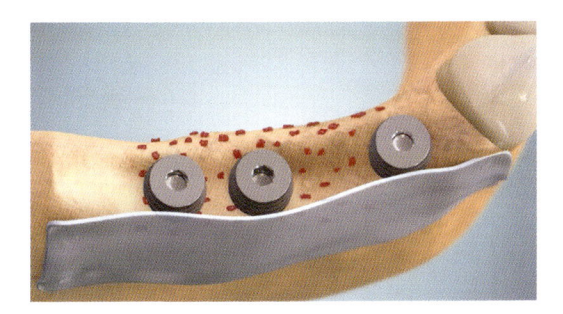

Fig. 17.8 Space maintenance quality of a membrane/bony wall

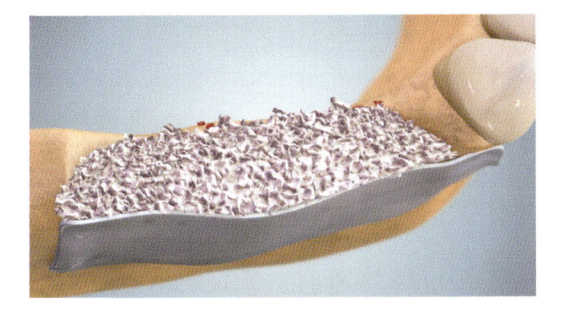

Fig. 17.9 Grafting with particulate material for enough bone potential (autogenous bone, growth factors, BMPs, vascularization has to be taken care of)

- Architecture of the defect
- Quality (bone potential) of the host bone
- Grafting envelope/space maintenance quality of the used membranes/techniques (Figs. 17.7, 17.8, and 17.9)

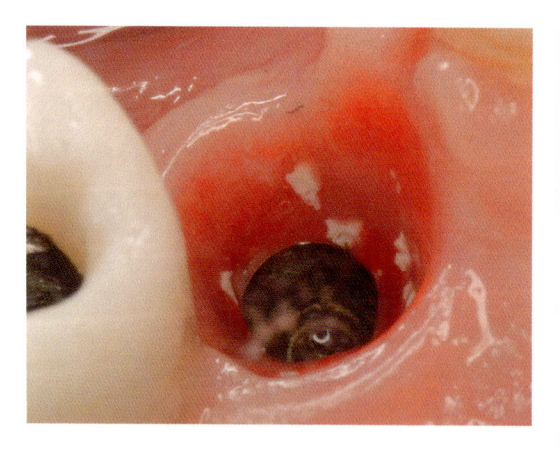

Fig. 17.10 Minimum 3–3.5mm tissue height

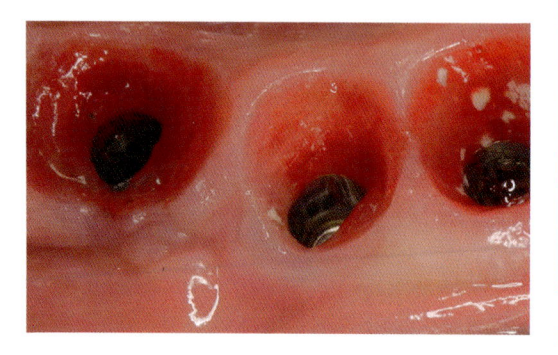

Fig. 17.11 Minimum 3 mm tissue thickness, otherwise there are discolorations

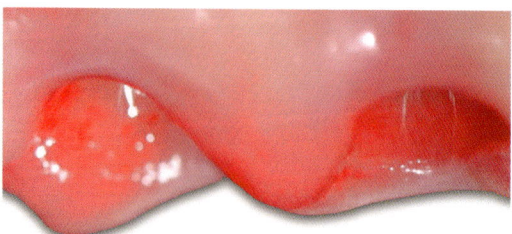

Fig. 17.12 We need at least 3 mm of attached gingiva around implants

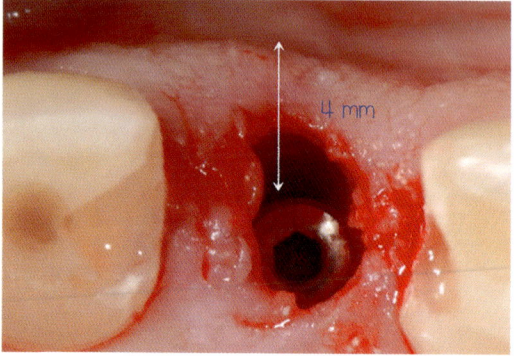

Fig. 17.13 Preventing the most tissue loss giving the maximum of volume stability (Capelli et al. 2013)

Three millimeters of attached gingiva around implants (Berglundh and Lindhe 1991, Hermann et al. 2007, Tarnow et al. 2000) (Figs. 17.10, 17.11, and 17.12)
3. *Implant position*
Parameters of ideal implant positions, predicting an ideal aesthetic outcome are:

- Two millimeters from the buccal level of the tissues. Nevertheless, grafting the gap between the implant and the buccal plate with bone substitute and grafting the tissues with connective tissue graft/membrane soft tissues will give us a distance of 4 mm from the buccal plane, which seems to prevent the most tissue loss and to give the maximum of volume stability (Capelli et al. 2013) (Fig. 17.13).

Implant design is essential for many reasons and relates to various aspects.

17.4.1 Collar Design

Older generations of implants showed a bone loss at the collar. In order to prevent bone and tissue loss, newer designs were implemented: rough surface on the shoulder of the implant, no polished collar, insertion technique under the level of the bone and special designs and textures at the collar of the implant or prosthetic parts (Norton 2013).

17.4.2 Platform Switching

A study of Hermann et al. (2001) shows that a micro-motion and bacterial endotoxins during masticatory forces may cause bone loss which occurs around implants. Platform switching/platform shifting design is employed to move the microgap from the position of the implant shoulder to a more medialized position. This seems to be beneficial for the bone level maintenance. A minimal platform switching of 0.45 mm seems to be enough to have this positive effect. In platform switching design implant concepts, bone loss will be reduced from 1.4–1.6 to 0.6 mm; this is supported by several articles confirming this beneficial effect (Al-Nsour et al. 2012).

17.4.3 Implant Connection

It is well accepted that a rigid implant connection will avoid micro-motion, screw loosening and eventually bacterial colonization. Therefore, using designs with a rigid connection seems to contribute to the maintenance of the bone level (Schmitt et al. 2014; Mangano et al. 2014a, b).

17.4.4 Surgical Technique

The most predictable situation in terms of volume maintenance, where we have the highest expectance of a natural outcome of the restoration on implants similar to the natural teeth, includes immediate implant placement, immediate loading, grafting of the gap, grafting of the soft tissue and immediate restoration with a provisional crown, ideally screw-retained. This is a conclusion of a multicenter study (Fig. 17.14) (Chu et al. 2012).

In other situations, where we need to raise a flap or to create an access point to facilitate a bone or soft tissue graft, we stay as minimally invasive as possible, at the same time not compromising the success of the grafting. These approaches require a sound knowledge of the bony and tissue structures and processes, advanced surgical skills and the creativity to be minimally invasive and create maximal aesthetic results.

It is important to design and execute the flap elevation in such a manner that it will preserve the hard and soft tissue environment in the manner which it existed prior to the implant placement procedures.

Principles:

(a) Avoid vertical releasing incisions, if possible, in the aesthetic zone. Vertical incisions may create a depression in the tissues, which, because of the lack of elastic fibers, will not have the same appearance as the adjacent soft tissue structures.
(b) Prefer incisions which are out of either the aesthetic zone or innovative grafting techniques as tunneling technique versus the more common envelope technique.

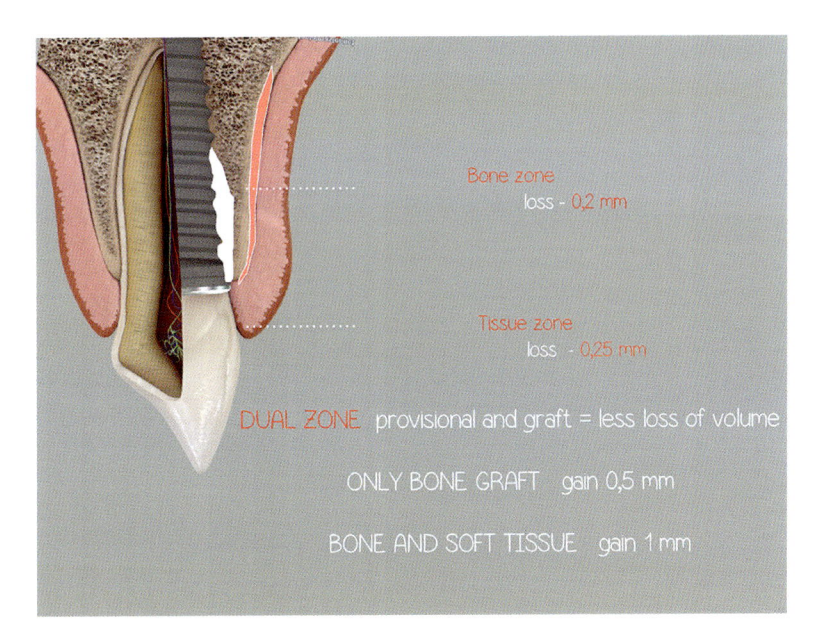

Fig. 17.14 Bone and soft tissue graft, provisional immediate restoration will avoid volume loss

(c) Prefer bone grafting methods which facilitate, with less invasive procedures (no secondary surgical field), less surgical sessions (simultaneously with implant placement) and the best aesthetic results. This is the art in contemporary implant dentistry.

(d) The suturing techniques and material selection are of primary importance. They give way to a traumatic suture using techniques that, advancing the flap coronally, facilitate to achieve the width and thickness as well as the height of the tissues required around implants in the first surgical session.

17.4.5 Provisional Abutment/ Provisional Crown

With every removal of the abutment, more than once, a certain volume of the surrounding structures will be lost (Rodríguez et al. 2013) through a destruction of the collagen fibers' adherence to the prosthetic collar. Therefore, techniques, procedures, or systems, which offer the possibility to avoid abutment disconnection using an individual final abutment from the very first or using the provisional abutment as a tool for impression coping or others, should be a criterion of choice. A concave profile of the running room, as well as a platform switching design of the provisional abutment, will create/maintain the tissue volume created (Fig. 17.15).

17.4.6 Final Abutment Design

It seems to have a decisive effect on the aesthetic success but also on the maintenance of the tissue volume, the papilla length, and the color. Many articles are confirming that a concave abutment design will conserve the tissue volume gained. Changing the emerging profile angle in the inter-implant space to a slight convex one, the papilla might gain 0.5 mm length. Several case studies show the possibility of gaining papilla length through manipulating and sculpting the gained peri-implant tissues and emergence profile of the final abutment and crown (Redemagni et al. 2009; Su et al. 2010; Lerner et al. 2012). The color of the abutment should be white, because according to a study, the human eye will notice the difference between a white and a black abutment (Fig. 17.16).

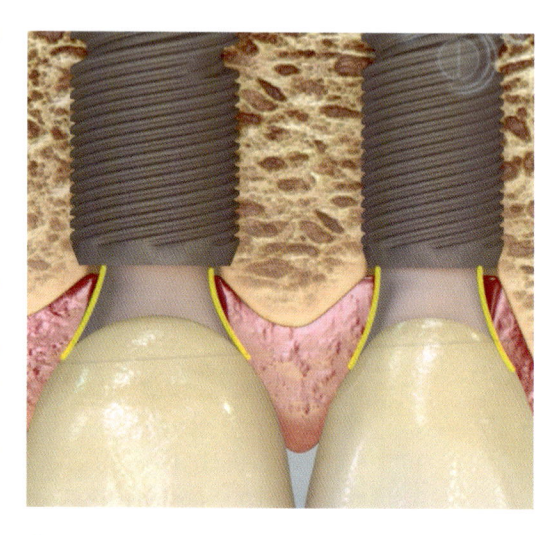

Fig. 17.15 Maintaining the tissue volume created using a concave profile of the running room

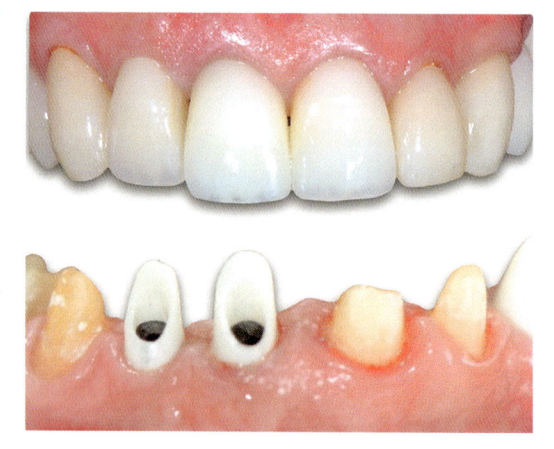

Fig. 17.16 *Black* or *white* abutment: The human eye will see the difference

17.4.7 Maintaining the Health and Volume of the Peri-implantary Tissues

Peri-implantitis is an inflammatory disease of the tissues surrounding the implant. This seems to be, today, the disease process which destroys through bacterial infection, inflammation, and subsequent bone loss the stability and health of the implant gingival and bony complex. Our purpose is to find solutions for preventing bone loss and infection. Cement in the sulcus around the restorative components (abutment and crown) seems to be one of the main reasons for this inflammatory process (Linkevicius et al. 2013). The solution and recommendation would be to place the cement margin at a maximal depth of 0.5 mm under the free gingival margin and cement using retraction cords in a manner similar to the cementation process of veneers. These will facilitate direct vision of residual retained cement in the sulcus environment.

The other option is a screw-retained restoration. This should be most preferred when the screw is not at a visible part of the tooth such as the incisal edge or on the direct facial surface.

In molar region, there are the same two options depending on the cleansability of the interdental spaces.

In the lateral zone, the maximal implant diameter is 4.3–5 mm. The mesio-distal dimension of the tooth is 10–12 mm. If the implant has been inserted deep enough in order to come out to an aesthetic gingival level, this will be the ideal situation to design the margin of the crown at an equigingival position (Fig. 17.17).

If the position of the implant is so near to the crestal bone, that an emergence profile would be too short to compensate the wide molar, then a screw-retained crown will be made in order to be able to clean professionally from time to time. This is preferred if the restoration has a ridge-lap modification to it.

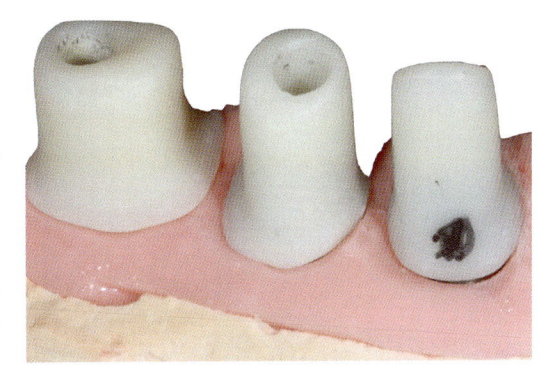

Fig. 17.17 Design and margin of the crown in the lateral zone

The materials, which seem to have the best affinity to the gingiva, are zirconia and e.max ceramics, which are the materials of choice in all restorations (Yamane et al. 2013). There is no singular "aesthetic zone," rather we consider the whole oral environment as an aesthetic zone.

Conclusion
Creating the necessary peri-implant tissues requires a profound scientific knowledge and understanding of the structures and processes in charge. To create this environment, a comprehensive, fast, effective but at the same time an aesthetic surgical and prosthetic concept and treatment are necessary including the protection of the existing tissues.

You need:
- A stable and aesthetic volume of bone around implants
- A stable soft tissue environment, i.e., 3 mm gingival height, 3 mm gingival thickness, and 3 mm attached gingiva around implants
- Tender manipulation of the soft tissues by creating the provisional/final abutments/crowns to get to the end result

Maintaining the peri-implant tissues is the best opportunity for long-term aesthetic and functional health and stability of the implant and reconstruction (Case 17.1 (Figs. 17.18 and 17.19), Case 17.2 (Figs. 17.20 and 17.21)).

298   H. Lerner

Case 17.1

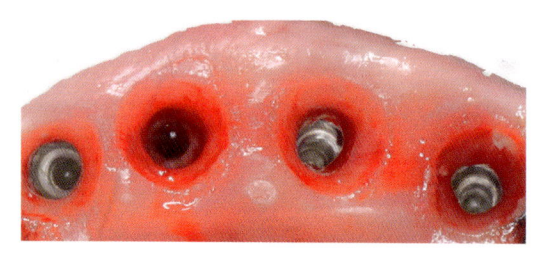

Fig. 17.18 Peri-implant tissues created

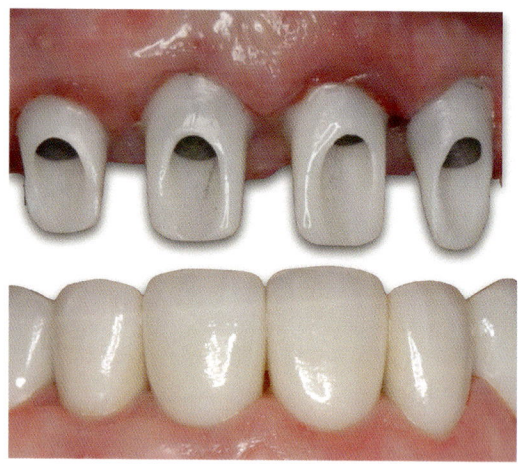

Fig. 17.19 Final abutments and crowns

Case 17.2

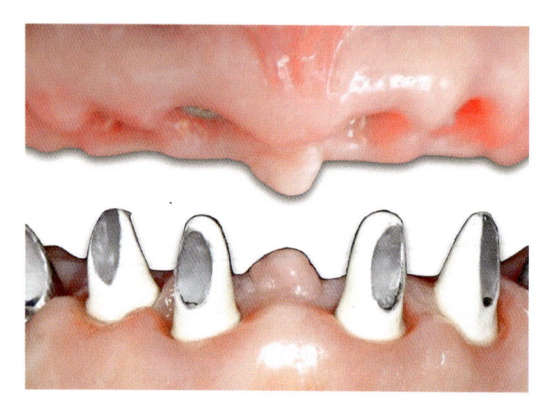

Fig. 17.20 Adjacent implants, tissue requirements fulfilled

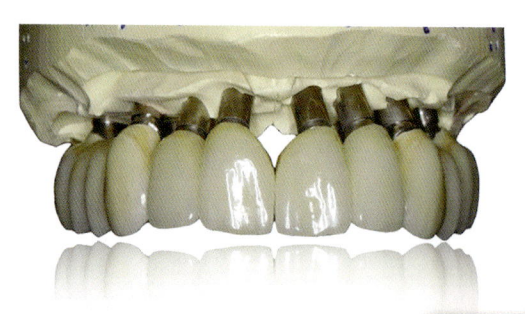

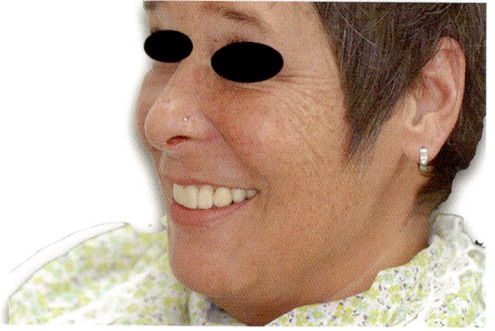

Fig. 17.21 Final aesthetic result pleasing the patient

References

Al-Nsour MM, Chan HL, Wang HL (2012) Effect of the platform-switching technique on preservation of peri-implant marginal bone: a systematic review. Int J Oral Maxillofac Implants 27(1):138–145

Araújo MG, Lindhe J (2005) Dimensional ridge alterations following tooth extraction. An experimental study in the dog. J Clin Periodontol 32(2):212–218

Belser UC, Grütter L, Vailati F, Bornstein MM, Weber HP, Buser D (2009) Outcome evaluation of early placed maxillary anterior single-tooth implants using objective esthetic criteria: a cross-sectional, retrospective study in 45 patients with a 2- to 4-year follow-up using pink and white esthetic scores. J Periodontol 80(1):140–151. doi:10.1902/jop.2009.080435

Berglundh T, Lindhe J (1991) Soft tissue barrier at implants and teeth. Clin Oral Implants Res 2:81–90

Buser D, Chappuis V, Bornstein MM, Wittneben JG, Frei M, Belser UC (2013) Long-term stability of contour augmentation with early implant placement following single tooth extraction in the esthetic zone: a prospective, cross-sectional study in 41 patients with a 5- to 9-year follow-up. J Periodontol 84(11):1517–1527. doi:10.1902/jop.2013.120635 Epub 2013 Jan 24

Cabello G, Rioboo M, Fábrega JG (2013) Immediate placement and restoration of implants in the aesthetic zone with a trimodal approach: soft tissue alterations and its relation to gingival biotype. Clin Oral Implants Res 24(10):1094–1100

Capelli M, Testori T, Galli F, Zuffetti F, Motroni A, Weinstein R, Del Fabbro M (2013) Implant-buccal plate distance as diagnostic parameter: a prospective cohort study on implant placement in fresh extraction sockets. J Periodontol 84(12):1768–1774. doi:10.1902/jop.2013.120474 Epub 2013 Mar 8

Caplanis N, Lozada JL, Kan JYK (2005) Extraction defect assessment, classification, and management. CDA J 33(11):853–863

Chu SJ, Salama MA, Salama H, Garber DA, Saito H, Sarnachiaro GO, Tarnow DP (2012) The dual-zone therapeutic concept of managing immediate implant placement and provisional restoration in anterior extraction sockets. Compend Contin Educ Dent 33(7):524–532 534

Cochran DL, Hermann JS, Schenk RK, Higginbottom FL, Buser D (1997) A histometric analysis of the implant-gingival junction around unloaded and loaded nonsubmerged implants in the canine mandible. J Periodontol 68:186–198

Fu JH, Wang HL (2011) Horizontal bone augmentation: the decision tree. Int J Periodontics Restor Dent 31(4):429–436

Fürhauser R, Florescu D, Benesch T, Haas R, Mailath G, Watzek G (2005) Evaluation of soft tissue around single-tooth implant crowns: the pink esthetic score. Clin Oral Implants Res 16(6):639–644

Hermann JS, Schoolfield JD, Schenk RK, Buser D, Cochran DL (2001) Influence of the size of the microgap on crestal bone changes around titanium implants. A histometric evaluation of unloaded non-submerged implants in the canine mandible. J Periodontol 72(10):1372–1383

Hermann F, Lerner H, Palti A (2007) Factors influencing the preservation of the peri-implant marginal bone. Implant Dent 11:162–169

Lerner H, Jacobson Z, Flax H (2012) Modified clinical approach for improved aesthetics in full-arch restoration. Cosmet Dent 4:34–37

Linkevicius T, Puisys A, Vindasiute E, Linkeviciene L, Apse P (2013) Does residual cement around implant-supported restorations cause peri-implant disease? A retrospective case analysis. Clin Oral Implants Res 24(11):1179–1184

Mangano C, Iaculli F, Piattelli A, Mangano F (2014a) Fixed restorations supported by Morse-taper connection implants: a retrospective clinical study with 10–20 years of follow-up. Clin Oral Implants Res 00:1–8. doi:10.1111/clr.12439

Mangano F, Macchi A, Caprioglio A, Sammons RL, Piattelli A, Mangano C (2014b) Survival and complication rates of fixed restorations supported by locking-taper implants: a prospective study with 1 to 10 years of follow-up. J Prosthodont 23(6):434–444. doi:10.1111/jopr.12152

Misch CE (1998a) Non-functional immediate teeth in partially edentulous patients: a pilot study of 10 consecutive cases using the Maestro Dental Implant System. Compendium 19:25–36

Misch CE (1998b) Non-functional immediate teeth. Dent Today 17:88–91

Misch CE, Hahn J, Judy KW, Lemons JE, Linkow LI, Lozada JL, Mills E, Misch CM, Salama H, Shaarawy M, Testori T, Wang H-L (2004) Workshop guidelines on immediate loading in implant dentistry. J Oral Implant 30(5):283–288

Norton M (2013) Primary stability versus viable constraint – a need to redefine. Int J Oral Maxillofac Implants 28(1):19–21

Redemagni M, Cremonesi S, Garlini G, Maiorana C (2009) Soft tissue stability with immediate implants and concave abutments. Eur J Esthet Dent 4(4):328–337

Rodríguez X, Vela X, Méndez V, Segalà M, Calvo-Guirado JL, Tarnow DP (2013) The effect of abutment dis/reconnections on peri-implant bone resorption: a radiologic study of platform switched and non-platform-switched implants placed in animals. Clin Oral Implants Res 24(3):305–311. doi:10.1111/j.1600-0501.2011.02317.x

Schmitt CM, Nogueira-Filho G, Tenenbaum HC, Lai JY, Brito C, Döring H, Nonhoff J (2014) Performance of conical abutment (Morse Taper) connection implants: a systematic review. J Biomed Mater Res A 102(2):552–574. doi:10.1002/jbmm.34709

Schnitman DA, Wohrle PS, Rubenstein JE, DaSilva JD, Wang NH (1997) Branemark implants immediately loaded with fixed prostheses at implant placement. Ten year results. Int J Oral Maxillofac Implants 12:495–503

Schwartz-Arad D, Chaushu G (1999) Full-arch restoration of the jaw with fixed ceramo-metal prosthesis: late implant placement. J Periodontol 70(1):90–94

Su H, González-Martín O, Weisgold A, Lee E (2010) Considerations of implant abutment and crown contour: critical contour and subcritical contour. Int Periodontics Restor Dent 30(4):335–343

Tarnow DP, Emtiag S, Classi A (1997) Immediate loading of threaded implants at stage one surgery in edentulous arches. Ten consecutive case reports with 1 to 5 year data. Int J Oral Maxillofac Implants 12:319–324

Tarnow DP, Cho SC, Wallace SS (2000) The effect of the interimplant distance on the height of the interimplant bone crest. J Periodontol 71:546–549

Vera C, De Kok IJ, Reinhold D, Limpiphipatanakorn P, Yap AK, Tyndall D, Cooper LF (2012) Evaluation of buccal alveolar bone dimension of maxillary anterior and premolar teeth: a cone beam computed tomography investigation. Int J Oral Maxillofac Implants 27(6):1514–1519

Wang HL, Ormianer Z, Palti A, Perel ML, Trisi P, Sammartino G (2006) Consensus conference on immediate loading: the single tooth and partial edentulous areas. Implant Dent 15:324–333

Wohrle P (1998) Single tooth replacement in the aesthetic zone with immediate provisionalization fourteen consecutive case reports. Pract Periodontics Aesthet Dent 9:1107–1114

Yamane K, Ayukawa Y, Takeshita T, Furuhashi A, Yamashita Y, Koyano K (2013) Bacterial adhesion affinities of various implant abutment materials. Clin Oral Implants Res 24(12):1310–1315. doi:10.1111/j.1600-0501.2012.02574.x

The Single Implant-Crown Complex in the Aesthetic Zone: Abutment Selection and the Treatment Sequencing

18

Stavros Pelekanos

Abstract

It is a great challenge for the clinician to choose a methodology, abutment design, and type of restoration in order to achieve optimal results and avoid complications in implant rehabilitations in the aesthetic zone. The great variety of materials that are coming in contact with the soft tissues (acrylic, base alloy, gold, titanium, zirconia, and recently lithium disilicate) further complicate the decision-making, and as they show different soft tissue response and color, they seem to affect the final result, especially in patients with thin biotype.

This chapter will focus on the methodology of the prosthetically driven single implant placement, especially in demanding aesthetic cases, on today's knowledge of the biology of different materials and abutment selection (customized vs. prefabricated abutments, screw vs cement retained) and provide some clinical guidelines to achieve optimum aesthetic results. Finally, new approaches regarding "immediate abutment placement," "intermediate abutment placement," and digital technology for impression in combination with prefabricated CAD lithium disilicate blocks will be discussed with the help of clinical case presentations.

Electronic Supplementary Material The online version of this chapter (doi:10.1007/978-3-319-50706-4_18) contains supplementary material, which is available to authorized users.

S. Pelekanos DDS, Dr. Med Dent
Department of Prosthodontics,
Dental School of Athens, University of Athens,
163b El. Venizelou Ave, Athens, Attica 176 72,
Greece
e-mail: pelekan@otenet.gr

18.1 Introduction

Successful implant restorations in the aesthetic zone require often demanding surgical and prosthetic therapeutic procedures in order to achieve long-term stable results. Anatomical factors such as the thin buccal bone plate, the thin soft tissues, and the high scalloping further complicate the decision-making and the treatment workflow. Several techniques have been implemented to reduce bone loss and preserve soft tissue architecture between extraction and implant restoration. Ridge preservation techniques, immediate or delayed implant placement and/or loading (Chen et al. 2004), and different guided bone regeneration procedures have been proposed and are at the same time still controversies in implant dentistry. Regarding prosthetics, different abutment materials and designs, new protocols like platform switching, the "one time-one abutment concept" (Degidi et al. 2014; Canullo et al. 2010; Pelekanos et al. 2013), and modern digital impression techniques combined with CAD-CAM procedures have been proposed in order to achieve optimal aesthetic results. Despite the clinical and scientific evidence, the clinical handling and the treatment sequence and workflow are of outmost importance determining the final outcome of the implant restoration.

This chapter aims to analyze and categorize different treatment modalities selecting the proper kind and placement timing of abutment, focus on the methodology and prosthetic treatment workflow in aesthetic implant cases, and give some guidelines to achieve optimum aesthetic results. A series of clinical cases and videos will also be presented.

18.2 Key Factors Affecting the Prosthetic Design

18.2.1 First Stage Surgery: Implant Positioning

It is evidenced that buccally placed implants tend to show three times more soft tissue recession than implants that are placed more palatally (Evans and Chen 2008). On the other hand, taking into consideration that the correct mesiodistal positioning of the implant is determining the presence or not of the papilla, it can be concluded that the most important factor for an optimal aesthetic result is the accurate implant placement (Grunder et al. 2005). The latter has to follow the axial inclination and position of the future clinical crown. The basic guidelines to be followed are:

- The implant shoulder should be placed at least 2 mm palatally (or lingually) of the labial surface of the future clinical crown as well as the buccal bone plate. This guideline affects in conjunction with the soft tissue biotype (thick or thin), the material, as well as the shape of the buccal transmucosal part of the abutment (convex, straight, or concave).
- The implant head has to be placed 3 mm (in machined/polished collars) to 4 mm (in rough to the top collars) below the zenith of the future crown in implants with a flat-to-flat abutment connection. In some implant systems, where an internal cone connection ("cold welding" type) in conjunction with rough to the top surface is provided (e.g. Astra, Ankylos), this distance can reach 4–5 mm. These guidelines affect the choice of the collar height and the diameter (platform switching) of the abutment.
- The axial inclination of the implant should meet the palatal or lingual surface of the future clinical crown for the anterior teeth and the center of the occlusal surface for the posterior teeth. This guideline affects mostly the choice of the retention type of the implant crown (cement- vs. screw-retained restorations).
- The minimum distance between the implant and the adjacent roots should be at least 2 mm if a non-platform-switching implant is used (Perez et al. 2012). This guideline affects the choice of the abutment diameter (platform switching) as well as the shape of the mesial and distal transmucosal contour (convex, straight, or concave).

Therefore, the use of guide stents could be very helpful in order to achieve the desired implant position (Fig. 18.1, Video 18.1).

18.2.2 Biological Considerations on Abutment Materials

There are fundamental differences regarding the biologic width between implants and teeth, with the most important being the presence of perpendicular fibers in the connective tissue inserted into the cementum of teeth. When placing an implant, those fibers are structured parallel to the titanium surface. Subsequently, better vascularity

Fig. 18.1 (**a**, **b**) Correct implant positioning (labial and mesiodistal view)

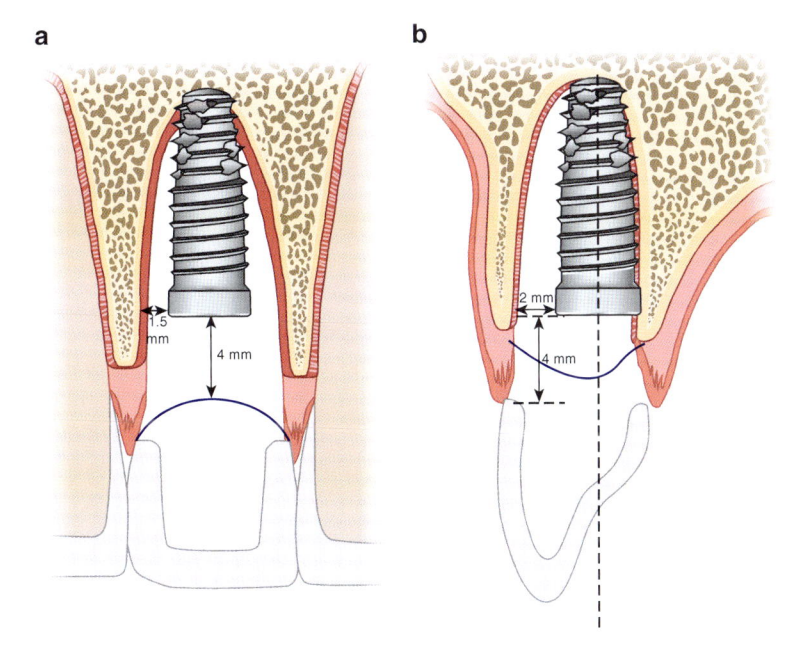

and smaller probing depths are found around teeth (Capelli 2013). Regarding quantitative data, biologic width (junctional epithelium + connective tissue) is expected to be around 3–4 mm in implant sites (Cochran et al. 1997), whereas in teeth the same measurements are around 2 mm (Gargiulo 1961; Vacek et al. 1994).

Based on the aforementioned data, peri-implant tissue could be more sensitive and prone to infection when compared to periodontal tissue, resulting in loss of attachment. Thus, the abutment materials coming in contact with the soft tissue might influence their condition.

Various materials have been proposed for abutment manufacturing. Acrylic, composite, titanium, gold, alumina, and zirconia abutments are the most commonly used. Recently, lithium disilicate and feldspathic ceramic abutment surfaces have been introduced in the dental market due to their advanced optical properties.

Titanium and alumina were initially considered the most biocompatible materials, presenting a mucosal attachment of around 1.5 mm in animal studies, where the abutments were placed one time (Abrahamsson 1998). With the appearance of zirconia in the dental market, studies showed similar results regarding biocompatibility (Welander et al. 2008). Recent data from a human study agree that 8 weeks after abutment connection, the soft tissue dimension was 3.6 mm, with 1.9 mm epithelium and 1.7 mm connective tissue (Tomasi et al. 2014).

Taking into consideration that dis- and reconnection of the abutment is common in everyday practice, the establishment of a mucosal barrier around an abutment cannot be predicted, and an apical displacement of the soft tissue is to be expected (Abrahamsson et al. 1997; Becker et al. 2012). The surface roughness and topography of the abutment material is very controversial issues affecting the quantitative histology of the soft tissue attached to it. It seems that increasing the surface Ra roughness might increase the connective tissue part of the mucosal attachment (Geurs et al. 2001), while excessive polishing leads to an increased epithelial part (Glauser et al. 2005). A threshold of Ra surface roughness value of around 0.2 μm does not affect the plaque accumulation (Quirynen et al. 1993; Bollen et al. 1996) and seems to be favorable for both titanium and zirconia regarding the soft tissue attachment (van Brakel et al. 2012). On the other hand, the surface micromorphology is a crucial factor affecting the quality of the bacterial colonization on the titanium surface (Barbour et al. 2007), thus further complicating the choice of the abutment material and processing. Although zirconia is a material very difficult to treat, specific laboratory polishing procedures are being followed in order to achieve optimum R_a values (0.2–0.4) (Happe et al. 2007).

Although acrylic and resin composites are the most frequently used materials for provisional restorations, there are almost no data available regarding their biocompatibility and soft tissue response as abutments.

One can understand that the prosthetic treatment workflow can influence the bone and soft tissue stability around an implant and the overall success of an implant restoration. This chapter focuses on the prosthetic workflow of different treatment modalities on the way to the definitive aesthetic single implant restoration.

18.3 From Implant Placement to Final Reconstruction

The restorative procedures in a single implant reconstruction can be influenced by the surgical treatment (one or two stages, use of *immediate* or *delayed placement* or loading protocols, bone or soft tissue augmentation procedures, etc.) and often can vary according to the clinician's and laboratory's experience. The following decision tree is proposed to clarify the steps of the prosthetic procedures (Fig. 18.2).

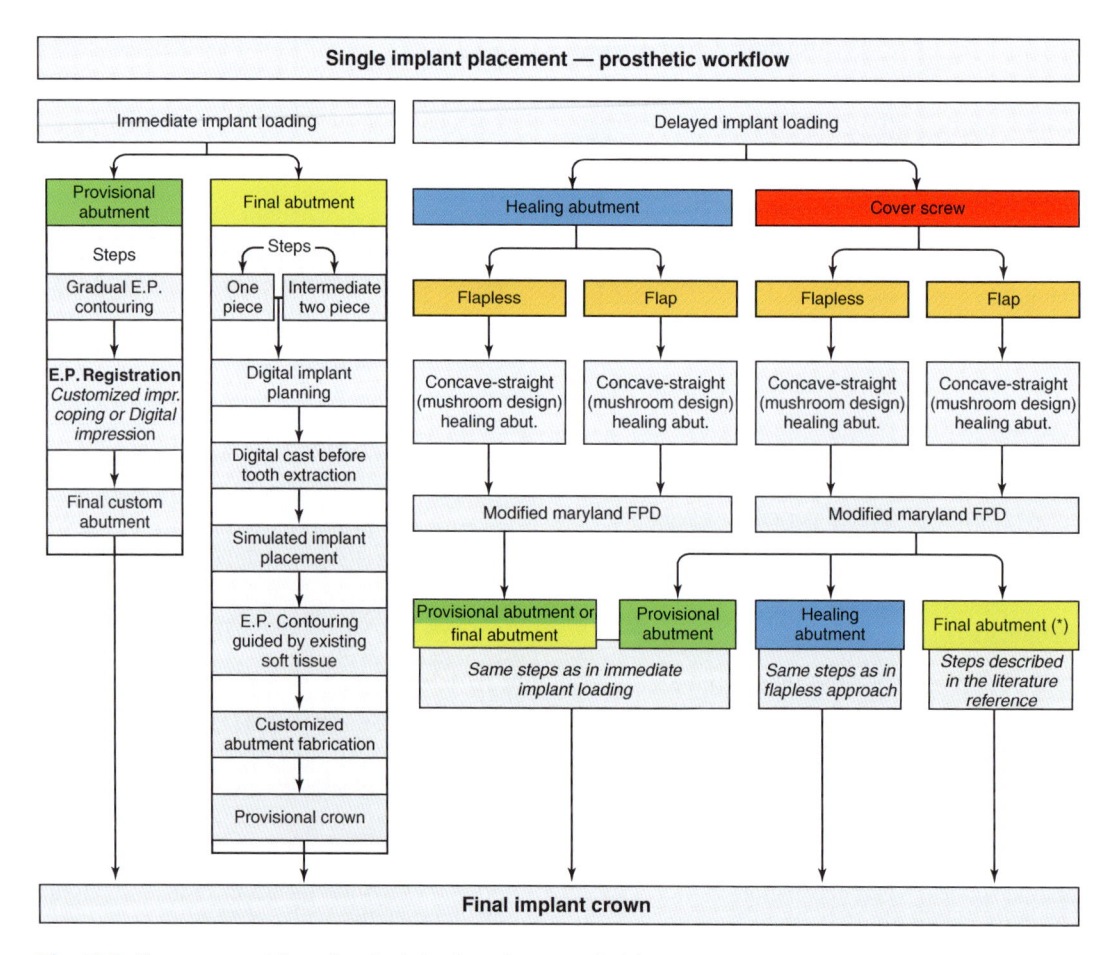

Fig. 18.2 Treatment workflow after single implant placement-decision tree

18.3.1 Immediate vs. Delayed Implant Loading

Depending mainly on the primary stability and the implant location, as well as on the bone and soft tissue conditions, the clinician should decide whether an immediate or a delayed loading would take place. The process of immediate loading on a single implant with a provisional or a final abutment should only be followed when the final insertion torque has reached at least 30 N/cm^2. In any other case, a delayed loading protocol should be followed. The decision for a healing abutment is made when the final torque exceeds 10 N/cm^2, which is approximately the number that a human hand can reach. In cases were the implant is inserted with a lower final insertion torque, a cover screw and a closed healing procedure is preferred.

18.3.1.1 Immediate Loading

Provisional Abutment
Immediate implant loading refers to the placement of a provisional or a final abutment immediately after the implant placement. When choosing a *provisional abutment* (acrylic or resin), the clinician should start in a concave design, and only in extraction sites, the profile should diverge gradually supporting the free gingival level (mushroom design). This is to ensure the stability of the graft material (autograft, allograft, or xenograft) which has been placed to fill the extraction socket and to stabilize the blood clot (Fig. 18.3a).

Only after the osseointegration period, the emergence profile can be contoured to the optimal shape gradually, by adding or removing material at the transmucosal contour. The abutment should be adapted every 10 days. After two to three appointments, the desired contour is usually achieved. The marginal soft tissue level should be stable for at least 4 weeks. Only then the final emergence profile can be captured with the use of a customized impression coping or with digital impression camera systems (see Cases 18.1 and 18.6). The final abutment is usually customized, fabricated by CAD/CAM systems. Considering the aforementioned method, although the emergence profile is controlled accurately, the repeated placement and removal of the abutment could lead to bone resorption and apical displacement of the soft tissue (Fig 18.3b) (Abrahamsson et al. 1997).

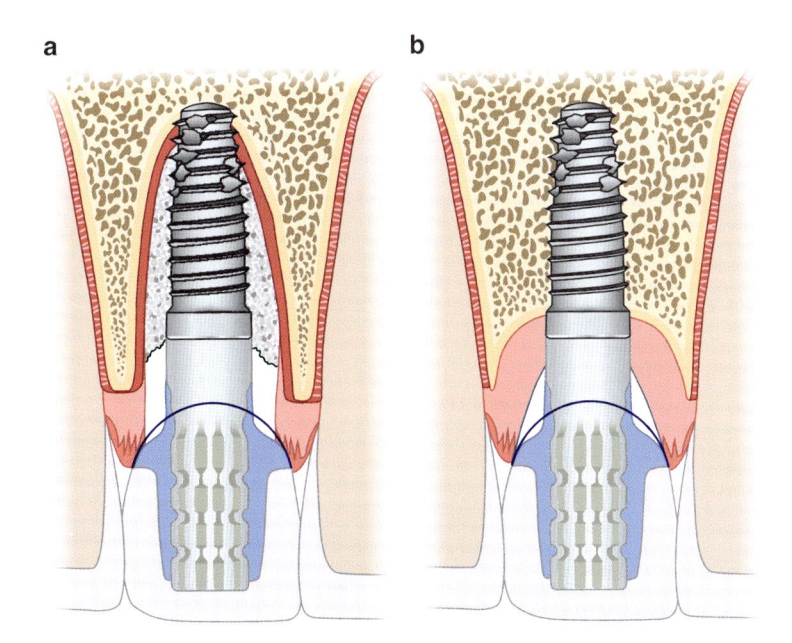

Fig. 18.3 (**a**, **b**) Immediate provisional abutment (mushroom design) before and after remodeling and EP development

Final Abutment ("One Time-One Abutment")

In order to avoid the abovementioned disadvantage, there is a tendency to place the *final abutment* immediately. There are two clinical studies (Degidi et al. 2014; Canullo et al. 2010) describing the one time-one abutment procedure in the premolar area, where the scalloping of soft tissue is usually low. Due to the round outline of the emergence profile in this area and the almost always-favorable quantity and quality of the bone, positioning of a final prefabricated abutment is usually aesthetically acceptable. Moving on to the anterior area, where the scalloping of the soft tissue is high, aesthetics become more demanding. In such cases, the use of customized abutments is mandatory.(Fig. 18.4a, b and Case 18.3).

The following procedure is indicated in cases of immediate implant placement following an extraction with a flapless approach. The dimensions and shape of the final abutment are guided by those of the extraction socket (Case 18.3 and Videos 18.5 and 18.6).

It is a prerequisite in the anterior area to use dental planning software in order to combine the soft tissue contour and the CBCT scan data.

Steps:

1. A cast is made before tooth extraction.
2. The cast is scanned and transformed to a digital one.
3. A 3D printed or stereolithographic cast is being fabricated.
4. The tooth to be extracted is cut, without damaging the soft tissue contour.
5. An implant or implant analog is inserted into the cast with the help of a guide stent.
6. The soft tissue contour is carefully prepared with the use of a diamond or carbide bur in order to achieve the optimal shape of the transmucosal contour. This procedure can be performed digitally as well.

Critical considerations during the preparation of the gingival mask (digitally or in the model):

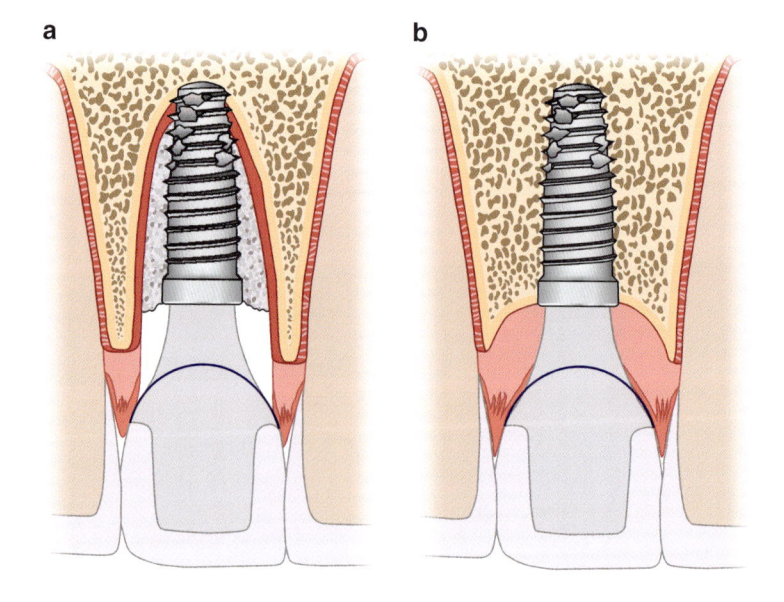

Fig. 18.4 (**a, b**) Immediate "one-time" customized final abutment before and after bone and soft tissue remodeling. Note the distance between the final abutment and the neighboring bony peaks (platform switching)

- To leave at least 2 mm of soft tissue thickness above the buccal bone plate in order to avoid gingival recession.
- To leave at least 2 mm of distance mesially and distally to the bony peaks of the adjacent roots to avoid bone resorption and future papilla loss (Perez et al. 2012). This precaution refers to the first 2–3 mm above to the implant head that is usually placed subcrestally mesially and distally and can be evaluated only by a periapical radiograph (see Fig. 18.4.).

7. A customized abutment usually made of zirconia or lithium disilicate is fabricated.
8. The customized abutment is inserted and torqued one time immediately after the implant placement, without any further removal.
9. The provisional crown is then inserted.
10. After the osseointegration period, the final crown is fabricated and inserted screw or cement retained. As far as a screw-retained version is concerned, one disconnection of the final abutment is needed (see Case 18.4 and Video 18.8).

There is another option in order to avoid the "pre-sculpturing" of the transmucosal contour all the way down to the implant level. In cases where an "immediate prefabricated intermediate" abutment is chosen, then the customization refers only to the coronal part of the transmucosal contour (see Fig. 18.5a, b, dotted lines).

The clinical procedure is described in Figs. 18.17, 18.18, 18.19, 18.20, and 18.21.

18.3.1.2 Delayed Loading

When delayed loading is chosen, usually due to reduced implant stability, a healing abutment or a cover screw is placed. Moreover, when extensive GBR and soft tissue grafting are necessary, a cover screw is the most common treatment of choice. Optionally, a healing abutment can be combined with GBR procedures.

Healing Abutment

The use of the healing abutment (one stage approach) is preferred due to the achievement of an open healing without distracting the mucco-

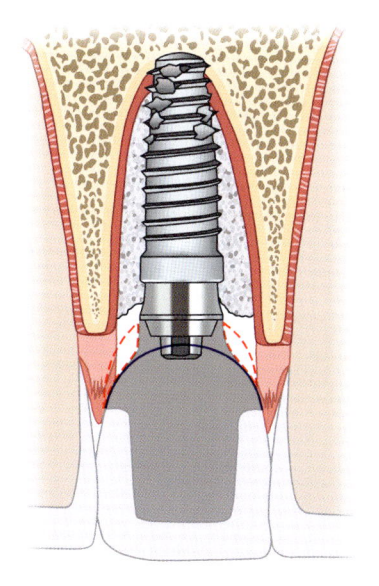

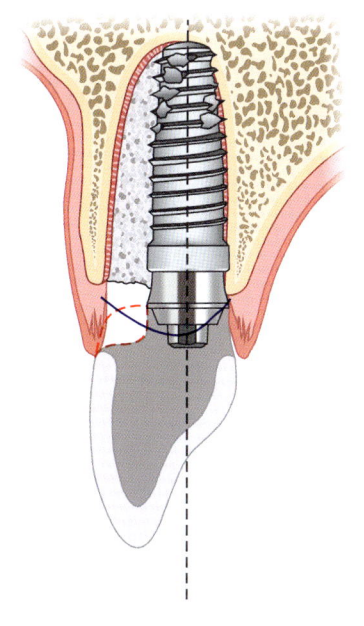

Fig. 18.5 "Immediate intermediate" abutment placement. *Dotted lines* show the contour borders allowed for profile intervention

gingival line and the width of the keratinized tissue in cases of immediate implant placement.

The flap approach dictates the shape of the healing abutment. When a *flapless approach* is chosen, the diameter of the healing abutment should be slightly smaller or equal to the diameter of the extraction socket only at the free gingival level in order to protect the xenograft placed between the implant and the buccal bone plate and simultaneously leave space for the blood clot. The contraction of the marginal soft tissue after the extraction and the immediate implant placement that varies from patient to patient should be taken into consideration. So starting from the implant platform level, the healing abutment should be divergent to implant platform (mushroom design). Otherwise the bone resorption can occur at a very early stage (see Figs. 18.6a, b and 18.7a, b).

In cases *where a flap is raised* (GBR or/and soft tissue grafting), a small concave healing abutment is preferred. The healing abutment should not exceed the diameter of the extraction socket (concave) in order to leave space for the blood clot and at the same time to provide space for the soft tissue growth. If a platform switching is performed at the same time with a GBR procedure, then a so-called double concavity is performed, thus protecting the particles of grafting material to stay on the implant level (Fig 18.8a, b and Case 18.6).

For provisionalization, a Rochette (acrylic) FPD is usually used mainly for the anterior region. After the osseointegration period, the healing abutment is removed, and a provisional or a final abutment is placed according to the aforementioned stages (1.1, 1.2) (see Cases 18.4 and 18.6).

Cover Screw

Depending mostly on the need of guided bone regeneration (GBR), a flap or flapless approach is chosen.

In case of a *flapless approach*, usually a free gingival graft, slightly wider than the extraction socket, is positioned in order to cover the cover screw and the xenograft. This procedure protects the distraction of the mucco-gingival line.

On the other hand, when extensive GBR and/or soft tissue are needed, *a flap is raised* in order to achieve a closed soft tissue healing. A Rochette-type FPD is usually chosen as a provisional. The provisional should be at a distance at least 2 mm from the soft tissue in order to avoid contact after postoperative swelling.

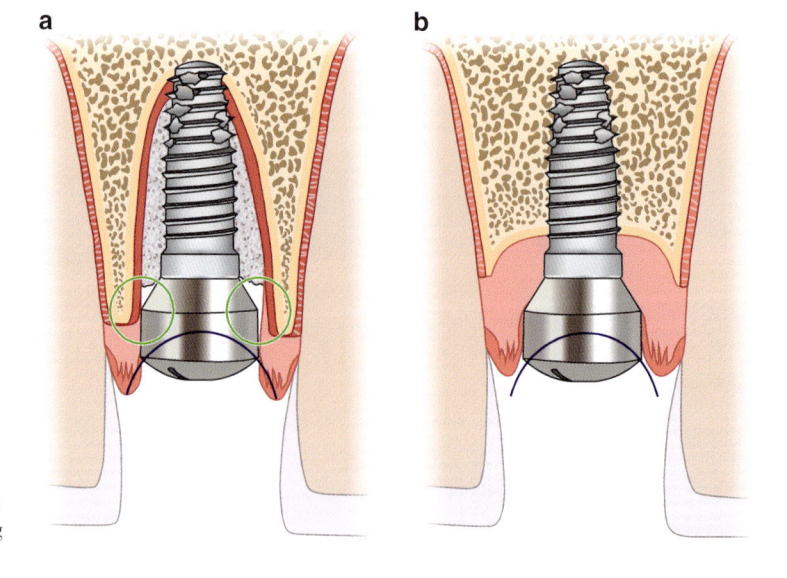

Fig. 18.6 (**a, b**) Immediate convex healing abutment positioning before and after bone and soft tissue remodeling. Flapless approach (incorrect design – note the distance between the abutment and the neighboring bone)

18 The Single Implant-Crown Complex in the Aesthetic Zone

Fig. 18.7 (**a, b**) Immediate "mushroom design" healing abutment before and after remodeling. Flapless approach (ideal design)

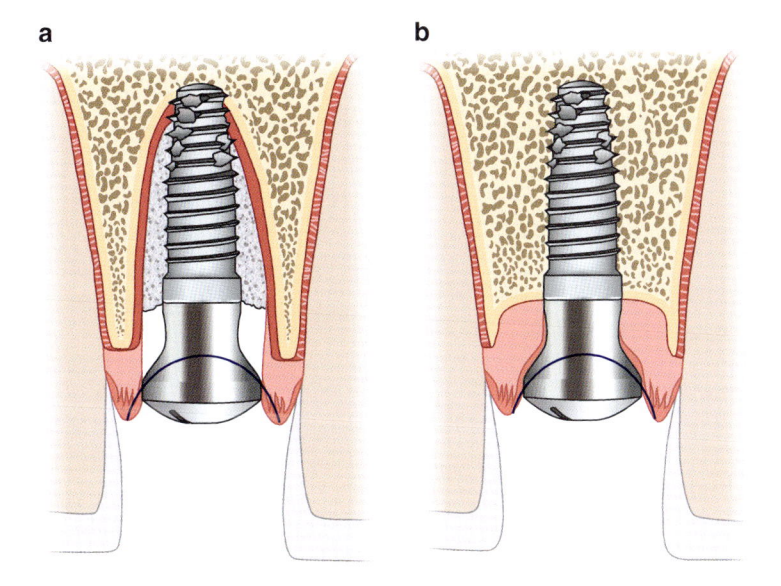

Fig. 18.8 (**a, b**) Immediate concave healing abutment positioning with platform switching before and after remodeling

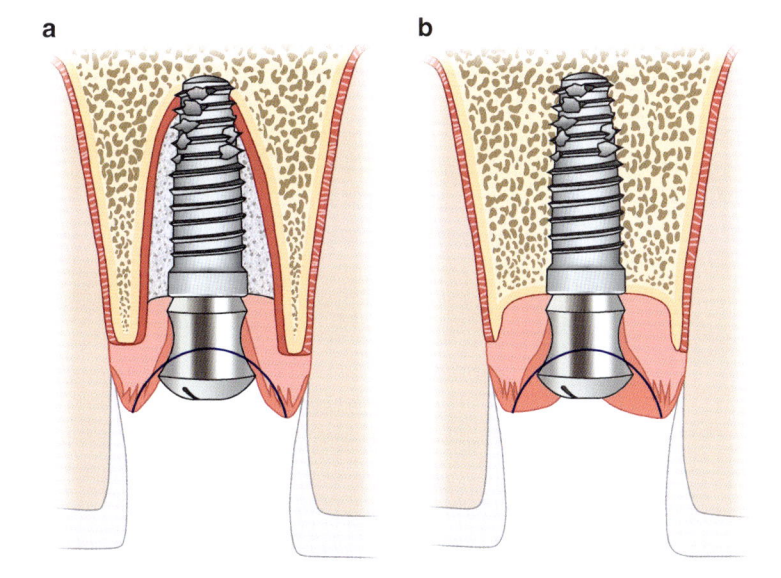

Following the osseointegration period, *a second-stage surgery* takes place. There are three options following the cover screw removal:

1. Placement of a healing abutment, which can have the dimensions close to those of the emergence profile of the definitive crown (slightly under-contoured), is the case when no flap is raised (enough soft tissue volume). In any other case (split thickness flap, additional subepithelial connective tissue grafting), a smaller or concave healing abutment is preferred.
2. Placement of a provisional abutment, which can be under-contoured in order to gradually achieve the optimal emergence profile as described in 1.1.
3. Placement of a final abutment, providing the definitive emergence profile contour as described in 1.2., is not always possible due to the closed healing and the fact that the

clinician cannot define the exact transmucosal contour of the future rehabilitation.

The following sequence of steps has been proposed in order to surpass the aforementioned difficulties (Pelekanos et al. 2013) (see Case 18.2 and Videos 18.3 and 18.4):

- Implant registration is performed directly after placement.
- Using an impression coping with low-shrinkage resin.
- Using digital impression of the implant head.
  - A cast containing the implant analog is fabricated.
  - After the osseointegration period, a full arch impression is made, including the edentulous space, to register the soft tissue contours of the healed ridge.
- The new soft tissue contours are transferred to the first implant cast with the use of a silicone key.
- The ideal labiogingival contour is marked according to the wax-up and neighboring teeth. A high-speed handpiece with a diamond bur is used to form an ideal transmucosal contour around the implant analog. This procedure does not differ from the one that is described in paragraph 1.2. It is a prerequisite for the implant to be place according to the basic rules as described in paragraph 1. Care should be taken to ensure the profile is under-contoured labially, starting almost parallel at the first 2 mm of the implant-abutment margin. In this manner, the abutment does not exert excessive pressure on the future overlaying soft tissue, and any possible gingival recession is reduced. The incisal part should diverge following the ideal emergence profile of the clinical crown. The mesial and distal transmucosal contours are designed customized in each case according to the distance of the implant head to the bony peaks of the adjacent roots (at least 2 mm) to avoid bone resorption and future papilla loss. This precaution refers to the first 2–3 mm above to the implant head that is usually placed subcrestally mesially and distally and can be evaluated only by a periapical radiograph. The prosthetic crown margin of the abutment should not extend more than 0.5–1.0 mm in the sulcus, thus protecting the flow of the cement into the sulcus in case on an intraoral cementation.
- A customized abutment usually made of zirconia or lithium disilicate is fabricated.
- In cases where an implant is placed closer than 2 mm to the neighboring teeth, a titanium prefabricated abutment (mesio-structure) is then indicated using platform switching and in a concave profile. The customization can follow in a higher level (2 mm)
- Uncovery consists of an incision offset palatally. The incision provides access to the implant platform without significant alteration of the soft tissue architecture.
- The customized abutment is placed one time with final torque without any further removal. A provisional crown is inserted.
- After soft tissue maturation, a final impression of the abutment is made using either soft tissue retraction with cord or pickup impression with a prefabricated coping. When using cord, the clinician should be gentle in order to avoid distraction of the soft tissue adherence around the abutment.
- The definitive crown is then either cemented intraoral (cement-retained restoration) or extraoral with one abutment removal and then screw retained onto the implant. The latter requires accurate positioning of the implant in order for the screw axis to meet the palatal or lingual surface of the crown. A hole to the final crown, for the screw insertion, is required (see also Case 18.4 and Video 18.8).

18.3.2 Immediate vs. Delayed Implant Placement

Following an extraction, the clinician faces the dilemma of placing an implant either immediately (type I) or delayed (types II, III) from 6 weeks up to 3 months (Chen et al. 2004). According to the literature, implant survival is not compromised by either choice (Chen et al. 2004). The principal parameters influencing this decision are bone quality, bone and soft tissue deficiency, the location of the implant, and last but not least clinicians' expertise.

18 The Single Implant-Crown Complex in the Aesthetic Zone

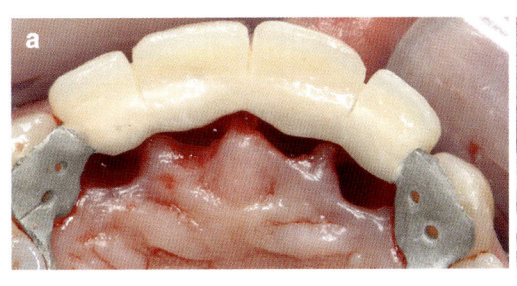

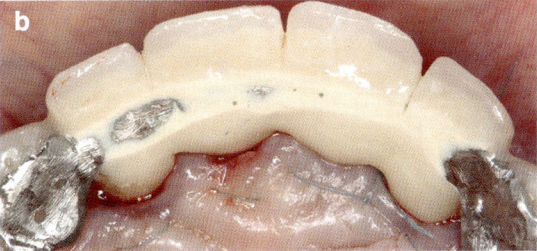

Fig. 18.9 (**a**, **b**) Extraction of four upper incisors. "Prosthetic socket preservation"

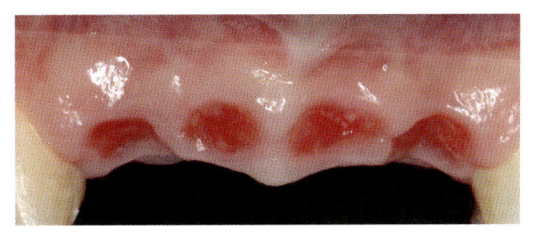

Fig. 18.11 Three weeks post-op

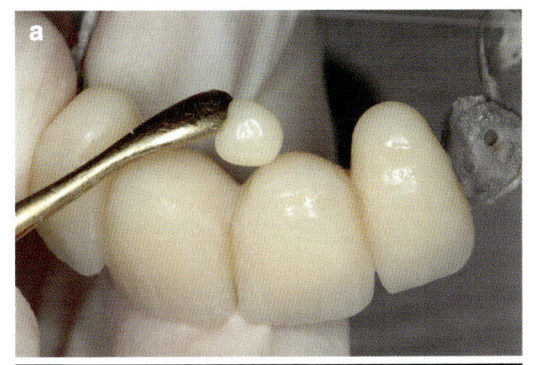

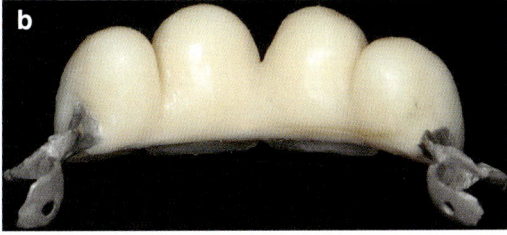

Fig. 18.10 (**a**, **b**) Shaping the pontic area by adding composite

Upon *delayed implant placement*, the uneventful wound healing is of utmost importance. The protection of the blood clot and the buccal bone plate can be supported by various surgical and prosthetic techniques. The term "socket preservation" usually used in the last years is probably inaccurate regarding its meaning. Surgically collagen sponge insertion into the extraction socket and the use of xenografts with or without free gingival grafts being the most popular could help to reduce bone resorption that will happen anyway regardless the procedure followed. Furthermore, prosthetically attention should be given regarding the pontic shape of the provisional especially in the aesthetic zone. An apically extended composite or acrylic bulk, positioned on the cervical side of the provisional, should cover the exact size of the socket, protecting the blood clot and thus inducing healing and meanwhile guiding the soft tissue regeneration ("prosthetic socket preservation") (Figs. 18.9a, b, 18.10a, b and 18.11).

After a delayed implant placement, the type of loading should be chosen (immediate vs. delayed). The steps regarding both procedures are mentioned in detail in part A.

18.3.3 Final Crown Reconstruction

The definitive implant crown can be categorized according the retention type, the material being made of, and the customization of the abutment. The single implant crown can be screw retained directly into:

- The implant
- A mesio-structure (prefabricated abutment) usually made out of metal (titanium)
- An abutment with horizontal screw
- The implant with screw access change

The crown can also be cement retained on a customized or a prefabricated abutment (straight or angled) made out of metal (titanium) or ceramics (zirconia, alumina, lithium disilicate, or feldspathic

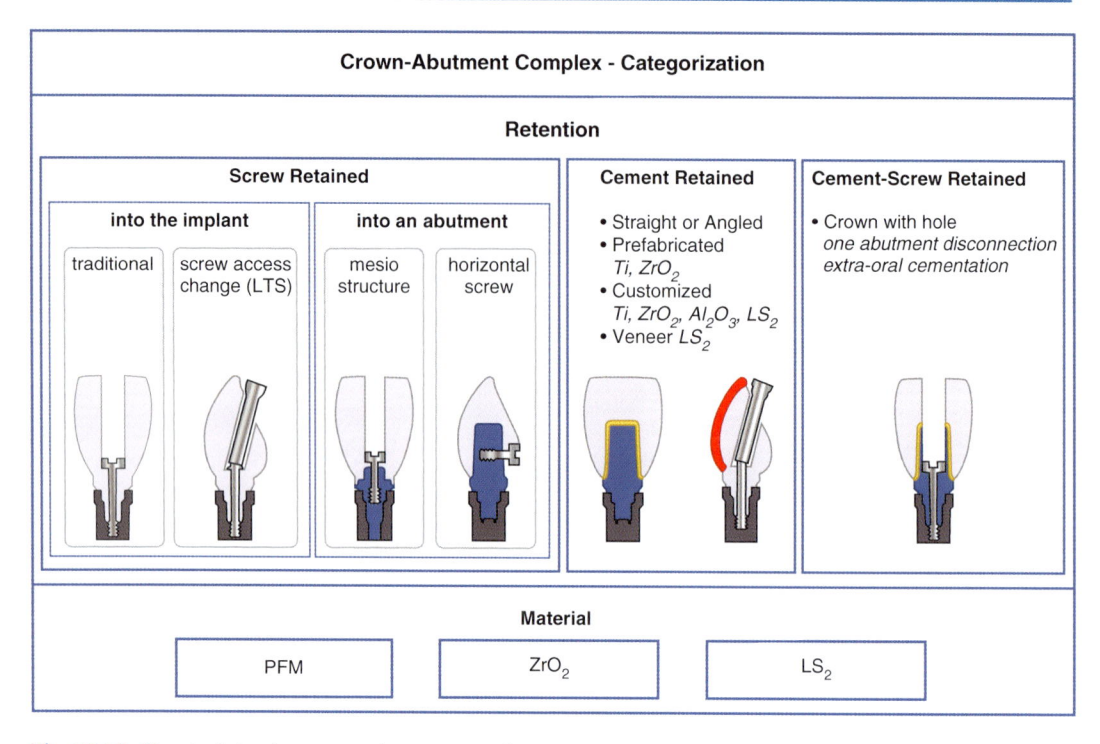

Fig. 18.12 The single implant crown-abutment complex

ceramic). Regarding the material, an implant crown in the aesthetic zone can be made out of PFM, zirconia, or lithium disilicate (e-max) (Fig. 18.12).

18.3.3.1 Cement- or Screw-Retained Implant Restorations

Cement-retained restorations, although might seem easier regarding the manufacturing procedures, can pose a critical disadvantage. Cement removal cannot be controlled after the cementation procedure given the anatomy of the abutment (concave areas) and the difference in the quality and quantity of peri-implant soft tissues (Agar et al. 1997). In a recent prospective study, excess cement was associated with peri-implant disease (Wilson 2009). In any case when an implant crown has to be cemented intraorally, it is mandatory a small retraction cord to be placed in the peri-implant sulcus protecting the cement penetration and facilitating an easy excess removal.

On the other hand, *screw-retained implant restorations* have become increasingly popular in the recent years as a method to overcome the problems associated with the cement overflow and providing accessibility to the implant platform whenever required. It is a prerequisite that the axial inclination of the implant should meet the palatal or lingual surface of the clinical crown, making the use of surgical guide stents a very important step. If the implant axis has an inclination of more than 15°, there is always a possibility to fabricate a screw-retained restoration by using a *small horizontal palatal or lingual screw* (Figs 18.13a, b and 18.14). Attention should be paid in the direction of the screw access in order for the clinician to be able to screw and unscrew the restoration.

Providing the fact that even in the hands of qualified and meticulous surgeons, in a large number of cases, the implant axis meets the incisal edge of the crowns, there is often a need of 10–12° angle correction. Usually most of the implant companies start with angulated abutments of 15°. Some companies (LTS, Nobel Biocare) provide special abutments and screw drivers that facilitate screw retention in the given angulation (10–12°), shifting palatal (or lingual) the screw access hole (see Case 18.5).

As previously mentioned in paragraphs A and B, the "one time-one abutment" concept is preferred especially in the aesthetic zone minimizing the risk of microbiological penetration into the implant and reducing the risk of apical soft tissue

18 The Single Implant-Crown Complex in the Aesthetic Zone

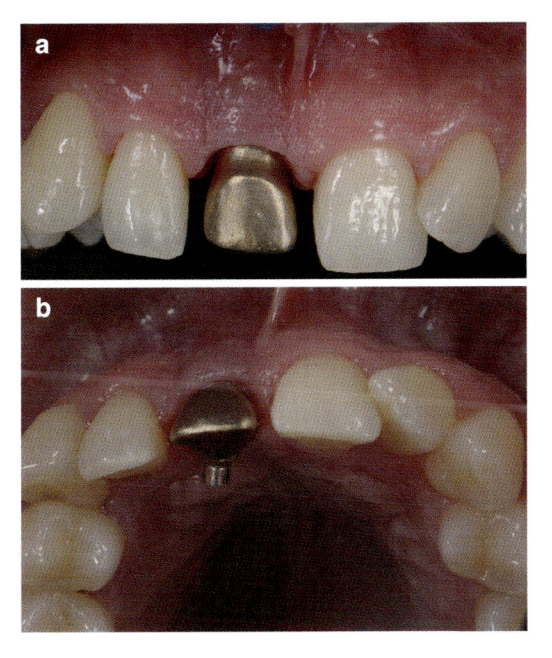

Fig. 18.13 (a, b) Fabrication of metal framework for the screw-retained final crown that contains a horizontal palatal screw access hole (labial and palatal view)

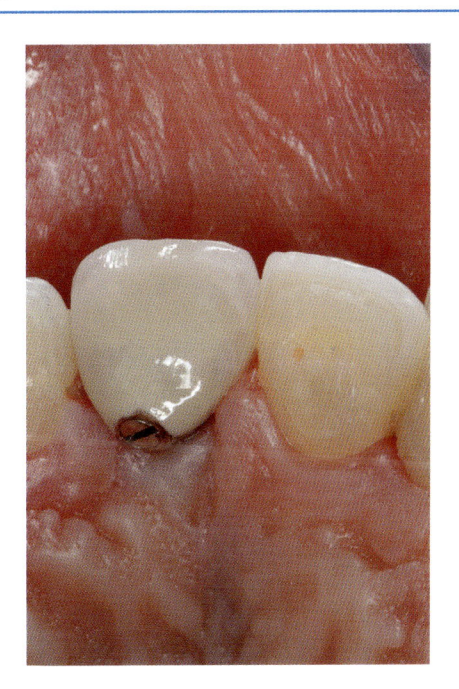

Fig. 18.14 The final crown is screw retained on the implant abutment through the horizontal screw (occlusal view)

gingival morphology - biotype		flat			scalloped			thick	thin
implant inclination		ideal	non-ideal		ideal	non-ideal			
			>15°	<15°		>15°	<15°		
retention	Cemented crown	prefabricated	✓	✓						
		customized	✓	✓		✓	✓	✓		
	Cemented veneer	customized	✓	✓	✓	✓	✓	✓		
	screw retained	into implant	✓		angle correction(2)	✓		angle correction(2)		
		into abutment	✓	horizontal screw		✓	horizontal screw			
	cement-screw retained		✓		angle correction(2)	✓		angle correction(2)		
abutment material		✓	Ti (>35°)	-	-	Ti (>35°)	-	Ti ZrO$_2$, LS$_2$	ZrO$_2$, LS$_2$
platform switching		Strongly indicated when implant-adjacent tooth distance < 1.5 mm							

(1) extra-oral cementation of crown with screw access hole
(2) LTS abutments / Dynamic abutments

Fig. 18.15 A prosthetic decision tree for the implant-abutment crown selection in the aesthetic zone

displacement (reduction of connection and disconnection of abutments). If such an abutment is already connected to the implant and the implant inclination allows the cementation to be performed outside of the mouth disconnecting the permanent abutment just one time, the removal of the excess cement can then easily and safely be performed, and the whole abutment-crown complex is transformed to a screw-retained restoration (cemented-screw-retained restoration (See Case 18.4).

In Fig. 18.15, below, a decision chart is made in order for the clinician to be able to select the proper abutment-crown design and material according to the case. The choice is differentiated according the gingival morphology and biotype (flat, scalloped, thick, thin), the implant inclination (ideal, nonideal >15° and nonideal<15°), and the implant proximity to the neighboring teeth-supporting bone (>1.5 mm, 1.5 mm).

The high scalloping of the soft and hard tissue usually seen in the aesthetic zone, in combination with higher aesthetic demands, makes the use of customized abutments almost obligatory when a cemented crown is chosen.

There are only two options where a prefabricated implant abutment can be chosen in the aesthetic zone. In cases with a flat gingival morphology, a prefabricated straight or angled abutment can be chosen combined with a cemented crown. But usually natural scallop of bone between midfacial and interproximal bone of maxillary anterior teeth varies from 2.1 to 4.1 mm (average 3 mm) (Becker et al. 1997). Taking that into consideration when a rough to the top implant is used, the implant platform can be sometimes located ≥4 mm subcrestally mesiodistally. In such cases, a cement retained or even a screw retained at the implant level restoration would jeopardize the bone stability around the implant neck. The close proximity of the implant (<2 mm) to the neighboring tooth (bone) further complicates the decision-making. According to the author in such cases, the combination of the following treatment steps could be beneficial for the hard and soft tissue stability:

- The use of a screw-retained crown on a 2 mm high prefabricated "intermediate" abutment (mesio-structure).
- The use of the above mentioned abutment "one time" so there would be no hard tissue irritation which could have a negative effect on the peri-implant gingival margin position.
- The combination of the above mentioned abutment with a screw-retained restoration (with customized emergence profile).
- The use of a platform-switching concept in combination with a customized abutment

("immediate intermediate" abutment concept) would minimize the bone and soft tissue resorption (Fig. 18.16a, b).

It should be emphasized that the abovementioned concept can be beneficial in cases where the implant is placed deep subcrestally (≥4 mm) in a mesiodistal direction and at the same time in a close proximity to the neighboring teeth (≤2 mm).

In the following clinical example, some steps are illustrated in a first premolar area (Figs. 18.17, 18.18, 18.19, 18.20, and 18.21).

18.3.3.2 Platform Switching: When Is Needed?

Platform switching to minimize peri-implant bone loss still seems to be a controversial issue in the literature (Romanos and Javed 2014). However, in a systematic review and meta-analysis showed that platform switching may preserve inter-implant bone height and soft tissue levels. The extent of the implant-abutment mismatch seems to determine the degree of the bone resorption (Atieh et al. 2010). These results were also confirmed in a randomized control trial (RCT) by Canullo et al. 2010. It is noteworthy that platform switching has to be differentiated in anterior and posterior areas due to the different anatomical conditions, like width of the bone and the flat gingival morphology, resulting in different outcomes and clinical relevance. So implant placement in wide ridges with a flat morphology do not significantly affect the buccal as well as the mesiodistal bone and soft tissue height whether a platform switching is performed or not.

In the aesthetic area, a very critical factor besides the buccal bone thickness around implants is the usually narrow spaces mesiodistally. Is was recommended to place the implant 1.5 mm from any adjacent tooth (Esposito 1993; Tarnow 2000). The high scalloping and the space limitations in the aesthetic zone further complicate the implant and abutment selection. It seems that the platform switching is mandatory when the implant-tooth distance is less than 1.5 mm (Vela et al 2012), and given the fact that implant-abutment connection is usually subcrestally in single implants, it is beneficial for the bone stability and the papilla preservation (Veis et al 2010).

18 The Single Implant-Crown Complex in the Aesthetic Zone

a

b

Fig. 18.16 (**a**, **b**) Immediate placement of a prefabricated abutment (mesio-structure) "one time before and after bone and soft tissue remodeling. Platform-switching and concave customized abutment design ("double concavity concept")

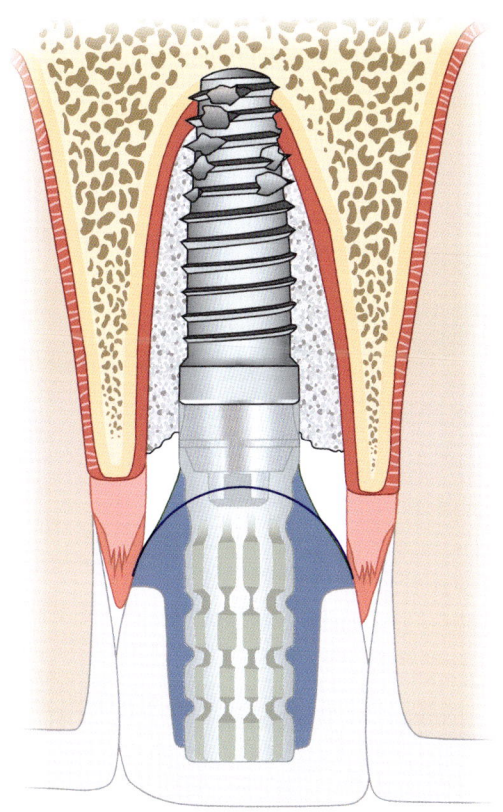

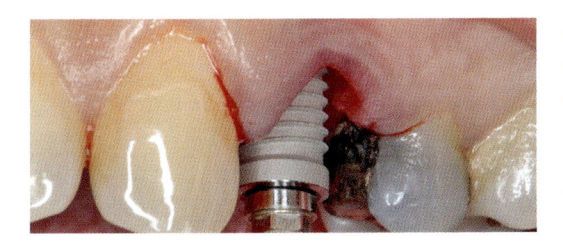

Fig. 18.17 Immediate implant placement (first upper premolar)

Since other factors such as function (micromovement of the implant-abutment junction), accurate 3D positioning of the implant (Grunder et al. 2005), and experienced prosthetic handling seem to be very critical for the hard and soft tissue stability as well, the combination of the platform switching with the "one abutment-one time" and the "double concavity" concept is highly recommended whenever possible (see Figs. 18.16, 18.17, 18.18, 18.19, 18.20, and 18.21).

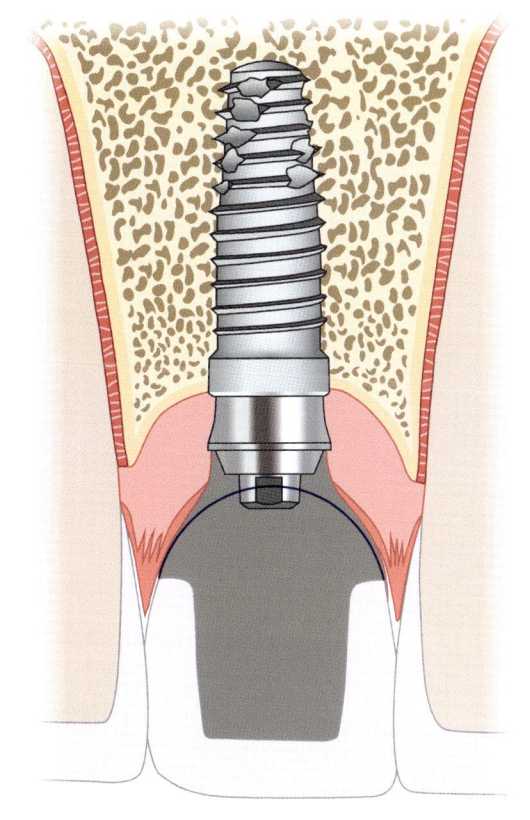

18.3.3.3 Metal or Ceramic Abutments

The choice of the abutment material is strictly guided by the gingival biotype and the implant angulation. With a thin biotype, a Zr or $LiSiO_2$ abutment would be preferable over the Ti abutment. The grayish color cannot be covered when the mucosal thickness is less than 2 mm (Jung et al. 2007).

On the other hand, Ti abutments were found to be beneficial in cases with a high unfavorable implant angulation (>35°) as they can be milled

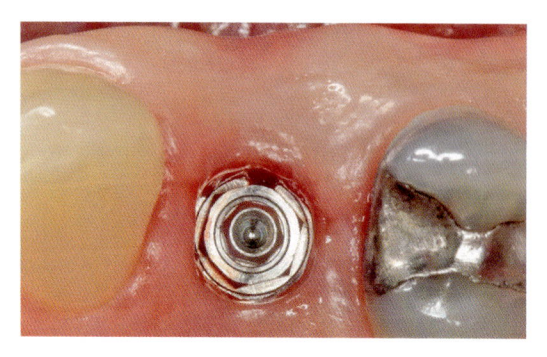

Fig. 18.18 Three months post-op after immediate "one time" prefabricated abutment placement

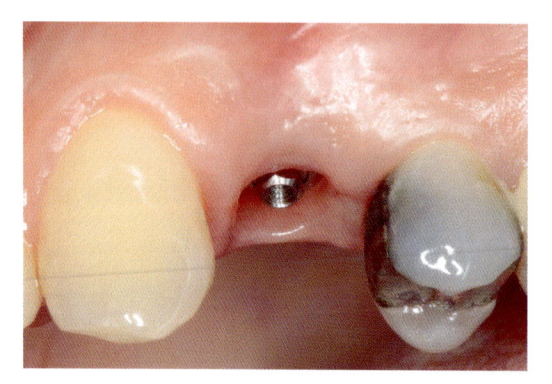

Fig. 18.19 Labial view

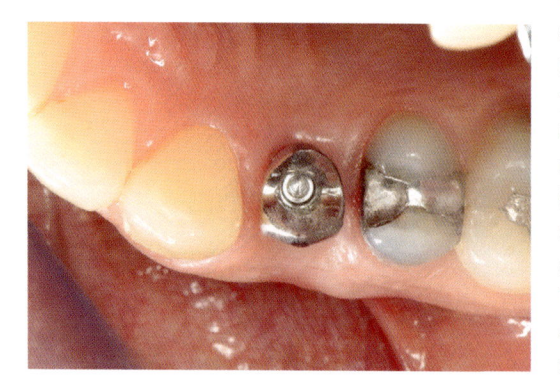

Fig. 18.20 Screw-retained mesio-structure try-in

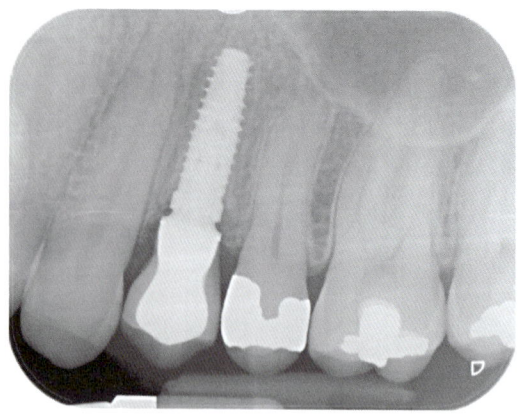

Fig. 18.21 Final screw-retained abutment showing the "immediate intermediate abutment concept" mesially (radiographic view)

in a small labial thickness in contrast to ceramic abutments (Fig. 18.15).

Comparing ceramic to metal abutments in a systematic review (Sailer et al. 2009), it appears that there is no difference in the long-term prognosis and survival rate (estimated 5 years 99.1% for ceramic abutments and 97.4% for metal abutments).

Regarding the stability of Zr and Ti abutment into the internal connection of the implant, it appears that when a Ti or Ti-base abutment is used, it might be beneficial in high loading (Leutert et al. 2012). On the Ti base, a ceramic abutment (Zr or LS_2) can be cemented with a dual-curing resin cement (see Case 18.6 and Video 18.15). The use of LiS_2 as an abutment which becomes more popular in recent years, is lucking long-term clinical and scientific evidence. According to the author's experience, there are two limitations in its use that have to be considered. The material itself is translucent, and sometimes the grayish appearance of the metal sleeve is shining through. The use of a more opaque dual-curing luting cement is indicated (i.e., multilink hybrid abutment cement, Ivoclar, Vivadent). Subsequently whenever LiS_2 is chosen as abutment material, it should be considered that the minimum strength according to the manufacturer's instructions is 0.6 mm, which is sometimes too much especially at the first 2 mm above the implant level in the mesiodistal aspect. Thus, careful case selection has to be performed for such abutments.

18.3.3.4 Digital Workflow in Aesthetic Single Implant Rehabilitation

The evolution in digital dentistry has allowed the use of intraoral scanners for capturing the emergence profile created. This must be done immediately after the removal of the provisional abutment to avoid size and shape changes due to the immediate soft tissue shrinkage (see Case 18.6, Video 18.12).

In the last case, an immediate implant is placed with open flap, and at the same time a GBR is performed. Due to satisfactory initial implant stability, a modified concave healing abutment was placed. Six months postoperative, the ideal emergence profile was created by means of a screw-retained implant provisional. After the digital impression of both the transmucosal contour and the implant (Bluecam, Sirona), the abutment was digitally formed in a reduced crown shape for cement-retained crown. A pre-crystalized lithium disilicate block (IPS e.max CAD, Ivoclar) with a pre-manufactured connection was chosen for the abutment fabrication. After the crystallization, this was luted, utilizing a dual-curing resin cement, to a titanium base with a pre-manufactured connection with perfect fit (Sirona). The whole prosthetic procedure of digital impression and abutment manufacturing is facilitated in a very precise and fast manner in the same day and is described with details in Case 18.6 and corresponding videos (Videos 18.12, 18.13, 18.14, 18.15, and 18.16).

Conclusion

The critical knowledge of both surgical and prosthetic procedures is required when a single implant is placed in the aesthetic zone. Minimizing the trauma and reducing the bone and soft tissue resorption are the ultimate goals of the treatment. Beside the implant choice, the accurate positioning, and the good management of the soft tissue, there are several prosthetic factors that influence the final outcome.

The prosthetic parameters determining the soft and the hard tissue stability around the implant-abutment connection are:

- The good interface seal between implant and abutment
- The reduced micro-movement of the abutment during function
- The distance between the abutment and the adjacent bone supporting the neighboring teeth
- The shape of the abutment
- The platform-switching concept when this is needed
- The selection of the proper design of the abutment-crown complex according to the case
- The standardized treatment workflow of the prosthetic procedures following a protocol (decision tree)

18.4 Clinical Cases

Case 18.1 Traditional approach of developing the transmucosal contour with a screw-retained provisional

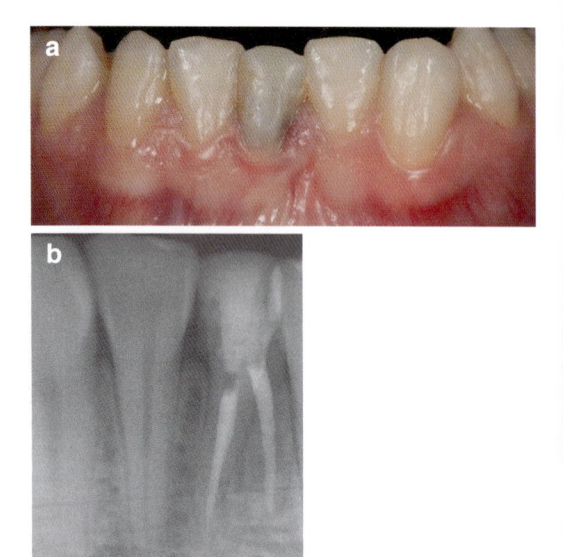

Fig. 18.22 (a, b) Upon initial clinical and radiographic evaluation, a vertical root fracture is diagnosed for the mandibular right central incisor

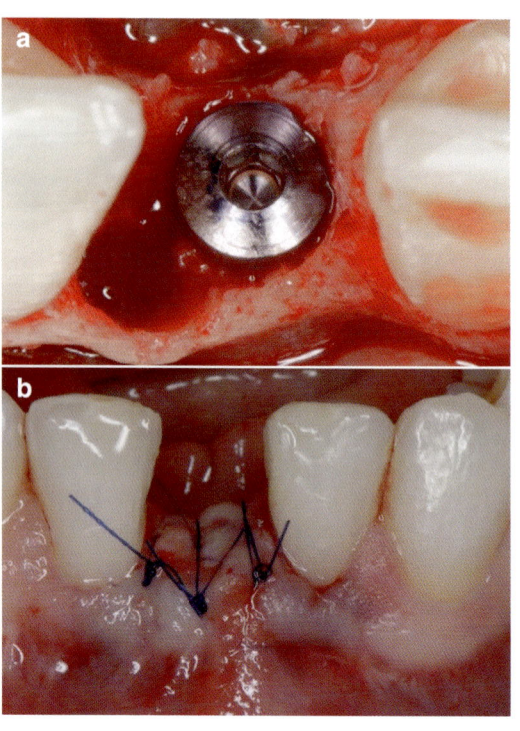

Fig. 18.23 (a, b) Immediate implant placement. The extraction socket is filled with xenograft and the flap is secured with a connective tissue graft

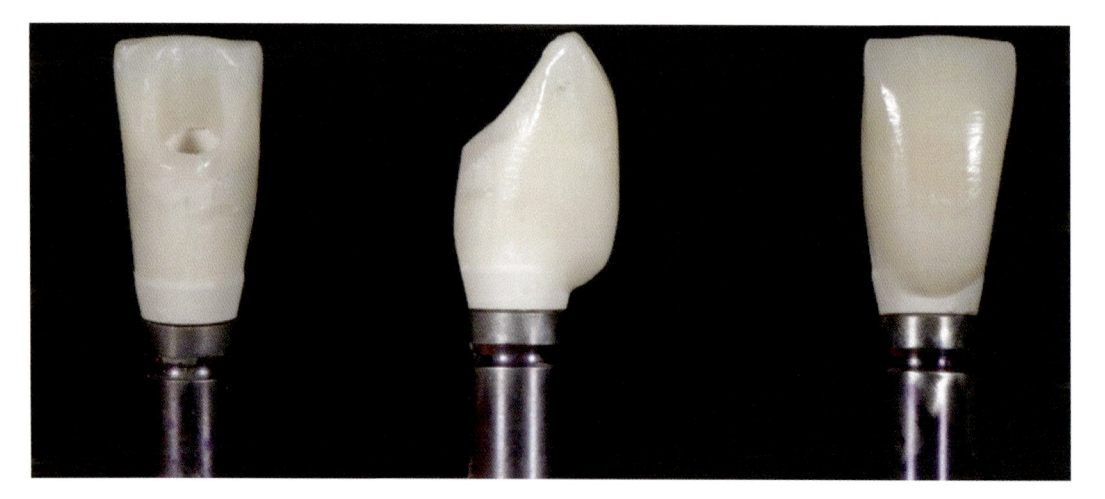

Fig. 18.24 The screw-retained provisional restoration is used for the emergence profile contouring by means of adding composite every 10 days

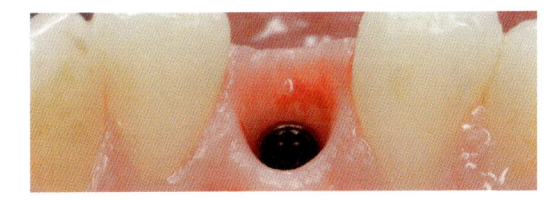

18 The Single Implant-Crown Complex in the Aesthetic Zone

Fig. 18.25 Achievement of the desired emergence profile

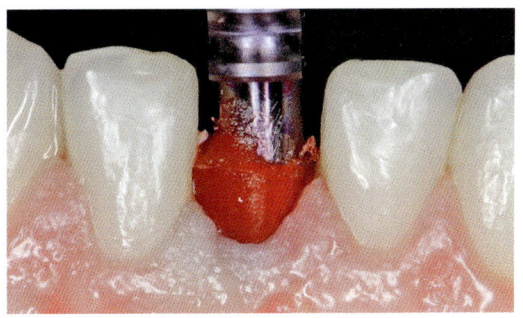

Fig. 18.26 Customization of the impression coping in order to transfer the achieved emergence profile to the final cast

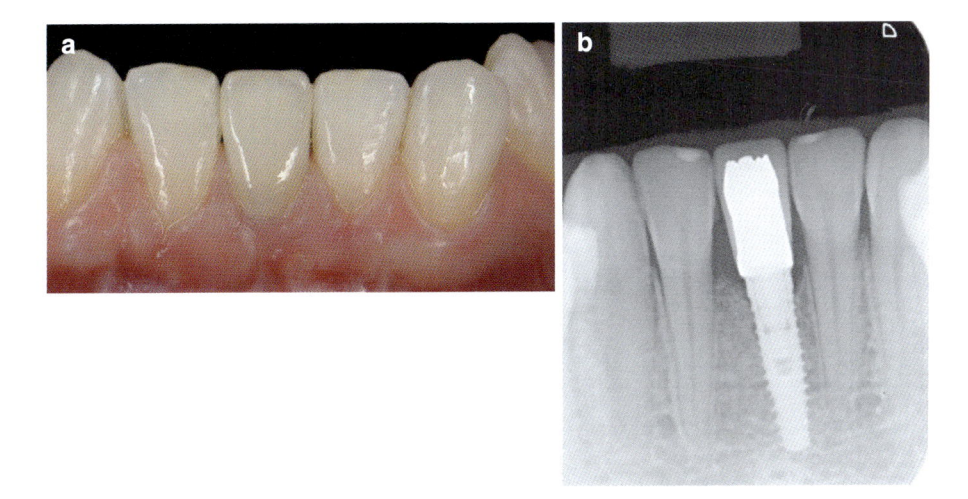

Fig. 18.27 (**a**, **b**) Final clinical and radiographic situation of the screw-retained crown

Case 18.2 Immediate definitive abutment connection at stage 2 surgery – "one abutment-one time"

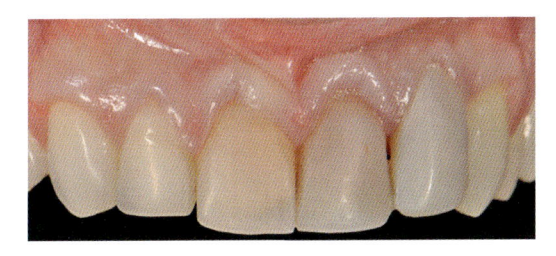

Fig. 18.28 Initial clinical situation

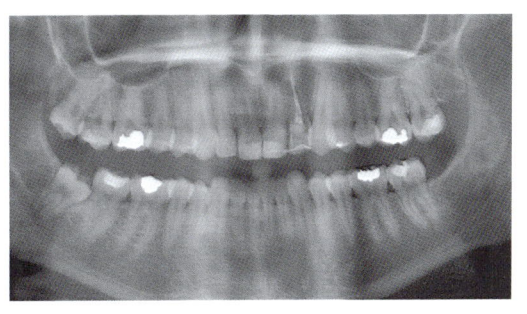

Fig. 18.29 Initial radiographic examination. The maxillary central incisors present periapical lesions, and the left lateral incisor presents root resorption

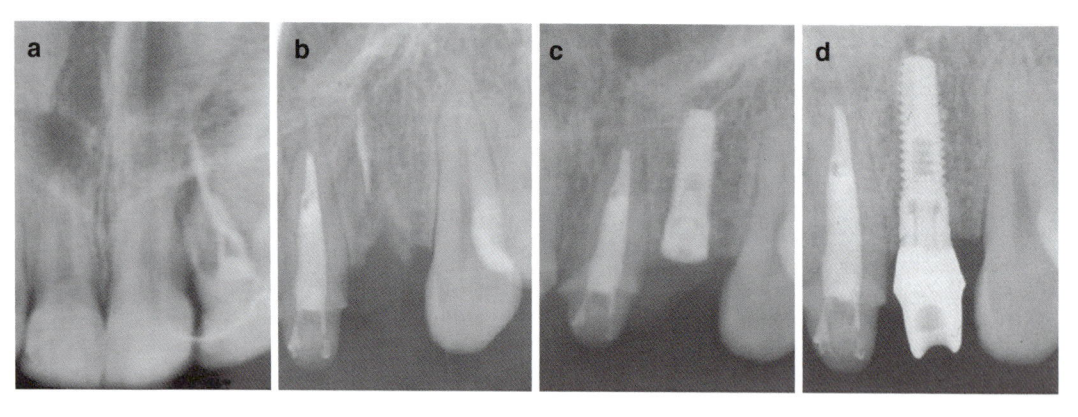

Fig. 18.30 (**a**) Initial clinical situation. Note the root resorption at the lateral incisor. (**b**) Extraction of the lateral incisor. (**c**) Implant placement, 2 months post-extraction. (**d**) Placement of the definitive abutment during second-stage surgery

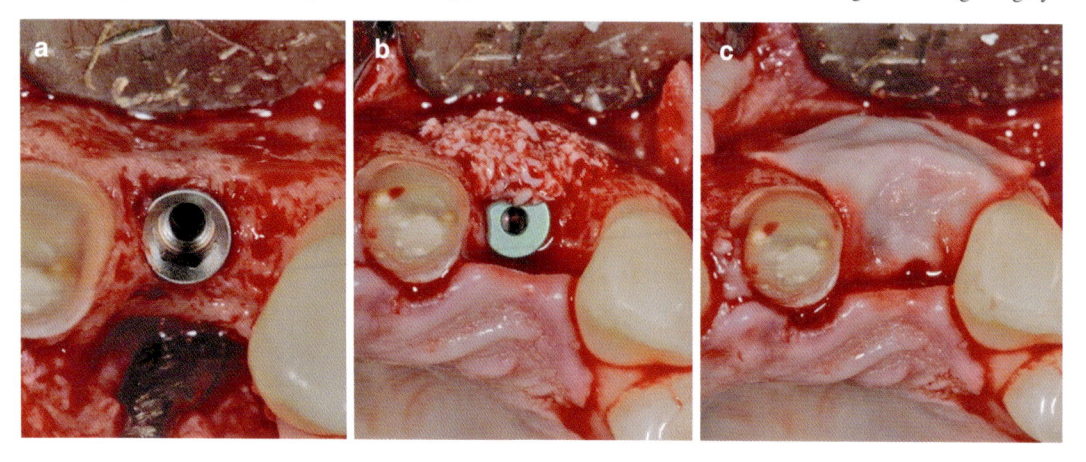

Fig. 18.31 (**a–c**) Implant placement. Due to the small thickness of the buccal bone (less than 2 mm), guided bone regeneration is performed with the use of a xenograft and a resorbable membrane

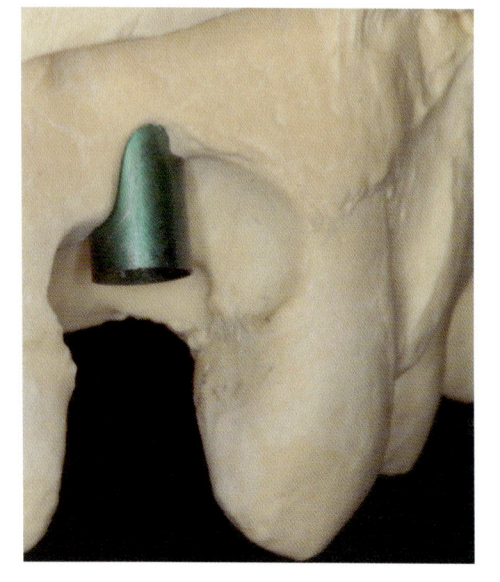

Fig. 18.32 The position of the implant is transferred to the initial cast with the use of a surgical stent. An implant analog is secured to this specific position

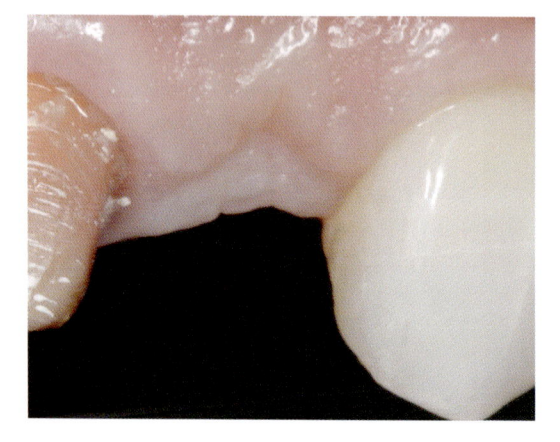

Fig. 18.33 Soft tissue maturation after the osseointegration period, *right* before second-stage surgery

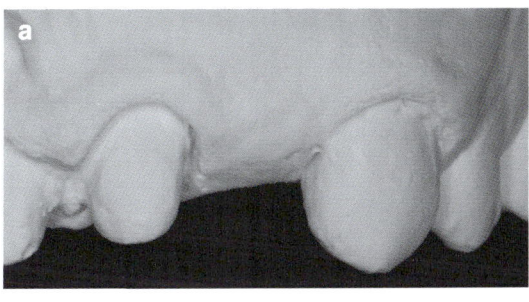

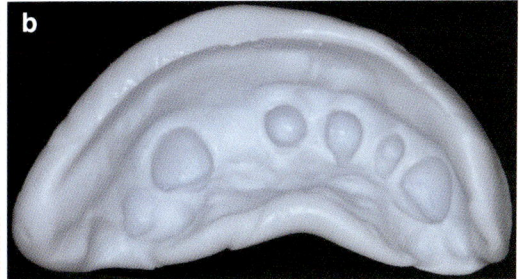

18 The Single Implant-Crown Complex in the Aesthetic Zone

Fig. 18.34 (**a, b**) The soft tissue morphology is registered with the use of a silicon index. This will be transferred to the initial cast with the use of gingival mask. The emergence profile will then be preprepared in order to customize the transmucosal contour in the laboratory

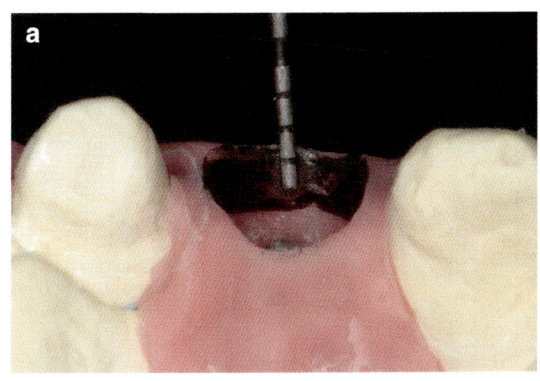

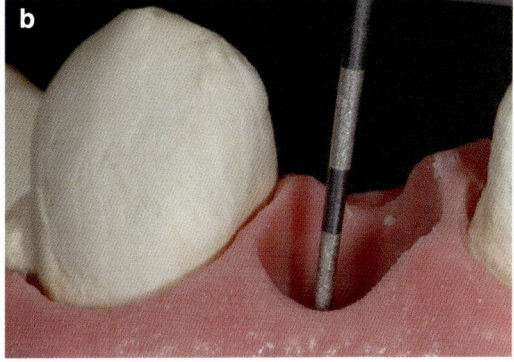

Fig. 18.35 (**a, b**) Customization of the transmucosal profile in the lab

Fig. 18.36 The metal sleeve in place after customization. The cast is scanned and the abutment is digitally designed and fabricated

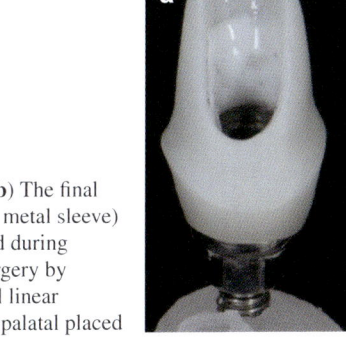

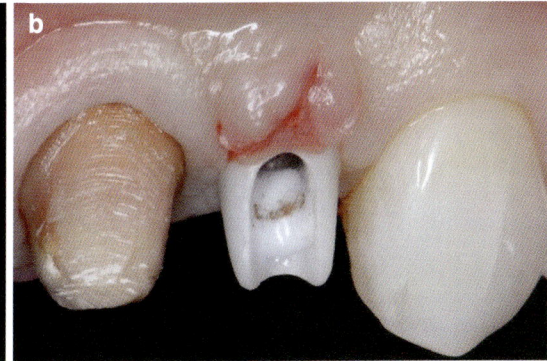

Fig. 18.37 (**a, b**) The final abutment (Zr on metal sleeve) that is positioned during second-stage surgery by means of a small linear incision slightly palatal placed

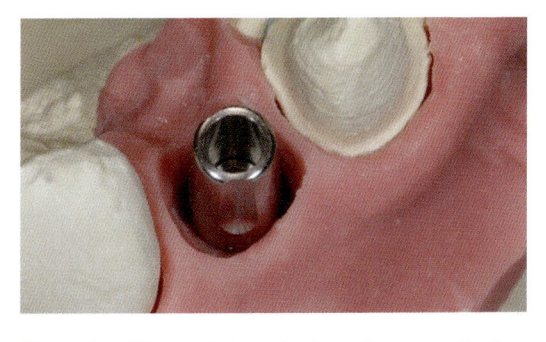

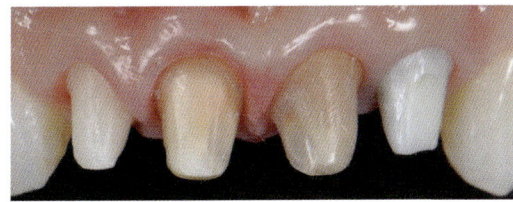

Fig. 18.38 Final preparations, 6 months after crown lengthening without further removal of the abutment

322   S. Pelekanos

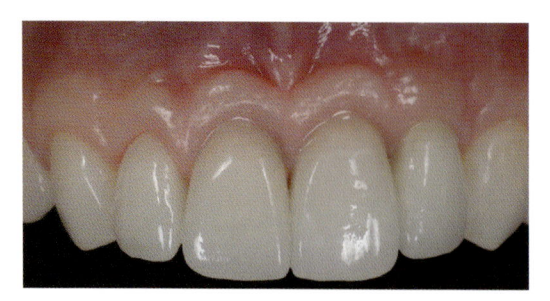

Fig. 18.39 Final clinical labial view of four single implant LS2 cemented crowns

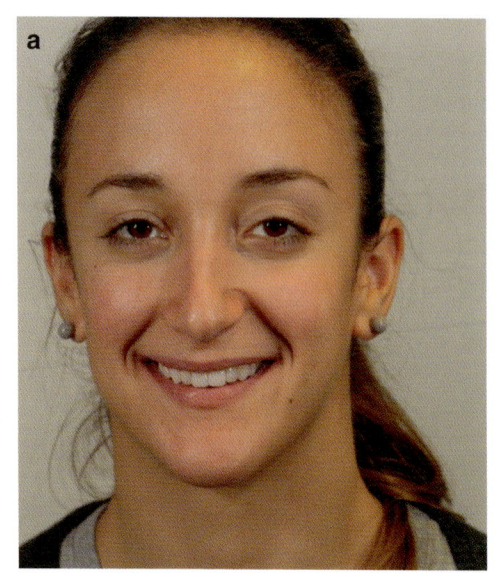

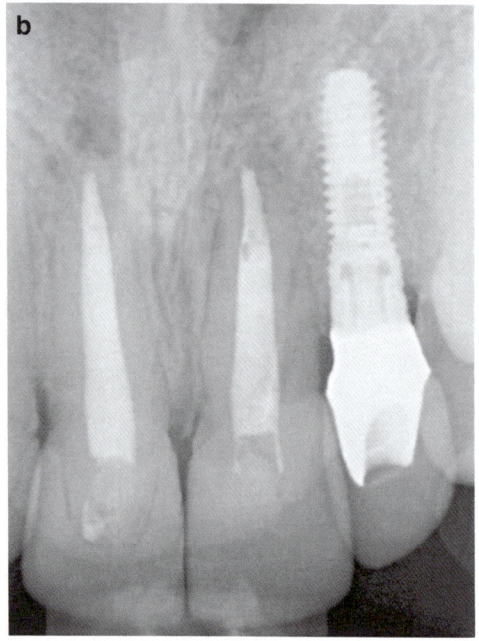

Fig. 18.40 (**a**, **b**) Smile and post-insertion radiographic

Case 18.3 Immediate implant placement combined with immediate definitive abutment connection

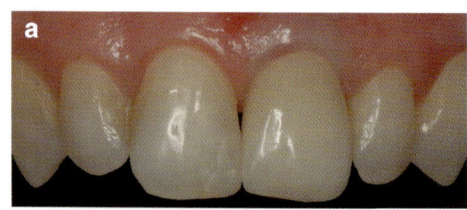

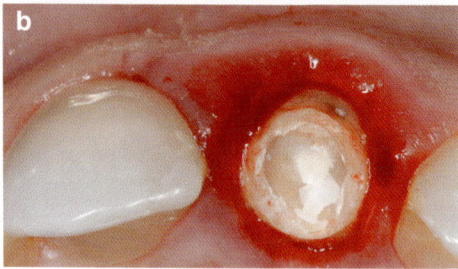

Fig. 18.41 (**a**, **b**) Initial clinical situation. Horizontal fracture of right lateral incisor

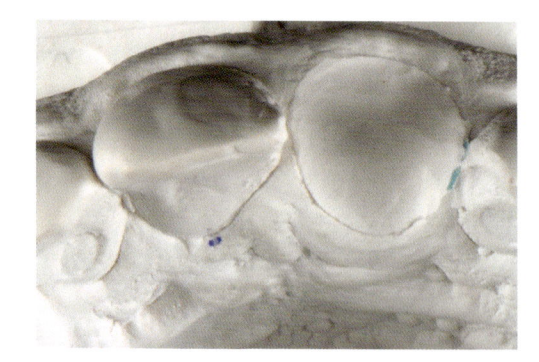

Fig. 18.42 Removal of the incisor on the cast

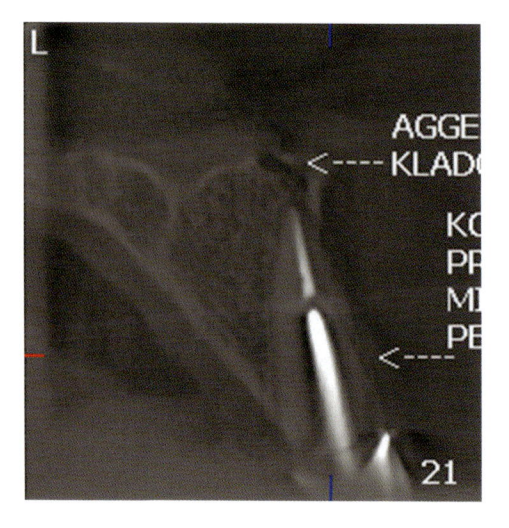

Fig. 18.43 Sagittal image from CBCT scan. Note the thin buccal bone plate

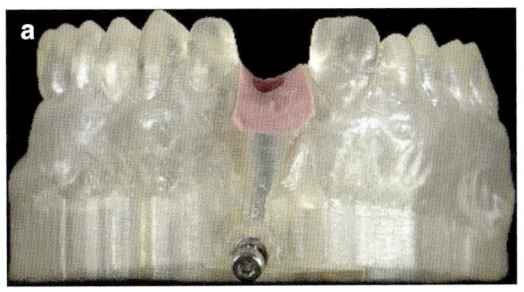

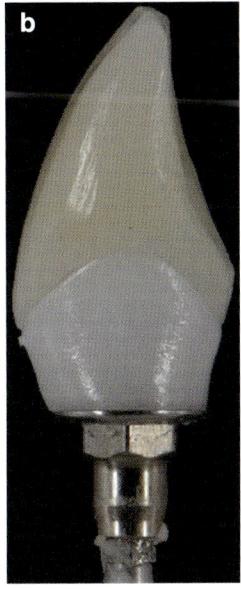

18 The Single Implant-Crown Complex in the Aesthetic Zone   323

Fig. 18.44 (**a**, **b**) After digital planning of the exact position of the implant, a stereolithographic cast (SimPlant, Materialise, Belgium) and the definitive abutment and provisional crown are fabricated

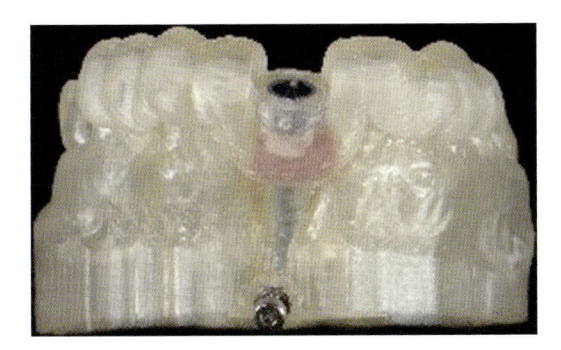

Fig. 18.45 The surgical guide stent (SimPlant, Materialise, Belgium)

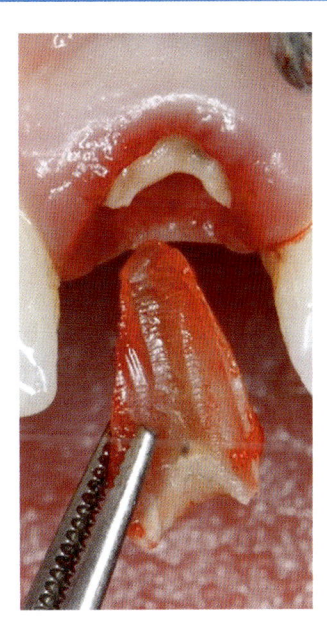

Fig. 18.46 The socket-shield technique (Huerzeler et al 2010) was utilized due to the thin buccal bone plate

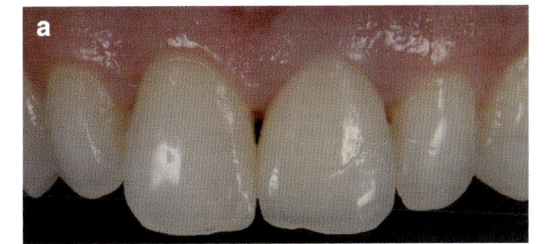

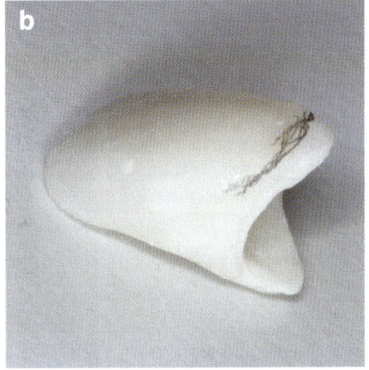

Fig. 18.47 (**a**, **b**) Clinical finding 3 months post-op. The cervical part of the provisional crown is altered to achieve a harmonic gingival outline

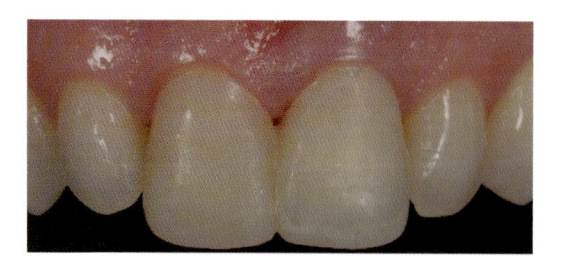

Fig. 18.48 Clinical appearance 6 months post-op. Splinted provisional (crown-veneer prep) of both central incisors

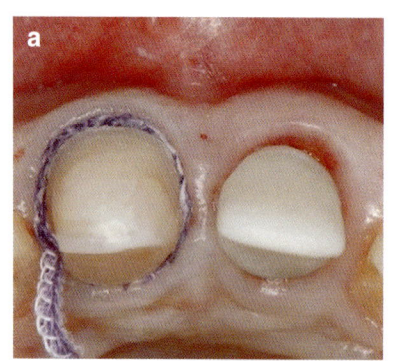

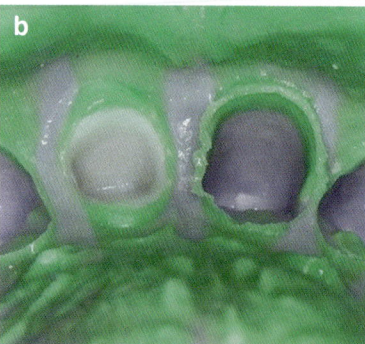

Fig. 18.49 (**a, b**) Veneer preparation of the right central incisor and final impression. Pickup impression using a lithium disilicate coping for the implant. The coping is fabricated from the preexisting STL file created to manufacture the abutment

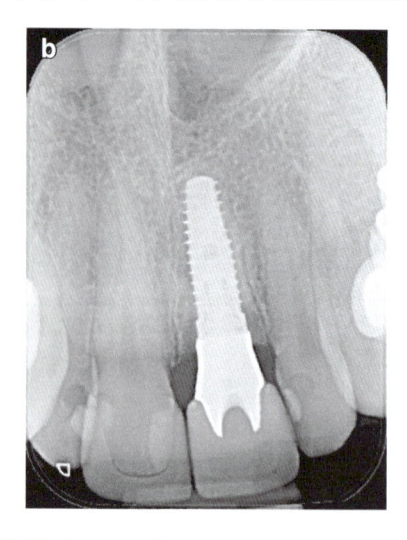

Fig. 18.50 (continued)

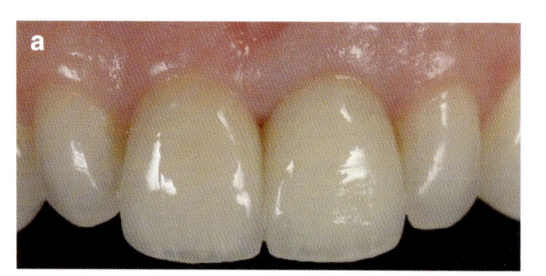

Fig. 18.50 (**a, b**) Final clinical (labial view) and radiographic situation

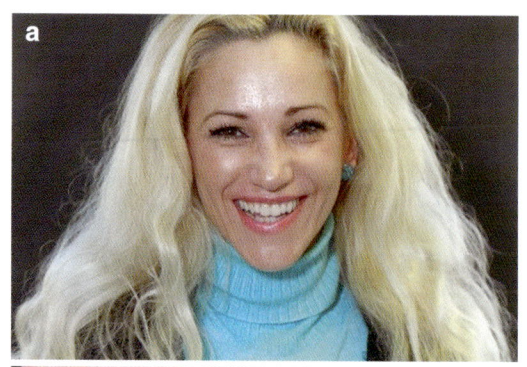

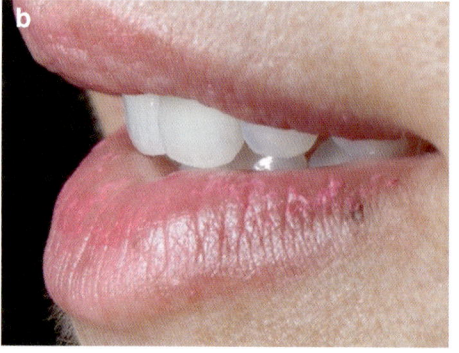

Fig. 18.51 (**a, b**) Face and lateral smile view

18 The Single Implant-Crown Complex in the Aesthetic Zone

Case 18.4 Immediate healing abutment connection combined with immediate implant placement

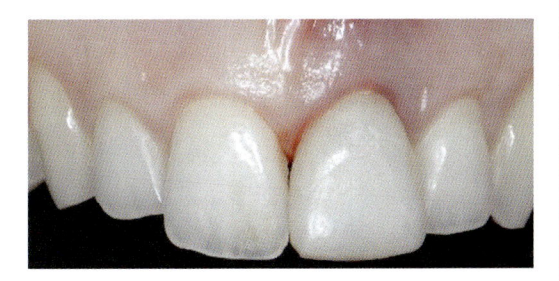

Fig. 18.52 Initial clinical situation

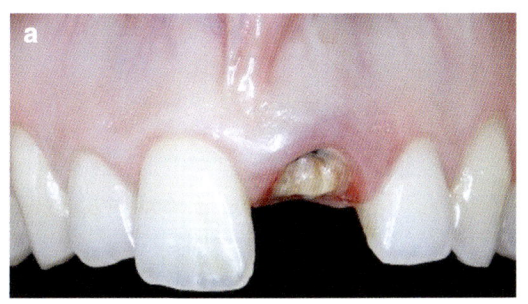

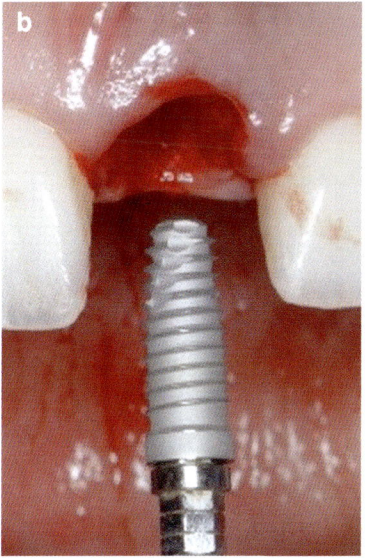

Fig. 18.53 (**a**, **b**) Inadequate amount of sound tooth structure. Tooth extraction and immediate implant placement

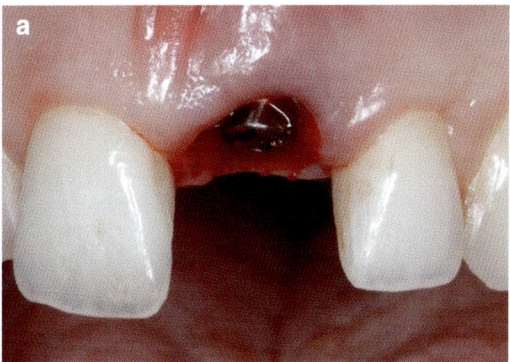

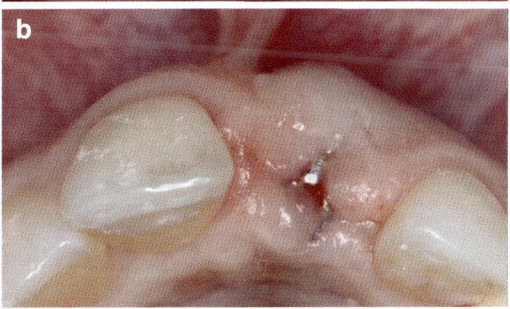

Fig. 18.54 (**a**, **b**) Clinical condition immediately (left) and 4 months post-op (right). Note the soft tissue growth around the concave healing abutment

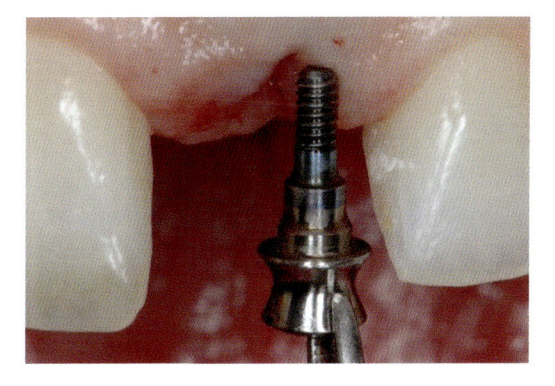

Fig. 18.55 Removal of the healing abutment, 4 months post-op

326 S. Pelekanos

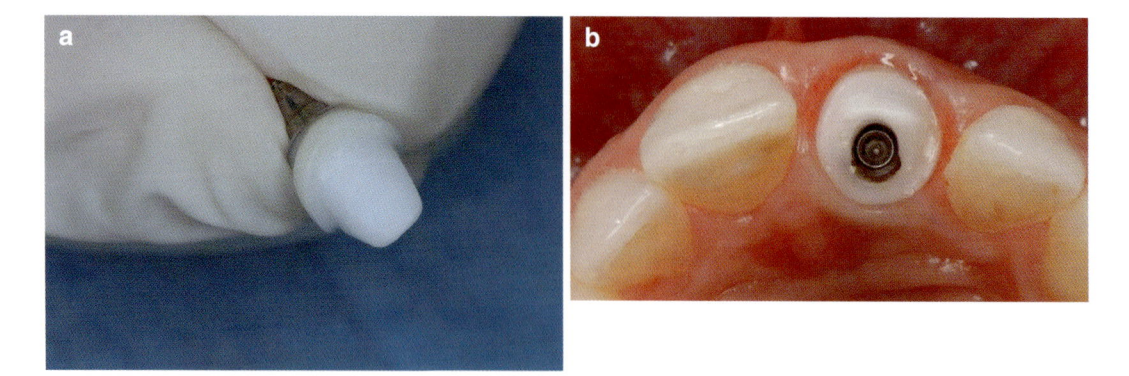

Fig. 18.56 (**a**, **b**) Fabrication of a zirconia final abutment luted on a metal sleeve and immediately inserted into the implant (no bacterial contamination into the implant)

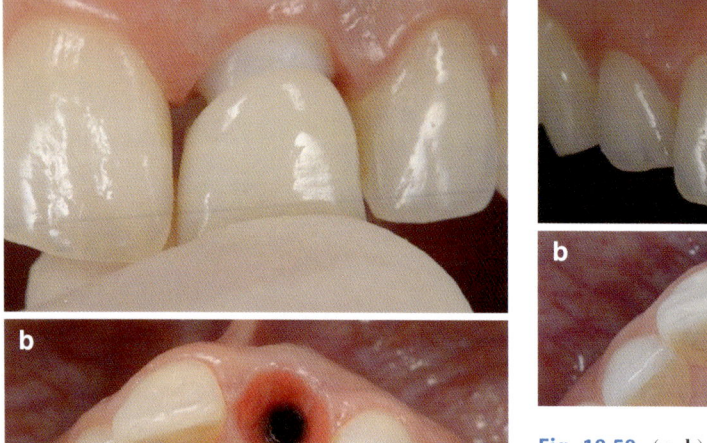

Fig. 18.57 (**a**, **b**) In order to avoid an intraoral cementation procedure and risk of excess cement remnants in the peri-implant tissues. The final abutment is removed once and the final crown is cemented with an extraoral technique. The restoration is screwed on the implant though an access hole that is prefabricated on the final crown

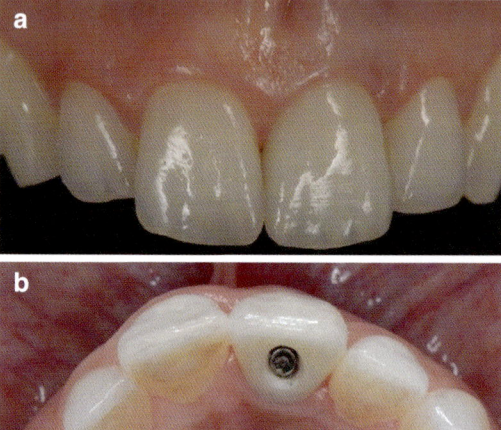

Fig. 18.58 (**a**, **b**) Final clinical appearance (labial and occlusal view)

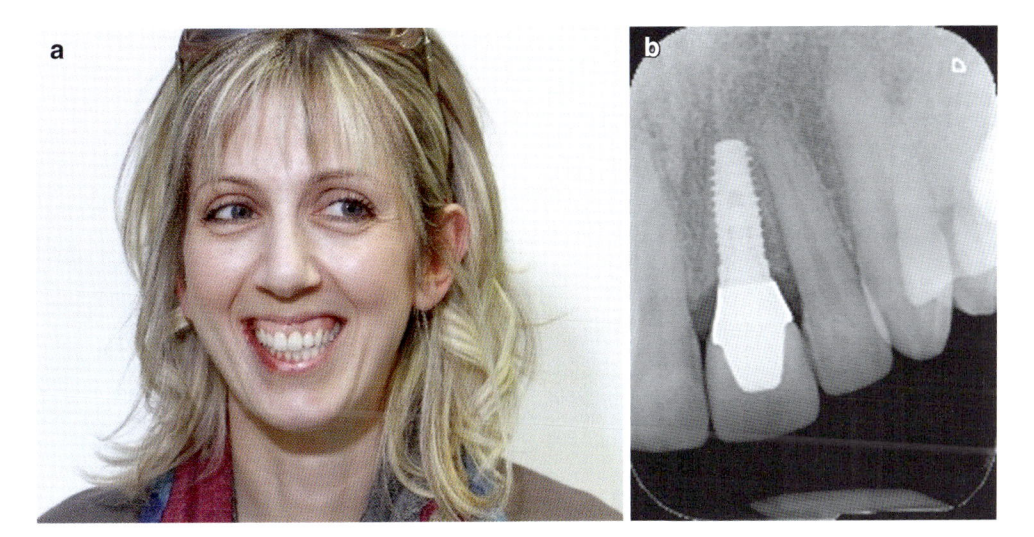

18 The Single Implant-Crown Complex in the Aesthetic Zone

Fig. 18.59 (**a, b**) Smile and final periapical radiograph

Case 18.5 Using an abutment with screw access correction

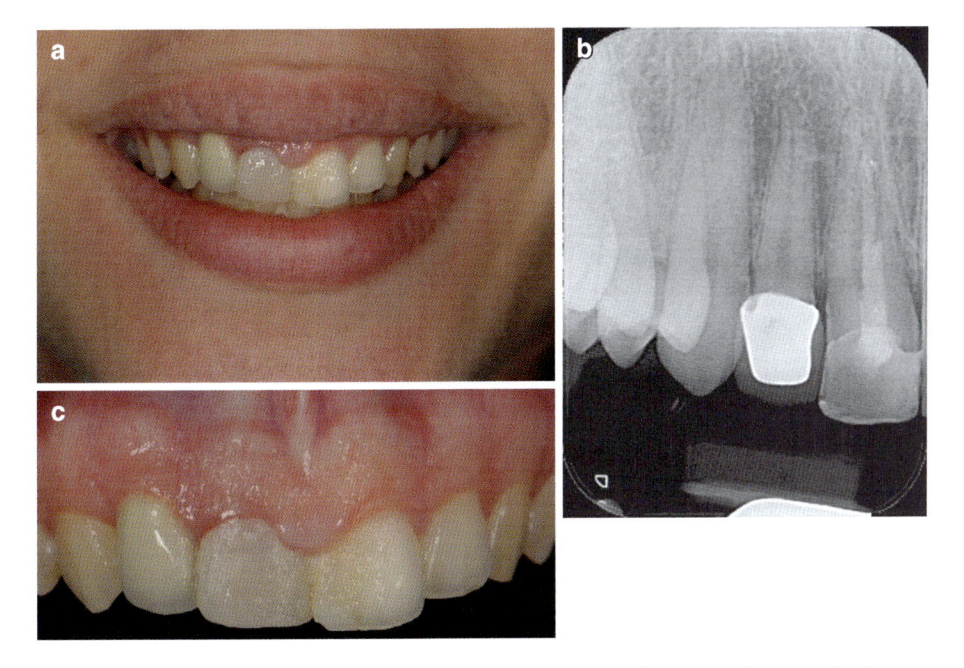

Fig. 18.60 (**a–c**) Initial clinical and radiographic situation. A vertical root fracture is diagnosed for the right central incisor. The tooth will be extracted

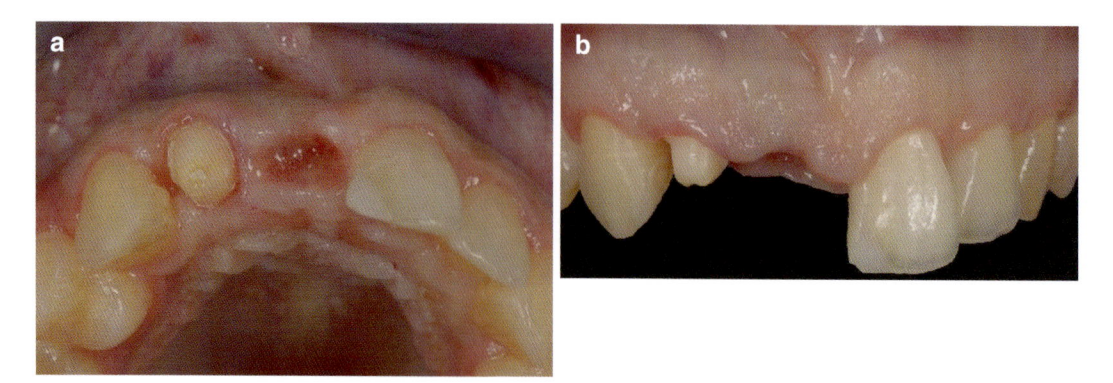

Fig. 18.61 (**a, b**) Clinical situation 1 month post-extraction

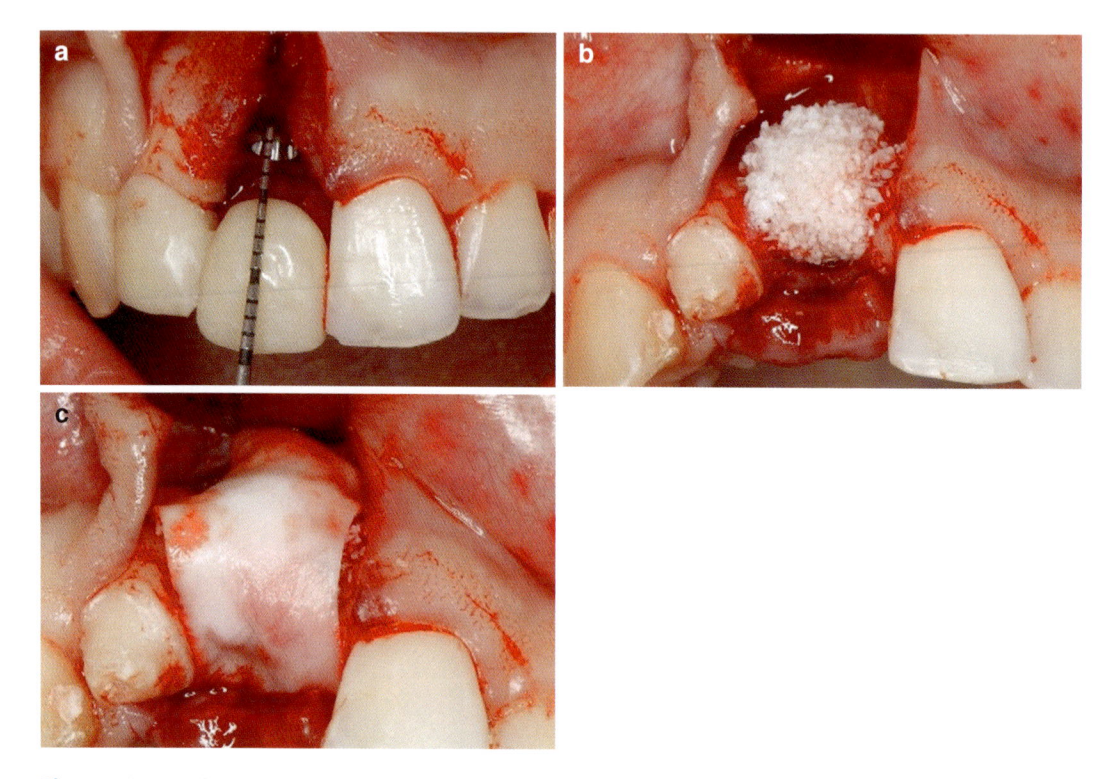

Fig. 18.62 (**a–c**) Implant placement and simultaneous guided bone regeneration due to the inadequate bone volume of the buccal plate

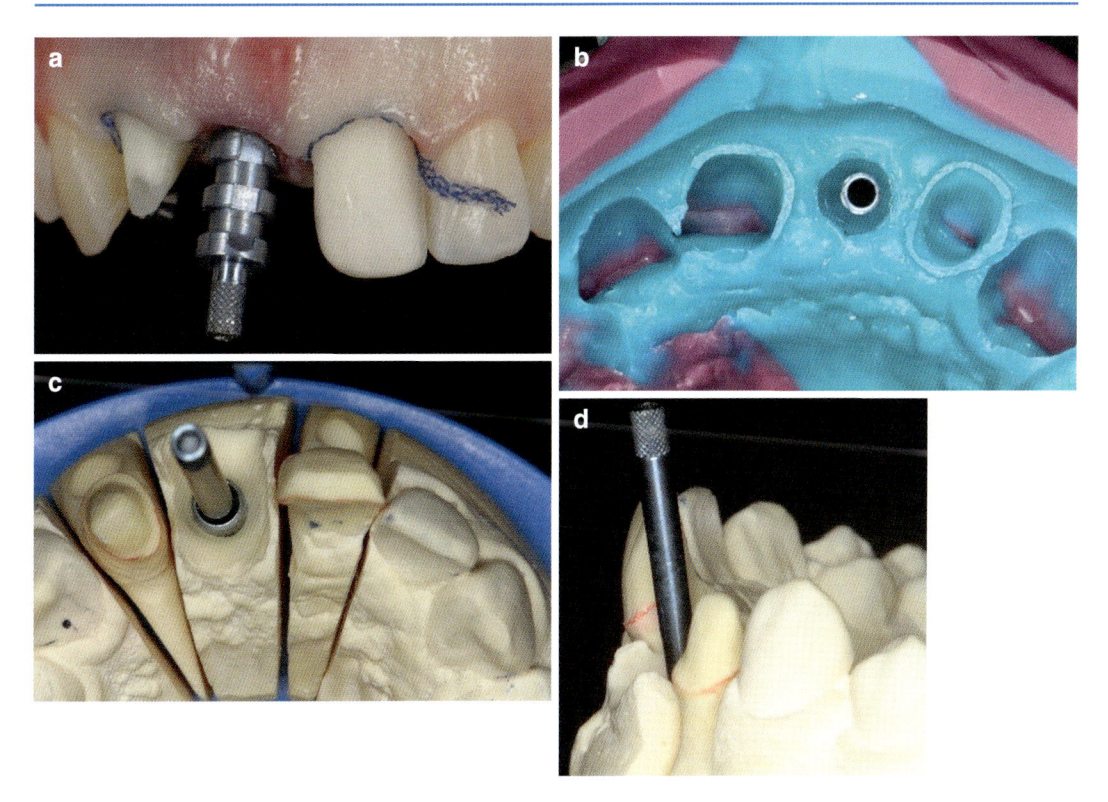

Fig. 18.63 (**a–d**) Final implant impression and fabrication of the study cast. The axis of the implant is unfavorable; however, it does not exceed 12°, making possible the use of a special abutment (LTS, Germany) in order to shift palatally the screw access hole

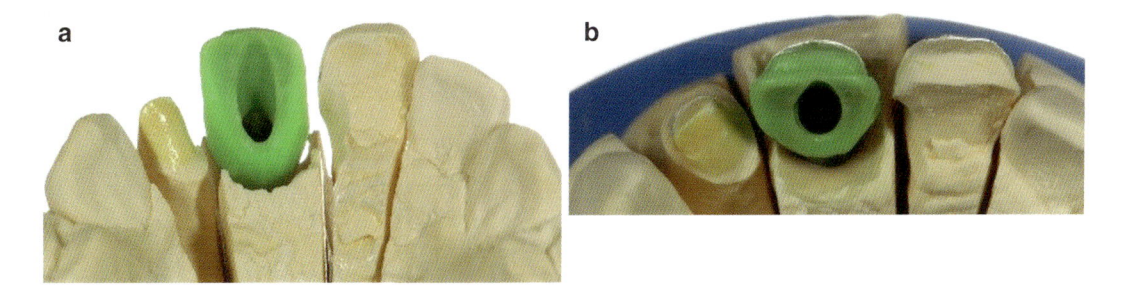

Fig. 18.64 (**a, b**) Waxing up of the implant crown. In order to achieve optimal color simulation, the wax-up is cut back in order to resemble to a veneer preparation, just like the adjacent teeth

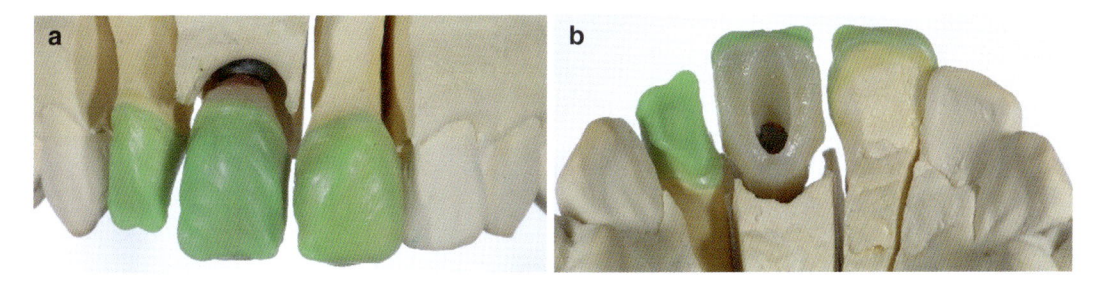

Fig. 18.65 (**a, b**) Wax-up of two veneers and an all-ceramic crown

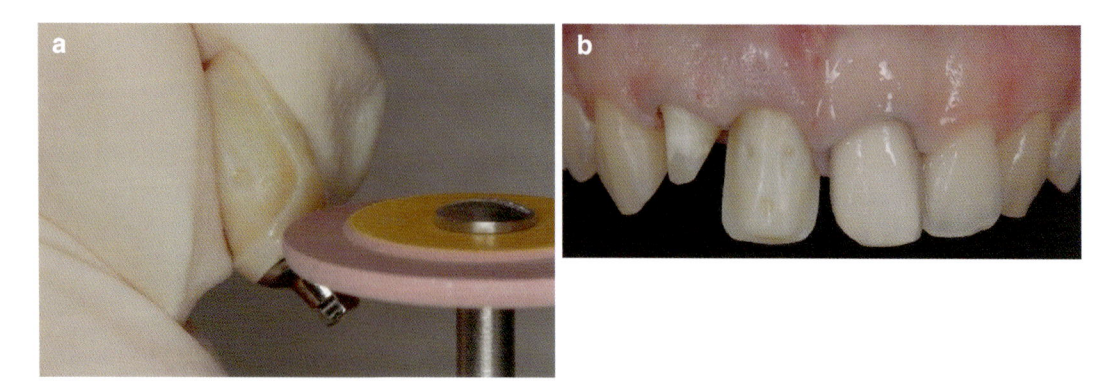

Fig. 18.66 (**a**, **b**) Polishing of the LS$_2$ implant abutment. And clinical view of the abutment

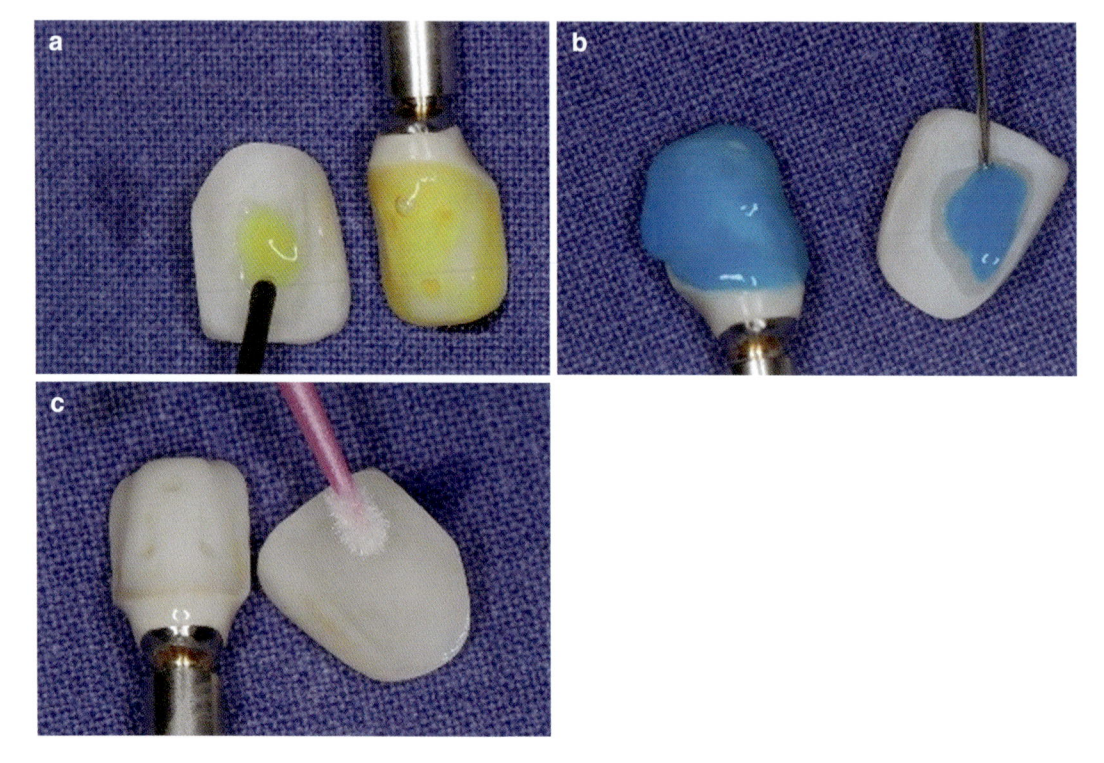

Fig. 18.67 Extraoral cementation of LS$_2$ veneer. (**a**) Etching of lithium disilicate ceramic with hydrofluoric acid 5% for 20 sec. (**b**) Cleaning of ceramic surface with H3PO4 for 2 min. (**c**) Ceramic primer application for 1 min

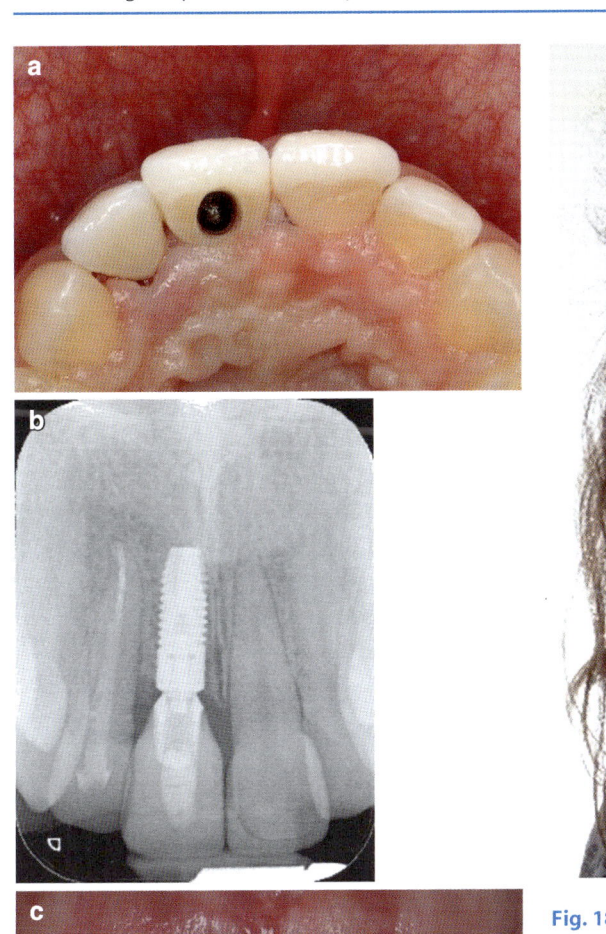

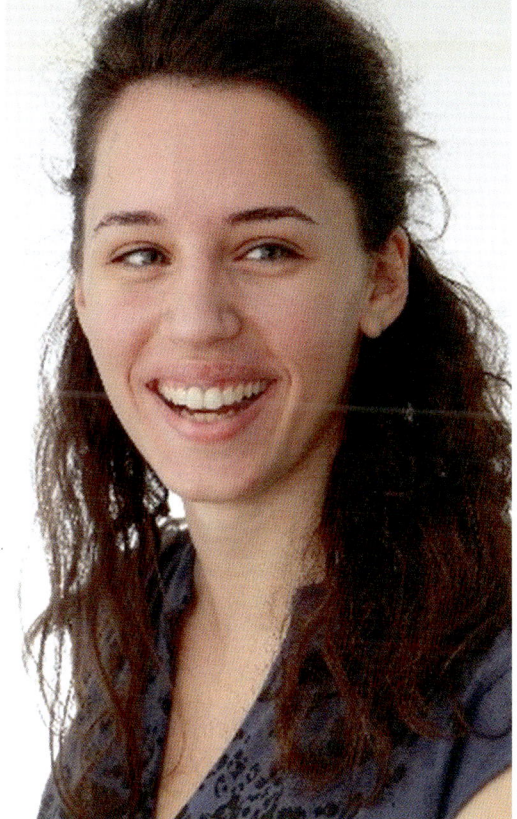

18 The Single Implant-Crown Complex in the Aesthetic Zone

Fig. 18.69 Final full-face picture

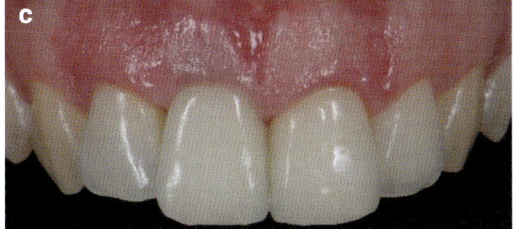

Fig. 18.68 (**a–c**) Final clinical and radiographic situation

Case 18.6 Prosthetic digital workflow, capturing the emergence profile and the implant intraoral, and using a prefabricated lithium disilicate ceramic block with a pre-manufactured connection geometry

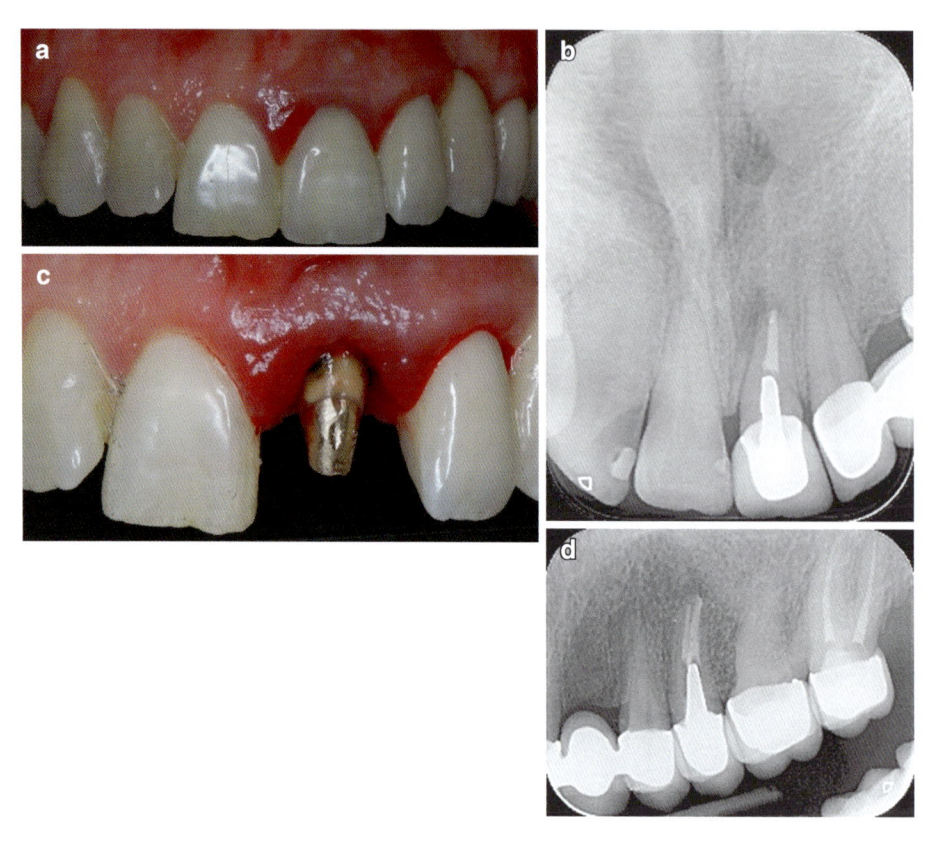

Fig. 18.70 (**a–d**) Initial clinical and radiographic evaluation. The prognosis of the *left* central incisor is poor and therefore will be extracted

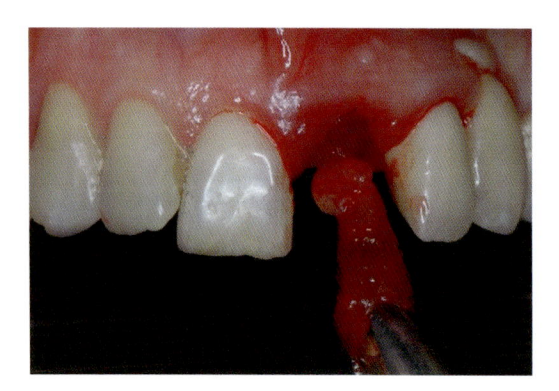

Fig. 18.71 Tooth extraction

18 The Single Implant-Crown Complex in the Aesthetic Zone

Fig. 18.72 (**a**, **b**) immediate implant placement followed by simultaneous guided bone regeneration with the use of bovine xenograft and a resorbable membrane

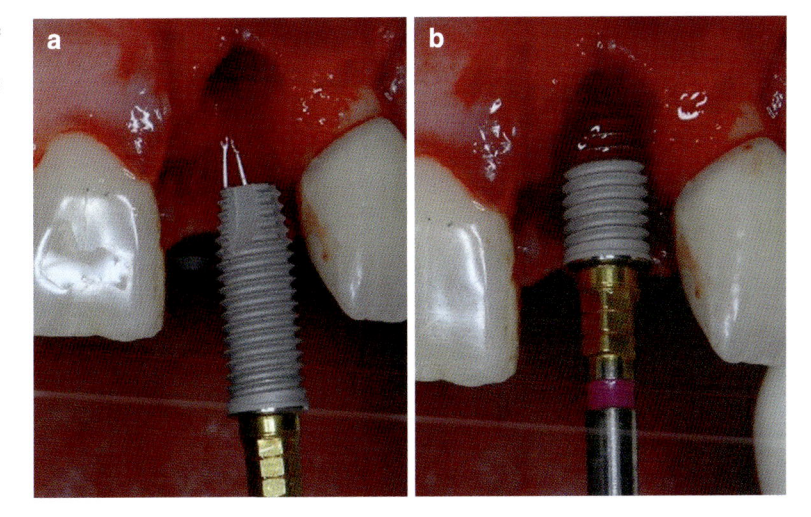

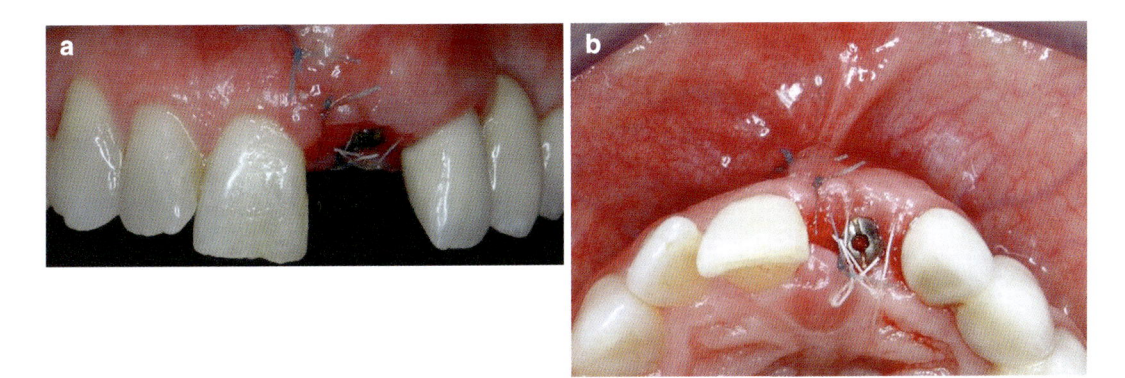

Fig. 18.73 (**a**, **b**) Since the initial stability is adequate a modified healing abutment is placed

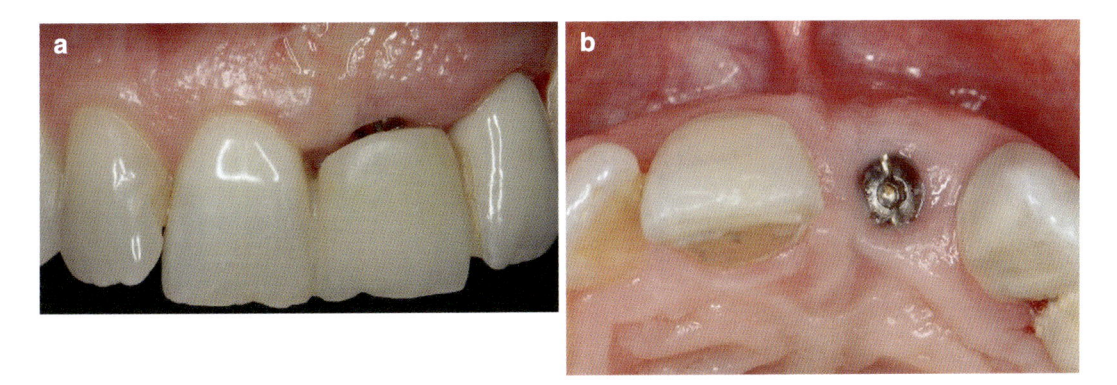

Fig. 18.74 (**a**, **b**) Clinical situation 6 months post-op

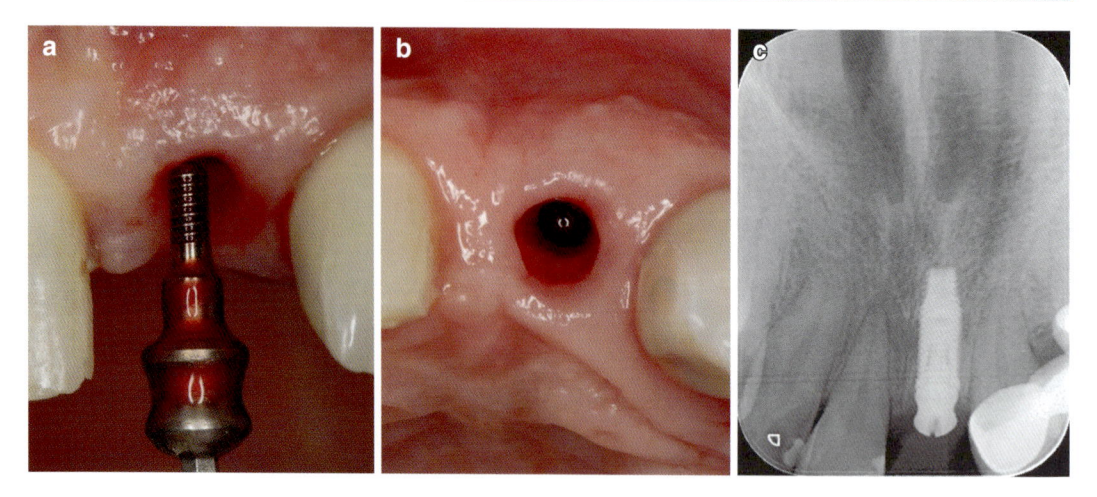

Fig. 18.75 (a–c) Radiographic evaluation and removal of the modified healing abutment. Note the good adaptation of the soft tissue around the healing abutment

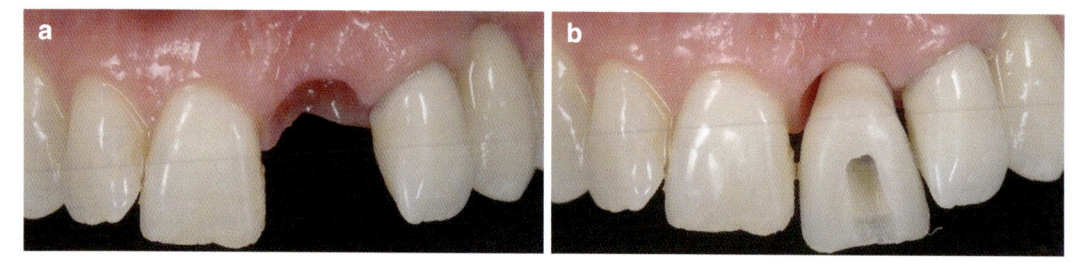

Fig. 18.76 (a, b) Placement of a screw-retained provisional restoration for the contouring of the desired emergence profile

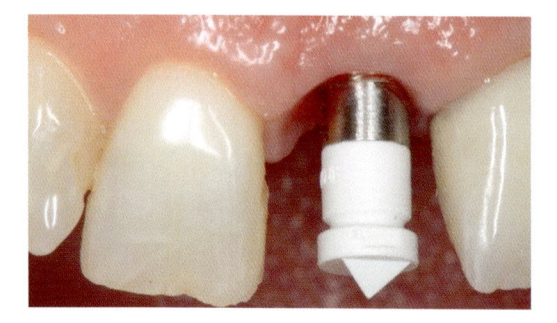

Fig. 18.77 Digital impression registration and the emergence profile

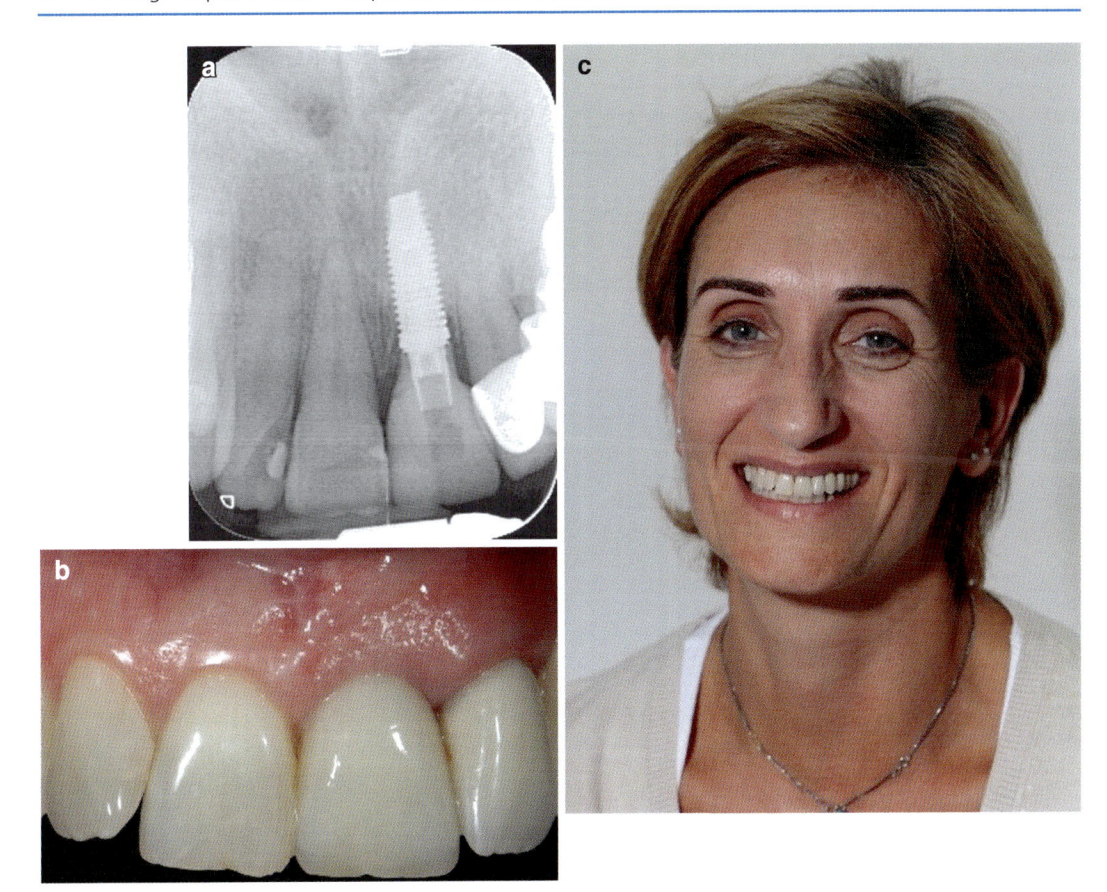

18 The Single Implant-Crown Complex in the Aesthetic Zone

Fig. 18.78 final clinical and radiographic situation

References

Abrahamsson I, Berglundh T, Lindhe J (1997) The mucosal barrier following abutment dis-reconnection. An experimental study in digs. J Clin Periodontol 24:568–572

Abrahamsson I, Berglundh T, Glantz P, Lindhe J (1998) The mucosal attachment at different abutments. An experimental study in dogs. J Clin Periodontol 25:721–727

Agar J, Cameron S, Hughbankc J, Parker H (1997) Cement removal from restorations luted to titanium abutments with simulated subgingival margins. J Prosthet Dent 78:43–47

Atieh M, Ibrahim H, Atieh A (2010) Platform switching for marginal bone preservation around dental implants: a systematic review and meta-analysis. J Periodontol 81:1350–1366

Barbour M, O'Sullivan D, Jenkinson H, Jagger D (2007) The effects of polishing methods on surface morphology, roughness and bacterial colonisation of titanium implants. J Mater Sci Mater Med 18:1439–1447

Becker W, Ochsenbein C, Tibbetts L et al (1997) Alveolar bone anatomic profiles as measured from dry skulls. Clinical ramifications. J Clin Periodontol 24:727–731

Becker K, Mihatovic I, Golubovic V, Schwartz F (2012) Impact of abutment material and dis-/re-connection on soft and hard tissue changes at implants with platform-switching. J Clin Periodontol 39:774–780

Bollen C, Papaioannou W, Van Eldere J et al (1996) The influence of abutment surface roughness on plaque accumulation and peri-implant mucositis. Clin Oral Implants Res 7:201–211

Canullo L, Bignozi I, Cocchetto R, Cristalli M, Ianello G (2010a) Immediate positioning of a definitive abutment versus repeated abutment replacements in post-extractive implants: 3-year follow-up of a randomized multicenter clinical trial. Eur J Oral Implantol 3:285–296

Canullo L, Fedele GR, Iannello G, Jepsen S (2010b) Platform switching and marginal bone-level alterations: the results of a randomized-controlled trial. Clin Oral Impl Res 21:115–121

Capelli M (2013) Surgical, biologic and implant-related factors affecting bone remodeling around implants. Eur J Esthet Dent 8:279–313

Chen S, Wilson T, Hammerle C (2004) Immediate or early placement of implants following tooth extraction: review of biologic basis, clinical procedures, and outcomes. Int J Oral Maxillofac Implants 19(suppl):12–25

Cochran D, Hermann J, Schenk R, Higginbottom F, Buser D (1997) Biologic width around titanium implants. A histometric analysis of the implanto-gingival junction around unloaded and loaded nonsubmerged implants in the canine mandible. J Periodontol 68:186–198

Degidi M, Nardi D, Daprile G, Piatelli A (2014) Nonremoval of immediate abutments in cases involving subcrestally placed postextractive tapered single implants: a randomized controlled clinical study. Clin Implant Dent Relat Res 16:794–805

Esposito M1, Ekestubbe A, Gröndahl K (1993 Sep) Radiological evaluation of marginal bone loss at tooth surfaces facing single Brånemark implants. Clin Oral Implants Res 4(3):151–157

Evans C, Chen S (2008) Esthetic outcomes of immediate implant placements. Clin Oral Implants Res 19:73–80

Gargiulo A, Wentz F, Orban B (1961) Dimensions and relations of the dentogingival junction in humans. J Periodontol 32:261–267

Geurs N, Vassilopoulos P, Reddy M (2001) Histologic evidence of connective tissue integration on laser microgrooved abutments. Clin Adv Periodontics 1:29–33

Glauser R, Schupbach P, Gottlow J, Hammerle C (2005) Periimplant soft tissue barrier at experimental one-piece mini-implants with different surface topography in humans: a light-microscopic overview and histometric analysis. Clin Implant Dent Relat Res 7(suppl 1):S44–S51

Grunder U, Gracis S, Capelli M (2005) Influence of the 3-D bone-to-implant relationship on Esthetics. Int J Periodontics Restor Dent 25(2):113–119

Happe A, Roling N, Schafer A, Rothamel D (2015) Effects of different polishing protocols on the surface roughness of Y-TZP surfaces used for custom-made implant abutments: a controlled morphologic SEM and profilometric study. J Prosthet Dent 113:440–447

Hürzeler MB1, Zuhr O, Schupbach P, Rebele SF, Emmanouilidis N, Fickl SJ (2010 Sep) The socket-shield technique: a proof-of-principle report. Clin Perinatol 37(9):855–862

Jung R, Sailer I, Hammerle C, Attin T, Schmidlin P (2007) In vitro color changes of soft tissues caused by restorative materials. Int J Periodontics Restorative Dent 27:251–257

Leutert C, Stawarczsky B, Truninger T, Hammerle C, Sailer I (2012) Bending moments and types of failure of zirconia and titanium abutments with internal implant-abutment connections: a laboratory study. Int J Oral Maxillofac Implants 27:505–512

Pelekanos S, Ntounis A, Jovanovic S, Euwe E (2013) Definitive abutment-driven stage-two surgery as a means to reduce peri-implant soft-tissue changes: introduction of a new concept. Int J Periodontics Restorative Dent 33:193–199

Perez F, Segalla JC, Marcantonio E Jr et al (2012) Gingival papilla dimensions in anterosuperior regions adjacent to single-tooth implants. Int J Periodontics Restorative Dent 32(1):93–100

Quirynen M, van der Mei H, Bollen C et al (1993) An in vivo study of the influence of the surface roughness of implants on the microbiology of supra- and subgingival plaque. J Dent Res 72:1304–1309

Romanos GE, Javed F (2014) Platform switching minimizes crestal bone loss around dental implants: truth or myth? J Oral Rehabil 41:700–708

Sailer I, Philipp A, Zembic A, Pjetursson B et al (2009) A systematic review of the performance of ceramic and metal implant abutments supporting fixed implant reconstructions. Clin Oral Implants Res 20(suppl4):4–31

Tarnow DP1, Cho SC, Wallace SS (2000 Apr) The effect of inter-implant distance on the height of inter-implant bone crest. J Periodontol 71(4):546–549

Tomasi C, Tessarolo F, Caola I, Wennstrom J, Nollo G, Berglundh T (2014) Morphogenesis of peri-implant mucosa revisited: an experimental study in humans. Clin Oral Implants Res 25:997–1003

Vacek J, Gher M, Assad D, Richardson A, Giambaressi L (1994) The dimensions of the human dentogingival junction. Int J Periodontics Restorative Dent 14:154–165

Van Brakel R, Meijer G, Verhoeven J et al (2012) Soft-tissue response to zirconia and titanium implant abutments: an in vivo within-subject comparison. J Clin Periodontol 39:995–1001

Veis A, Parissis N, Tsirlis A, Papadeli C, Marinis G, Zogakis A (2010 Dec) Evaluation of peri-implant marginal bone loss using modified abutment connections at various crestal level placements. Int J Periodontics Restorative Dent 30(6):609–617

Vela X1, Méndez V, Rodríguez X, Segalá M, Tarnow DP (2012 Apr) Crestal bone changes on platform-switched implants and adjacent teeth when the tooth-implant distance is less than 1.5 mm. Int J Periodontics Restorative Dent. 32(2):149–155

Welander M, Abrahamsson I, Berglundh T (2008) The mucosal barrier at implant abutments of different materials. Clin Oral Implants Res 19:635–641

Wilson T (2009) The positive relationship between excess cement and peri-implant disease: a prospective clinical endoscopic study. J Periodontol 80:1388–1392

Implant Provisionalization: The Key to Definitive Aesthetic Success

19

Edward Dwayne Karateew

Abstract

Developing implant aesthetics can be elusive to many clinicians. Too often we see practitioners jumping from the implant uncovery to the definitive restoration, only to be questioned by themselves, the patient or their referring colleague: 'why does it not look correct' or 'why does it not feel right when I bite?' There is no doubt that the fabrication of a provisional implant-supported restoration is a costly procedure both in clinical time and additional cost to the patient. However, when it is avoided, for any reason, there often are complications with the final prosthesis. One must think of the provisional restoration as the prototype from which the definitive restoration evolves; ideally the only difference being is the material from which each is fabricated. Aesthetics and function are always established in this relatively inexpensive plastic material prior to the investment of time and effort being put into the definitive restoration.

19.1 Introduction

A long-recognized complication in implant dentistry and most notably having the greatest effect on the aesthetic potential of dental implants in the 'anterior aesthetic zone' is the coronal loss of the bone. Common sequelae to this is the loss of gingival tissues most notably in the papillary area and on the direct facial. This 'cupping' effect begins at the time of implant uncovering and at removal of the cover screw and proceeds through the healing abutment phase, placement of the impression abutment, provisional abutment and definitive prosthetic abutment connection. This progressive loss carries through to the early stages of functional loading until it eventually stabilizes at a position 1–2 mm apical to its initial position (Hermann et al. 1997a; Abrahamson et al. 1997). It has been postulated that this bone remodelling is the establishment of a 'biologic width' around the implant-abutment interface which is similar to that which is found around a natural tooth (Hartman and Cochran 2004). More specifically, the observed 1–2 mm of apical bone remodelling along with the sulcular epithelial and connective

E. Dwayne Karateew, DDS
Advanced Education in Periodontics,
University of Illinois at Chicago,
801 South Paulina Avenue,
Chicago, IL 60612, USA
e-mail: karateew@uic.edu

tissue attachment demonstrates a strong correlation with the dimension of a 'biologic width' which has been described around the natural dentition in humans (Gargiolo et al. 1961).

There are many factors which have been demonstrated to influence the volume of peri-implant bone loss as well as the time at which it occurs. These implant design influencers are well defined, and their clinical and/or histological consequences are documented.

19.2 Implant Design Influencers

19.2.1 The Platform Switch

Initially wide-diameter implants were introduced to the marketplace, and due to a lack of matching prosthetic components, these implants were restored with standard-diameter abutments. The terms platform switched and platform shifted can be used interchangeably. The key principle of a platform-switch/switched implant and abutment connection is that the abutment diameter is of a narrower dimension than that of the implant shoulder. Thus, the peri-implant biologic width is established in more of a horizontal dimension, rather than being strictly established along the vertical axis of the implant body. Biologically, this will reduce the net bone remodelling effect in both lateral and vertical dimensions and act to preserve the biologic width in a more coronal position (Rodriguez-Ciurana et al. 2006). Long-term radiological observation suggested that these 'platform-switched' implant-abutments had a previously unknown beneficial effect as they demonstrated a positive effect on crestal bone maintenance. This positive effect of the bone being apposed up to and over the shoulder of the implant (Degiudi et al. 2009) has been described in numerous publications over the years, and the 'platform-switch' concept is widely accepted (Vela et al. 2012; Al-Nsour et al. 2012). The marginal bone loss around platform-switched implants has been demonstrated to be significantly less than around platform-matched implants (Annibali et al. 2012; Cumbo et al. 2013). Many theories exist to explain this phenomenon including the transference of the stress concentration from the cortical bone to the cancellous bone during loading (Chang et al. 2010) as well as containment of the implant-abutment junction and resultant microgap to a spatial position further removed from the osseous tissues.

This configuration has many advantages particularly in the aesthetic zone, not only with the osseous structures but with the overlying soft tissue components as well. In canine studies (Cochran et al. 2013), the volume of connective tissue was found to be positioned in a more coronal location than in platform-matched implant-abutment connections. Wang et al. (2015) have recently demonstrated that there is a statically significant difference between platform-switched and non-platform-switched implants at the healing intervals of 0–12 months and 3–12 months with respect to bone remodelling. The marginal bone response was greater (demonstrated greater bone loss) in non-platform-switched implants than to their platform-switched counterparts. Earlier, Donovan et al. (2010) were able to clinically demonstrate that there is limited bone modelling in platform-switched implants.

Of importance to implant treatment planning and subsequent implant placement, it has been noted that with the use of platform-switched implants, both the implant-implant distance and the implant-tooth distance may be decreased from the standard allowances. Elian et al. (2014) have proposed that the inter-implant distance, for two adjacent implants, may be safely reduced to less than 3 mm when utilizing implants with this design feature. Additionally, Vela et al. (2012) have suggested the implant-tooth dimension may be reduced to less than 1.5 mm.

19.2.2 The Microgap

The microgap is a factor which has been implicated in the cratering of the bone around coronal aspect dental implant (Jansen et al. 1997). The microgap has been defined as the interface between the implant and the abutment in standard two-piece arrangements (Hermann et al. 2001).

The presence of the microgap has been implicated in the presence of bacterial contamination. It is this bacterial contamination and their associated toxins which have been directly implicated in a localized chronic inflammation and the subsequent loss of the crestal bone vertically (Quiryen and Van Steenberghe 1993) and horizontally (Tarnow et al. 2000). More specifically, it is the aggregate concentration of inflammatory cells below the bone crest and adjacent to the microgap which has a high correlation to the saucerization or cuplike bone loss (Broggini et al. 2006).

The microgap which is resultant of the implant-abutment connection, irrespective of its spatial position, has been theorized to be a contributing factor in the distancing of the peri-implant bone from this junction. In most contemporary 'two-piece' implant systems, the microgap or implant-abutment interface is placed in an equi-crestal (at the same level as the crest of the bone) or slightly supra-crestal (coronal to the crest of the bone). It has been found that in traditional two-piece implant systems, there is an apical migration of the bone to implant contact. This represented a dimensional change of 2 mm from the microgap location to the most coronal peri-implant bone when the implant is placed in either a submerged or non-submerged manner (Hermann et al. 1997b).

Implant designs which feature long Morse taper connections have been associated with less peri-crestal bone loss during function. Weng et al. (2011) were able to demonstrate in the dog model that differing microgap configurations and spatial positioning had varying results in bone loss around implants placed in a submarginal spatial position. In this study, the Morse taper internal connection was associated with the lesser amount of linear bone loss irrespective of equi-crestal or subcrestal placement of the microgap at monthly intervals for the initial 6 months of healing.

Differences in implant design have also been shown to have a direct effect on the bacterial colonization of the microgap structures. In an in vitro study, Koutouzis et al. (2011a) were able to demonstrate significantly less bacterial colonization of the internal aspects of implant-abutment connection with a Morse taper system than conical internal connection. One can conclude that the configuration of the implant-abutment microgap plays a role in the ability of bacteria to invade (Feitosa et al. 2013) and establish a favourable environment for subsequent increase in bacterial cell numbers and an increase in the production of exotoxins which may have an additional negative influence on the peri-implant tissues.

19.2.3 The Implant-Abutment Connection

The architecture and engineering of the connection between the implant and the abutment is of critical importance. Multiple connection configurations exist and have been used with varying results in both stability (Mangano et al. 2009) and prosthetic complications (Krebs et al. 2013) and with maintenance of the peri-implant soft and hard tissues (Tesmer et al. 2009). From an engineering perspective, a 'Morse taper' is one which is defined as two mated conical surfaces, which in turn lends the term 'conical cone connection' to this style of interface. The precision fit of this single component of the overall implant design influences the ability of bacteria to colonize the microgap area during occlusal load (Koutouzis et al. 2011a, b). The absence of colonizing bacteria is directly correlated with minimizing the volume of peri-implant bone loss (Mangano et al. 2009). Additionally, this connection type is integral in the efficiency of the occlusal load transfer from the prosthesis, through the abutment and into the implant body and ultimately the surrounding bony structure. The high mechanical stability of the 'Morse taper/conical cone connection' significantly reduces prosthetic complications (Mangano et al. 2008, 2011) (Fig. 19.1).

19.2.4 The Provisional Restoration

Clinicians are continually seeking both established and new protocols which aid with increasing the predictability of clinical procedures.

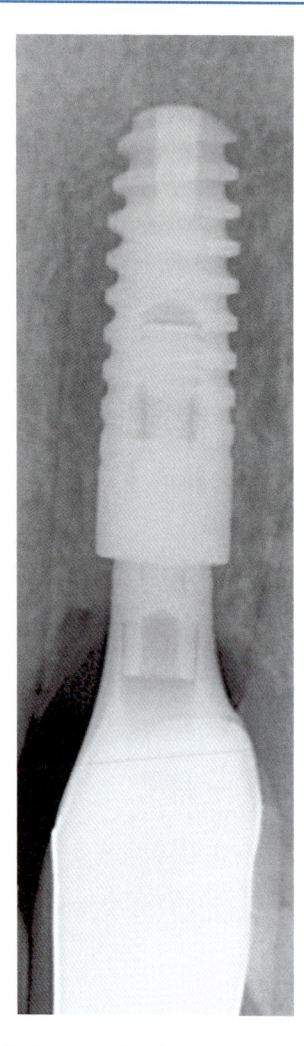

Fig. 19.1 Radiograph of a Morse taper/conical cone connection implant demonstrating a platform shift. Note the bone growth which is up and over the shoulder of this implant which has been in function for 6 years

These protocols establish both idealized functional form and creating and managing stable soft tissue contours. When dealing with implant placement and the subsequent restoration of endosseous implants in the 'anterior aesthetic zone', any advantage to establish harmony between the hard/soft tissue profile and the prosthesis is welcomed.

Although there are alternative methods by which one can provisionalize an area in which an implant has been inserted, such as an Essix appliance, a Provisional (acrylic) PRDP or 'Maryland'-type Provisional FDP, amongst others, none of these alternatives offer similar development and control of the soft tissue contours and hence the ultimate aesthetics of the peri-implant tissues as the implant-supported provisional restoration. These secondary methods can be recognized as simple space fillers, where ultimately the aesthetics are created strictly by the level of skill of our laboratory partners.

Provisional restorations supported by dental implants are a critical and exacting aspect of our clinical practice. These interim restorations not only function to stabilize relative adjacent and opposing tooth positions but also allow the clinician to test varying restorative designs and observe their influence on the soft tissue contours. They give us the necessary biologic parameters for ideal gingival contouring and aesthetics. The purported role of the implant-supported provisional abutment/crown complex is to provide some level of function to the underlying endosseous implant as well as to develop superlative soft tissue contours and therefore maximal aesthetics prior to the fabrication of the definitive prosthesis. Once these contours have been established, the sole distinction between the provisional and final restoration is the material from which each is fabricated.

Minimizing a disturbance to the underlying bony structures is the biological basis to flapless surgery or a minimally invasive surgical protocol. The evidence suggests that these protocols may preserve bony vascularization as this style procedure does not disturb the periosteum of the alveolar bone (Al-Juboori et al. 2012). This can ultimately lead to a decreased volume of surgical trauma-related bone resorption, and there also have been suggestions of enhanced osseointegration (Jeong et al. 2007).

A second technique which has been utilized successfully and is supported in the literature is the installation of an immediate provisional restoration on the implant at the time of Stage 1 surgical placement. In studies, 'immediate non-occlusal loading' of dental implants has demonstrated no biologic or prosthetic complications when compared to 'early loading' groups (Testori et al. 2007).

19.2.5 The Provisional Abutment

When treatment planning is a provisional implant-supported restoration, several decisions must be made with respect to not only the material from which the abutment is fabricated but also will the provisional restoration be cement or screw retained and will the provisional abutment/restorative unit be fabricated directly in the oral environment or in the laboratory via an indirect technique.

Study of the occlusion is paramount, as one chooses the appropriate interim abutment material. Plastic (PEEK) may not be able to tolerate prolonged resistance to occlusal function and lateral/protrusive excursive forces in patients with a deep overbite (Angle Class II Division 2). Conversely, a solid titanium provisional abutment not only increases the cost of the provisional restoration significantly, but it is difficult to modify with rotary instruments so that the submergence profile of the provisional restoration may be altered to effect a desired change in the gingival margin position.

Perhaps it is the metal cylinder or chimney is the provisional abutment which can provide the foundation for the optimal provisional restoration. Not only are they cost-effective, but PMMA and bis-acryl restorative materials can be mechanically 'locked' to the cylinders for the provision of a screw-retained direct or indirectly fabricated interim implant-supported restoration.

Screw-retained provisional restorations should be attempted whenever possible. As the PMMA or bis-acryl material is easy to remove and replace, access to the prosthetic screw is easily facilitated, and repair subsequent to the restoration replacement on the implant is virtually seamless. Screw retention avoids the perils of excess cement overflow and its recognized deleterious effect on the peri-implant tissues. Gross cement overflow has been demonstrated to have a positive correlation with (1) occlusal displacement of the provisional restoration, (2) inadequate access to clean up the overflowed cement and (3) establishment of an environment around the implant and restoration which is not conducive to the long-term health of the peri-implant hard and soft tissues (Wadhwani et al. 2012) (Fig. 19.2).

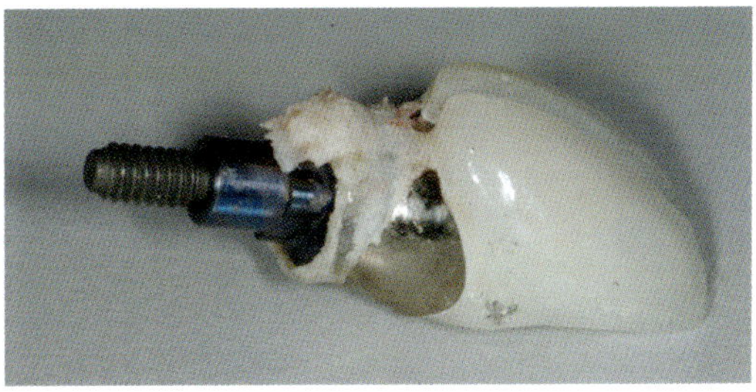

Fig. 19.2 Extreme excess of cement circumferentially around implant-abutment and abutment/crown interfaces. This was the culprit for a suppurating lesion. This restorative complex was replaced

Due to difficulty of controlling the spatial positioning (depth) of the abutment/restorative interface on the provisional abutment, cement retention should be avoided. However, there exist those rare clinical situations when one cannot utilize screw retention, and thus cement must be utilized. Diligent technique must be used not to overfill the intaglio surface of the provisional restoration, visualization of the restorative margin is critical to aid in the post cementation clean-up and clean-up protocols are employed so that leaving residual cement is avoided.

19.3 Conventional Provisional Protocol

Delayed sequencing of the provisional restoration can be provided as either an early or conventional technique as described by Buser et al. (2013a). Both early and conventional provisional loading approaches have been shown to be equally successful when making observations relative to long-term outcome assessments (Buser et al. 2013a). These are perhaps the most challenging implant-supported provisional restorations to clinically fabricate; the implants which are provisionalized after uncovering, as often hard and soft tissue landmarks have been lost. Therefore, the provisional restoration may require multiple modifications prior to ideal soft tissue form is achieved.

Whether or not the staged (either early or conventional) provisional restoration is lab processed or fabricated chairside, the material of choice must be one which allows for easy facilitation of future modifications. These modifications may either be additive or subtractive in nature and will facilitate the fine-tuning of the soft tissue profile. It has been suggested that the initial provisional restoration be fabricated in a manner in which it is under-contoured so that the dynamic compression method (Wittneben et al. 2013) be utilized to obtain the peri-implant tissue shaping. Over-contouring is to be avoided as this may give the appearance of facial soft tissue recession or cause blunting of the interproximal papillae.

The purpose of the conventional provisional prosthesis, as with all implant-supported provisional restorations, is to translate to the restorative complex, the submergence profile of the tooth being replaced. The coronal aspect of the integrated implant is circular; contrary to this, however, the cross-sectional anatomy of the dentition in the anterior aesthetic zone is either triangular or ovoid. The linear distance between the shoulder of the implant and the gingival margin (running distance) and degree of customization of the provisional abutment/crown complex will determine how seamless this transition is and whether or not the illusion of a natural tooth is achieved.

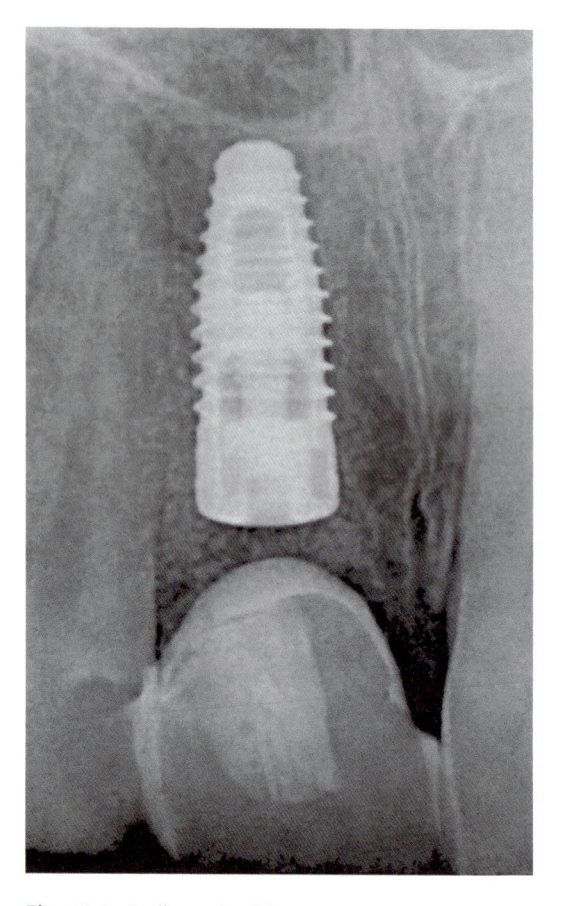

Fig. 19.3 Radiograph of integrated implant at time of consultation for final restoration. Existing 'healing provisional' was an acrylic Maryland-type restoration

19.4 Traditional Immediate Provisionalization Protocol: Example Case #1 (Figs. 19.3, 19.4, 19.5, 19.6, 19.7, 19.8, 19.9 and 19.10)

As described, there are traditional protocols which exist for the fabrication of provisional abutment/crown complexes. These often result in multiple removal events of the interim prosthetic components. Abrahamson et al. have shown that with the average clinical case there are five (5) abutment dis-/reconnections events (Abrahamson et al. 1997). For each of these abutment changes, there is the establishment of a local inflammatory process which eventually can lead to the

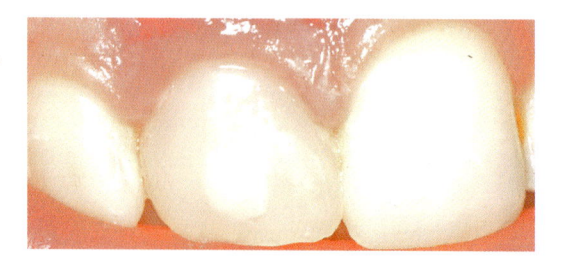

Fig. 19.4 Initial under-contoured implant-supported provisional restoration. The stated goal of this stage of treatment is to create an excess of tissue

establishment of a 'biologic width' and the concurrent apical migration of the alveolar bone and subsequent loss of vertical soft tissue profile.

The fabrication and connection of the provisional restoration at the time of implant placement (immediate 'non-functional' loading) is

19 Implant Provisionalization: The Key to Definitive Aesthetic Success

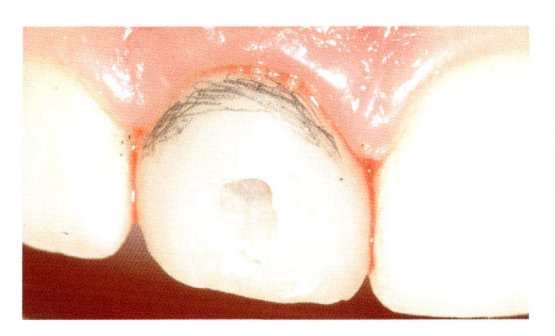

Fig. 19.5 The gingival margin is scribed onto the provisional restoration. This serves as a landmark for altering the submergence profile when the restoration is removed and is manipulated on the benchtop

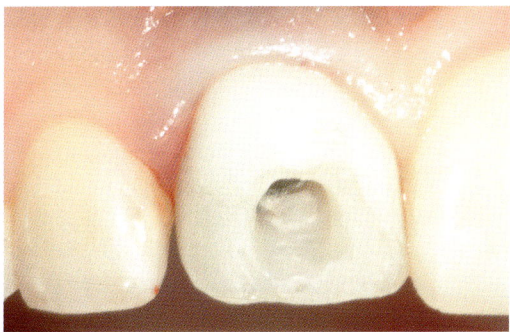

Fig. 19.8 Augmented provisional restoration replaced on the implant. Will evoke blanching of the soft tissues

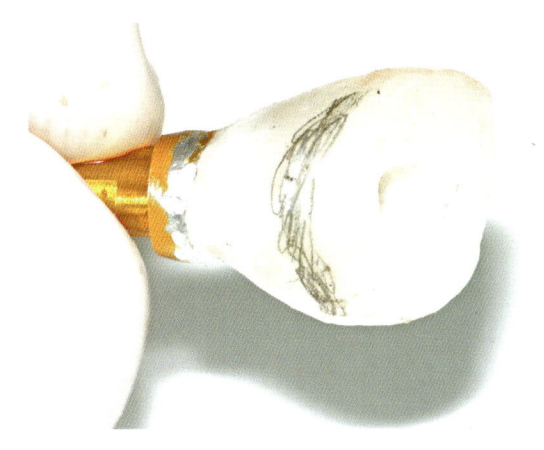

Fig. 19.6 The provisional restoration and abutment. The scribed line identifying the gingival margin is clearly visible

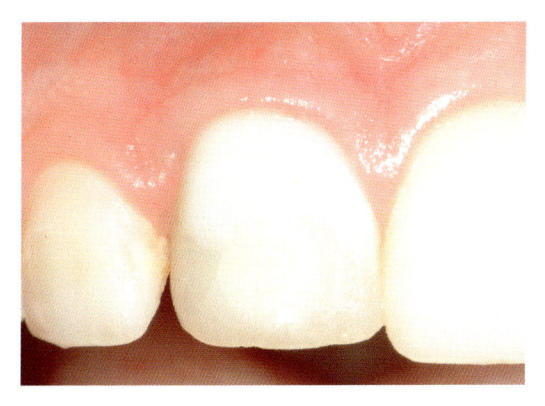

Fig. 19.9 Idealized gingival contour established by additive strategy of provisional modification

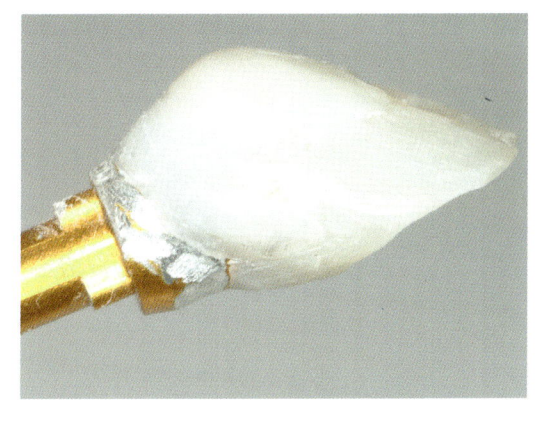

Fig. 19.7 Lateral view of the provisional restorative complex. Acrylic has been added to increase the submergence profile. This will relocate the gingival margin to a more apical position

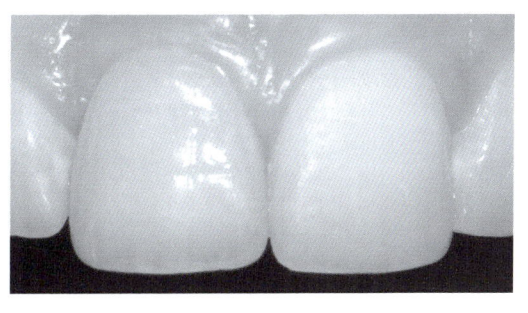

Fig. 19.10 Definitive restoration demonstrating gingival health and contour which mimics the contralateral maxillary central incisor

considered to be a safe treatment methodology and will not deleteriously effect the process of osseointegration (Grütter and Belser 2009). It has been suggested that the fabrication of the provisional restoration at the time of immediate implant placement into the fresh extraction socket may be the most predictable method to maintain soft tissue aesthetic contours. Although the long-term stability of the hard and soft tissue contours is controversial, there remains opinion which supports the judicious use of an immediate provisional restoration affixed to an immediately placed implant (Block et al. 2009). Although the use of a concomitant bone allograft and/or xenograft may improve the long-term prospective tissue contours (Buser et al. 2013b), zero to minimal volumes of grafting materials should be considered when also immediately loading. When considering immediate provisional protocols in a clinical situation, it behoves the practitioner to exercise extreme caution. Implant length (>8 mm), insertional torque (or corresponding ISQ value), implant design, ability to provide screw retention which is preferred, avoidance of physiological function and clinician experience are all factors which should be considered prior to the fabrication of an immediate provisional restoration.

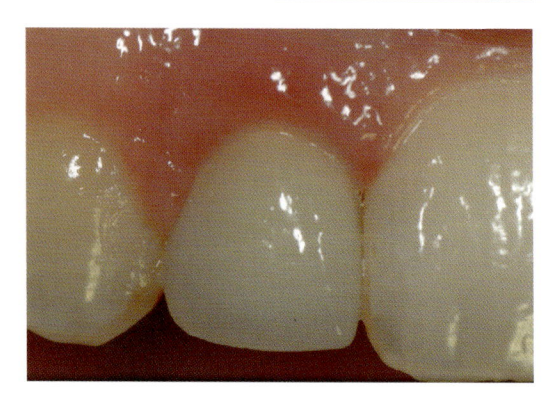

Fig. 19.11 Clinical appearance of fractured tooth #7

19.5 The Minimal Abutment Change (MAC) Protocol and Example Case #2

The minimal abutment change (MAC) technique (Karateew 2014) has been designed to enhance the retention of the supporting bony structures and thereby enhance the maintenance of the soft tissue profile specifically in the anterior aesthetic zone in immediate placement with immediate non-occlusal loading of a provisional restoration on a single tooth implant.

Once the tooth has been diagnosed and treatment planned to be removed and replaced with a single implant (Figs. 19.11 and 19.12), and the patient is medically cleared for such a procedure, the MAC protocol can be successfully utilized to maximize the outcome with a relatively simple procedure. Adhering to the principles of ALARA, initial radiographs and CBCT scan is obtained (Fig. 19.13). Further assessment of the potential implant receptor site can be verified utilizing tertiary diagnostic and virtual implant planning software.

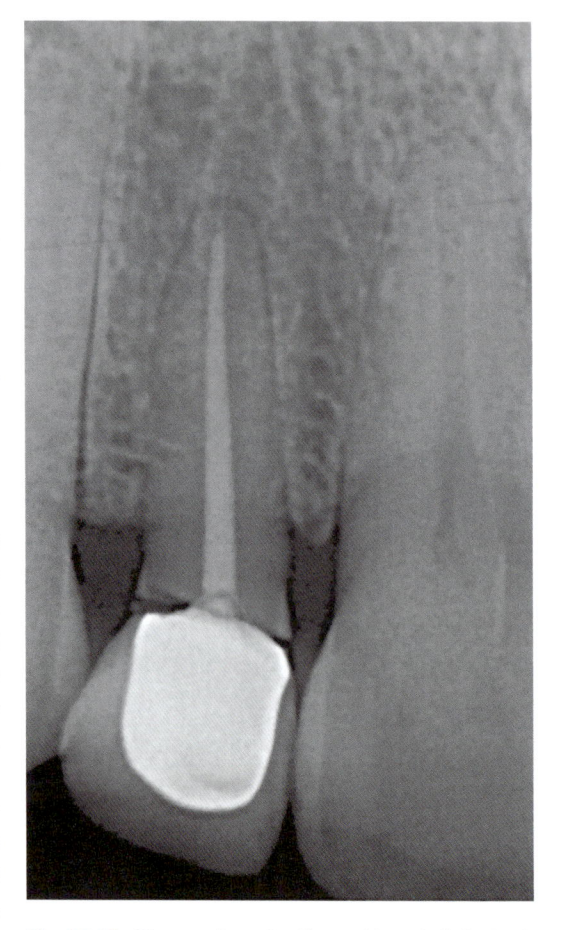

Fig. 19.12 Upon review of radiographic and clinical evidence, and upon consultation with the patient, this fractured tooth has been determined to be hopeless and will be replaced with a single tooth implant (STI)

Prior to the tooth being extracted, an incisal edge record is fabricated with pattern resin (Fig. 19.14); this will allow the clinical crown

19 Implant Provisionalization: The Key to Definitive Aesthetic Success 345

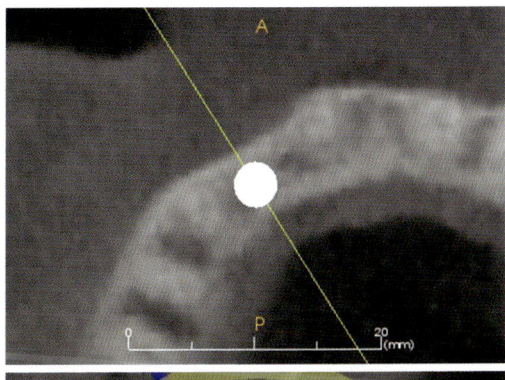

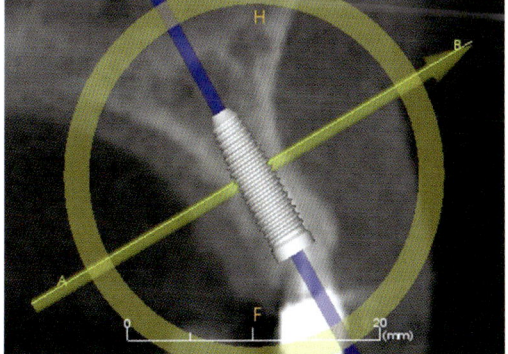

Fig. 19.13 CBCT analysis of immediate implant placement to replace the failed tooth #7.14

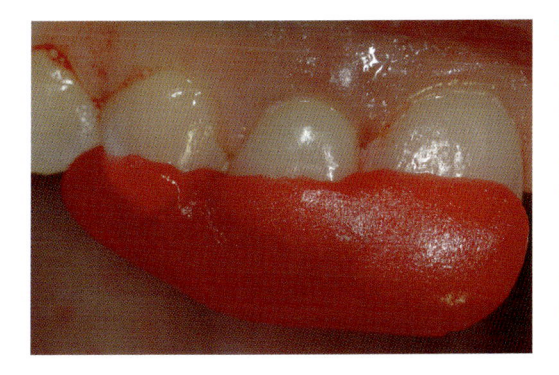

Fig. 19.14 Incised edge index is fabricated prior to the extraction of the hopeless tooth. This will facilitate exact spatial replacement of the clinical crown on the immediate implant-abutment complex

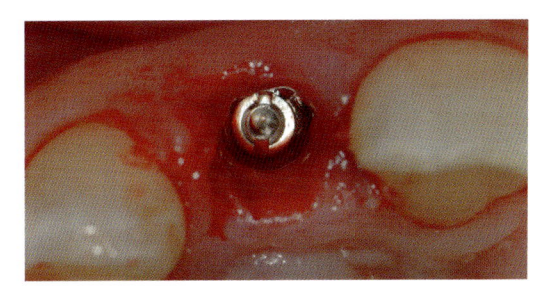

Fig. 19.15 Immediate implant placed with a flapless technique once the tooth has been extracted

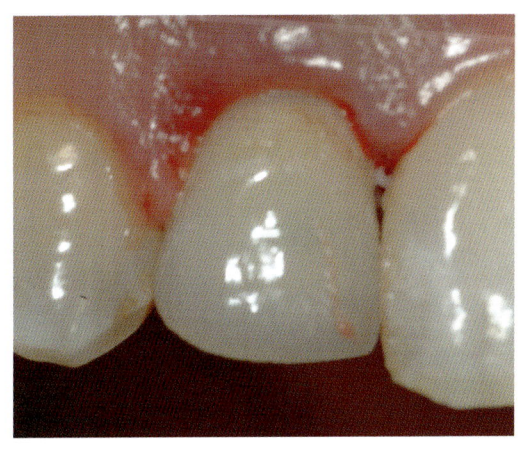

Fig. 19.16 Immediate implant and immediate nonfunctional provisional restoration utilizing the MAC technique. Patients' clinical crown was repositioned with the incisal edge index and its relation to the abutment secured with acrylic. The submergence contours of the provisional/abutment complex are idealized and polished prior to placement on the implant

to be carefully indexed in the mouth and then relined and margins finished with bis-acryl or a self-curing acrylic resin outside of the oral cavity, on the benchtop. This resin jig will ensure that the provisional restoration (hollowed clinical crown) will be in the same spatial position on the provisional abutment once the implant has been placed as it was during the initiation of the procedure (Figs. 19.15 and 19.16). Once the osteotomy is completed, the implant is immediately placed into the extraction socket and a provisional abutment is affixed to which the provisional restoration can be placed. This Morse taper implant-abutment system has now become an immediate implant placement and immediate non-functional provisional restoration (Romanos 2004). It is critical to evaluate the occlusion during this procedure to ensure that there is no functioning contact between the immediate implant restoration and the opposing occlusion. This is not only confirmed in the habitual occlusion (maximal intercuspal position) but also in all excursive pathways. If this provisional restoration is to be retained with cement, considerable care must be utilized during the cementation procedure in order to avoid the inadvertent trapping of subgingival excess material. Conversely, the provisional restoration can be designed to be screw retained with some additional alterations.

After the appropriate healing time for this newly placed implant/provisional restoration, the first abutment dis-/reconnection occurs during the impression procedure. The provisional restoration/abutment units are removed, an impression coping is placed and an impression of the area is recorded with the preferred impression material. Once the implant impression, bite registration and opposing dentition have been recorded, any supporting information, such as photograph, should be obtained. This will allow the laboratory to mimic the characteristics of the adjacent natural dentition. At this time the provisional abutment and restoration are replaced, and once again the area is checked for excess cement and potential occlusal prematurity. The impressions and ancillary documentation will be sent to the laboratory for the fabrication of the definitive restoration.

The placement of the final restoration will follow as per regular protocols, once the definitive abutment and crown have been fabricated. A verification radiograph should be taken at this time to ensure complete seating of the abutment as well as the restoration and to ensure there is no excess cementation material on the visible portion of the circumference of the restoration (Fig. 19.17). This can either be cement or screw retained whichever is the clinician's preference. This final step constitutes the second and final abutment dis-/reconnection. As with all implant-supported restorations, yearly clinical and radiographic examinations should be considered to monitor the health of the fixture (Zarb and Schmitt 1990) (Fig. 19.18).

The MAC protocol, as has been described, has the distinct advantage of decreasing the abutment dis-/reconnection procedures from an average of five to only two. This has a dramatic effect on the health of the peri-implant hard and soft tissue health. It is the maintenance of this tissue health which in turn will have a positive influence on the aesthetics of the implant restoration.

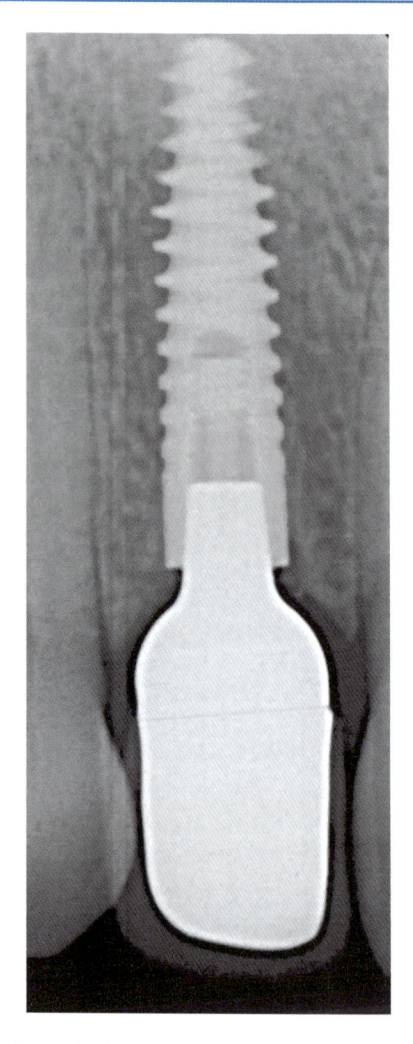

Fig. 19.17 Radiograph of the final abutment/restorative complex of a 5-year post insertion

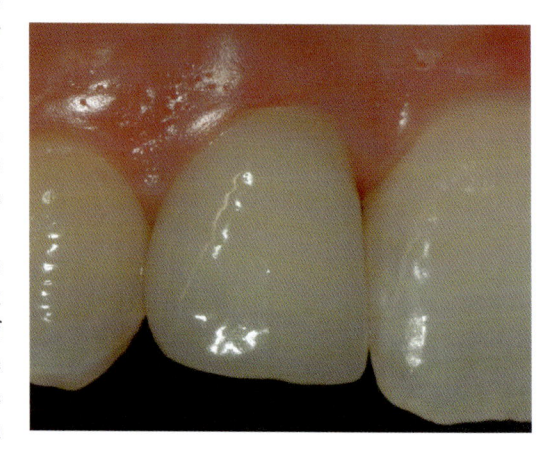

Fig. 19.18 Clinical appearance of the soft tissue complex and final restoration at a 5-year post insertion

19 Implant Provisionalization: The Key to Definitive Aesthetic Success

The Zero Abutment Change (ZAC) technique (Karateew 2014) is a novel and contemporary approach to the 'one abutment/one time' concept described by Salama (2011) and the 'one abutment at one time' technique of Degiudi et al. (2011). As described in the corresponding literature, these OAOT protocols utilize stock prosthetic abutments as provided by the corresponding implant companies. This can present the clinician with problem notably if the placement of the implant necessitates either a deep subgingival or subcrestal position or has a significant angulation. Additionally, stock prosthetic abutments all have a round profile when view from the incisal, and this can lead to a discrepancy between the prosthesis and the true cross-sectional anatomical shape of the tooth which is being replaced, such as the proverbial round peg in a square hole. The ZAC technique improves on these previously described techniques as it allows for the pre-surgical fabrication of a customized, patient-specific, CAD/CAM abutment. Salama states that the 'significant advantage to this evolving protocol, is that there is less chance of traumatizing the stability and position of the peri-implant soft tissue' (Salama 2011).

19.6 The Zero Abutment Change (ZAC) Protocol and Example Case #3

When contemplating the Zero Abutment Change (ZAC) protocol technique, the health of the patient must be initially assessed and then the replacement of the failing tooth with a dental implant, patient-specific abutment and restoration can be treatment planned. Initial radiographs are reviewed and a CBCT scan is mandatory, as is a digital intra-oral scan or digital model scan to make an STL file of the dentition. Tertiary software is used to treatment plan the implant placement and the rapid prototype fabrication of a custom surgical guide. This unique software can now be used to 'merge' the DICOM data of the CBCT scan and the STL files of the digital intra-oral scan so that a patient-specific, CAD/CAM abutment can be produced prior to the surgical appointment (Figs. 19.19 and 19.20).

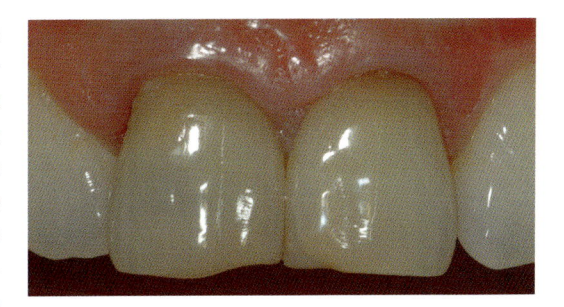

Fig. 19.19 Clinical appearance of hopeless tooth #8

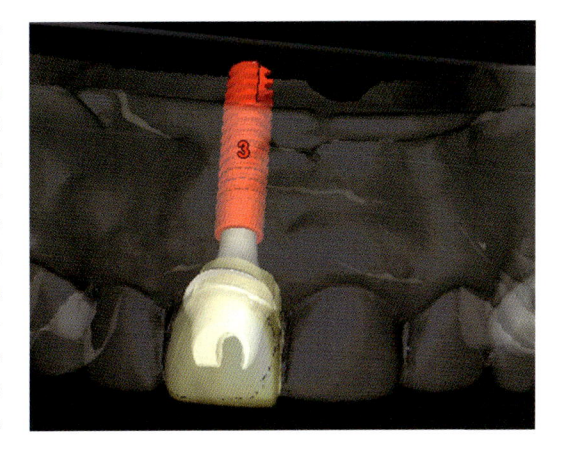

Fig. 19.20 By merging the DICOM and STL data sets, a digital treatment plan is created including the proposed patient-specific titanium abutment and provisional restoration which are to be fabricated prior to the implant being placed

Once treatment planning has been completed and the surgical guide and custom abutment ordered and received, the surgical appointment can be set (Fig. 19.21). At the start of the surgery, again a resin index is obtained of the incisal edge position (Fig. 19.22). This will facilitate the exact spatial replacement of the hollowed anatomic crown (provisional) on the patient specific, custom pre-surgically fabricated titanium abutment; which will be relined in the same manner as in the previously described MAC protocol.

The tooth can now be atraumatically removed and the implant immediately placed into the fresh socket environment. The precision of placement with the surgical guide is not only in the buccal-lingual, mesial-distal and coronal-apical dimensions but also can predict the timing of the implant in 360° of rotation, which is critical as

Fig. 19.21 Surgical guide, final titanium abutment and acrylic provisional restoration are fabricated and delivered prior to the implant placement surgery; for this case the acrylic provisional provided was provided as a backup in case his own clinical crown could not be utilized as the provisional restoration

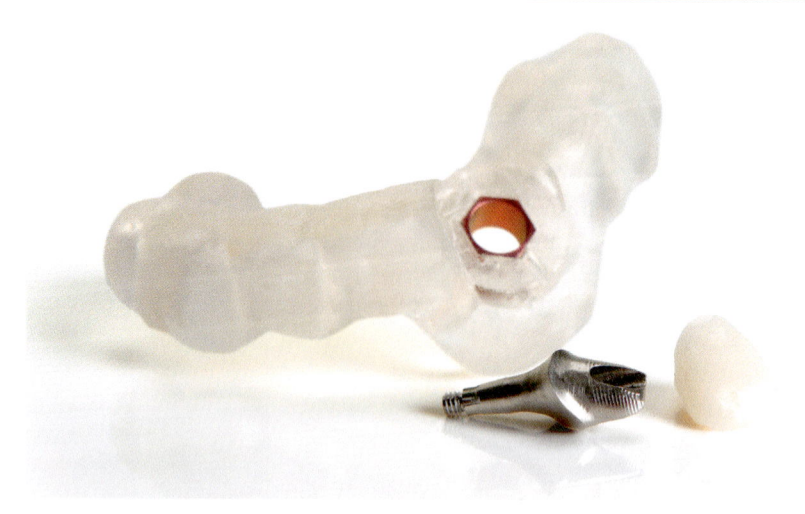

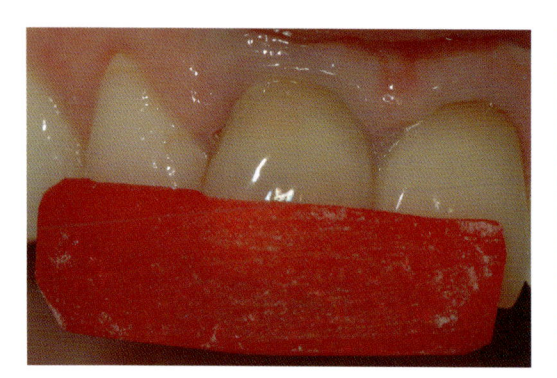

Fig. 19.22 Incised edge index created so that his own clinical crown can be repositioned on the final titanium abutment in the same spatial relation as it was pretreatment

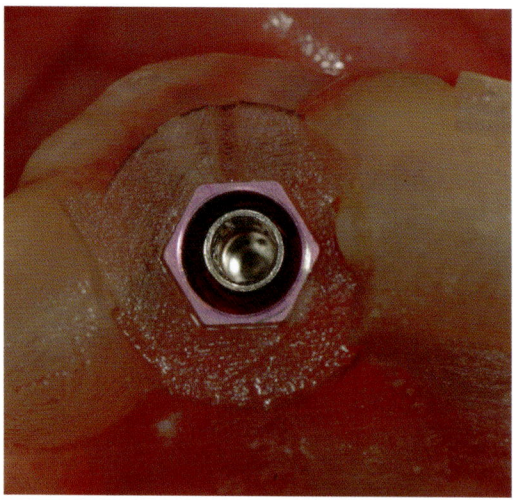

Fig. 19.23 Occlusal view of implant transfer abutment viewed through the surgical guide. The osteotomy and implant placement were all accomplished through this surgical guide, making this a fully guided surgery

the implant and the abutment are indexed and these indices must mate with precision to facilitate the exact abutment positioning and hence the exact provisional position. The insertional resistance to torque must be evaluated as this will determine whether or not immediate non-functional loading of the implant can be considered. This ideal value is specific for each implant system (Degiudi et al. 2006). In this case being demonstrated, the patient's own tooth is being utilized as the provisional restoration; however, it is possible to have an acrylic provisional milled by the same digital laboratory as is designing the custom abutment.

Once the implant has been positioned with the custom surgical guide (Fig. 19.23), the patient-specific titanium (or zirconium) abutment (Fig. 19.24) affixed and torqued to the appropriate value for the prosthetic screw, this implant-abutment configuration will never be disassembled. This is the significant biologic advantage to this protocol. The provisional restoration must be cement retained as the abutment is not to be removed again; however, the cementation may either be an intra-oral or extra-oral procedure (Figs. 19.25, 19.26, and 19.27).

After the appropriate healing time (Fig. 19.28), only the provisional restoration can be removed

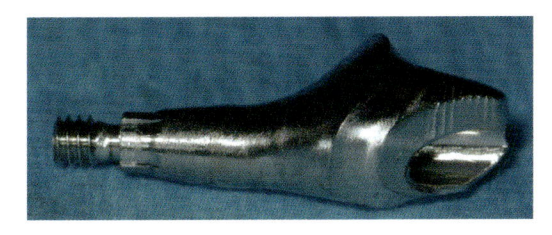

Fig. 19.24 Patient-specific titanium abutment prior to affixing onto the immediately placed implant

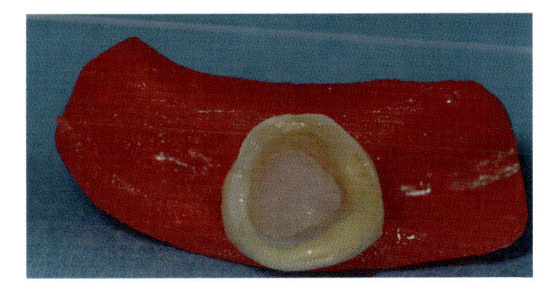

Fig. 19.25 Intaglio of hollowed clinical crown in resin incisal edge index prior to placement in vivo on the custom abutment

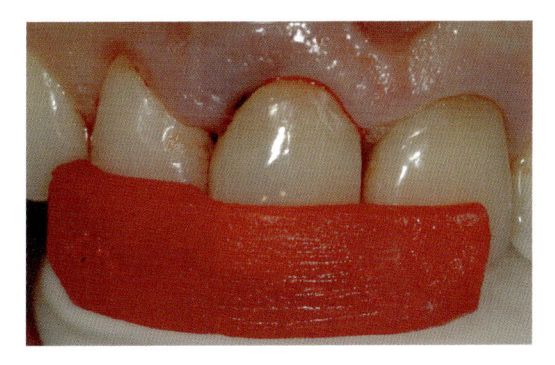

Fig. 19.26 Patient-hollowed clinical crown is related to the custom abutment utilizing the incisal edge index

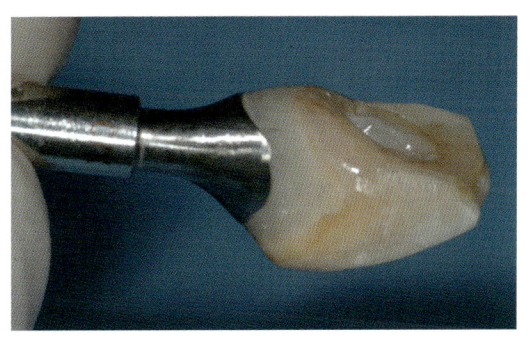

Fig. 19.27 Finished 'screw-mentable' retained provisional restoration/abutment complex. The patients' own clinical crown served as the provisional 'shell' which was filled with composite restorative material to provide strength

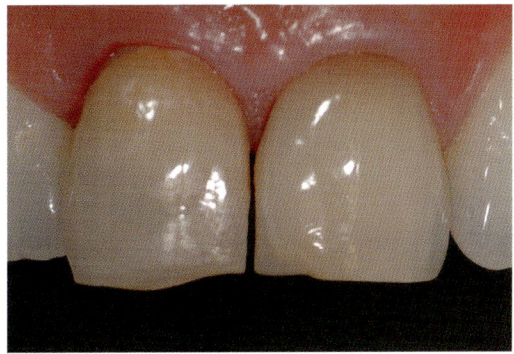

Fig. 19.28 Healed provisional complex prior to changing the crown for the definitive restoration

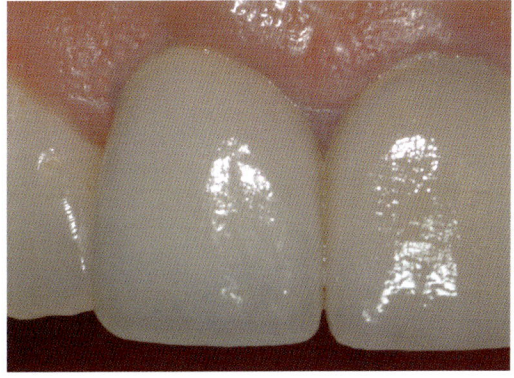

Fig. 19.29 Final restoration #8

and a record of the coronal aspect of the abutment in relation to the adjacent dentition can be obtained. This may be done in an analogue or a digital technique. Once the laboratory has the impressions and models, however, produced, along with the occlusal registration and opposing model, the definitive restoration can be fabricated. When completed this final restoration is inserted by only removing the provisional restoration and replacing this with the newly created prosthesis (Fig. 19.29).

The ZAC protocol gives the clinician a tremendous biologic advantage by never removing the patient-specific abutment once it has been affixed to the implant at the surgical appointment.

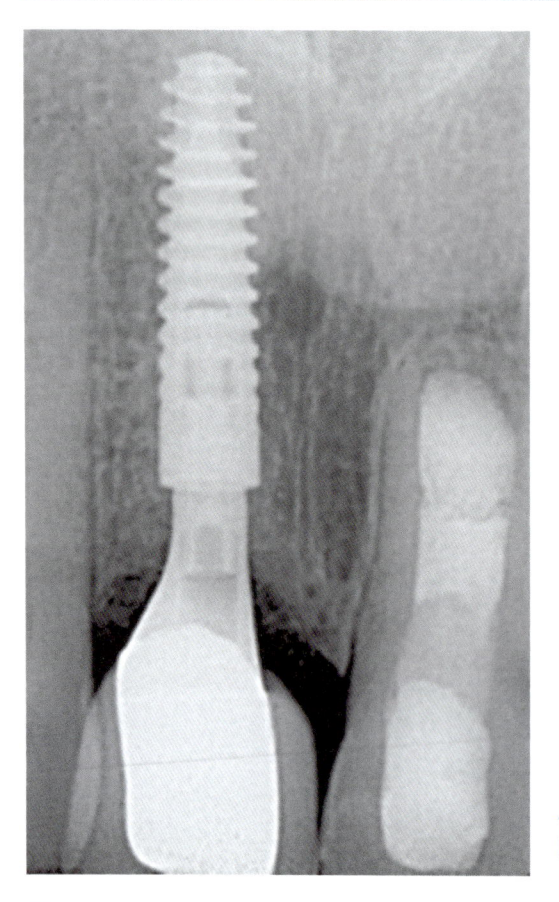

Fig. 19.30 Radiograph of implant-abutment-restoration at 3 years

When executed with a platform shift, conical cone connection implant, there is no opportunity for a microgap to exert a negative influence on the surrounding tissues. The subsequent radiographic evaluations will demonstrate the establishment of a small, lateralized 'biologic width' at a more coronal position than we are used to observing (Fig. 19.30). There is no vertical saucerization as is witnessed in standard protocols.

Conclusions

Provisional restorations, whether conventionally staged or of the immediate type, allow the clinician to preserve and ultimately control the peri-implant hard and soft tissues by mastering the restorative material stacked between the implant shoulder and that portion of the restoration which is visible supragingivally. Therefore, control of the submergence profile of the tissues gives the clinician the opportunity to position the gingival margin precisely where it is wanted for maximal aesthetic effect. This is best appreciated when the patient becomes an active participant in the aesthetic discussion. Fabrication and manipulation of the provisional restoration give both the clinician and patient an opportunity to slowly manipulate the peri-implant tissues for the benefit of contours and ultimately the aesthetic advantage. The provisional restoration is a critical component of an overall treatment plan as it affords the opportunity to critically evaluate the function and aesthetics in a material which is easily manipulated. Once functional surfaces, restorative contours, tissue margins and dento-gingival complex profiles are established to both the patients and clinician's approval, then they are able to proceed with the definitive restoration.

References

Abrahamson I, Berglundh T, Lindhe J (1997) The mucosal barrier following abutment dis/reconnection. An experimental study in dogs. J Clin Periodontol 24(8):568–572

Al-Juboori MJ, Bin Abdulrahaman S, Jassan A (2012) Comparison of flapless and conventional flap and the effect on crestal bone resorption during a 12-week healing period. Dent Implantol Updat 23(2):9–16

Al-Nsour MM, Chan HL, Wang HL (2012) Effect of the platform- switching technique on preservation of peri-implant marginal bone: a systematic review. Int J Oral Maxillofac Implants 27(1):138–145

Annibali S, Bignozzi I, Cristalli MP, Graziani F, La Monaca G, Polimeni A (2012) Peri-implant marginal bone level: a systematic review and meta-analysis of studies comparing platform switching versus conventionally restored implants. J Clin Periodontal 30(11):1097–1113

Block MS, Mercante DE, Lirette D, Mohamed W, Ryser M, Castellon P (2009) Prospective evaluation of immediate and delayed provisional single tooth restorations. J Oral Maxillofac Surg 67(11 Suppl):89–107

Broggini N, McManus LM, Hermann JS, Medina R, Schenk RK, Buser D, Cochran DL (2006) Peri-implant inflammation defined by the implant-abutment interface. J Dent Res 85(5):473–478

Buser D, Chappuis V, Bornstein MM, Wittneben JG, Frei M, Belser UC (2013) Long-term stability of contour augmentation with early implant placement following single tooth extraction in the esthetic zone: a prospective, cross-sectional study in 41 patients with a 5- to 9-year follow-up. J Periodontol 84(11):1517–1527

Chang CL, Chen CS, Hsu ML (2010) Biomechanical effect of platform switching in implant dentistry: a three-dimensional finite element analysis. Int J Oral Maxillofac Implants 25(2):295–304

Cochran D, Mau LP, Higginbottom F et al (2013) Soft and hard tissue histologic dimensions around dental implants in the canine restored with smaller-diameter abutments: a paradigm shift in peri-implant biology. Int J Oral Maxillofac Implants 28:494–502

Cumbo C, Marigo L, Somma F, La Torre G, Minciacchi I, D'Addona A (2013) Implant platform switching concept: a literature review. Eur Rev Med Pharmacol Sci 17(3):392–397

Degiudi M, Nardi D, Piattelli A (2011) One abutment at one time: non-removal of an immediate abutment and its effect on bone healing around subcrestal tapered implants. Clin Oral Implants Res 22(11):1303–1307

Degiudi M, Piattelli A, Gehrke P, Felice P, Carinci F (2006) Five-year outcome of 111 immediate nonfunctional single restorations. J Oral Implantol 32(6):277–285

Degiudi M, Piattelli A, Shibli JA, Strocchi R, Iezzi G (2009) Bone formation around a dental implant with a platform switching and another with a tissue care connection: a histologic and histomorphometric evaluation in man. Titanium 1(1):8–15

Donovan R, Fetner A, Koutouzis T, Lundgren T (2010) Crestal bone changes around implants with reduced abutment diameter placed non-submerged and at subcrestal positions: a 1-year radiographic evaluation. J Periodontol 81(3):428–434

Elian N, Bloom M, Dard M, Cho SC, Trushkowsky RD, Tarnow D (2014) Radiological and micro-computed tomography analysis of the bone at dental implants inserted 2, 3 and 4 mm apart in a mining model with platform switching incorporated. Clin Oral Implants Res 25(2):22–29

Feitosa PP, de Lima AB, Silva-Concilio LR, Brandt WC, Neves AC (2013) Stability of external and internal implant connections after a fatigue test. Eur J Dent 7:267–271

Gargiolo AW, Wentz FM, Orban B (1961) Dimensions and relations of the dentogingival junction in humans. J Periodontol 32:261–267

Grütter L, Belser UC (2009) Implant loading protocols for the partially edentulous esthetic zone. Int J Oral Maxillofac Implants 24 Suppl:169–179

Hartman GA, Cochran DL (2004) Initial implant position determines the magnitude of crestal bone remodeling. J Periodontol 75:572–577

Hermann JS, Cochran DL, Nummikoski PV, Buser D (1997) Crestal bone changes around titanium implants. A radiographic evaluation of unloaded non-submerged and submerged implants in the canine mandible. J Periodontol 68:1117–1130

Hermann JS, Schoolfield JD, Nummikoski PV, Buser D, Schenk RK, Cochran DL (2001) Crestal bone changes around titanium implants: a methodologic study comparing linear radiographic with histometric measurements. Int J Oral Maxillofac Implants 16(4):475–485

Jansen VK, Conrads G, Richter EJ (1997) Microbial leakage and marginal fit of the implant-abutment interface. Int J Oral Maxillofac Implants 12:527–540

Jeong SM, Choi BH, Li J, Kin HS, Ko CY, Jung JH, Lee HJ, Lee SH, Engelke W (2007) Flapless implant surgery: an experimental study. Oral Surg Oral Med Oral Pathol Oral Radiol Endod 104(1):24–28

Karateew ED (2014) Mac and Zac: clinical protocols for predictable implant aesthetics. Dentistry Today 33(9):90–98

Koutouzis T, Wallet S, Calderon N, Lindgren T (2011) Bacterial colonization of the implant-abutment interface using an in vitro dynamic loading model. J Periodontol 82(4):613–618

Krebs M, Schmenger K, Meumann K, Weigl P, Moser W, Nentwig GH (2013) Long-term evaluation of Ankylos dental implants, part 1: 20-year life table analysis of a longitudinal study of more than 12,500 implants. Clin Implant Dent Relat Res 17:e275

Mangano C, Mangano F, Piattelli A, Iezzi G, La Colla L, Mangano A (2008) Single-tooth Morse taper connection implants after 1 year of functional loading: a multicenter study on 302 patients. Eur J Oral Implatol 1(4):305–315

Mangano C, Mangano F, Piattelli A, Iezzi G, Mangano A, La Colla L (2009) Prospective clinical evaluation of 1920 Morse taper connection implants: results after 4 years of functional loading. Clin Oral Implants Res 20(3):254–261

Mangano C, Mangano F, Shibli JA, Tettamanti L, Figliuzzi M, d'Avila S, Sammons RL, Piatelli A (2011) Prospective evaluation of 2,549 Morse taper connection implants: 1- to 6-year data. J Periodontol 82(1):52–61

Quiryen M, Van Steenberghe D (1993) Bacterial colonization of the internal part of two stage implants. An in vivo study. Clin Oral Implants Res 4:158–161

Rodriguez-Ciurana X, Rodado-Alonso C, Selala-Torres M (2006) Benefits of an implant platform modification technique to reduce crestal bone resorption. Implant Dent 15:313–320

Romanos GE (2004) Present status of immediate loading of oral implants. J Oral Implantol 30(3):189–197

Salama H. One abutment/one time. dentalXP.com, May 2011.

Tarnow DP, Cho SC, Wallace SS (2000) The effect of inter-implant distance on the height of inter-implant bone crest. J Periodontol 71:546–549

Tesmer M, Wallet S, Koutouzis T, Lundgren T (2009) Bacterial colonization of the dental implant fixture-abutment interface: an in vitro study. J Periodontol 80(12):1991–1997

Testori T, Galli F, Capelli M, Zuffetti F, Esposito M (2007) Immediate nonocclusal versus early loading of dental implants in partially edentulous patients: 1-year results from a multicenter randomized controlled clinical trial. Int J Oral Maxillofac Implants 22(5):815–822

Vela X, Mendez V, Rodriguez X, Segala M, Tarnow DP (2012) Crestal bone changes on platform-switched implants and adjacent teeth when the tooth-implant distance is less than 1.5 mm. Int J Periodontics Restor Dent 32(2):149–155

Wadhwani C, Hess T, Pineyro A, Opler R, Chung K-H (2012) Cement application techniques in luting implant-supported crowns: a quantitative and qualitative survey. Int J Oral Maxillofac Implants 27:859–864

Wang Y, Kan J, Rungcharassaeng K, Roe P, Lozada J (2015) Marginal bone response of implant with platform switching and non-platform switching in posterior healed sites: a 1-year prospective study. Clin Oral Implants Res 26(2):220–227

Weng D, Nagata MJH, Bosco AF, de Melo LGN (2011) Influence of microgap location and configuration on radiographic bone loss around submerged implants: an experimental study in dogs. Int J Oral Maxillofac Implants 26:941–946

Wittneben JG, Buser D, Belser UC, Brägger U (2013) Peri-implant soft tissue conditioning with provisional restorations in the esthetic zone: the dynamic compression technique. Int J Periodontics Restor Dent 33(4):447–455

Zarb GA, Schmitt A (1990) The longitudinal clinical effectiveness of osseointegrated dental implants: the Toronto study. Part 1: surgical results. J Prosthet Dent 63:451–457

Biomaterials Used with Implant Abutments and Restorations

20

Toru Sato, Kazuhiro Umehara, Mamoru Yotsuya, and Michael L. Schmerman

Abstract

In the aesthetic zone, the implant superstructure and abutment are key determinants for stability and durability. In this chapter, we describe the materials and the selection criteria for the abutment and the superstructure. Additionally, complications are reviewed which may be caused by the selected material post operatively.

20.1 Introduction

In the aesthetic zone, the implant superstructure and abutment are key determining factors for stability and durability (Martin et al. 2014), they are influenced by material tolerance to para-functional habits. Their compatibility is also related to forces placed in the axial direction on the superstructure (Kois 2001). Also of importance is the form of implant being utilized. Any residual bony defect may have an effect. Finally, the color, tone, and the diaphaneity of natural teeth and soft tissues are contributory to acceptable outcomes. Zirconium is increasingly being used as a solution to the inherent implant prosthodontic problems which occur in many situations. This material has relevance as an abutment for definitive restoration in the anterior aesthetic zone. However, it should be noted that complications have been observed with zirconia as a restorative material (Takano et al. 2012) (Fig. 20.1).

Prosthetic restorations utilizing occlusal screw-retained superstructures are the treatment of choice, if possible. The restorative planning should be simple, aesthetically appealing, and provide for ease of maintenance. All these factors will minimize the total number of complications. In the aesthetic zone, however, the implant position may be influenced by anatomic limitations. In those clinical situations where the implant must be restored with an angled abutment, to compensate for off-axis

T. Sato, DDS, PhD (✉)
Department of Crown and Bridge Prosthodontics,
Tokyo Dental College, 2-9-18 Misaki-cho,
Chiyoda-ku, Tokyo 101-0061, Japan
e-mail: torusato@tdc.ac.jp

K. Umehara, DDS, PhD
Umehara Dental Office, 123 Dotemachi Hirosaki,
036-8182 Aomori, Japan
e-mail: ume1@cocoa.ocn.ne.jp

M. Yotsuya, DDS, PhD
Department of Fixed Prosthodontics,
Tokyo Dental College, 2-9-18 Misaki-cho,
Chiyoda-ku, Tokyo 101-0061, Japan
e-mail: yotsuyam@tdc.ac.jp

M.L. Schmerman, DDS
Department of Periodontics, University of Illinois
College of Dentistry, Chicago, IL 60612, USA

Illinois Masonic Hospital, Chicago, IL, USA
e-mail: drkool@uic.edu

placement, the prosthetic design often dictates a cement-retained restoration. The selection of the type of implant fixtures (style and material), to be used for the abutment and the prosthesis, demands undivided attention (Smith 1997; Belser et al. 2000; Weber and Sukotjo 2007; Salvi and Bragger 2009; Sailer et al. 2012; Shadid and Sadaqa 2012).

Moreover, the constant change and improvement in material science, i.e., prosthetic materials designed and fabricated by CAD/CAM technology, gives the restorative dentist more choices and dilemmas. Computer assistance allows the use of a ceramic puck and veneering pressed or layered porcelain, and the resultant choice of the adhesive systems is nothing less than remarkable (Welander et al. 2008).

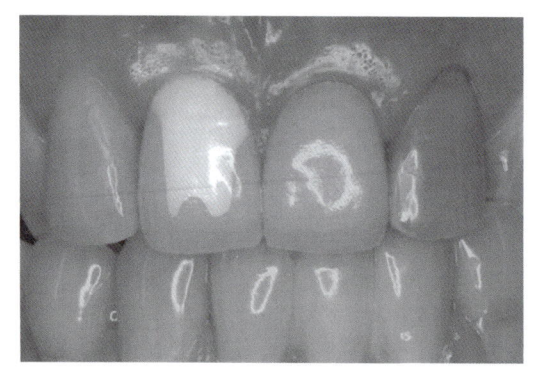

Fig. 20.1 Zirconia has relevance as an abutment for definitive restoration in the anterior aesthetic zone

20.2 Biological Aspects

Personal and professional care must be meticulous in attaining and maintaining the biological success of the restoration (Giannopoulou 2003). This cannot be overemphasized. It is important to understand that the success of an implant restoration is dependent on the interface of the implant and the abutment (Lazzara and Porter 2006). Its influence is reflected in the health of the surrounding bone and peri-implant soft tissues. The extent of a micro-gap between an implant and the abutment may be the cause of bacterial collection and invasion in the the peri-implant region (Piattelli et al. 2003) (Fig. 20.2).

The existence of a micro-gap in the two-piece implant is related to movement between the abutment and the implant body. This movement, which is precipitated by mastication or parafunctional habits, causes flexure in the abutment. This allows for a space to open and close between itself and the relatively static implant body. This opening and closing between the abutment and implant body facilitates the collection of bacteria, their by-product exotoxins and saliva (Koutouzis et al. 2011). It is theorized that this pumping of a toxic pool of materials initiates and/or promotes the inflammatory response surrounding the abutment/implant

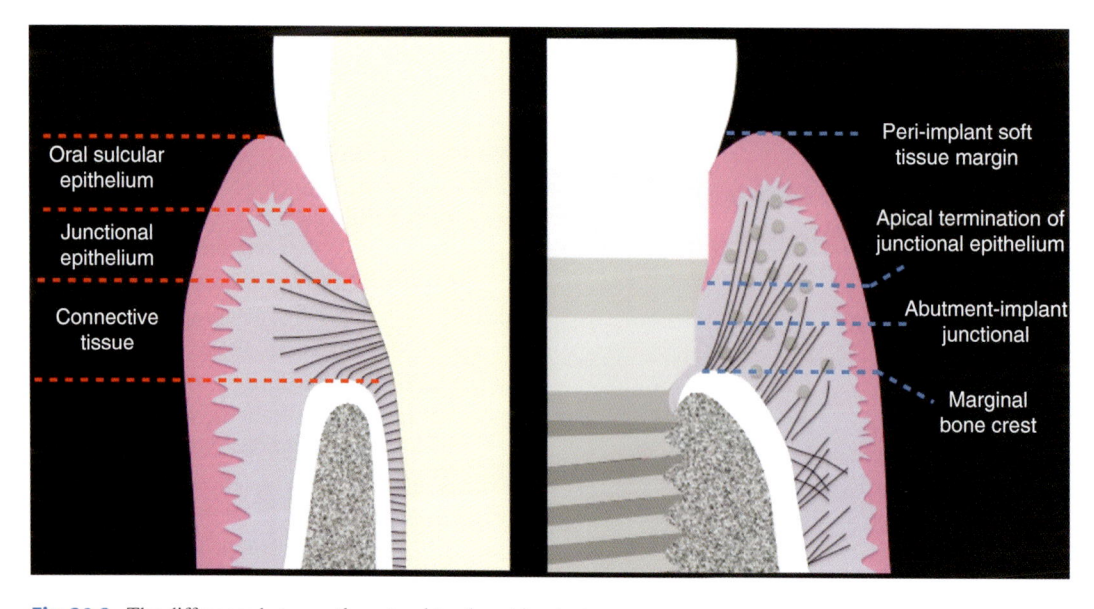

Fig. 20.2 The difference between the natural tooth and implant

20 Biomaterials Used with Implant Abutments and Restorations

junction and leads to further peri-implant bone loss (Harder et al. 2012).

20.3 Materials of the Abutment

Materials used in crowns include (1) metals (precious and non-precious), (2) ceramics, and (3) resins. The principle types of metals utilized are titanium and titanium alloys because of their mechanical strength, biocompatibility, and biostability. Ceramics such as alumina and zirconia are used for cosmetic purposes and may be fused to a metal surface (metal ceramic) or used alone (all ceramic). Resins, like ceramics are used for cosmetic purposes. Types of resins used include composite and hybrids as the provisional restoration. The material used for an abutment may influence the position of the soft tissue attachment.

Most notably, that attachment is less prone to form when abutments made from a gold alloy are used (Fig. 20.3). This can lead to eventual bone resorption. The soft tissue attachment sometimes does not form on these abutments and may instead form directly on the implant body (Abrahamsson et al. 1998).

Although titanium (Fig. 20.4) offers excellent osseointegration, oral bacteria readily adhere to it (Bürgers et al. 2010). Regardless of whether the surface is polished or rough, any small quantitative difference leads to an increase in bacterial adhesion and consequent plaque formation. Bacterial adherence to titanium is related to the material's success in osseointegration. Substances such as calcium phosphate and serum proteins preferentially layer onto the surface of titanium, thereby increasing the osseointegration potential (Hanawa and Ota 1991). Accordingly, bacteria in an oral environment may also create a biofilm upon which to adhere (Fig. 20.5).

Zirconia is a ceramic material that has excellent dimensional stability and mechanical strength because of its chemical structure. It is also known to be able to self-repair crazing (Vagkopoulou et al. 2009; Canullo et al. 2014). Zirconia should be prepared with copious amounts of water as the crystalline surface structure can fracture in its absence. (Tables 20.1 and 20.2).

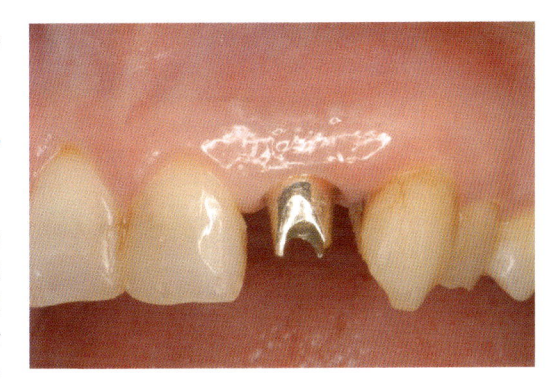

Fig. 20.3 Gold alloy abutment

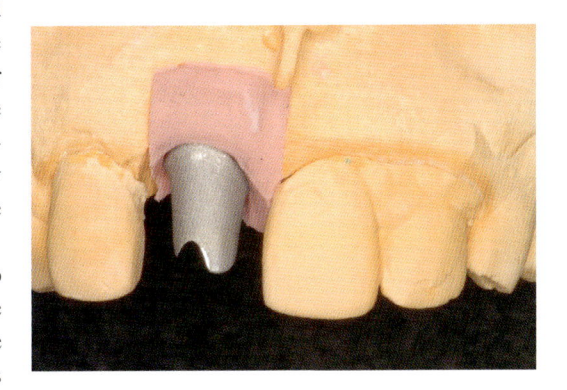

Fig. 20.4 Titanium abutment

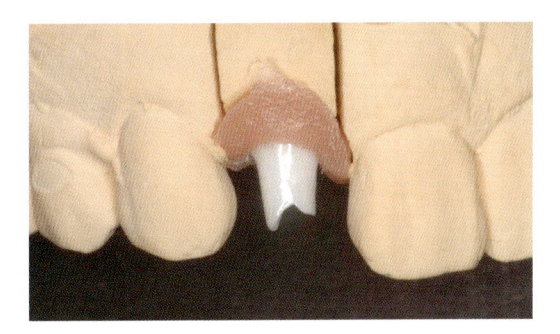

Fig. 20.5 Zirconia ceramic abutment

20.4 Abutment Selection

As the superstructures which are secured to dental implants have superstructures which may also be in contact with the peri-implant gingival tissues, biologically compatible materials must be selected. Their functionality must fulfill jaw motion requirements. In addition their appearance must satisfy aesthetic requirements. The most important factor influencing abutment selection is whether an abutment is compatible with the soft tissue while insuring complete connection between the implant body and the superstructure (Annibali et al. 2012; Benic et al. 2012; Gehrke et al. 2013) (Fig. 20.6).

Table 20.1 Positive and negative characteristics of zirconia

Positive	Negative
Hypoallergenic	Access to technology is necessary for fabrication (i.e., CAD/CAM system, sintering furnace, etc.)
Better reproduction of the color of the root surface	Not possible to solder as a metal framework
Less fluctuation in pricing of zirconium as opposed to noble metals	Difficult to remove veneering material after cementation
Thermal conductivity similar to a natural tooth	No long-term data on material

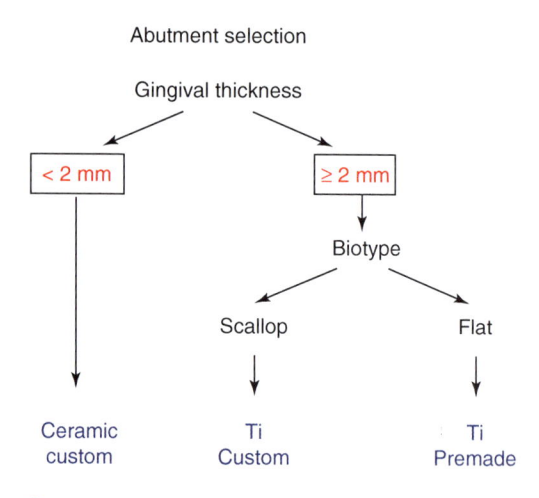

Fig. 20.6 Selection of abutment material correlates to soft tissue thickness and form

Table 20.2 Classification of ceramics for fixed prosthetics according to their clinical use with required mechanical and chemical properties (ISO6872 2015)

Class	Recommended clinical indications	Mechanical and chemical properties	
		Flexural strength [MPa] Minimum value for mean (see 7.3.1.4)	Chemical solubility [µg/cm²]
1	(a) Monolithic ceramic for single-unit anterior	50	<100
	(b) Ceramic for coverage of a metal framework or a ceramic substructure	50	<100
2	(a) Monolithic ceramic for single-unit anterior or posterior prostheses adhesively cemented	100	<100
	(b) Partially or fully covered substructure ceramic for single-unit anterior or posterior prostheses adhesively cemented	100	<2000
3	(a) Monolithic ceramic for single-unit anterior or posterior prostheses and for three-unit prostheses not involving molar restoration adhesively or nonadhesively cemented	300	<100
	(b) Partially or fully covered substructure for single-unit anterior or posterior prostheses and for three-unit prostheses not involving molar restoration adhesively or nonadhesively cemented	300	<2000
4	(a) Monolithic ceramic for three-unit prostheses involving molar restoration	500	<100
	(b) Partially or fully covered substructure for three-unit prostheses involving molar restoration	500	<2000
5	Monolithic ceramic for prostheses involving partially or fully covered substructure for four or more units or fully covered substructure for prostheses involving four or more units	800	<100

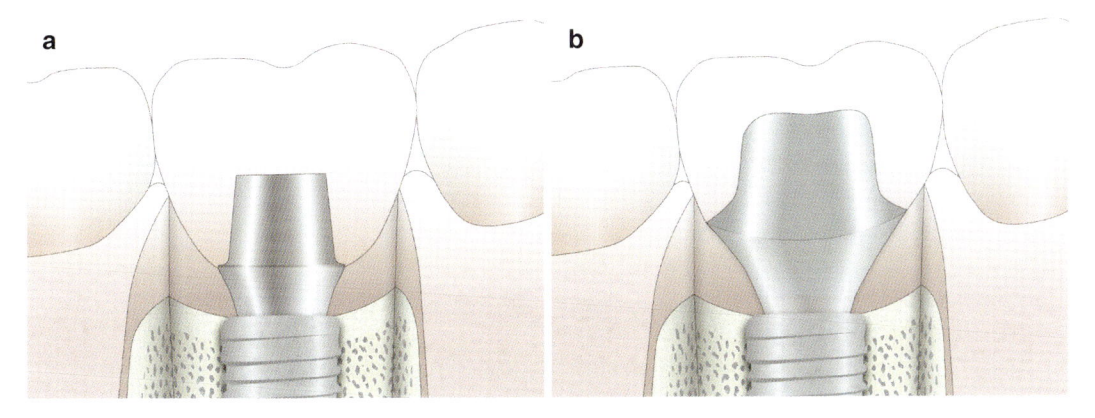

Fig. 20.7 (**a**) Pre-fabricated abutment: It is difficult to obtain a natural aesthetic appearance. (**b**) Custom abutment: It is easier to make an ideal curvature to adapt to the natural gingival sulcus

A natural aesthetic appearance is difficult to obtain with a pre-fabricated or "stock" abutment (Fig. 20.7a). To attain an aesthetic and natural appearance, an abutment that conforms to anatomical standards must be used. A shoulder shape with a curve which conforms to the natural gingival sulcus may help to achieve this goal (Fig. 20.7b). It is important to develop the soft tissue around the implant to mimic the soft tissue around the natural tooth (Gehrke et al. 2013; Levine et al. 2014).

20.5 The Custom Abutment

20.5.1 Form and Function of the Custom Abutment

Prosthetic treatment is ideally a custom-fabricated solution. In dental practice, technicians customize prostheses to work in the mouths of specific patients with individual attention to detail. This is done using standardized equipment provided by various dental manufacturers before final prosthetic placement (Gehrke et al. 2013).

The primary standard by which implant success is judged, is by how well soft tissue integrates with the prosthetic components. Success is influenced by factors which vary from patient to patient. Superstructures may be either screw retained or cemented to abutments. The advantage of screw retention is that superstructures can be removed, cleaned, and serviced outside of the oral environment (Michalakis 2003). Cementing the superstructure minimizes the size of the joint area, thus improving the fit and aesthetics. This also reduces the time and effort required for installation. The related disadvantage of cementing is thorough removal of excess cement, which is the leading cause of peri-implantitis (Linkevicius et al. 2011; Linkevicius et al. 2013). The potential problem may be minimized by using custom abutments.

20.5.2 Supragingival Contour

There exists no clinical evidence to support the "gull wing" supragingival shape preference of Kay (1985). The "gull wing" refers to the concept of the alternating rise and fall in the gingival margins of adjacent teeth (i.e., in the span of teeth 6, 7, 8, 9, 10, 11). This shape resembles a gull's wing when observed from the adjacent surface. In both tooth implant-supported restorations, with or without pontics, a provisional restoration should be placed to sculpt the supragingival contour to that of the surrounding gingival soft tissues. The contour of the final prosthesis is determined after observing the outcome. However, in the case of pontics and implants, it must be kept in mind that it is common to encounter situations where ancillary procedures must be performed prior to prosthetic placement (i.e., connective tissue grafting) on the gingival tissues. This may be done in accordance with the gull wing aesthetic concept.

20.5.3 Subgingival Contour

The subgingival contour of the abutment and crown complex can either have a straight or positive profile or conversely a concave profile. The theoretical advantage in producing a negative or concave profile is that the tissue maintains a certain amount of thickness superior to the shoulder of the implant (Hidaka and Minami 2003). When possible, it is preferable that an area from 0.5 to 1.0 mm subgingival to the implant body be made concave as described by Rompen et al. (2007). However, a straight profile is more realistic (Hidaka 2012) (Fig. 20.8a). The author believes that a concave shape apical to the gingival margin is ideal for implant restorations (Suese et al. 2009; Hidaka 2012) (Fig. 20.8b).

Contours of adjacent surfaces should be handled in the same manner as with the restoration of natural teeth. Observations made by Tarnow et al. (1992) and Cho et al. (2006), indicate that when the distance between the roots in natural teeth is about 1-2 mm and the distance between the contact point and the bone crest is 5 mm or less, soft tissue fills the gingival embrasure. This helps to avoid the so-called black triangle (Hidaka and Minami 2003). If the distance between roots is 2 mm or greater, either orthodontic treatment is performed or a half pontic shape should be used to strengthen the contour of the adjacent surface from about 1 mm below the gingival margin (Hidaka 2012). A similar approach can be used for implant restorations. Furthermore, in implant restorations, the target distance from the alveolar crest to the adjacent contacts should be 6.5 mm between natural teeth and implants and 4.5 mm between implants according to a study by Garber et al. (2001).

20.5.4 Abutment Coloration

Depending on the type of abutment (metal, zirconia etc.), the coloration of the gingival tissues may be influenced (Jung et al. 2007). It is particularly important to keep this in mind when working with custom abutments for implants in the anterior aesthetic zone. A large variety of coloration is available for zirconia abutments. As a result, translucent materials within a very small range of value can be selected (Gehrke et al. 2013).

20.5.5 Advantages of Custom Abutments

The area of transition to the gingiva is an especially important part, which determines the quality of the custom abutment. The approximation of the soft tissues around implants will resemble, soft tissue around natural teeth depends on tissue distribution in the supra-alveolar fiber apparatus. This would be difficult to achieve with pre-

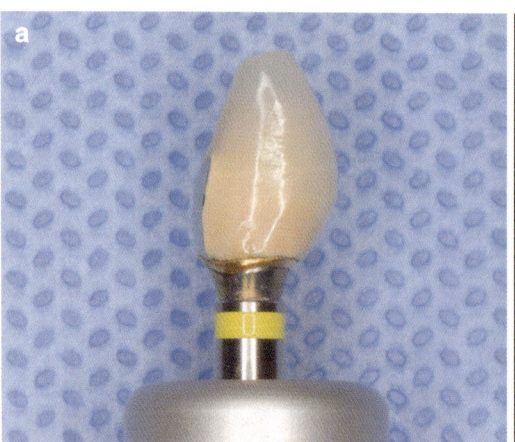

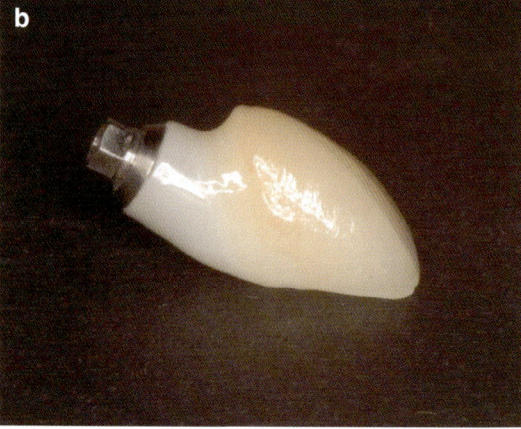

Fig. 20.8 Subgingival contour of the abutment/restorative complex. (**a**) Thin type. (**b**) Thick type

Table 20.3 The merits of the custom abutment (Modified of Gehrke et al. 2013)

The merit of the custom abutment
An improved ability to clean the cement gap
The portion of the abutment under the veneering material can be relatively small without affecting the long-term survival of the restoration. The inherent strength of the material and the thickness of the base of the structure ensure this
Emergence angle of the implant/abutment can be altered The custom abutment can secure the retention of an ideal superstructure
When produced by milling center, quality is carefully maintained

fabricated abutments. Custom abutments are advantageous in that "the thickness of the frame (core) can be reduced because the form of the crown is supported by the diminished tooth shape of the abutments." In addition, "the positioning and angle of the implants can be adjusted to a certain extent" (Table 20.3), so they can be made to fit individual patients (Gehrke et al. 2013).

20.5.6 Treatment of Abutment Surfaces

The surface texture of abutments, particularly that of the base, plays an important role in achieving and maintaining the health of soft tissue around implants. To take advantage of the benefits benefits of custom abutments produced with CAD/CAM, soft tissue attachment should be promoted through proper surface treatment. The surface shape of pre-made abutments and custom abutments produced with CAD/CAM differs greatly with respect to texture uniformity (Gehrke et al. 2013; Gehrke et al. 2015).

20.5.7 Treatment of Base Surfaces

When performing surface treatments for titanium abutments produced with CAD/CAM, it is recommended that a diamond rubber polisher with a narrow grain diameter be used for zirconia structures. A small brush and diamond polishing paste specific for zirconia are used for polishing.

Palladium is a milling residue of titanium abutments, while sulphuric acid is a milling residue of zirconia abutments. These particles are almost invisible to the unaided eye. Recent studies (Clementini et al. 2013; Canullo et al. 2012a) have evaluated the problems that these residual compounds cause in practice and their effect on the soft tissues surrounding the implants (Canullo and Gotz 2011). It is suspected that they may have some influence on the long-term prognosis of the soft tissue around the implants (Canullo and Gotz 2012).

It is recommended that abutments that are as clean as possible be used. Superstructures should be cleaned in an ultrasonic cleaner after polishing (Canullo et al. 2012b, c). A mixture of acetone and alcohol works well as an antimicrobial solution.

Plasma treatment is another method of cleaning the contaminants off the abutment proper, prior to the abutment leaving the lab. The plasma treatment generates an ionic bombardment with argon gas, which detaches the contaminants from the surface of the prosthetic product and converts them into their gaseous phase, which is ejected at the same time, removing any residue (Canullo et al. 2012a, c) (Fig. 20.9).

20.6 Selection of the Retention Method and Superstructure Characteristics

Crown superstructures can be classified as (1) cement-retained or (2) screw-retained based on the method of retention. In cement retention, superstructures are attached using a luting cement (i.e., glass ionomer cement, zinc phosphate cement, or adhesive resin cement) and cannot be removed by the patient nor easily by the dentist. In screw retention, superstructures are attached with prosthetic screws which can be removed by a dentist when necessary.

20.6.1 Cement Retention
(Fig. 20.10a–d)

The method of production of the superstructure differs greatly for cement-retained and screw-retained

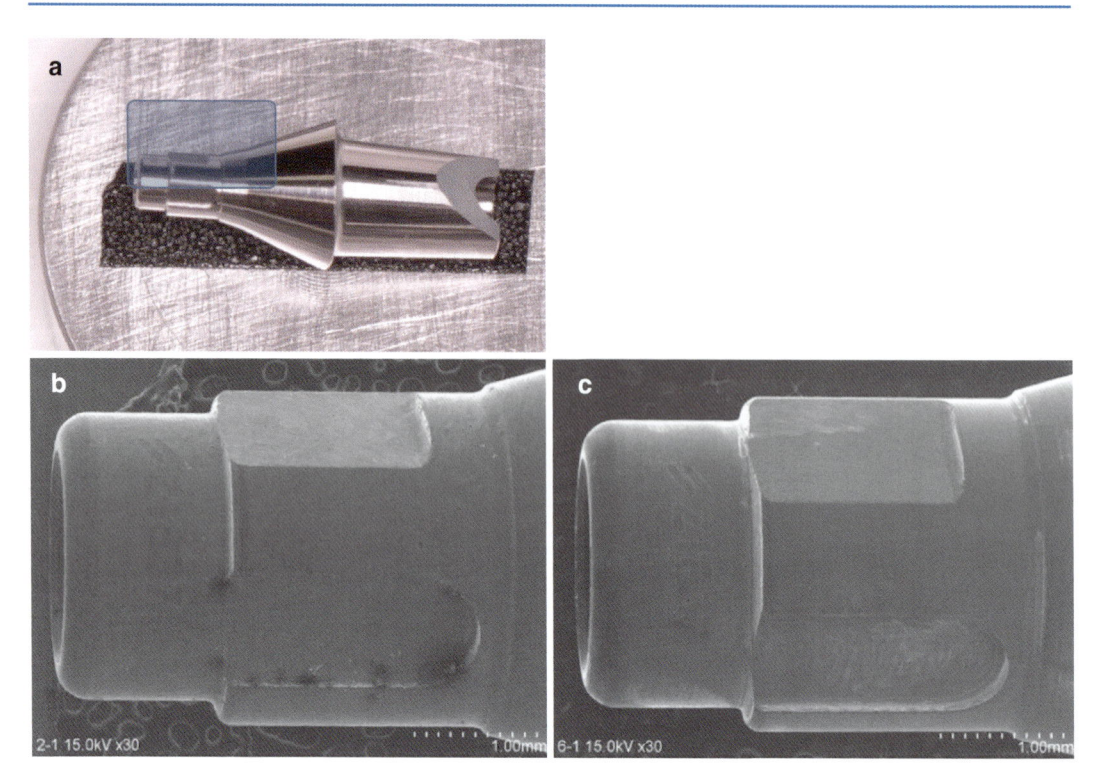

Fig. 20.9 Electronic microscope image of abutment leaving the laboratory after usual preparation procedures. (**a**) Abutment. (**b**) Before treatment with plasma cleaner. (**c**) After treatment with plasma cleaner

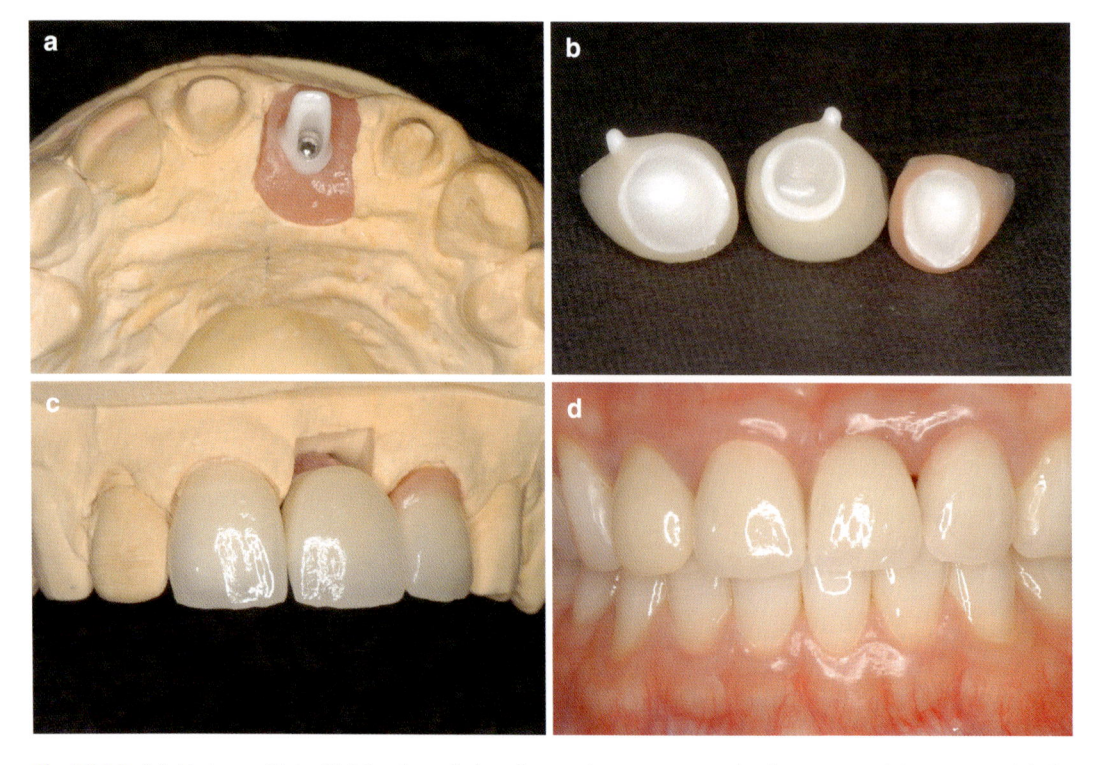

Fig. 20.10 (**a**) Abutment (Zn) which has been designed to receive a cement retained crown on a laboratory model. (**b**) Intaglio surface of Zircobond crowns. (**c**) Zircobond crowns on model. (**d**) Zircobond crown retained on the zirconia abutment with provisional cement

prostheses. Impressions for cement-retained superstructures may be taken with the abutments affixed to the implants. The superstructures are produced using similar techniques to those used for prostheses of natural teeth.

The advantage of cement retention is that the technique is relatively simple. There is no need for access holes as with screw retention and thus ensures freedom of aesthetics and design. The prime disadvantage of cement retention is that the veneering restoration must be physically separated from the substructure in order to be removed. A common disadvantage to cement retention is that the prosthetic screw may loosen and subsequently lead to inflammation in the surrounding tissues as a result of the ensuing bacterial invasion of the implant/abutment microgap. Damage to the screw and internal threads of the implant itself may also occur (Hebel and Gajjar 1997; Michalakis 2003; Wilson 2009).

20.6.2 Screw Retention
(Figs. 20.11a–d and 20.12a–d)

Screw-retained super-structures, on the other hand, must be produced with an access hole. This makes impression taking more complicated. With screw retained restorations, it is relatively easy to separate the superstructures from the bases, and it is possible to clean abutments and superstructures

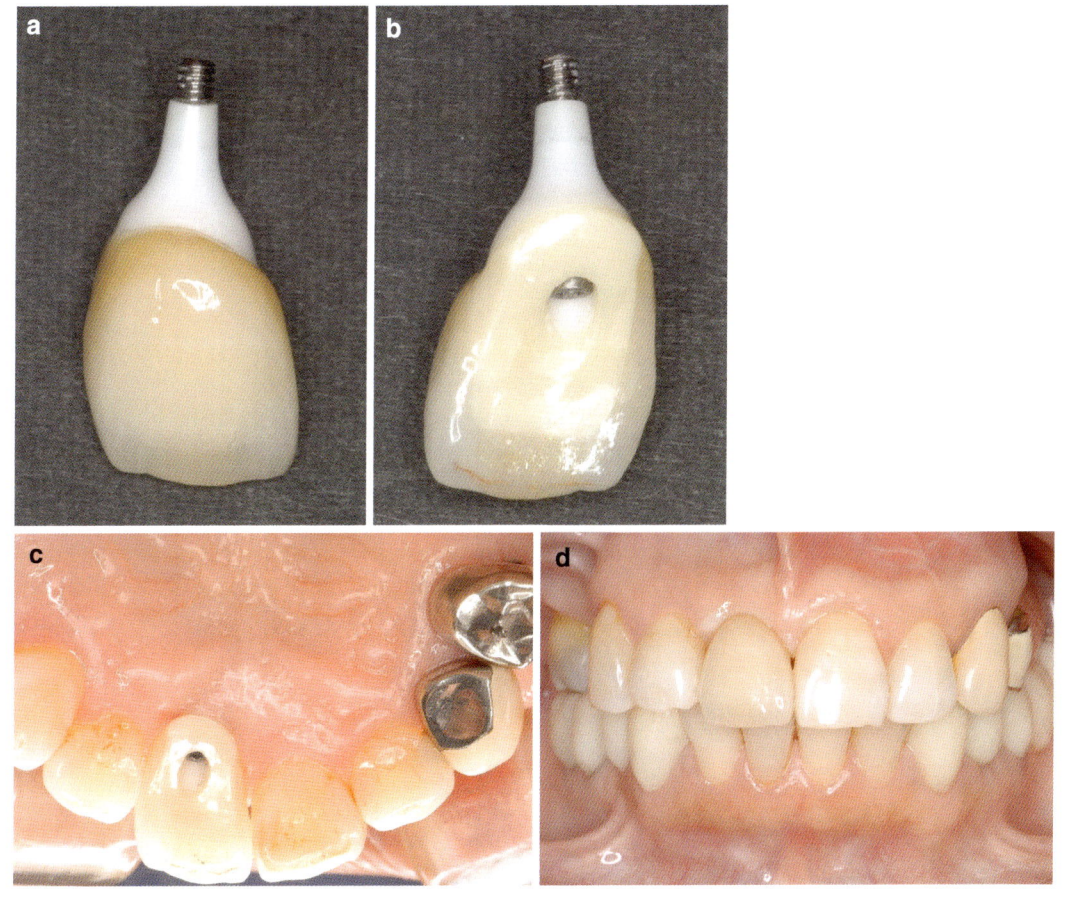

Fig. 20.11 (a) Zirconia abutment with Zircobond crown (facial view). (b) Zirconia abutment with Zircobond crown (palatal view). (c) Final restoration (palatal view). (d) Final restoration (frontal view)

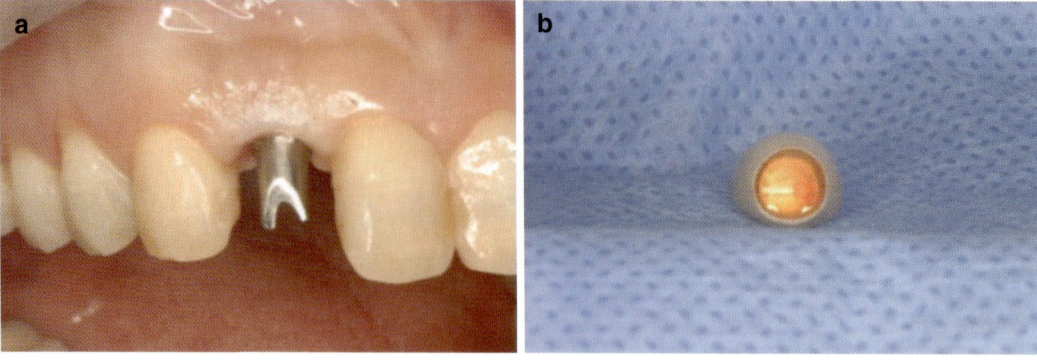

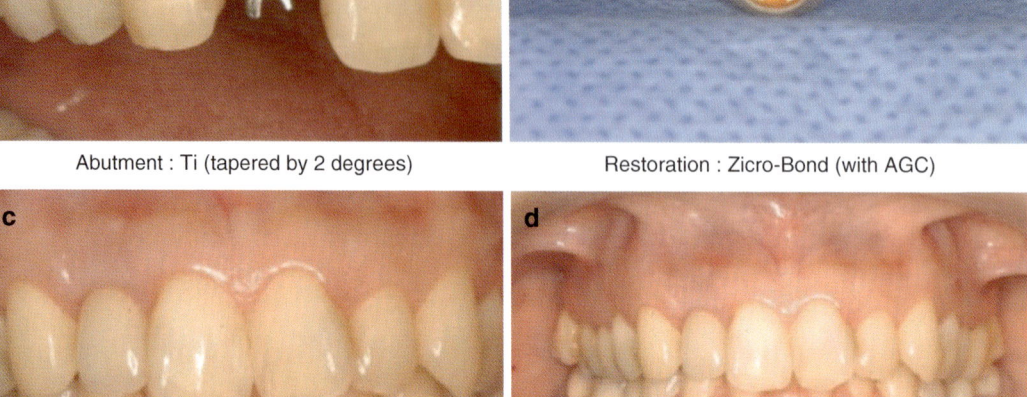

Fig. 20.12 Non-cement-retained restoration. Auro Galva Crown (AGC)-electroformed gold crown. (**a**) Abutment: Titanium with a precise 2° taper. (**b**) Restoration: Zircobond crown with AGC coping. (**c**) Final restoration (frontal view). (**d**) Final restoration (full retracted dentition)

extraorally. When the access hole is positioned on the occlusal surface, the result can be aesthetically unappealing (Michalakis 2003)

Dental professionals have varying opinions regarding the prosthetic designs in implant therapy. These opinions arise from the different perspectives of each individual. More specifically, dentists think about the precision of occlusion and design. Dental hygienists think about the ease of maintenance, while dental technicians think about the ease of making superstructures that are aesthetically pleasing. Therefore, although these opinions may be in disagreement, they should be considered along with the patient's desires. It is sensible for the dentist to make the final decision after thorough discussion between the three professionals (dentist, dental technician, and dental hygienist) along with consideration of the patient's wants and desires.

Care should be taken to have this discussion prior to the start of treatment so the patient is aware. If done so after treatment begins (implant has been placed and integrated), any limitation on the design or materials used in the prosthesis may lead to the dissatisfaction of the patient.

Once the definitive prosthetic design of the superstructure has been determined, a decision on the material it is to be fabricated from must be made. The material that is selected can also influ-

20 Biomaterials Used with Implant Abutments and Restorations

Table 20.4 Selection criteria of the restorative material in accordance with the case type (Modified of Sogo 2010)

	Strength	Aesthetic/function
Ceramics	Modern ceramics demonstrate low abrasive characteristics. (Older types of ceramics may cause wear to the opposing natural dentition).	Aesthetics are easy to maintain in the long term
	May be fractured by sudden trauma	Low plaque retention
Hybrid resin	Minimal wear to opposing natural dentition	Retrograde wear and change of color common findings – material is more porous and softer than ceramics
	Adhesive strength with metal frame decreases with age	High plaque retention
	Material absorbs saliva, causing staining and material deterioration	
	Repair of fracture made with relative ease	
Metal	Excellent resistance to wear, kind to opposing dentition	Not tooth colored leading to consideration of inferior aesthetics
		Less adhesion of the plaque than a hybrid resin

ence the selection of the materials to be used for abutments and frameworks at a later date. The crown material is typically selected from three categories: ceramics, hybrid resins, and metals. Selection criteria for different patients are listed below (Sogo 2010) (Table 20.4).

20.6.3 Complications of Abutment Materials: Fracture of the Implant Abutment

Destructive testing of the implant abutment (Kim et al. 2013) and wear testing of zirconia and titanium abutments (Hara et al. 2014) have been reported. Figure 20.13 shows the fracture of the Zirconium custom abutments in a clinical situation. Ultimately, custom titanium abutments were fabricated anew for this patient and the clinical outcome thus far has been good. SEM images of the fractured zirconia abutments were taken, and elemental analysis was performed with an electron-probe microanalyzer (JXA-8200, JEOL, Tokyo), after which detected elements were compared. Observation of a cross section of a fractured abutment with a SEM revealed that three fractures had arisen in the area where buccal stress had concentrated. In addition, the elemental analysis detected Ti in the fractured area. The reason for these fractures occurred in succession was likely that tensile stress was focused on the buccal abutment junctions. Furthermore, the Ti detected in the fractured abutments in elemental analysis was probably detected in the internal wall of the implant itself. In essence, zirconia abutments may be made of more aesthetically pleasing material, but they can fracture due to insufficient strength when adequate abutment thickness cannot be achieved. Moreover, because zirconia is a hard material, it may scrape off the internal wall of the implant itself (Figs. 20.13 and 20.14).

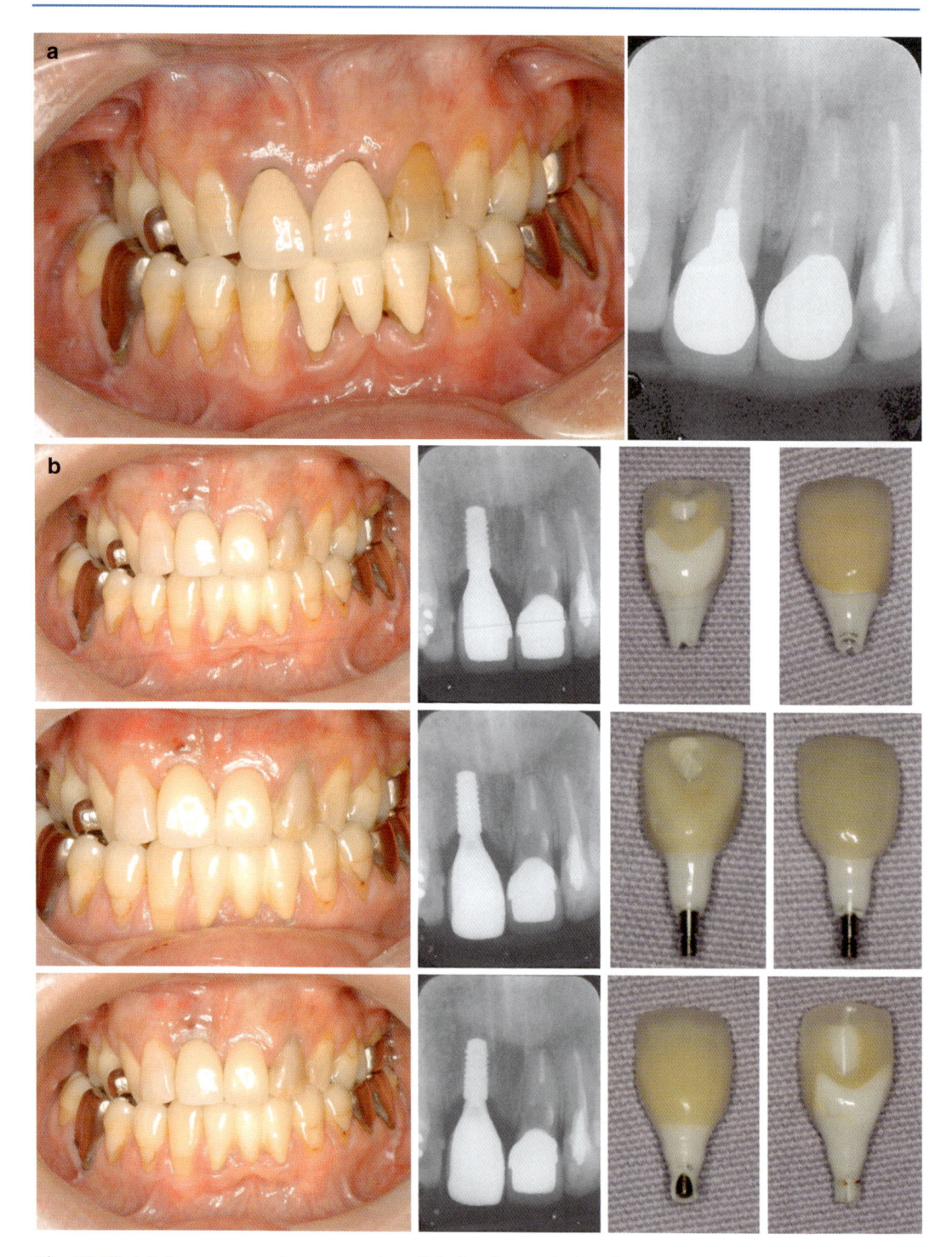

Fig. 20.13 (**a**) Demonstrates the preoperative clinical and radiographic findings. (**b, c**) Three different fractures in CARES zirconia abutments of Straumann bone-level system over a span of 5 months. These images represent the outcome after 2 years of initial function of the original Zr abutment. It was realized that the abutment had fractured when the superstructure was removed after a fistula was noted on the labial side of the maxillary right central incisor. A new abutment was created. However, additional fractures in the abutments were observed in August and September of the same year

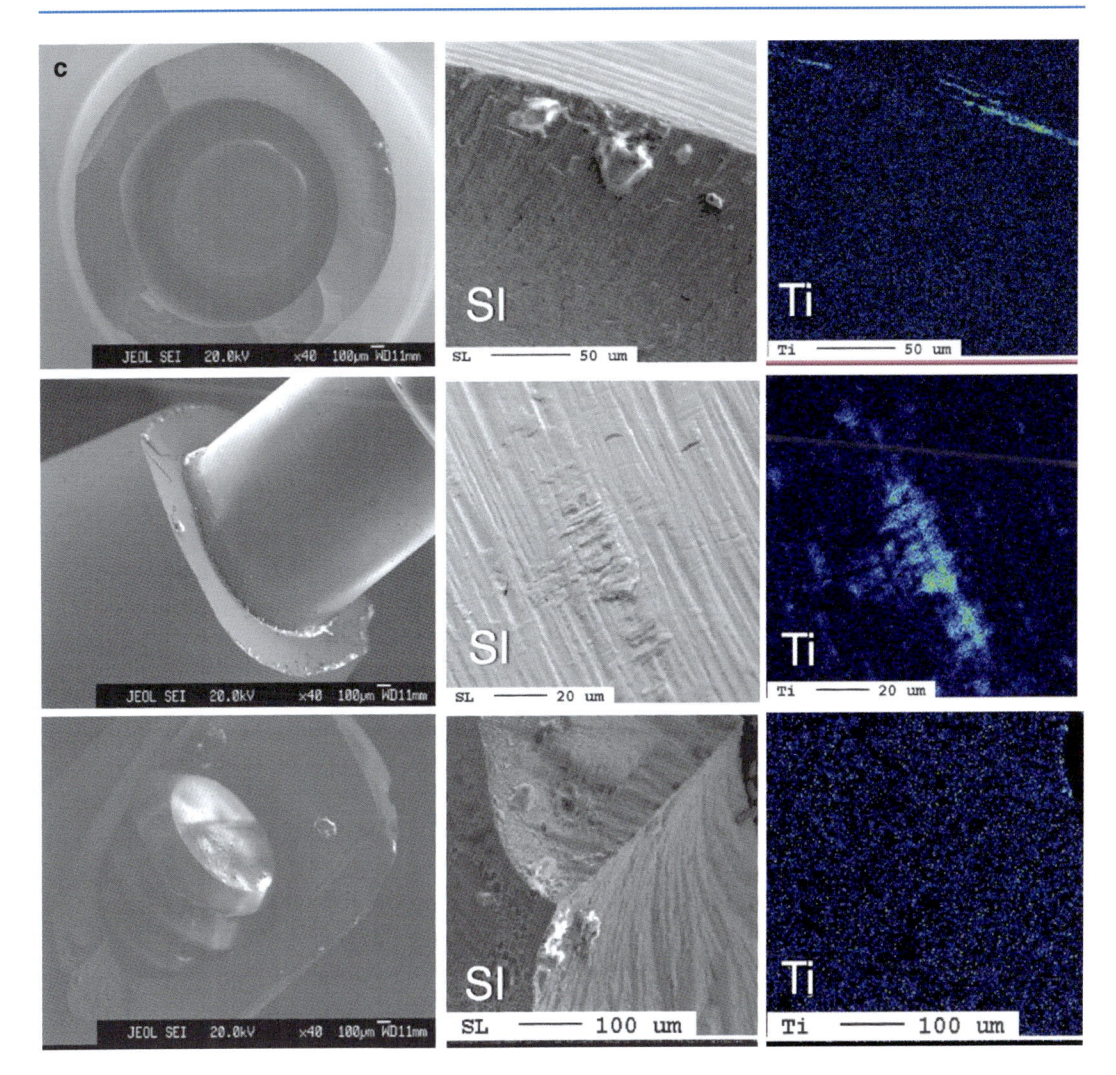

20 Biomaterials Used with Implant Abutments and Restorations

Fig. 20.13 (continued)

Pre-made Titanium   **Zirconia custom**   **Titanium sleeve**

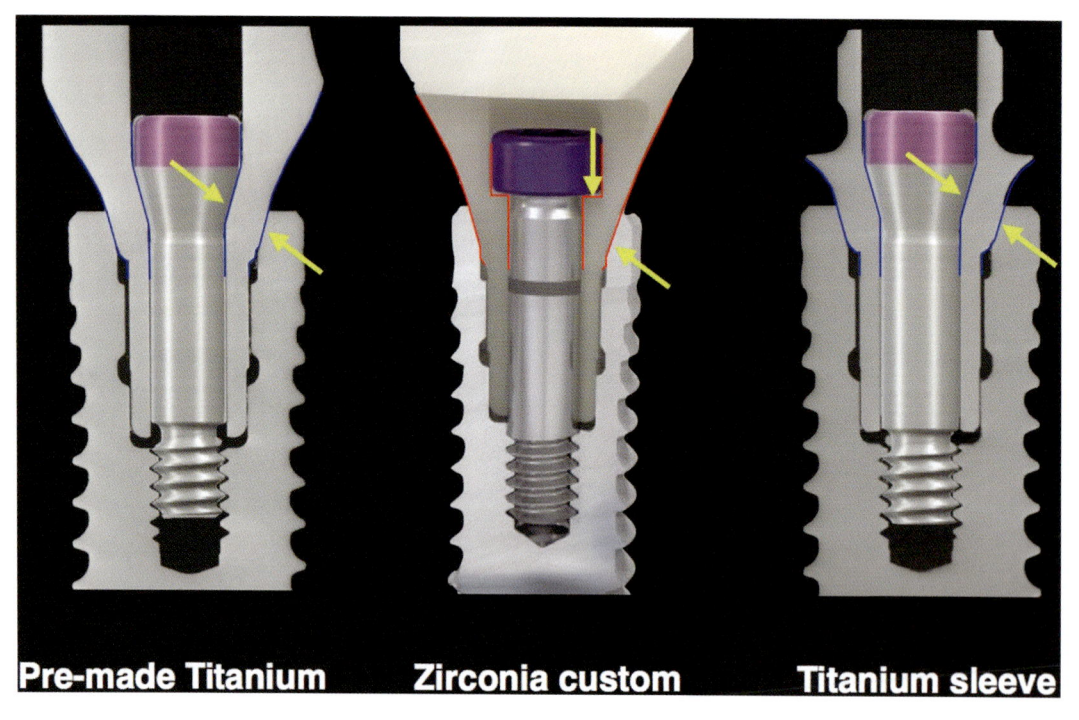

Fig. 20.14 Demonstrates the internal structure of the various abutments (Modified quotation by Institut Straumann AG, 2013). As is the case with pre-made titanium and titanium sleeve-type abutment/implant combinations, the taper of wall receiving the screw surface and intaglio surface of the implant receiving the abutment are matched so that upon tightening, the loads will be matched. However, as with the case of zirconia abutments (Kitagawa et al. 2005; Norton 1999), the screw head is a flat topography as the abutment is not elastic. It is considered necessary that the clinician must pay attention to the torque values generated as to avoid excessive tightening

Summary

Superstructures and abutments of dental implants must be designed and manufactured with tolerances of high stability, durability, resistance to chemicals, and must be biocompatible. In the aesthetic zone, zirconia has been used in various situations as abutments of implant superstructures or for crowns. It is often unknown what effect the physical changes which occur with age will have on this material. In addition, various factors such as the type of implant, the design or material of abutments, the degree of plaque control, and occlusal forces influence cosmetic prostheses. Not only must we perform evidence-based treatments but also select the appropriate treatment for each patient. This is based on their individual characteristics while referencing long-term outcome observations and case studies.

References

Abrahamsson I, Berglundh T, Glantz PO, Lindhe J (1998) The mucosal attachment at different abutments. An experimental study in dogs. J Clin Periodontol 25(9):721–727

Annibali S, Bignozzi I, La Monaca G, Cristalli MP (2012) Usefulness of the aesthetic result as a success criterion for implant therapy: a review. Clin Implant Dent Relat Res 14:3–40

Benic GI, Wolleb K, Sancho-Puchades M, Hammerle CH (2012) Systematic review of parameters and methods for the professional assessment of aesthetics in dental implant research. J Clin Periodontol 39(suppl 12):160–192

Belser UC, Mericske-Stern R, Bernard JP, Taylor TD (2000) Prosthetic management of the partially dentate patient with fixed implant restorations. Clin Oral Implants Res 11(suppl 1):126–145

Bürgers R, Gerlach T, Hahnel S, Schwarz F, Handel G, Gosau M (2010) In vivo and in vitro biofilm formation on two different titanium implant surfaces. Clin Oral Implants Res 21:156–164

Bundy KJ (1994) Corrosion and other electrochemical aspects of biomaterials. Crit Rev Biomed Eng 22(3/4):139–251

Canullo L, Gotz W (2011) Cell growth on titanium disks treated by plasma of argon: experimental study. Clin Oral Implants Res 22(9):1082–1083

Canullo L, Gotz W (2012) Peri-implant hard tissue response to glow – discharged abutment: prospective study. Preliminary radiological results. Ann Anat 194:174–478

Canullo L, Micarelli C, Clementini M, Carinci F (2012a) Cleaning procedures on customized abutment: microscopical, microbiological and chemical analysis. Clin Oral Implants Res 23(Suppl 7):55–56

Canullo L, Micarelli C, Iannello G (2012b) Microscopical and chemical surface characterization of the gingival portion and connection of an internal hexagon abutment before and after different technical stages of preparation, Clinical Oral Implant Research, Early View, First publishing online; 16 May 2012

Canullo L, Micarelli C, Lembo-Fazio L, Iannello G, Clementini M (2012c) Microscopical and microbiologic characterization of customized titanium abutments after different cleaning procedure, Clinical Oral Implant Research, Early View, First publishing online; 5 Dec 2012

Canullo L, Micarelli C, Lembo-Fazio L, Iannello G, Clementini M (2014) Microscopical and microbiologic characterization of customized titanium abutments after different cleaning procedures. Clin Oral Implants Res 25:328–336

Cho HS, Jang HS, Kim DK, Park JC, Kim HJ, Choi SH et al. (2006) The effects of interproximal distances between roots on the existence of interdental papillae according to the distance from the contact point to the alveolar crest. J Periodontol 77:1651–1657

Clementini M, Canullo L, Micarelli C (2013) Fibroblast growth on titanium disks treated by argon plasma: an in vitro triple-blinded study. Eur J Oral Implantol 6(Suppl. Spring):S29–S30

ISO 6872 (2015) Dentistry-ceramic material International Standard ISO 6872 4th edn, 2015-06-1, Switzerland

Garber D, Salama M, Salama H (2001) Immediate total tooth replacement. Compendium 22:210–217

Gehrke P, Ludwigshafen FC (2013) Join the (r)evolution, individual, CAD/CAM-supported implant setups part 1. Team work. J Cont Dent Educ 4:330–337

Gehrke P, Tabellion A, Fischer C (2015) Microscopical and chemical surface characterization of CAD/CAM zircona abutments after different cleaning procedures. A qualitative analysis. J Adv Prosthodont 7:151–159

Giannopoulou C (2003) Effect of intracrevicular restoration margins on peri-implant health: clinical, biochemical, and microbiologic findings around esthetic implants up to 9 years. Int J Oral Maxillofac Implants 18:173–181

Hanawa T, Ota M (1991) Calcium phosphate naturally formed on titanium in electrolyte solution. Biomaterials Oct 12(8):767–774

Harder S, Quabius ES, Ossenkop L, Mehl C, Kern M (2012) Surface contamination of dental implants assessed by gene expression analysis in a whole-blood in vitro assay: a preliminary study. J Clin Periodontol 39(10):987–994

Hara M, Takuma Y, Sato T, Koyama T, Yoshinari M (2014) Wear performance of bovine tooth enamel against translucent tetragonal zirconia polycrystals after different surface treatments. Dent Mater J 33(6):811–817

Hebel KS, Gajjar RC (1997) Cement-retained versus screw-retained implant restorations: achieving optimal occlusion and esthetics in implant dentistry. J Prosthet Dent 77:28–35

Hidaka T, Minami M (2003) The basic coronal restoration treatment. Ishiyaku Publication Inc., Tokyo, pp 67–68

Hidaka T (2012) Protocol in esthetic implant restoration. Ann Jpn Prosthodont Soc 4:35–42

Jung RE, Sailer I, Hämmerle CH, Attin T, Schmidlin P (2007) In Vitro color changes of soft tissues caused by restorative materials. Int J Periodontics Restorative Dent 27(3):251–257

Kay HB (1985) Criteria for restorative contours in the altered periodontal environment. Int J Periodontics Restor Dent 5(3):42–63

Kim J, Raigrodski A, Flinn B, Rubenstein J, Chung K, Mancl L (2013) In vitro assessment of three types of zirconia implant abutments under static load. J Prosthet Dent 109:255–263

Kitagawa T, Tanimoto Y, Odaki M, Nemoto K, Aida M (2005) Influence of implant/abutment joint designs on abutment screw loosining in a dental implant system. J Biomed Mater Res B Appl Biomater 75B:457–463

Kois JC (2001) Predictable single tooth peri-implant esthetics: five diagnostic keys. Compend Contin Educ Dent 22(3):199–206

Koutouzis T, Wallet S, Calderon N, Lundgren T (2011) Bacterial colonization of the implant-abutment interface using an in vitro dynamic loading model. J Periodontol 82(4):613–618

Lazzara RJ, Porter SS (2006) Platform switching as a means to achieving implant dentistry for controlling post-restorative crestal bone levels. Int J Periodontics Restor Dent 26:9–17

Levine RA, Huynh-Ba G, Cochran DL (2014) Soft tissue augmentation procedures for mucogingival defects in esthetic sites. Int J Oral Maxillofac Implants 29(suppl):155–185

Linkevicius T, Vindasiute E, Puisys A, Peciuliene V (2011) The in uence of margin location on the amount of undetected cement excess after delivery of cement-retained implant restorations. Clin Oral Implants Res 22:1379–1384

Linkevicius T, Vindasiute E, Puisys A, Linkeviciene L, Maslova N, Puriene A (2013) The infuence of the cementation margin position on the amount of undetected cement. A prospective clinical study. Clin Oral Implants Res 24:71–76

Martin WC, Pollini A, Morton D (2014) The infuence of restorative procedures on esthetic outcomes in implant dentistry: a systematic review. Int J Oral Maxillofac Implants 29(suppl):142–154

Michalakis KX, Hirayama H, Garefis PD (2003) Cement-retained versus screw-retained implant restorations: a critical review. Int J Oral Maxillofac Implants 18:719–728

Norton MR (1999) Assessment of cold-welding properties of the conical interface of two commercially available implant systems. J Prosthet Dent 81(2):159–166

Piattelli A, Vrespa G, Petrone G, Iezzi G, Annibali S, Scarano S (2003) Role of the microgap between implant and abutment : a retrospective histologic evaluation in monkeys. J Periodontol 74:346–352

Rompen E, Raepsaet N, Domken O, Touati B, van Dooren E (2007) Soft tissue stability at the facial aspect of gingi-vally converging abutments in the esthetic zone: a pilot clinical study. J Prosthet Dent 97(6Suppl): S119–S125

Sailer I, Muhlemann S, Zwahlen M, Hammerle CH, Schneider D (2012) Cemented and screw-retained implant reconstructions: a systematic review of the survival and complication rates. Clin Oral Implants Res 23(suppl 6):163–201

Salvi GE, Bragger U (2009) Mechanical and technical risks in implant therapy. Int J Oral Maxillofac Implants 24(suppl):69–85

Shadid R, Sadaqa N (2012) A comparison between screw- and cement-retained implant prostheses. A literature review. J Oral Implantol 38:298–307

Smith RB (1997) Cemented vs screw-retained implant prostheses: the controversy continues. Alpha Omegan 90:58–63

Sogo A (2010) Implant prosthesis for young dentists and technicians Introduction to technical experts – Step by step from examination and diagnosis to superstructure installation, Quintessence of Dental Technology Art & Practice (suppl), Tokyo pp 57–66

Suese K, Sato T, Minami M, Kawazoe T (2009) Stress analysis of the design of zirconia copings and abutments on implant restorations: a 3-D finite element method. J Jpn Soc Oral Implantol 22:461–470

Takano T, Tasaka A, Yoshinari M, Sakurai K (2012) Fatigue strength of Ce-TZP/AL2O3 nanocomposite with different surfaces. J Dent Res 91:800–804

Tarnow DP, Magner AW, Fletcher P (1992) The effect of the distance from the contact point to the crest of bone on the presence or absence of the interproximal dental papilla. J Periodontol 63:995–996

Vagkopoulou T, Koutayas SO, Koidis P, Strub JR (2009) Zirconia in dentistry: part1. Discovering the nature of an upcoming bioceramic. Eur J Esthet Dent 4(2):130–151

Weber HP, Sukotjo C (2007) Does the type of implant prosthesis affect outcomes in the partially edentulous patient? Int J Oral Maxillofac Implants 22(suppl): 140–172

Welander M, Abrahamsson I, Berglundh T (2008) The mucosal barrier at implant abutments of different materials. Clin Oral Implants Res 19(7):635–641

Wilson TG Jr (2009) The positive relationship between excess cement and peri-implant disease: A prospective clinical endoscopic study. J Periodontol 80:1388–1392

Digital Implant Abutment and Crowns in the Aesthetic Zone

21

Nesrine Z. Mostafa, Chris Wyatt, and Jonathan A. Ng

Abstract

The use of digital technology has revolutionized implant dentistry by enhancing diagnostics, streamlining treatment planning, increasing the accuracy of implant placement and optimizing the design of abutments and crowns. This chapter describes the digital workflow in terms of the following aspects: (1) digital impression, (2) digital implant treatment planning and (3) digital abutment and crown design and manufacturing. Advances in digital technology are also discussed including (1) current range of materials available for implant abutment fabrication using computer-aided design and computer-aided manufacturing (CAD/CAM) and (2) CAD/CAM provisional crown at the time of implant placement.

21.1 Introduction

Replacement of missing anterior teeth with implant-supported restorations is a challenging procedure due to high aesthetic and functional demands of patients. The provision of an aesthetic restoration requires ideal implant placement, properly designed abutments and crowns as well as proper material selection (Fig. 21.1). The introduction of digital technology for three-dimensional radiography, implant planning, abutment and crown fabrication offers more control and potentially enhances aesthetic result for today's patients (Fig. 21.1).

N.Z. Mostafa, BDS, MSc Dip Pros, PhD, FRCD(C) (✉)
C. Wyatt, BSc, DMD, MSc, Dip Pros, FRCD(C)
Division of Prosthodontics & Dental Geriatrics,
Department of Oral Health Sciences,
University of British Columbia, 2199 Wesbrook Mall,
Vancouver, BC V6T1Z3, Canada
e-mail: nmostafa@dentistry.ubc.ca; cwyatt@dentistry.ubc.ca

J.A. Ng, BMedSc, DDS, MSc FRCD(C)
#1403-805 West Broadway,
Vancouver, BC V5Z1K1, Canada
e-mail: dr.ng@prosthodontist.ca

21.2 Digital Treatment Planning (CBCT and Digital Impressions)

The planning for all implant reconstructions needs to be driven by the dental professional who is placing the final prosthesis (Hinckfuss et al. 2012). Implant treatment planning in the aesthetic

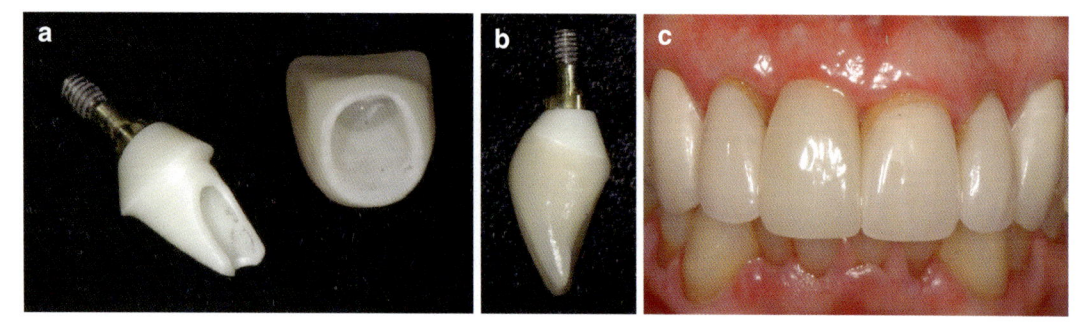

Fig. 21.1 Restoration of a single missing anterior tooth with an all ceramic crown and abutment: (**a**) ceramic abutment and crown, (**b**) ceramic abutment and crown emergence profile and (**c**) ceramic abutment and crown replacing the maxillary right central incisor

zone (maxillary incisors, canines and premolars) poses a particular challenge. The position, depth and angulation of the implant determines the abutment design, which can only be determined if the final crown has been envisioned.

Diagnostic records for treatment planning implant reconstructions include extra-oral and intraoral photographs, articulated study casts and cone beam computed tomography (CBCT). Diagnostic visualization of the proposed crown (wax-up) provides information on the available restorative space, appropriate emergence profile and the selection of abutment and crown materials (El Askary 2001; Karunagaran et al. 2014).

The use of CBCT has significantly improved the diagnostic information available for clinicians and has facilitated surgical guidance for the accurate surgical placement of implants based on the planned restoration (Fanning 2011). CBCT allows the visualization of the height and width of the remaining bone, root morphology of adjacent teeth and proximity to important anatomical structures (Fig. 21.2). Implant planning software allows for accurate selection of implant size, position and angulation based on the planned restoration and patient's anatomy determined from the CBCT scan (Orentlicher et al. 2012) (Fig. 21.2).

Fusion of digital data from the CBCT (DICOM files) data and digital data (STL files) from the scanned wax-up of the restoration on a dental cast or digital impression with a virtual wax-up is possible (Fig. 21.3). The use of a virtual wax-up saves laboratory time and cost by removing manual wax-up reproduction of the missing teeth. Moreover, this virtual setting enables clinicians to virtually articulate the maxillary and mandibular dentition, to restore missing teeth in functional positions and to fabricate the surgical guide (Worthington et al. 2010). It is now possible to digitally plan implant surgery, fabricate surgical guides and fabricate CAD/CAM abutments and crowns (Bornstein et al. 2014) (Fig. 21.3).

Currently, there are several implant planning programmes using virtual implant placement and subsequent fabrication of surgical guides including Nobel Clinician (Nobel Biocare), In Vivo (Anatomage) and SIMPLANT (Materialize). Each software platform differs in the type of guides which can be fabricated and hosts a library of compatible implant system. Software systems have allowed for increased efficiency and accuracy in planning implant treatment. The majority of the third-party planning software render cone beam CT (CBCT) information into an image that can be moved, rotated and enlarged on the monitor, which offers a more realistic evaluation of the available bone and structural limitations. Proposed implants are digitally positioned in the software and are chosen from a complete library of available implant types, diameters and lengths. With the ability to annotate vital structures such as nerves and other bone limitations, the software is capable of providing warnings when planned implant positions are unfavourable. This software also allows for the ability to merge DICOM data obtained from the CBCT with the STL file created

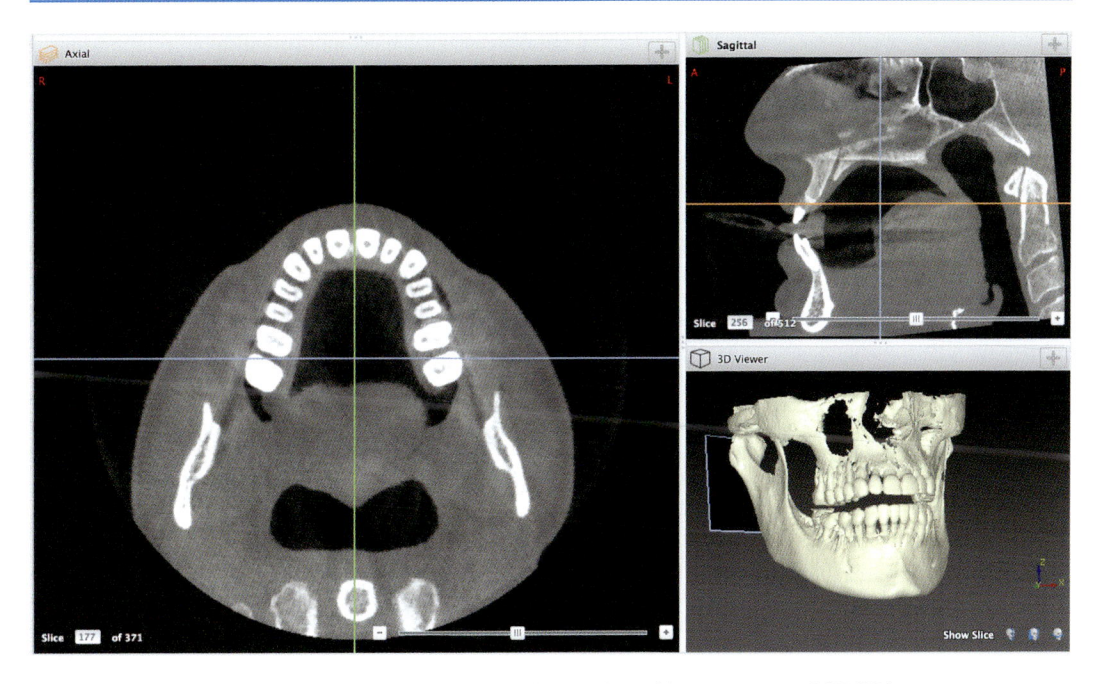

21 Digital Implant Abutment and Crowns in the Aesthetic Zone

Fig. 21.2 Axial cross section, sagittal cross section and frontal view of 3D reconstructed CBCT images

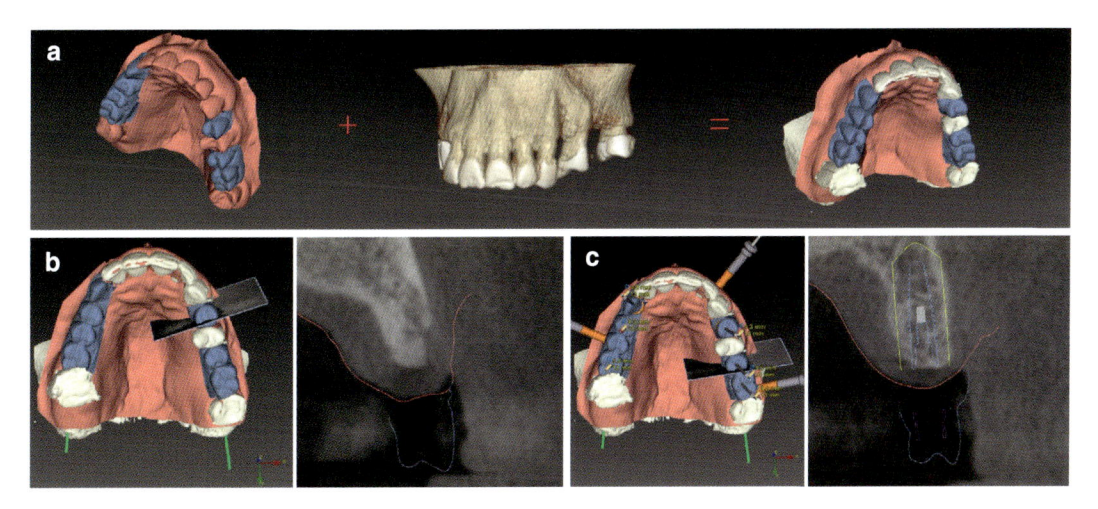

Fig. 21.3 Digital implant planning: (**a**) fusion of the data from an STL file of the digital cast with the wax-up and the DICOM data from the CBCT, (**b, c**) prosthetically driven implant surgical planning

from the digital scan of a dental cast with an idealized wax mock-up to create a unified image that can then facilitate even more precise planning of the implants position and angulation (Fig. 21.4). The ability to do this not only provides digital visualization of planned restorative positions, but can now more adequately and more predictably anticipate necessary adjunctive surgical procedures such as bone grafting and even soft tissue augmentation. With the ability to exchange this information digitally, it facilitates an advanced treatment planning interaction between the restoring clinician and surgeon. The ability to plan more accurately is the prerequisite for more appropriate

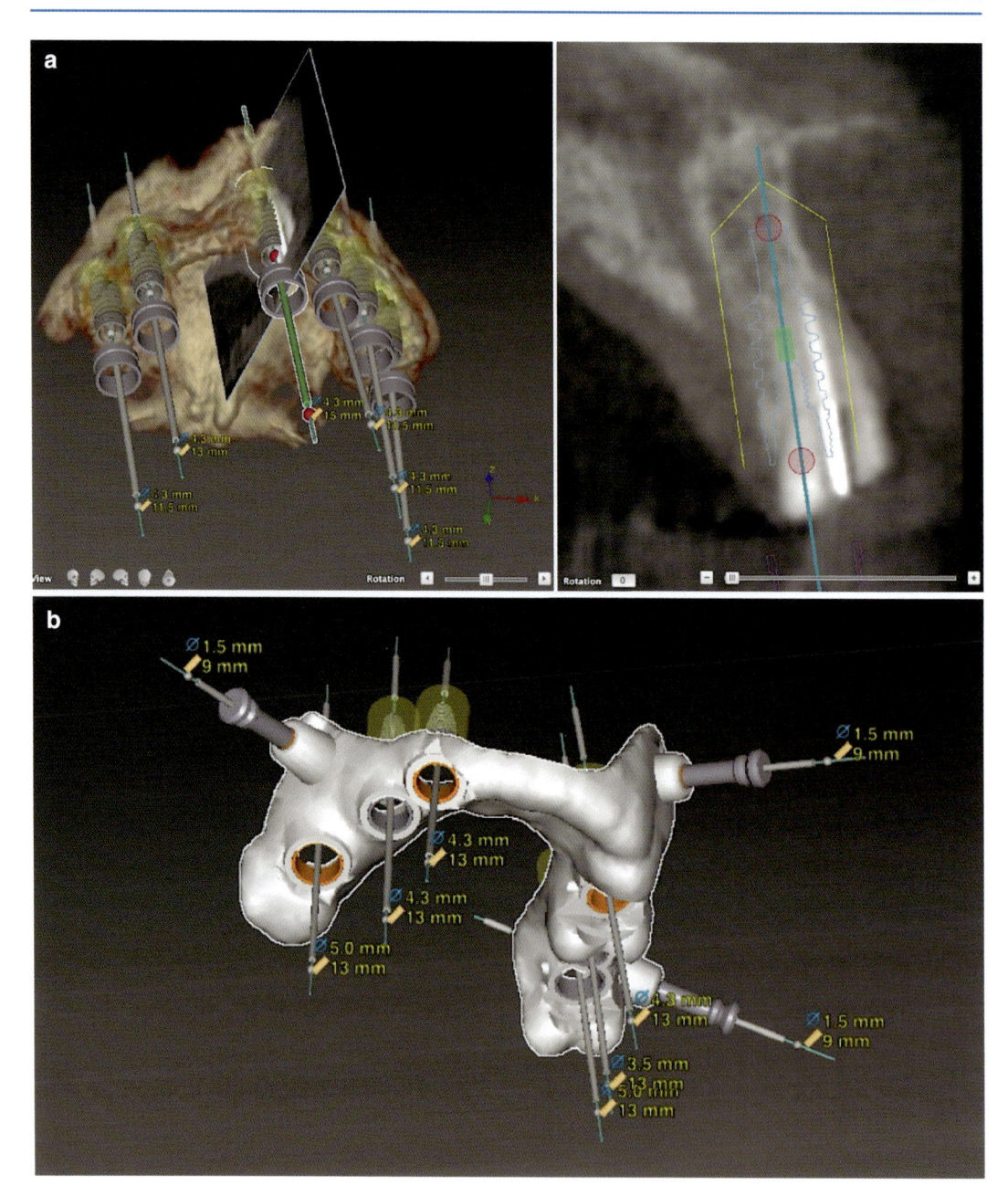

Fig. 21.4 Planning of the implant surgery utilizing Nobel Clinician: (**a**) virtual implant planning and placement and (**b**) CAD/CAM surgical guide design

and accurate delivery of implant therapy. Digital treatment planning is easily converted to clinical reality with the click of a button for the fabrication of a surgical template by CAD/CAM printing of a surgical guide (Fig. 21.5). This type of guide offers a high level of precision for the placement of the planned implant, which in turn affords predictable surgical outcomes. Most systems have bone-, mucosa- or tooth-supported guides and are compatible with virtually any implant system. The accurate digitalization of the soft tissue remains a challenge; however in the partially edentulous patient, surgical guides can be fabricated on stable adjacent teeth (Figs. 21.4 and 21.5).

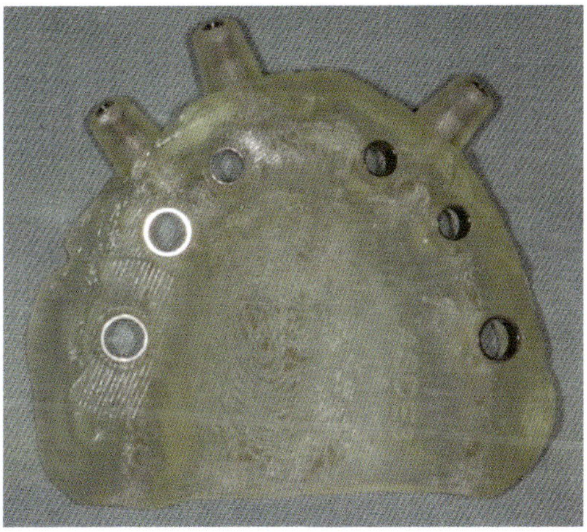

21 Digital Implant Abutment and Crowns in the Aesthetic Zone

Fig. 21.5 CAD/CAM surgical guide with guided sleeves for optimal implant position and angulation

21.3 CAD/CAM Manufacturing for Implant Abutments and Crowns

CAD/CAM is increasingly being utilized by dental laboratories in the manufacturing of crowns and fixed dental prostheses (van Noort 2012). The implementation of this digital methodology has decreased manufacturing costs by reducing technician time and material costs while increasing productivity (Beuer et al. 2008).

All CAD/CAM systems have three components: scanning device to capture data regarding the oral environment (tooth preparation, implant position and angulation as well as adjacent teeth and occluding tooth geometry), CAD system to design the dental restoration and CAM device to construct the restoration.

21.3.1 Digital Scanner

There are two methods for digital scanning: (1) intraoral scanning (Fig. 21.6) and (2) extra-oral (dental laboratory) scanning (Fig. 21.7). Today's intraoral digital scanners can capture 3D information on the restorative space, adjacent tooth position, angulation, size and shape. Scanners exist in various shapes and sizes with the iTERO (Align Technologies), True Definition (3M) and TRIOS (3Shape) as free-standing units, while some scanners such as the CS3500 (Carestream) and TRIOS (3Shape) offer a USB connection to any desktop or laptop computers. Units that allow for in-office milling of restorations include the Omnicam (CEREC) and E4D (Planmeca). Advantages of digital scanning are evident on maintenance of record and the ability to fabricate surgical guides and working casts at any time in the future. Moreover, there are wands as small as a dental handpiece (i.e. 3M True Definition) and can be scanned with the patient in any position. The CEREC® 1 (Sirona Dental Systems, Charlotte, NC) was the first commercially available system for direct digital impressions and after 25 years is now in its fourth generation (Seelbach et al. 2013). Today, three-dimensional video capture offers a much greater image quality. The LAVA COS (3M ESPE, Lexington, USA) system is based on the use of active optical wavefront sampling (Rohaly et al. 2008). The technology captures three-dimensional images with a single lens; the images, through complex proprietary algorithms, are used to create data sets, at a rate of 20 sets per second, while capturing over 10,000 data points in each set. This process results in a scan consisting of 2,400 data sets which amount to 24 million data points per scan (Kachalia and Geissberger 2010). However, TRIOS three scanner from 3Shape scanner uses a parallel Confocal imaging technique for taking 3D images with a fast scanning time (Hong-Seoka and Chintala 2015). The digital methodology involves the capture of an image of the prepared tooth, adjacent and opposing teeth, as well as a bite registration to create a three-dimensional data file (STL). An alternative method would involve digitalization of the master casts generated from conventional impression techniques, using an extra-oral scanner to obtain a three-dimensional data file (STL). The STL data set is then utilized to design the crown in the virtual realm. The crown is fabricated by a subtractive milling method, utilizing an industrially fabricated block of ceramic or composite material. The combination of state of the art intraoral digital scanning and dental laboratory digital milling should provide "perfectly" fitting restorations (Figs. 21.6 and 21.7).

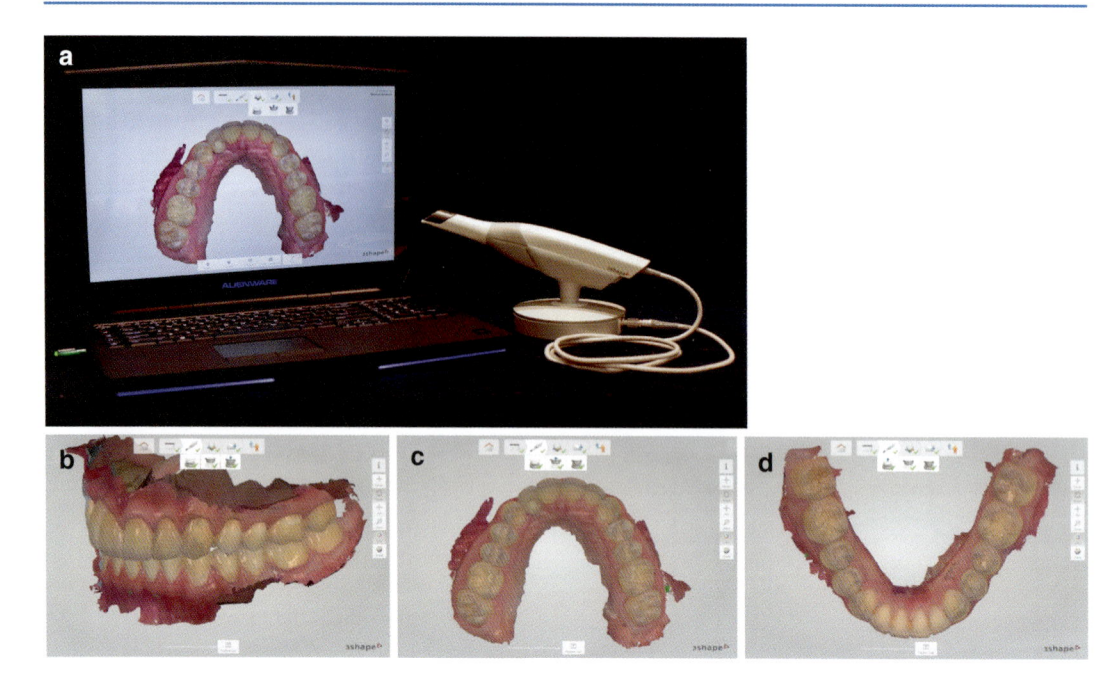

Fig. 21.6 3 Shape TRIOS Digital Impression System showing intraoral scanner and computer screen (**a**), digital impression of maxillary arch (**b**), digital impression of mandibular arch (**c**), and bite scan (**d**)

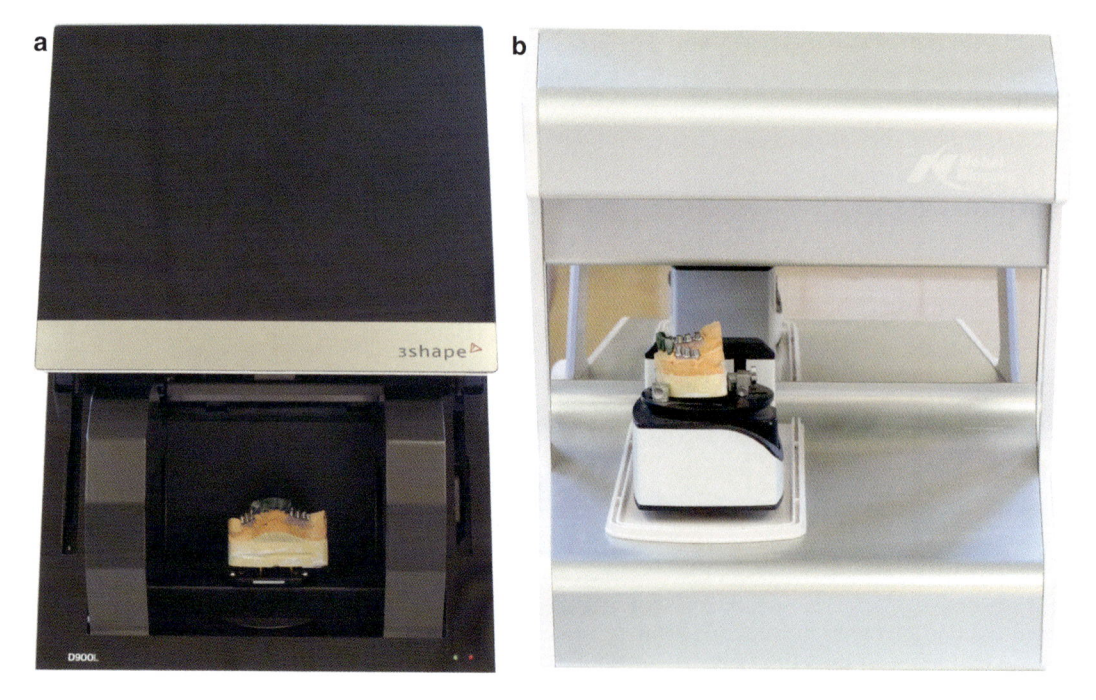

Fig. 21.7 Bench top scanners and cast: (**a**) 3Shape D900L scanner and (**b**) NobelProcera 2G scanner

The obvious advantages to the digital impression are patient comfort and cleanliness, virtually instantaneous 3D visualization of the scans, electronic transfer to the dental laboratory, ability to interact with the laboratory on design of the implant surgical guides, abutments and crowns in virtual space and finally storage of information for future use in abutments and crown fabrica-

21 Digital Implant Abutment and Crowns in the Aesthetic Zone

tion. Moreover, the transfer of digital information does not require disinfection, land transportation or fabrication of a gypsum cast for articulation. Thus, the potential for dimensional inaccuracies could be eliminated, or at least dramatically reduced (Syrek et al. 2010).

However, the use of digital impression equipment and software can pose some particular challenges. There can be a steep learning curve to master the software and can be time consuming at first, lack of standardization of file type for transfer and storage and cost of the scanners. Moisture control remains an issue with both conventional and digital impressions; this is compounded with scanners that require the use of powder to visualize teeth and other structures.

Digital impressions can be used to either produce casts by milling or printing (stereolithography) plastic materials (Kachalia and Geissberger 2010). Cast milling is usually performed by large dental laboratories or by dental manufacturing companies (Miyazaki and Hotta 2011). Both in-office milling and laboratory milling of crowns have demonstrated acceptable clinical crown accuracy (May et al. 1998; Akbar et al. 2006).

It is important to mention that the production of casts is not necessary, and in fact virtual casts from digital impressions have been found to be accurate (Hwang et al. 2013). Fabrication of dental restorations in virtual space offers many advantages over traditional techniques. The data file is available almost instantaneously for the lab technician to evaluate, and can provide feedback to the dentist (Craddock 2011). Digital technology can also help reduce the environmental impact of the dental practice and laboratory by reducing the waste of traditional impression materials (Christensen 2009), not requiring extra materials for remakes (Lee and Gallucci 2013), and by removing the need for disinfection and transportation (Brawek et al. 2013) of intraoral impressions.

21.3.2 Design Software

Different manufacturers provide CAD software that is utilized for designing different types of dental restorations (Fig. 21.8). The design data can be stored in several data formats. Standard transformation language (STL) is the main format used for CAD/CAM technology. 3Shape software produces STL files that can be used with several implant systems. Conversely, several manufacturers utilize other data formats that are

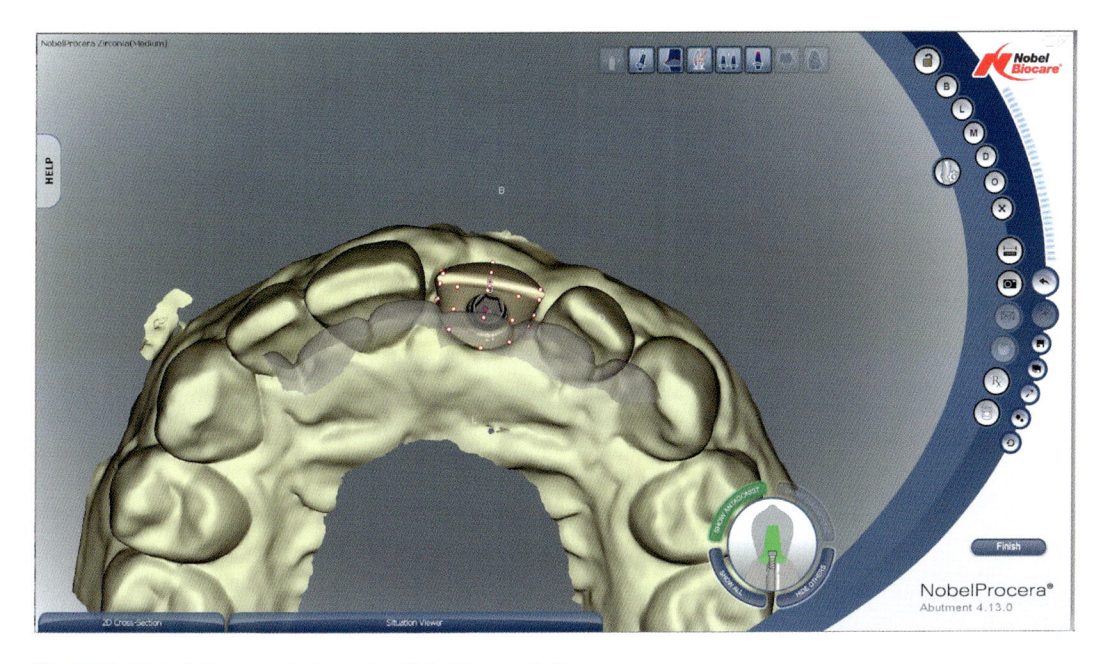

Fig. 21.8 Digital abutment design using NobelProcera Software

specific to that particular manufacturer (i.e. closed systems) such as 3D design software by Nobel Biocare (Procera), Straumann (CARES) and ASTRA TECH (ATLANTIS VAD) (Beuer et al. 2008) (Fig. 21.8).

21.3.3 Processing Devices

The design data produced with the CAD software is sent for CAM-processing and loaded into the milling machine. Milling machines can be divided based on the number of milling axes: 3-axis, 4-axis and 5-axis devices. Three-axis milling devices control bur movement along three planes (X, Y and Z). They mill the stock material from the top or bottom, but are not able to mill undercuts. Therefore, they are acceptable for single crowns and short-span fixed dental prostheses. Four-axis mills have a tension bridge (fourth axis) in addition to the three spatial axes; hence, its mill undercuts in only one direction, while five-axis mills can control their tool paths in five motions simultaneously (i.e. X, Y and Z axes plus tension bridge (fourth axis) and milling spindle (fifth axis)). The use of five-axis mills is beneficial in milling custom implant abutments and long-span fixed dental prosthesis which can be rotated to fit in shorter stock material (Beuer et al. 2008).

21.4 Digital Impression of Implants

Digital impressions of implants can be undertaken with the use of specific implant scan body impression copings (Fig. 21.9). Implant companies have created one- and two-piece scan bodies, but the mono block one-piece design is more common. The digital impression may be a segment or a complete arch depending upon the complexity of the case. The dental laboratory can create an implant master cast from the digital impression file by either milling or 3D printing of a urethane material (Hinds 2014) (Fig. 21.9).

21.5 CAD/CAM Implant Abutments

Several abutments are available for implant-supported restorations including prefabricated, cast metal alloy and CAD/CAM abutments. The selection of an implant abutment is based on several factors including the smile line, exposure of the crown and adjacent mucosal tissue, mucosal thickness over the abutment, implant angulation, restorative space, clinician's preference, patient expectations, and cost (Bidra and Rungruanganunt 2013). Implant crowns can be directly connected to the implant via an abutment screw, but this requires a cast metal alloy interface. The ideal prosthetic space height needed for a cemented implant crown is 8–10 mm (Misch et al. 2005), which accounts for 3 mm needed for emergence profile, 3–5 mm for the abutment height (crown retention and resistance form), and 2 mm for the appropriate porcelain incisal or functional surface thickness. Alternately, it is challenging to achieve ideal tooth proportions if the inter-occlusal distance exceeds 15 mm (Misch et al. 2006).

The first CAD/CAM implant abutments were fabricated using ATLANTIS custom abutments and described by Kerstein (Kerstein et al. 2000).

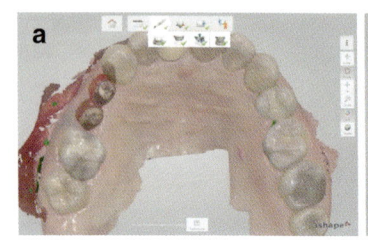

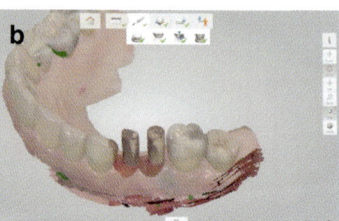

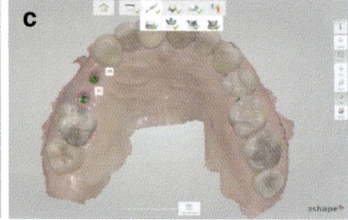

Fig. 21.9 Occlusal and lateral view of full arch scan digital impression using implant scan bodies attached to the implants (**a**, **b**) and implant position relative to the adjacent teeth (**c**)

The ATLANTIS system used a bench top scanner to digitize the master cast including the implant analogue head and the opposing cast. A digital library of teeth was used as a basis to create a custom digital abutment design. The final design was then exported to an industrial milling machine to create the custom titanium or zirconia abutment. Nobel Biocare expanded its Procera technology to scan wax patterns of abutments, which were then milled out of an Alumina ceramic material (Andersson et al. 1998). ASTRA TECH (ATLANTIS VAD), Nobel Biocare (Procera), Straumann (CARES) and others have developed more sophisticated digital abutment design software which can be used with several implant systems (3Shape), but the digital workflow from scanning to fabrication remains the same.

The use of CAD/CAM allows for the creation of a custom titanium or ceramic abutments which engage the implant head with built-in antirotational features and has an anatomical profile and interface for the definitive crown. The fabrication of the abutment can be the result of a wax-up on a laboratory abutment analogue or created on a digital scan. In either case, the laboratory technician has control over the emergence profile and crown margin spatial location with respect to the soft tissue and form (height and taper) to support the planned crown. In addition, CAD/CAM custom abutments are more cost effective to fabricate than cast custom metal abutments (Priest 2005). Milled titanium or zirconia abutments are better fitting to the implant interface and have better mechanical properties compared to cast alloy abutments. The CAD software has a built-in biomechanical failsafe design for appropriate thickness, height and implant head interface connection and crown margin width. The laboratory technician with the dentist's input has control of the emergence profile of the abutment with respect to the soft tissue. Abutments can be created from passive cylinders to tissue supporting/displacing conical structures depending upon the desired tissue profile. Clinically, up to 1 mm of tissue compression is possible without risking ischaemia. This creates the optimal emergence profile for the final aesthetic crown. The end result should be an abutment that mimics the natural tooth root in profile, size and curvilinear shape to create an ideal interface for the final cemented crown (Fig. 21.10). The CAD software allows for designing abutments and subsequent digital transfer to a CAM milling centre to create the abutment from a solid block of the selected material (Fig. 21.10).

21.6 Material Selection for CAD/CAM Implant Abutments

Several materials are available for CAD/CAM custom abutments including titanium, gold/pink hue titanium and zirconia (Fig. 21.11). The CAD software allows for designing abutments and the digital transfer to a CAM milling centre to create the abutment from a solid block of the selected material. The zirconia is milled in the green state (lightly sintered) with CAD software programming to compensate for the 20 % final sintering shrinkage (Manicone et al. 2007). Titanium alloy is recommended for use in high occlusal load areas of the mouth such as the replacement of canines and bicuspids. The use of white zirconia is recommended for incisors to maximize aesthetics by preventing display of metal at the crown interface and discolouration of the overlaying mucosa. However, zirconia is white relative to natural teeth and roots, which led to the development of tooth-coloured tinted zirconia abutments (Shah et al. 2008; Nakamura et al. 2010). Advantages and disadvantages of commercially available CAD/CAM materials are presented in Table 21.1 (Fig. 21.11).

Titanium is a grey metal alloy that can create a blue-grey discolouration of the overlying mucosa, especially in patient's mouths that have thin gingival biotype (Yildirim et al. 2000; Glauser et al. 2004). Gingival and/or connective tissue grafting has been suggested to increase the thickness of the mucosa to mask this problem. However, this additional surgical procedure may not be accepted by many patients (Kois 2001, 2004). Gold-coloured, nitride-coated, titanium abutments have also been produced as an alternative option to meet aesthetic and functional requirements in the anterior maxilla. Bressan et al. (2011) assessed the influence of

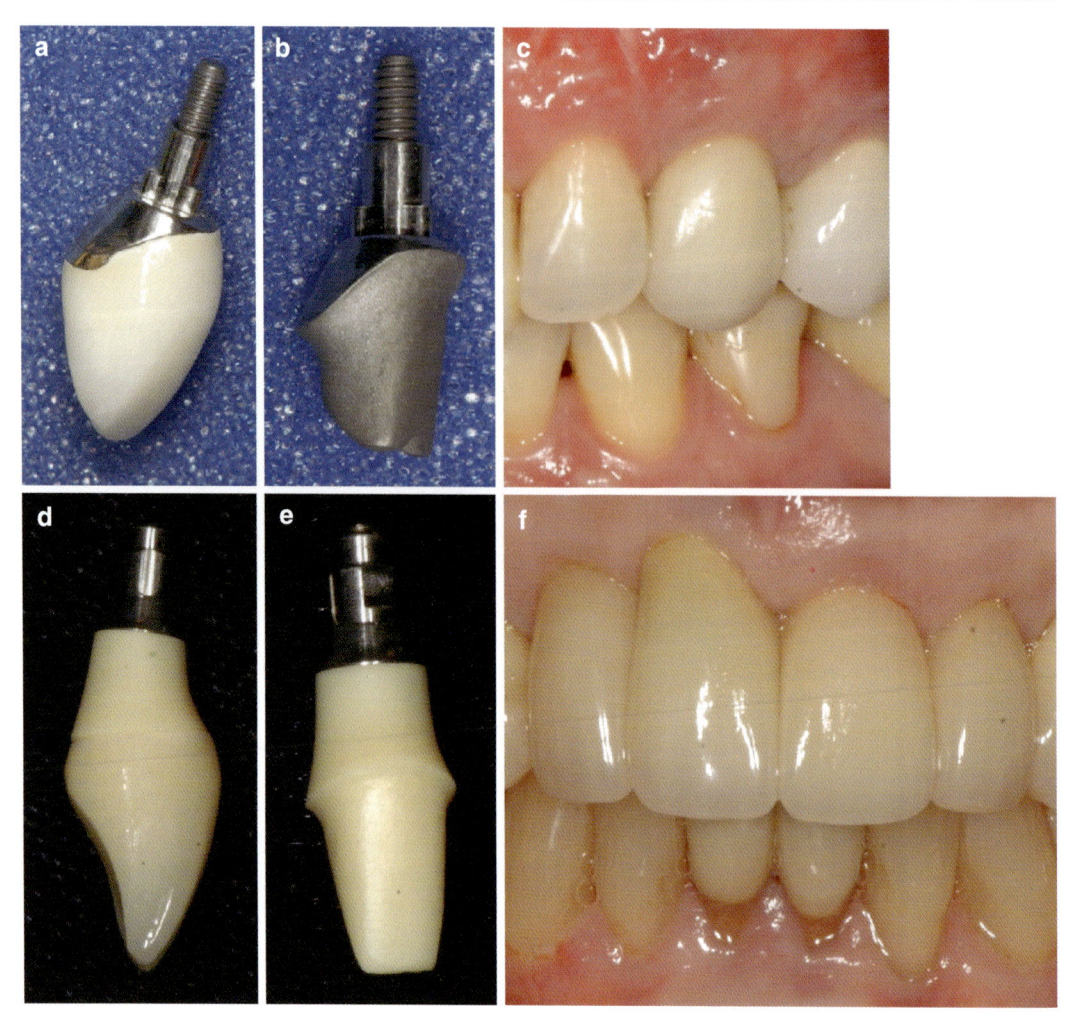

Fig. 21.10 Restoration of missing anterior teeth with different abutment and crown materials. (**a**) CAD/CAM titanium abutment and metal-ceramic crown, (**b**) CAD/CAM titanium abutment, (**c**) CAD/CAM titanium abutment and metal-ceramic crown replacing the maxillary left canine, (**d**) CAD/CAM zirconia abutment and crown, (**e**) CAD/CAM zirconia abutment and (**f**) CAD/CAM zirconia abutment and crown replacing the maxillary left central incisor

three different abutments (titanium, gold and zirconia) on peri-implant mucosal discolouration in the anterior maxilla. All the abutments resulted in colour change in the peri-implant tissues when compared to mucosal tissues adjacent to a contralateral natural tooth. Interestingly, there were no significant differences in the colour performance of gold and zirconia abutments, but titanium abutments resulted in significantly higher colour differences.

The increased demand for highly aesthetic restorations led to the development of tooth-coloured ceramic implant abutments. Densely sintered alumina ceramic was the first aesthetic abutment to be introduced (Prestipino and Ingber 1993a, b). Although alumina abutments have favourable aesthetic (tooth-like colour) and are biologically compatible, they are prone to fracture (Boudrias et al. 2001). Glauser et al. (2004) developed zirconia (yttrium oxide-stabilized zirconia) abutments to address this weakness.

Zirconia is a significantly stronger material than alumina, although fracture of zirconia abutments at the implant-abutment interface has been described both clinically (Aboushelib and Salameh 2009) and in vitro (Kim et al. 2013).

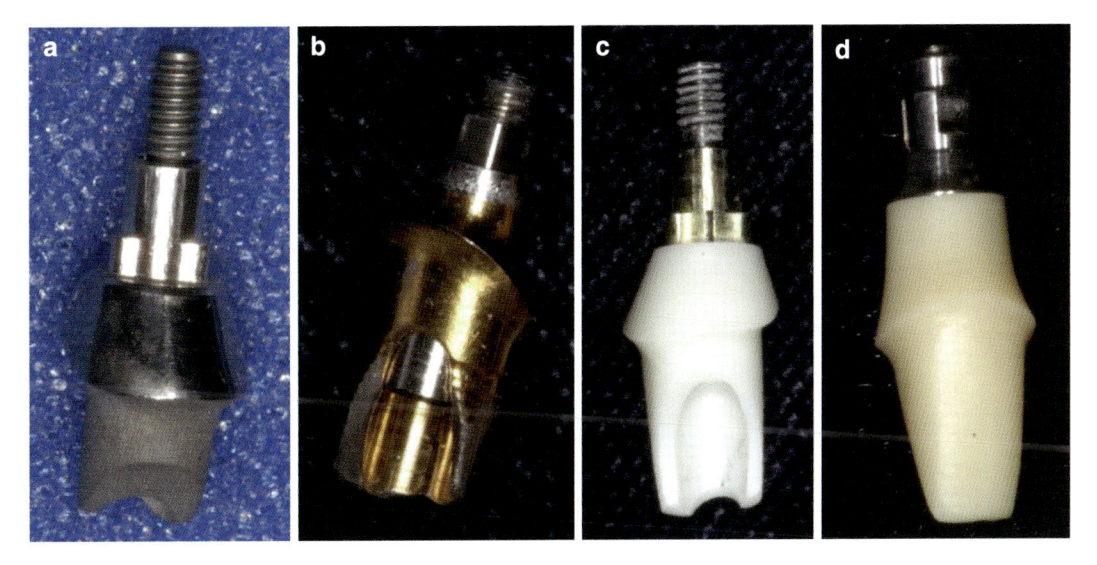

Fig. 21.11 Implant abutments made from different materials: (**a**) titanium abutment, (**b**) gold hue titanium abutment, (**c**) white zirconia abutment and (**d**) coloured zirconia abutment

Table 21.1 Advantages and disadvantages of the available CAD/CAM materials

	Advantages	Disadvantages
Titanium	Biocompatibility	Blue-greyish colour can show through thin gingival biotype and all-ceramic restorations except zirconia
	Good physical properties	
	Easily modified	
Gold or pink hue titanium	Gold coating provides good aesthetics for thin tissue biotypes and all-ceramic restorations	Abutment alteration can damage aesthetic coating
	Biocompatibility	More expensive
	Good physical properties	
Zirconia	Indicated for anterior zone	Increased risk of fracture at implant-abutment interface
	Good aesthetics (coloured zirconia)	Over-preparation can compromise strength (technique sensitive)
	Strong	White opaque colour can show through thin biotypes (if coloured zirconia is not available)

Most implant manufacturers have moved to a two-piece hybrid titanium-zirconia abutment with a prefabricated metal interface to address this problem. The CAD zirconia abutments can either be friction-fitted titanium bases with screw retention onto the implant or simply bonded to the titanium base (Kim et al. 2013). Hybrid titanium/ceramic abutments demonstrated similar mechanical behaviour to titanium abutments and improved mechanical performance when compared to zirconia abutments (Canullo 2007; Sailer et al. 2009; Carvalho et al. 2014). Recently, shaded zirconia abutments were introduced to the market to further enhance aesthetics of implant abutments in the aesthetic zone. However, the addition of pigments prior to final sintering has allowed for more natural coloured zirconia abutments; however coloured zirconia has less favourable mechanical properties (Shah et al. 2008).

21.6.1 CAD/CAM Ceramic Crowns

Once implant abutments are fabricated, optimally fitting crowns can be designed and fabricated. Although it is possible to mill titanium, chrome cobalt or other dental alloys, their use as crown copings to support ceramics is limited by aesthetics. Crowns can be milled entirety out of lithium disilicate (Ivoclar e.max) and surface stained. More commonly, dental laboratories will mill zirconia or lithium disilicate as cores to be covered with feldspathic porcelains. The resulting product has varying degrees of translucency and strength.

The fit of crowns fabricated using completely digital technologies has been assessed, and the results of this study have suggested that the vertical marginal gap of lithium disilicate crowns fabricated by the fully digital methodology (i.e. digital impression and CAD/CAM fabrication) was significantly smaller than that measured in crowns fabricated by the conventional methodology (Ng et al. 2014). The mean vertical marginal gap for crowns fabricated by the digital methodology was 48 μm, which was similar to the values reported in other studies (Luthardt et al. 1999; Tinschert et al. 2001; Lee et al. 2008). The fully digital technique of impression and crown fabrication provides a better fitting margin than the conventional method.

21.6.2 Immediate Implant and CAD/CAM Provisional Crown Placement

Taking CBCT-guided technology to the next step involves the fusion of CBCT and optically scanned diagnostic casts to allow for guided implant placement and to fabricate a patient specific CAD/CAM abutment and provisional restoration in one appointment with appropriate contours to maintain tissue architecture. Steps for SIMPLANT immediate smile concept are summarized in Table 21.2. The abutment could be utilized as the final abutment "one-abutment, one-time". However, it is challenging to develop aesthetically acceptable margin when delivering a CAD/CAM abutment at the time of surgery due to the associated changes in the surrounding bone and soft tissues following tooth extraction and/or implant placement. Alternatively, the immediate CAD/CAM abutment can be replaced with a new digital abutment to achieve best aesthetic results (Mandelaris and Vlk 2014).

Table 21.2 Steps for SIMPLANT immediate smile concept

1. Dentition and soft tissue scan (intraoral scan or model scan)
2. Virtual wax-up or model scan with wax-up (STL file)
3. CBCT scan (DICOM files)
4. Implant planning using computer software
5. Fabrication of Facilitate surgical guide and implant definitive ATLANTIS abutment
6. Design and fabrication of interim crown
7. Guided implant surgery on patient
8. Insertion of definitive abutment and interim crown

Conclusions

The use of digital technology is revolutionizing dentistry and in particular implant surgery and prosthetics. At the present time, it is possible to plan implant placement, design both titanium and ceramic abutments and fabricate provisional and definitive crowns. As clinicians and dental technicians adopt the digital workflow into their professional practice, the companies that produce the scanners and software will no doubt enhance the user experience and reduce the costs.

References

Aboushelib MN, Salameh Z (2009) Zirconia implant abutment fracture: clinical case reports and precautions for use. Int J Prosthodont 22(6):616–619

Akbar JH, Petrie CS, Walker MP, Williams K, Eick JD (2006) Marginal adaptation of cerec 3 CAD/CAM composite crowns using two different finish line preparation designs. J Prosthodont 15(3):155–163

Andersson M, Razzoog ME, Oden A, Hegenbarth EA, Lang BR (1998) Procera: a new way to achieve an all-ceramic crown. Quintessence Int 29(5):285–296

Beuer F, Schweiger J, Edelhoff D (2008) Digital dentistry: an overview of recent developments for CAD/CAM generated restorations. Br Dent J 204(9):505–511

Bidra AS, Rungruanganunt P (2013) Clinical outcomes of implant abutments in the anterior region: a systematic review. J Esthet Restor Dent 25(3):159–176

Bornstein MM, Al-Nawas B, Kuchler U, Tahmaseb A (2014) Consensus statements and recommended clinical procedures regarding contemporary surgical and radiographic techniques in implant dentistry. Int J Oral Maxillofac Implants 29(Suppl):78–82

Boudrias P, Shoghikian E, Morin E, Hutnik P (2001) Esthetic option for the implant-supported single-tooth restoration – treatment sequence with a ceramic abutment. J Can Dent Assoc 67(9):508–514

Brawek P, Wolfart S, Endres L, Kirsten A, Reich S (2013) The clinical accuracy of single crowns exclusively fabricated by digital workflow—the comparison of two systems. Clin Oral Investig 17:2119–2125 1–7

Bressan E, Paniz G, Lops D, Corazza B, Romeo E, Favero G (2011) Influence of abutment material on the gingival color of implant-supported all-ceramic restorations: a prospective multicenter study. Clin Oral Implants Res 22(6):631–637

Canullo L (2007) Clinical outcome study of customized zirconia abutments for single-implant restorations. Int J Prosthodont 20(5):489–493

Carvalho MA, Sotto-Maior BS, Del Bel Cury AA, Pessanha Henriques GE (2014) Effect of platform connection and abutment material on stress distribution in single anterior implant-supported restorations: a nonlinear 3-dimensional finite element analysis. J Prosthet Dent 112:1096–1102

Christensen GJ (2009) Impressions are changing: deciding on conventional, digital or digital plus in-office milling. J Am Dent Assoc 140(10):1301–1304

Craddock MRWRJ (2011) Is the US army dental corps ready for the digital impression? USA Army Med Dep J 1:38–41

El Askary AS (2001) Multifaceted aspects of implant esthetics: the anterior maxilla. Implant Dent 10(3):182–191

Fanning B (2011) CBCT – the justification process, audit and review of the recent literature. J Ir Dent Assoc 57(5):256–261

Glauser R, Sailer I, Wohlwend A, Studer S, Schibli M, Scharer P (2004) Experimental zirconia abutments for implant-supported single-tooth restorations in esthetically demanding regions: 4-year results of a prospective clinical study. Int J Prosthodont 17(3):285–290

Hinckfuss S, Conrad HJ, Lin L, Lunos S, Seong WJ (2012) Effect of surgical guide design and surgeon's experience on the accuracy of implant placement. J Oral Implantol 38(4):311–323

Hinds KF (2014) Intraoral digital impressions to enhance implant esthetics. Compend Contin Educ Dent 35(3 Suppl):25–33

Hong-Seoka P, Chintala S (2015) Development of high speed and high accuracy 3D dental intra oral scanner. Proc Eng 100:1174–1181

Hwang YC, Park YS, Kim HK, Hong YS, Ahn JS, Ryu JJ (2013) The evaluation of working casts prepared from digital impressions. Oper Dent 38:655–662

Kachalia PR, Geissberger MJ (2010) Dentistry a la carte: in-office CAD/CAM technology. J Calif Dent Assoc 38(5):323–330

Karunagaran S, Markose S, Paprocki G, Wicks R (2014) A systematic approach to definitive planning and designing single and multiple unit implant abutments. J Prosthodont 23:639–648

Kerstein RB, Castellucci F, Osorio J (2000) Utilizing computer generated titanium permanent healing. Abutments to promote ideal gingival form and anatomic restorartions on implants. Comendium 21(10):793–802

Kim JS, Raigrodski AJ, Flinn BD, Rubenstein JE, Chung KH, Mancl LA (2013) In vitro assessment of three types of zirconia implant abutments under static load. J Prosthet Dent 109(4):255–263

Kois JC (2001) Predictable single tooth peri-implant esthetics: five diagnostic keys. Compend Contin Educ Dent 22(3):199–206 quiz 208

Kois JC (2004) Predictable single-tooth peri-implant esthetics: five diagnostic keys. Compend Contin Educ Dent 25(11):895–896 898, 900 passim; quiz 906–897

Lee SJ, Gallucci GO (2013) Digital vs. conventional implant impressions: efficiency outcomes. Clin Oral Implants Res 24(1):111–115

Lee KB, Park CW, Kim KH, Kwon TY (2008) Marginal and internal fit of all-ceramic crowns fabricated with two different CAD/CAM systems. Dent Mater J 27(3):422–426

Luthardt RG, Sandkuhl O, Reitz B (1999) Zirconia-TZP and alumina – advanced technologies for the manufacturing of single crowns. Eur J Prosthodont Restor Dent 7(4):113–119

Mandelaris GA, Vlk SD (2014) Guided implant surgery with placement of a presurgical CAD/CAM patient-specific abutment and provisional in the esthetic zone. Compend Contin Educ Dent 35(7):494–504

Manicone PF, Rossi Iommetti P, Raffaelli L (2007) An overview of zirconia ceramics: basic properties and clinical applications. J Dent 35(11):819–826

May KB, Russell MM, Razzoog ME, Lang BR (1998) Precision of fit: the Procera AllCeram crown. J Prosthet Dent 80(4):394–404

Misch CE, Goodacre CJ, Finley JM, Misch CM, Marinbach M, Dabrowsky T et al (2005) Consensus conference panel report: crown-height space guidelines for implant dentistry-part 1. Implant Dent 14(4):312–318

Misch CE, Goodacre CJ, Finley JM, Misch CM, Marinbach M, Dabrowsky T et al (2006) Consensus conference panel report: crown-height space guidelines for implant dentistry-part 2. Implant Dent 15(2):113–121

Miyazaki T, Hotta Y (2011) CAD/CAM systems available for the fabrication of crown and bridge restorations. Aust Dent J 56(Suppl 1):97–106

Nakamura K, Kanno T, Milleding P, Ortengren U (2010) Zirconia as a dental implant abutment material: a systematic review. Int J Prosthodont 23(4):299–309

Ng J, Ruse D, Wyatt C (2014) A comparison of the marginal fit of crowns fabricated with digital and conventional methods. J Prosthet Dent 112(3):555–560

Orentlicher G, Goldsmith D, Abboud M (2012) Computer-guided planning and placement of dental implants. Atlas Oral Maxillofac Surg Clin N Am 20(1):53–79

Prestipino V, Ingber A (1993a) Esthetic high-strength implant abutments. Part I. J Esthet Dent 5(1):29–36

Prestipino V, Ingber A (1993b) Esthetic high-strength implant abutments. Part II. J Esthet Dent 5(2):63–68

Priest G (2005) Virtual-designed and computer-milled implant abutments. J Oral Maxillofac Surg 63(9 Suppl 2):22–32

Rohaly J, Hart DP, Brukilacchio TJ (2008) Three-channel camera systems with non-collinear apertures. USA. 7,372,642

Sailer I, Sailer T, Stawarczyk B, Jung RE, Hammerle CH (2009) In vitro study of the influence of the type of connection on the fracture load of zirconia abutments with internal and external implant-abutment connections. Int J Oral Maxillofac Implants 24(5):850–858

Seelbach P, Brueckel C, Wöstmann B (2013) Accuracy of digital and conventional impression techniques and workflow. Clin Oral Investig 17(7):1759–1764

Shah K, Holloway JA, Denry IL (2008) Effect of coloring with various metal oxides on the microstructure, color, and flexural strength of 3Y-TZP. J Biomed Mater Res B Appl Biomater 87(2):329–337

Syrek A, Reich G, Ranftl D, Klein C, Cerny B, Brodesser J (2010) Clinical evaluation of all-ceramic crowns fabricated from intraoral digital impressions based on the principle of active wavefront sampling. J Dent 38(7):553–559

Tinschert J, Natt G, Mautsch W, Spiekermann H, Anusavice KJ (2001) Marginal fit of alumina-and zirconia-based fixed partial dentures produced by a CAD/CAM system. Oper Dent 26(4):367–374

van Noort R (2012) The future of dental devices is digital. Dent Mater 28(1):3–12

Worthington P, Rubenstein J, Hatcher DC (2010) The role of cone-beam computed tomography in the planning and placement of implants. J Am Dent Assoc 141(Suppl 3):19S–24S

Yildirim M, Edelhoff D, Hanisch O, Spiekermann H (2000) Ceramic abutments – a new era in achieving optimal esthetics in implant dentistry. Int J Periodontics Restor Dent 20(1):81–91

Challenging Maxillary Anterior Implant-Supported Restorations: Creating Predictable Outcomes with Zirconia

22

Michael Moscovitch

Abstract

The restoration of form and function with dental implants often presents challenges to the most experienced clinician. Each case category has requirements, whether it is a single tooth or a complete arch in need of restoration. The anterior zone, especially the maxilla, can present issues beyond our traditional knowledge of tooth-supported restorations. The high lip line accompanied by irregular bone loss patterns has challenged the practice of implant dentistry since the inception of reliable osseointegrated implants. In the ensuing years, the advancement of implant technology along with regenerative technologies has provided the backbone of improving treatment outcomes. Developments such as 3D radiography, advanced treatment planning software and high-performance ceramics have opened new possibilities in treatment objectives and greater understanding of the requirements for successful management of the complex anterior aesthetic zone. This chapter will explore a series of cases from the single tooth to multi-unit restorations in both the maxilla and mandibular zones. Explanation of the differential treatment choices and subsequent restorative results will be presented along with pertinent supporting evidence.

The restoration of form and function with fixed restorations on dental implants often presents challenges to the most experienced clinician (Goodacre et al. 2003; Walton 2014a). The maxillary anterior zone is particularly sensitive to a myriad of gnathological and biological complications effecting outcomes with respect to occlusion and aesthetics beyond our traditional knowledge of tooth-supported restorations. Lip line position and bone loss patterns associated with tooth loss exacerbate our abilities to provide predictable results.

Advancements in treatment planning technologies, computer-aided design/computer-assisted manufacturing (CAD/CAM) software for the

M. Moscovitch, DDS, (Prosthodontist)
Assistant Clinical Professor, Division of Restorative Sciences, Boston University, Residency Program, McGill University, Montreal, QC, Canada

Private Practice, 4150 St. Catherine St. West, Suite 210, Montreal, QC H3Z 2Y5, Canada
e-mail: drmoscovitch@mospros.com

restorative workflow and high-strength ceramics, specifically zirconia, give the clinician the ability to visualize and control the many variables in executing treatment (Kapos and Evans 2014; Wismeijer et al. 2014). Developments in digital radiography, especially cone beam computed tomography (CBCT), and various associated planning software for implant placement and restoration design provide the restorative community with a reliable protocol for visualizing the requirements for successful management of the anterior fixed implant-supported restoration (Harris et al. 2012; Cassetta et al. 2013). The information obtained from the diagnostic data allows for the ability to coordinate the accurate placement of implants with or without regenerative hard and soft tissue technologies to produce proper support of the proposed restoration. The data from planning software is used to create the polymethyl methacrylate (PMMA) provisional restoration (Güth et al. 2012; Moscovitch and Saba 1996). The functional and aesthetic aspects can be then refined and used in the design of the definitive zirconia restoration (Moscovitch 2015a, b). The purpose of this chapter is to explore and present the clinical experience of the author in cases from single tooth to multi-unit fixed implant-supported zirconia restorations in the maxilla.

22.1 Clinical Considerations

Tooth loss patterns in the maxilla can range from one tooth to multiple teeth and associated aetiologies are well documented in the literature (Cohen 2008). The soft and hard tissue changes, specifically those patients who present with advanced periodontitis or advanced bone loss with existing removable prosthetics, have been shown to be the most challenging scenarios in achieving conditions for successful osseointegration (Wood and Vermilyea 2004).

The management of implant placement for the various clinical situations described above has also been well documented (Pjetursson et al. 2012).

The challenges in establishing predictable function and aesthetics in fixed implant-supported maxillary restorations are related to the variations in available healthy bone and soft tissue conditions. It is incumbent upon clinicians to be able to visualize the restorative outcome before beginning treatment. The beginning of this journey starts with the gathering of records to aid in the design of the definitive prosthesis. This includes a complete clinical and radiographic assessment to arrive at an appropriate diagnosis for the fixed restorative possibilities (Dym 2015). The workflow (Fig. 22.1) for zirconia restorations starts with coordinating available support for an adequate amount of implants to support the proposed prosthesis. The choice of an implant system should reflect current evidence-based parameters with respect to soft and hard tissue response as well as prosthetic stability (Jokstad et al. 2004; Lang et al. 2004). The visualization of the proposed restoration is accomplished through a diagnostic mock-up using wax-ups or denture teeth on the pretreatment study casts. This procedure allows for both analogue and digital pathways in

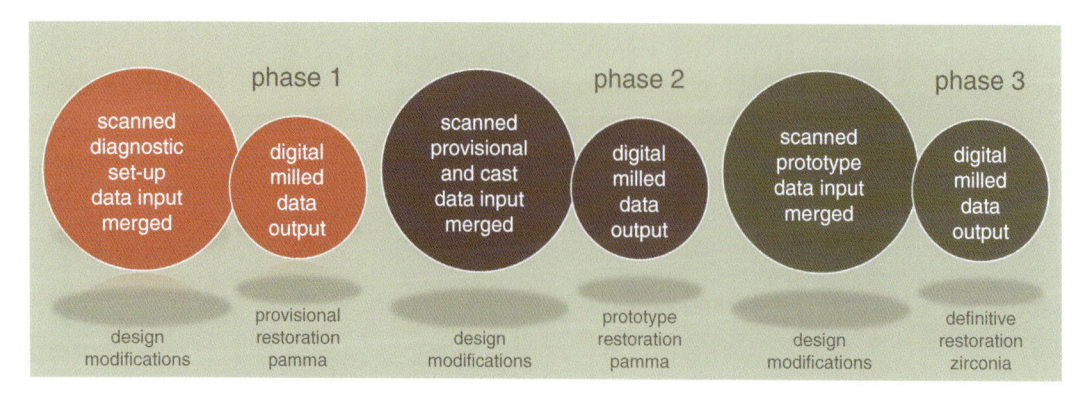

Fig. 22.1 Restorative workflow

planning the placement and number of implants to support the proposed restoration. The objective of this exercise is to have the implants fall within the mesial-distal and facial-lingual dimensions of the proposed restoration. Sometimes, this is not possible and there is a need to know if this guideline is exceeded, i.e. implants outside the restoration borders will allow for the successful execution of a definitive zirconia fixed restoration. All of this is done in consultation with the treatment team, this being the restorative clinician and the surgical clinician as well as the laboratory technician (Moscovitch 2015a).

22.2 Zirconia Technology

22.2.1 Introduction

Zirconia has been used for many years in dental applications for framework designs in fixed prosthodontics as a substitute for metallic frameworks as well as copings for single crowns and veneered with feldspathic ceramics to obtain function and aesthetics (Conrad et al. 2007; Guess et al. 2012; Hisbergues et al. 2009). Unfortunately, these restorations suffered from excessive chip-off fractures from the zirconia substrate in all but maxillary anterior applications (Raigrodski et al. 2012). To compensate for this phenomenon, restorative dentists generally prescribed protective acrylic (PMMA) appliances to protect the restorations (Alqahtani 2013; Klasser et al. 2010; Schmitter et al. 2014). Patients' lack of compliance with wearing these appliances resulted in the above complications with the veneering feldspathic materials. In response to these issues, a monolithic and/or minimally veneered approach to the use of zirconia was developed by Keren (Keren and Caro 2009). The results of this development provided for no feldspathic porcelain in function to avoid the damage and wear associated with zirconia-based restorations. According to a clinical study by the author (Moscovitch 2015c), the outcomes over a 68-month period in a private practice clinical environment reported no complications with respect to damage and wear. This created a new opportunity in fixed prosthodontics to provide patients with aesthetics and durable restorations in all clinical applications. The laboratory procedures to fabricate monolithic and minimally veneered zirconia restorations were initially performed by manual milling procedures and subsequently replaced by computer numerically controlled (CNC) machinery and CAD/CAM software resulting in greater efficiency in the manufacturing process and in the clinical workflow. These zirconia restorations were equally precise whether manually or digitally milled (Karl et al. 2012).

22.2.2 Dental Zirconia

Structural ceramic zirconia materials provide excellent erosion, corrosion and abrasion resistance along with temperature resistance, fracture toughness and strength. This ceramic alloy is used in extreme service applications that take advantage of its superior wear and corrosion resistance (Christensen 2012; Kelly and Denry 2008; Ozkurt and Kazazoğlu 2010).

Zirconia is a monoclinic crystal structure at room temperature and transitions to tetragonal and cubic forms at higher temperatures. The transformation from the monoclinic to the tetragonal phase commences at 980 °C and is complete at 1,173 °C. The tetragonal phase changes into the cubic modification at 2,370 °C. However the tetragonal and cubic forms are metastable as they cool to room temperature. The volume expansion caused by the cubic to tetragonal to monoclinic transformation induces large stresses, and these stresses cause ZrO_2 to crack upon cooling from high temperatures. This behaviour destroys the mechanical properties of fabricated components during cooling and makes pure zirconia useless for any structural or mechanical application. Several oxides, which dissolve in the in the zirconia crystal structure can slow down or eliminate these crystal structure changes. Commonly used effective additives are MgO, CaO and Y_2O_3. When the zirconia is doped with these various oxides, the tetragonal and/or cubic phases can be maintained at room temperature. The significant mechanism of the microscopic transformation of tetragonal to monoclinic crystalline form under stress at the surface of dental zirconia is known as *transformation toughening* (Chevalier and Gremillard 2009). The stabilized forms of zirconia are useful in many industrial, medical and dental applications (Hisbergues et al. 2009).

The use of tetragonal zirconia has the potential to revolutionize the performance outcomes of dental restorations. The properties of this material help in creating time-efficient workflows, aesthetics and durability for tooth and implant-supported restorations as well as implants and abutments.

Dental zirconia is typically known as tetragonal zirconia polycrystal stabilized with 3% yttrium oxide and is commonly abbreviated to 3YTZP. Aluminum oxide is also added to increase strength. The exact formula for dental zirconia is not published and varies by manufacturer. The properties to maximize strength and aesthetics have been a challenge for the producers of this material. Experienced technicians are able to evaluate and choose reliable materials based solely on subjective evaluation. The development of quantifiable standards in the formulae and processing is necessary for the reliable performance of zirconia dental restorations (Al-Amleh et al. 2010).

In spite of these limitations, zirconia has been used routinely as copings and frameworks to support feldspathic porcelain for the past decade. Inconsistencies in clinical reporting of outcomes have further confounded the professions' understanding of the appropriate parameters for reliable fabrication of dental restorations (Larsson and Wennerberg 2014).

Many long-term clinical trials confirm the clinical success of functionally veneered zirconia in the anterior zone and selected posterior applications. However, unacceptable chipping of the feldspathic veneer continues to be an issue with bilayered zirconia restorations (Sagirkaya et al. 2012).

More recently the use of monolithic zirconia (no veneer of feldspathic porcelain) and minimally veneered zirconia with feldspathic porcelain on the facial surface to enhance aesthetics or replace gingival structures with pink feldspathic porcelain is becoming popular due to the development of zirconia materials with enhanced aesthetic properties and efficient digital milling procedures (Rojas-Vizcaya 2011; Thalji and Cooper 2014).

The properties associated with dental zirconia are high strength, toughness, wear resistance, nonabrasive, acid resistant, thermal insulator, high biocompatibility, aesthetics, low plaque adhesion and adaptable to all restoration designs in both tooth- and implant-supported fixed restoration (Hisbergues et al. 2009; Alghazzawi et al. 2012; Flinn et al. 2012; Gökçen-Röhlig et al. 2010; Ko et al. 2014; Janyavula et al. 2013; Jung et al. 2010; Park et al. 2014). All of these enable this material to be a serious consideration as a substitute for traditional restorative materials in all applications. There is a greater demand today for aesthetic, reliable and cost-effective materials from our patients (Walton 2014b). The availability of monolithic and minimally veneered zirconia is proving to be the best choice for enhancing the prosthetic outcomes of our patients (Moscovitch 2015c).

22.2.3 Restorative Workflow

The clinical and laboratory procedures follow a three-phase protocol. Phase 1 involves the production of a fixed provisional (PMMA). Phase 2 incorporates the information developed in the functional trial of the provisional restoration in the fabrication of a prototype (PMMA) of the definitive restoration. Phase 3 is the milling, colouring and application of white and pink feldspathic ceramics to the non-functional facial surfaces of the zirconia restoration (Moscovitch 2015b).

22.2.4 Phase 1

The objective of this phase of treatment is twofold: first, to generate an analogue or digital guide for the placement of the implants (Cassetta et al. 2013; Reyes et al. 2015), and, second, to scan the diagnostic mock-up or to use the virtual mock-up to mill a fixed PMMA provisional restoration (see Case 22.2, Fig. 22.3d, and Case 22.5, Fig. 22.6h–j). The timing of the insertion of a fixed provisional is determined when the implants are placed based on an immediate or a delayed loading protocol

(Barewal et al. 2012). When a delayed loading protocol is used, a removable provisional may or may not be provided depending on functional and aesthetic requirements. Sometimes, a fixed provisional can be used for this protocol, if (1) there are adjacent teeth to the surgical site that are going to receive tooth-supported restorations in conjunction with the implant-supported restorations and (2) teeth are strategically kept during the healing phase of the implants and subsequently removed when the implants are ready to be loaded (see Case 22.5, Fig. 22.6d, e).

Existing fixed provisionals as described above are adapted to the supporting implants by either connecting the cylinders directly to screw-retained abutment(s) or implant(s) intraorally or relined to cement-retained abutment(s). Routinely, however, a new PMMA provisional is milled to refine the adjustments of the previous working provisionals (see Case 22.2, Fig. 22.3d, and Case 22.5, Fig. 22.6n, o).

When a removable provisional is initially used, the fabrication of the fixed provisional is carried out on the scanned master casts of the existing implant(s), directly or with screw or cemented retained abutment(s) (see Case 22.6, Fig. 22.7h, i) (Moscovitch 2015a, b, c).

22.2.5 Phase 2

After an appropriate clinical trial and adjustment of the provisional restoration or modification of the implant abutment(s), analogue impressions are made from the modified provisionals and supporting abutment(s) (see Case 22.5, Fig. 22.6m, and Case 22.6, Fig. 22.7g) (Cho et al. 2015). The casts are poured with high-quality die stone from both impressions, scanned and merged with existing data to produce a PMMA prototype for the definitive zirconia restoration (see Case 22.1, Fig. 22.2d; Case 22.2, Fig. 22.3d; Case 22.5, Fig. 22.6n). This prototype can be managed in two ways: (1) simply adjusted for function and aesthetics and (2) left in place as a further clinical trial to evaluate the changes incorporated (see Case 22.5, Fig. 22.6p). It is worthy to note that if the changes are extensive, then a secondary prototype may be necessary to maintain design control. When the completed prototype is ready, it is scanned and merged with existing files to produce the definitive zirconia restoration (see Case 22.5, Fig. 22.6r, and Case 22.6, Fig. 22.7j–l) (Moscovitch 2015a, b, c).

22.2.6 Phase 3

The scanned data from the prototype and the master cast is analysed for integrity of design with regard to function and aesthetics (see Case 22.5, Fig. 22.6n). This analysis includes the verification of abutment design, selection and inclination. Virtual modifications are carried out as necessary, i.e. contour, strength, hygiene access, occlusal form and facial cutbacks for white or pink feldspathic ceramics in the non-functioning anterior facial surfaces or gingival areas (to meet patient-specific aesthetic requirements). If the changes need intraoral modification of the abutments, they are carried out at this time and require a new master cast which can be then merged to the existing data file. These procedures preclude any significant errors in the design of the definitive zirconia restoration due to the fact that only minor adjustments to the facial surfaces or occlusion can be made once the zirconia restoration is completed.

The completed file is then used with the CAD/CAM software to mill the definitive zirconia restoration according to the manufacturer's specifications (see Case 22.5, Fig. 22.6r, and Case 22.6, Fig. 22.7j–l). The zirconia restoration is coloured with stains before sintering. The feldspathic white and pink ceramics are added as described above where required (see Case 22.4, Fig. 22.5e; Case 22.5, Fig. 22.6s; and Case 22.6, Fig. 22.7m) and then staining and glazing finish the process. Post-delivery minor occlusal adjustments are carried out with fine high-speed diamonds and copious water spray. The adjusted surfaces are finished with a zirconia polishing system (Moscovitch 2015a, b, c). Where necessary, the screw access channels are then sealed with composite and polytetrafluoroethylene (PTFE) tape (see Case 22.6, Fig. 22.7n, 22.7q) (Moráguez and Belser 2010).

22.3 Clinical Cases

Case 22.1: Single Tooth, Facial Veneered

A female patient aged 33 presented with the following clinical considerations: internal resorption of the left maxillary central incisor, a significant diastema between the right and left maxillary central incisors as well as a high lip line. The patient's expectation was to have the tooth replaced with a dental implant to avoid a removable or tooth-supported fixed restoration and to maintain the original diastema.

In consideration of the above conditions, the treatment that was carried out was the placement of a 15 mm implant at the time of extraction of the left maxillary incisor and immediately loaded with a screw-retained provisional restoration. After a healing period of 6 months, the provisional restoration was replaced with a definitive minimally veneered zirconia screw-retained restoration, incorporating a titanium base into the implant. During treatment, the patient decided that she no longer wanted to maintain the diastema between the two central incisors. To effect closure of the diastema, the left central incisor was fabricated with a wider mesial-distal dimension, and composite material was added to the right central incisor to complete the closure of the space (Fig. 22.2).

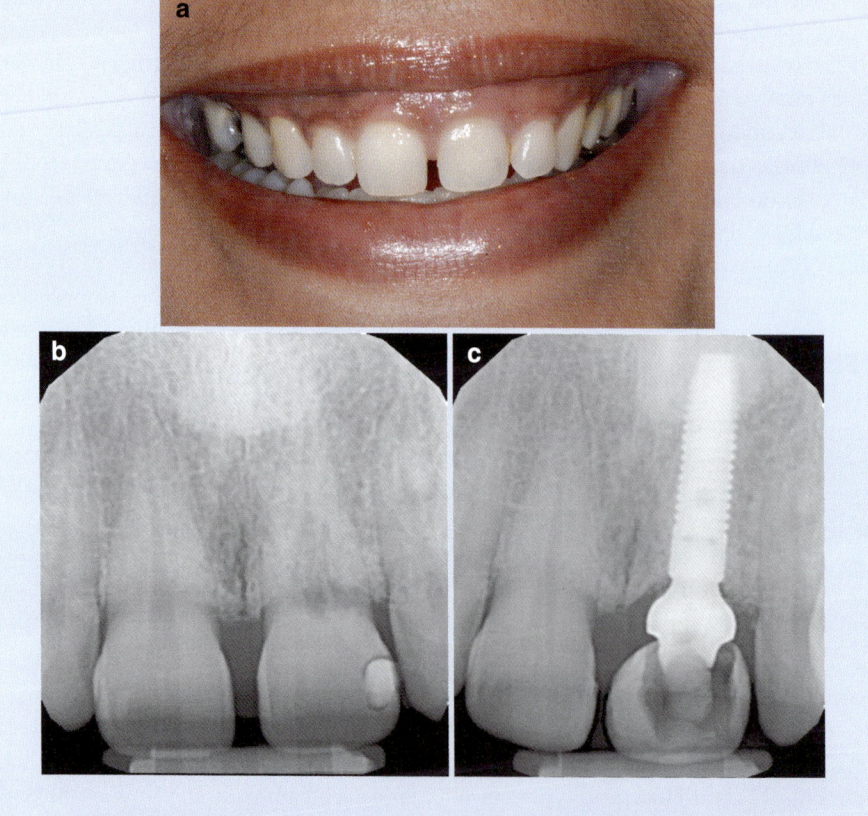

Fig. 22.2 Case 22.1: Single tooth, facial veneered. (**a**) Pretreatment full smile. (**b**) Pre-treatment radiograph. (**c**) Working radiograph of provisional restoration. (**d**) Digital design of the PMMA prototype and the zirconia restoration. (**e**) Zirconia restoration with facial porcelain (not in function) and titanium base. (**f**) Soft tissue site and implant at time of delivery. (**g**) Facial intraoral view of zirconia restoration with facial porcelain (not in function) maxillary left central incisor and full facial composite restoration of maxillary right central incisor. (**h**) Post-treatment full smile. (**i**) Post-treatment radiograph

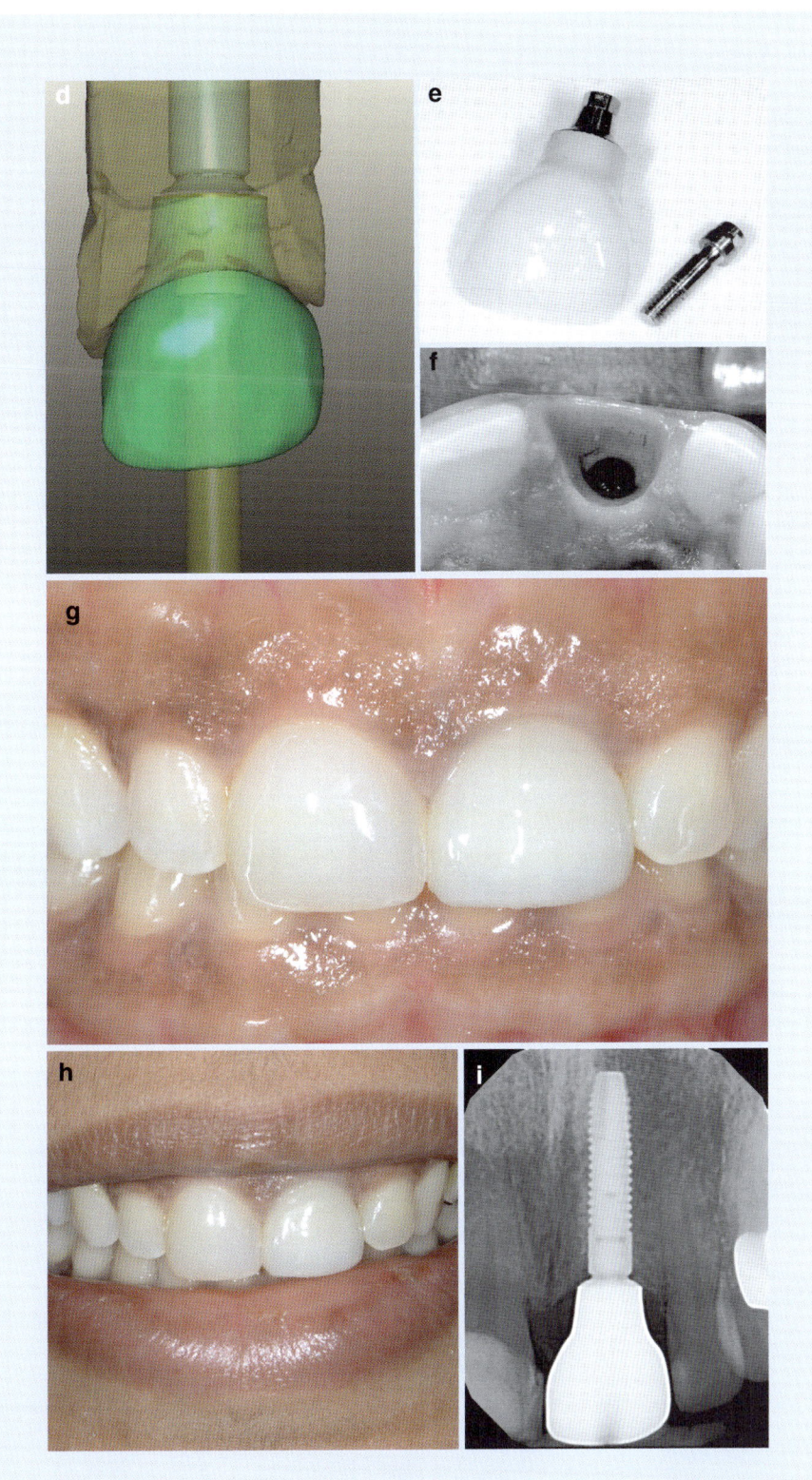

22 Challenging Maxillary Anterior Implant-Supported Restorations

Fig. 22.2 (continued)

Case 22.2: Multi-tooth, Facial Veneered and Pink Papillae

A male patient aged 22 presented with the following clinical considerations: the maxillary right central and lateral incisors being avulsed and the left maxillary central incisor and its mesial-incisal aspect being fractured through the pulp chamber as a result of a traumatic hockey injury sustained 1 week prior. As well, there was a small chip of enamel from the distal aspect of the mandibular right central incisor. Facial trauma was minimum and healed uneventfully. The patient's expectation was to have the missing and damaged teeth restored with implants and fixed restorations to match the original aesthetics as closely as possible.

In consideration of the above conditions, the treatment that was carried out was the placement of a dental implant along with soft and hard tissue grafting in the position of the right central incisor. Due to space considerations, the right lateral incisor was to be restored with a pontic attached to the right central incisor. The left central incisor underwent endodontic therapy. During this treatment, the edentulous space was managed with a removable acrylic partial denture. Subsequently, this was replaced with a fixed provisional: lateral incisor pontic, central incisor cement-retained abutment in the implant to support the full crown and the left central incisor, a full crown. The mandibular central incisor was restored with composite material. The definitive restoration was splinted to provide maximum stability (Fig. 22.3).

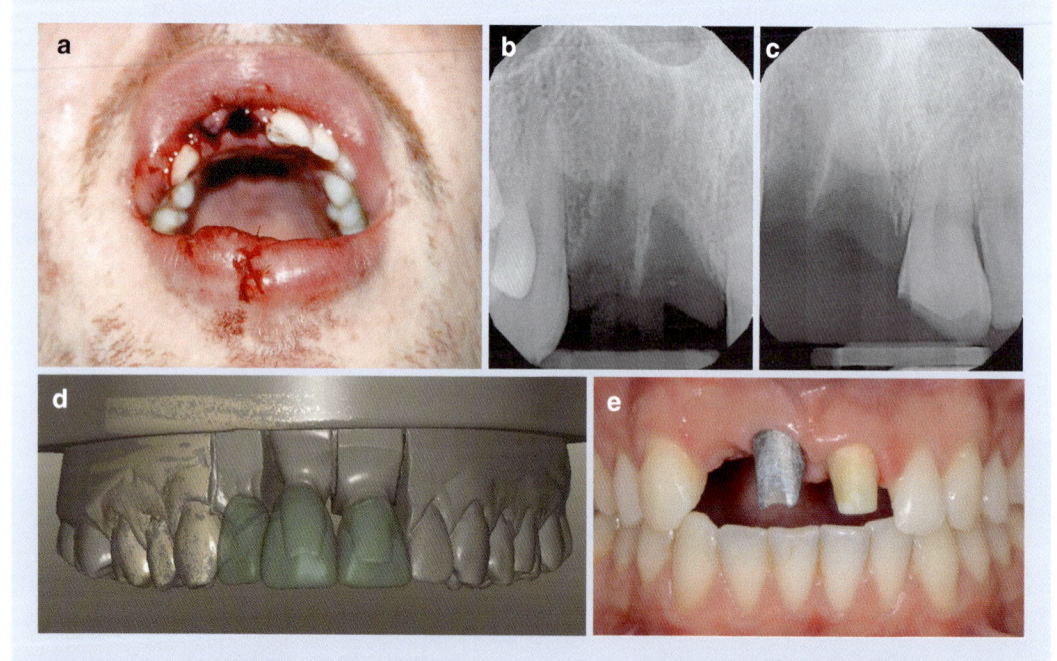

Fig. 22.3 Case 22.2: Multi-tooth, facial veneered and pink papillae. (**a**) Pretreatment extra-oral view. (**b**, **c**) Pretreatment radiographs. (**d**) Digital view for the provisional-prototype and zirconia restoration. (**e**) Posttreatment facial intraoral view of abutments. (**f**) Posttreatment facial intraoral view of zirconia restoration with facial porcelain (not in function) and pink feldspathic papillae. (**g**) Posttreatment full smile. (**h–j**) Posttreatment radiographs

22 Challenging Maxillary Anterior Implant-Supported Restorations 391

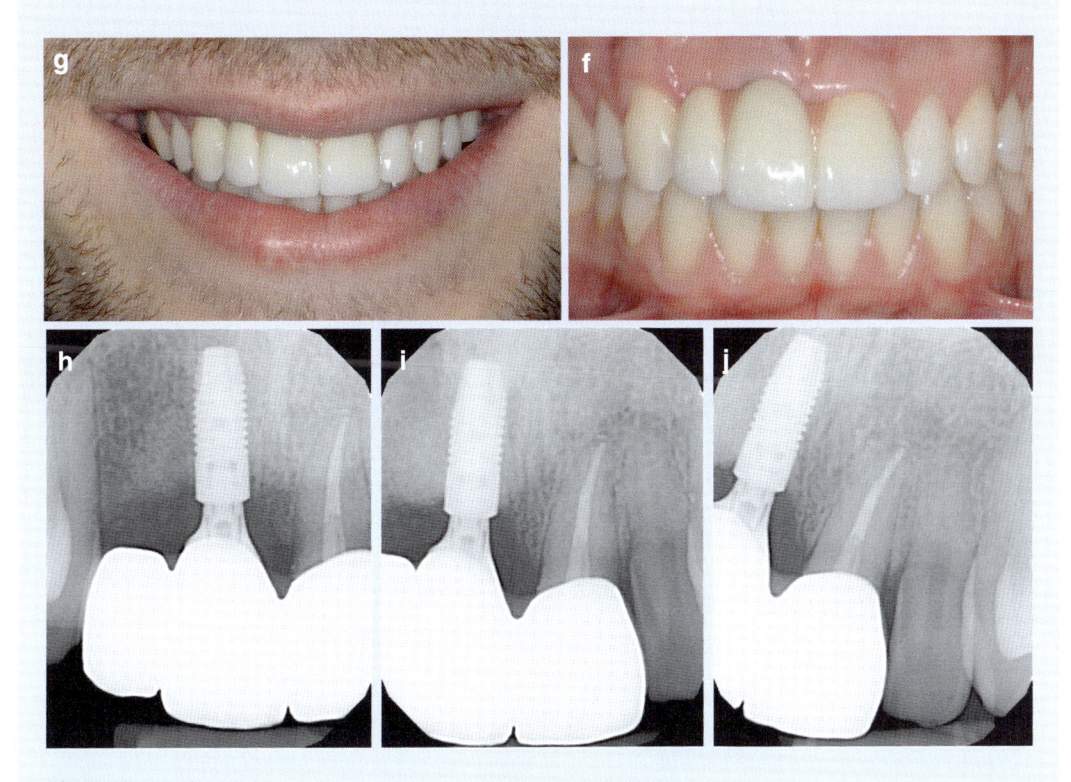

Fig. 22.3 (continued)

Case 22.3: Multi-tooth, Facial Veneered and Pink Gingivae

A female patient aged 49 presented with the following clinical considerations: a maxillary removable partial denture replacing the lateral and central incisors as well as a significant malocclusion. In addition, the upper left second bicuspid was missing. The patient's expectation was to have the missing teeth replaced with implant-supported restorations in conjunction with full orthodontic treatment to correct the malocclusion.

In consideration of the above conditions, three implants were placed in the maxillary anterior edentulous space to aid in orthodontic anchorage. Upon completion of orthodontic treatment, an implant was placed in the maxillary second bicuspid position. The restoration of all implants and additional direct and indirect restorations were carried out on the anterior and posterior teeth as required. Specifically, the definitive four-unit maxillary anterior implant-supported fixed restoration (screw retained) consisted of a minimally veneered zirconia restoration with white and pink feldspathic porcelain. The pink ceramic was required to compensate for the compromised ridge form as a result of wearing a removable prosthesis for 27 years (Fig. 22.4).

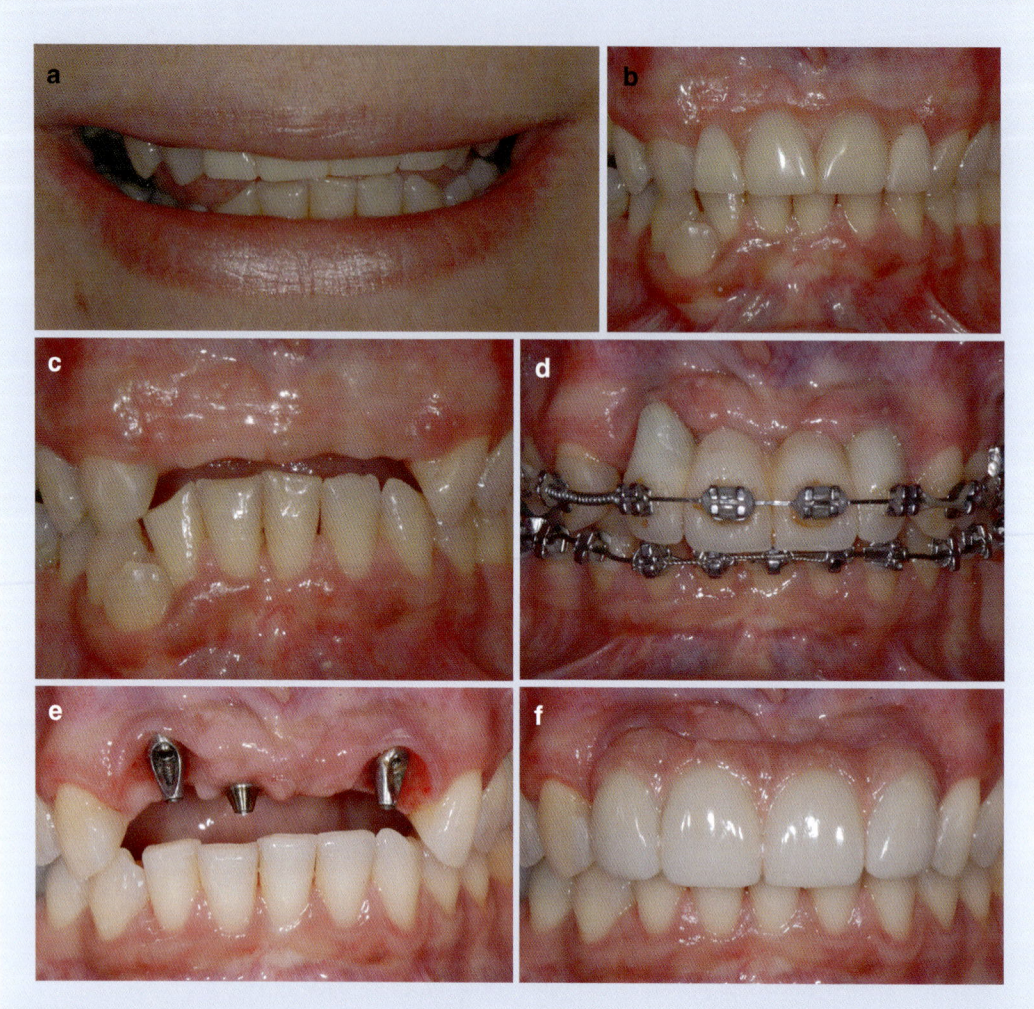

Fig. 22.4 Case 22.3: Multi-tooth, facial veneered and pink gingivae. (**a**) Pretreatment full smile. (**b**) Pretreatment intraoral view. (**c**) Pretreatment intraoral view without maxillary removable partial denture. (**d**) Intraoral facial view of provisional maxillary anterior restoration and orthodontic treatment. (**e**) Posttreatment intraoral facial view of abutments and completed orthodontic treatment. (**f**) Posttreatment facial intraoral view of zirconia restoration with feldspathic facial porcelain (not in function) and pink feldspathic gingivae. (**g–i**) Posttreatment radiographs. (**j**) Posttreatment full smile

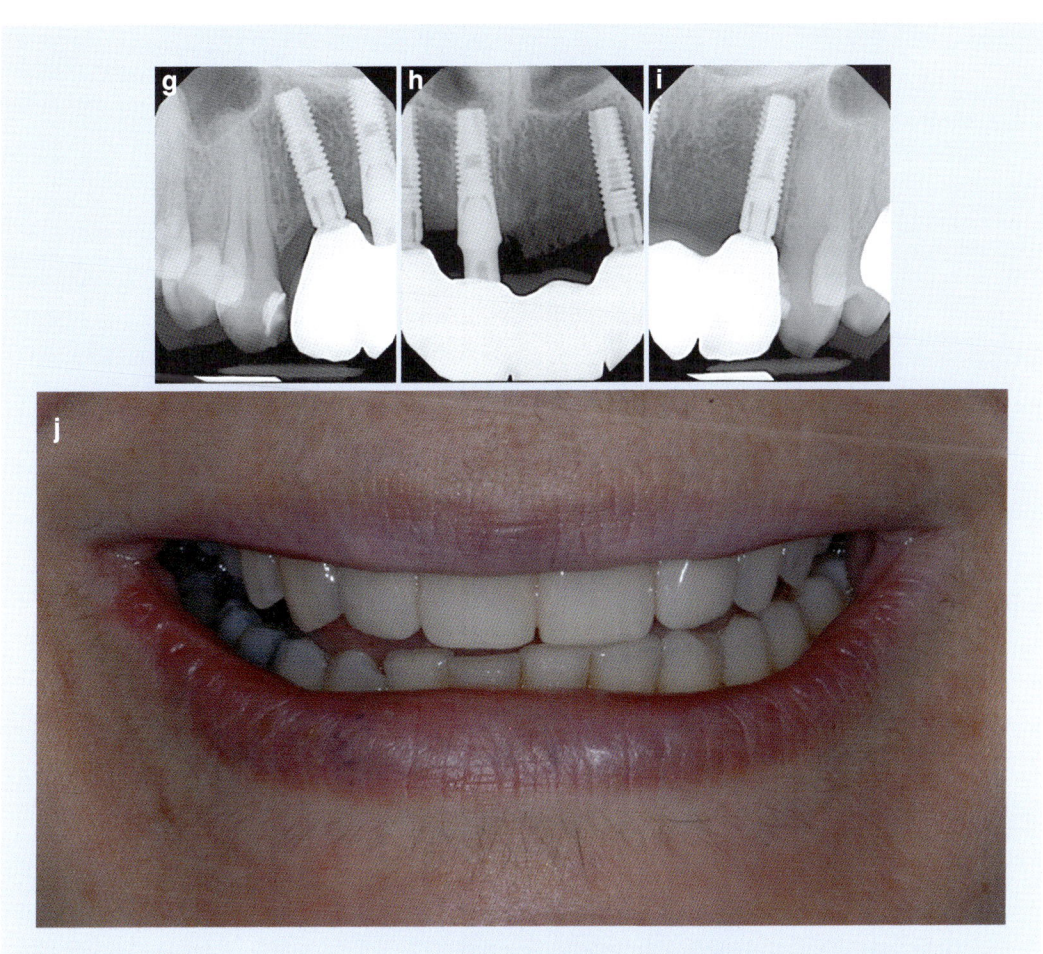

Fig. 22.4 (continued)

Case 22.4: Multi-tooth, Facial Veneered

A female patient aged 62 presented with the following clinical considerations: a failing fixed maxillary tooth-supported anterior porcelain-metal restoration supported by the maxillary left and right canines with four pontics replacing the maxillary incisors. The existing bridge exhibited porcelain fractures as well as a framework fracture. In addition, the left endodontically treated maxillary canine was fractured supragingivally. The patient's expectation was to have a new fixed maxillary anterior restoration.

In consideration of the above conditions, two implants were placed in the maxillary right central and left lateral incisor positions. A cast gold post and core was placed in the left maxillary canine. The definitive restorations were as follows: single minimally veneered zirconia crowns for the left and right maxillary canines and a four-unit minimally veneered zirconia maxillary anterior implant-supported fixed restoration (screw retained) replacing the incisors (Fig. 22.5).

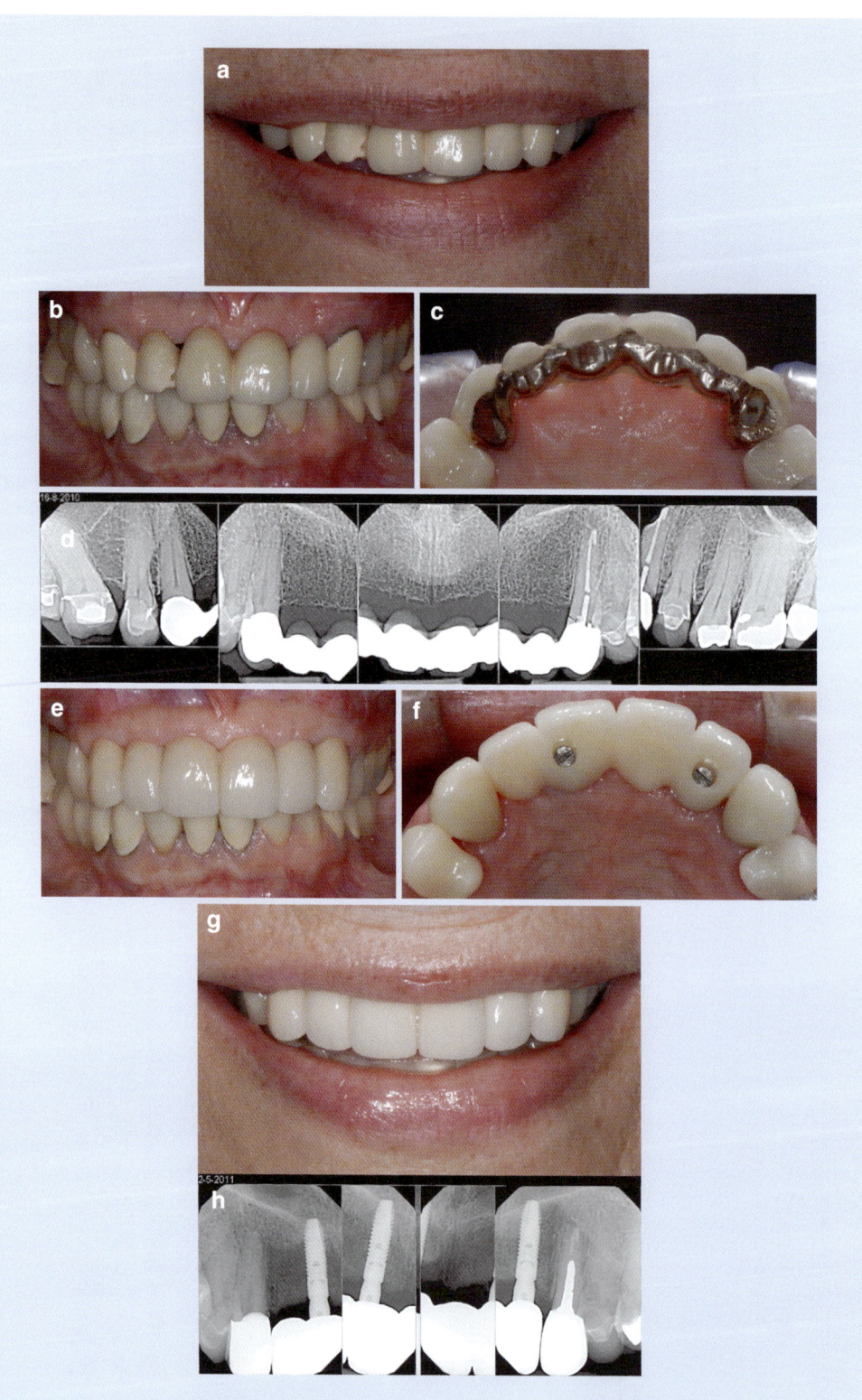

Fig. 22.5 Case 22.4: Multi-tooth, facial veneered. (**a**) Pretreatment full smile. (**b**) Pretreatment intraoral facial view. (**c**) Pretreatment intraoral lingual view. (**d**) Pretreatment radiographs. (**e**) Posttreatment intraoral facial view. (**f**) Posttreatment intraoral lingual view. (**g**) Posttreatment full smile. (**h**) Posttreatment radiographs

Case 22.5: Full Arch, Anterior Facial Veneered

A female patient aged 58 presented with the following clinical considerations: a damaged and worn maxillary tooth-supported fixed full-arch restoration. The remaining supporting abutment teeth were periodontally compromised and were not good candidates to support a new reconstruction. The patient's expectation was to have a full-arch implant-supported reconstruction and to avoid the use of a removable interim restoration.

In consideration of the above conditions, a sequential approach was used to reconstruct the maxillary arch. Strategic, tooth abutments were retained initially to support a fixed provisional restoration utilizing the original porcelain-metal bridge. During this phase, five implants were placed as follows: maxillary right first and second bicuspids, maxillary left first and second bicuspids and maxillary right lateral incisor positions. Following appropriate healing time for the implants, a second fixed provisional was fabricated in PMMA supported by the originally maintained teeth and the new implants. In the next phase, the remaining teeth were extracted and four additional implants were placed as follows: maxillary right first molar and canine and maxillary left canine and second molar positions. Upon the completion of the integration of the previous implants, a maxillary full-arch minimally veneered (six anterior teeth) zirconia restoration was fabricated supported by the nine implants. The posterior implants used screw-retained abutments (6) and the anterior implants used cement-retained abutments (3) due to the facial inclination of the implants. Following the maxillary reconstruction, the patient elected to replace the existing 12 mandibular porcelain-metal crowns with zirconia restorations (Fig. 22.6).

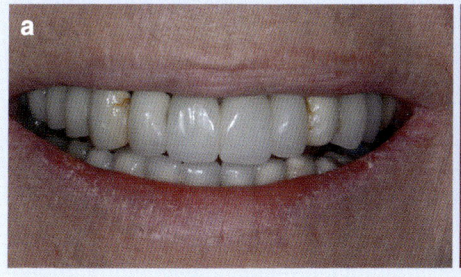

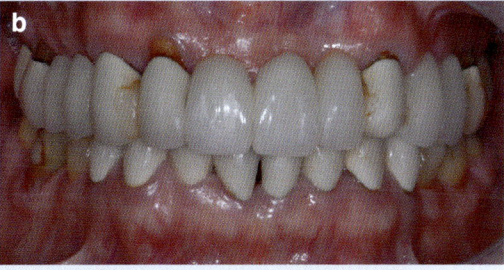

Fig. 22.6 Case 22.5: Full arch, anterior facial veneered. (**a**) Pretreatment full smile. (**b**) Pretreatment intraoral view. (**c**) Pretreatment radiographs. (**d**) Intraoral view of retained abutments for the initial provisional restoration. (**e**) Intraoral view of the initial provisional restoration (modified original bridge) with the first five implants in place. (**f**) Intraoral view with the retained abutments and the five implants with transferred copings in preparation for the impression to fabricate the secondary provisional restoration. (**g**) Digital view of the scanned master cast for the secondary provisional restoration. (**h–j**) Digital views of the Standard Tessellation Language (STL) files for the milling of the secondary PMMA provisional. (**k**) Laboratory view of the completed secondary PMMA provisional. (**l**) Intraoral view of the secondary provisional after placement of the additional four implants. (**m**) Laboratory view of the master cast of the nine implants with abutments. (**n**) Digital view of the master cast with the virtual design of the PMMA prototype-provisional used in the development of the zirconia restoration. (**o**) Laboratory view of the master cast with PMMA prototype-provisional. (**p**) Intraoral view of the adjusted PMMA prototype. (**q**) Digital view of the master cast. (**r**) Digital view of the master cast with the STL file for the zirconia restoration. Note the facial cutbacks of the maxillary anterior teeth for the feldspathic porcelain (not in function). (**s**) Laboratory view of the completed zirconia restoration with anterior facial porcelain (not in function). (**t**) Intraoral occlusal view of the soft tissue and implant abutments. (**u**) Intraoral facial view of the soft tissue and implant abutments. (**v**) Intraoral view of the maxillary zirconia restoration with facial porcelain (not in function). (**w**) Intraoral view of the maxillary and mandibular zirconia restorations. (**x**) Posttreatment full smile. (**y**) Posttreatment radiographs of the maxillary zirconia restoration

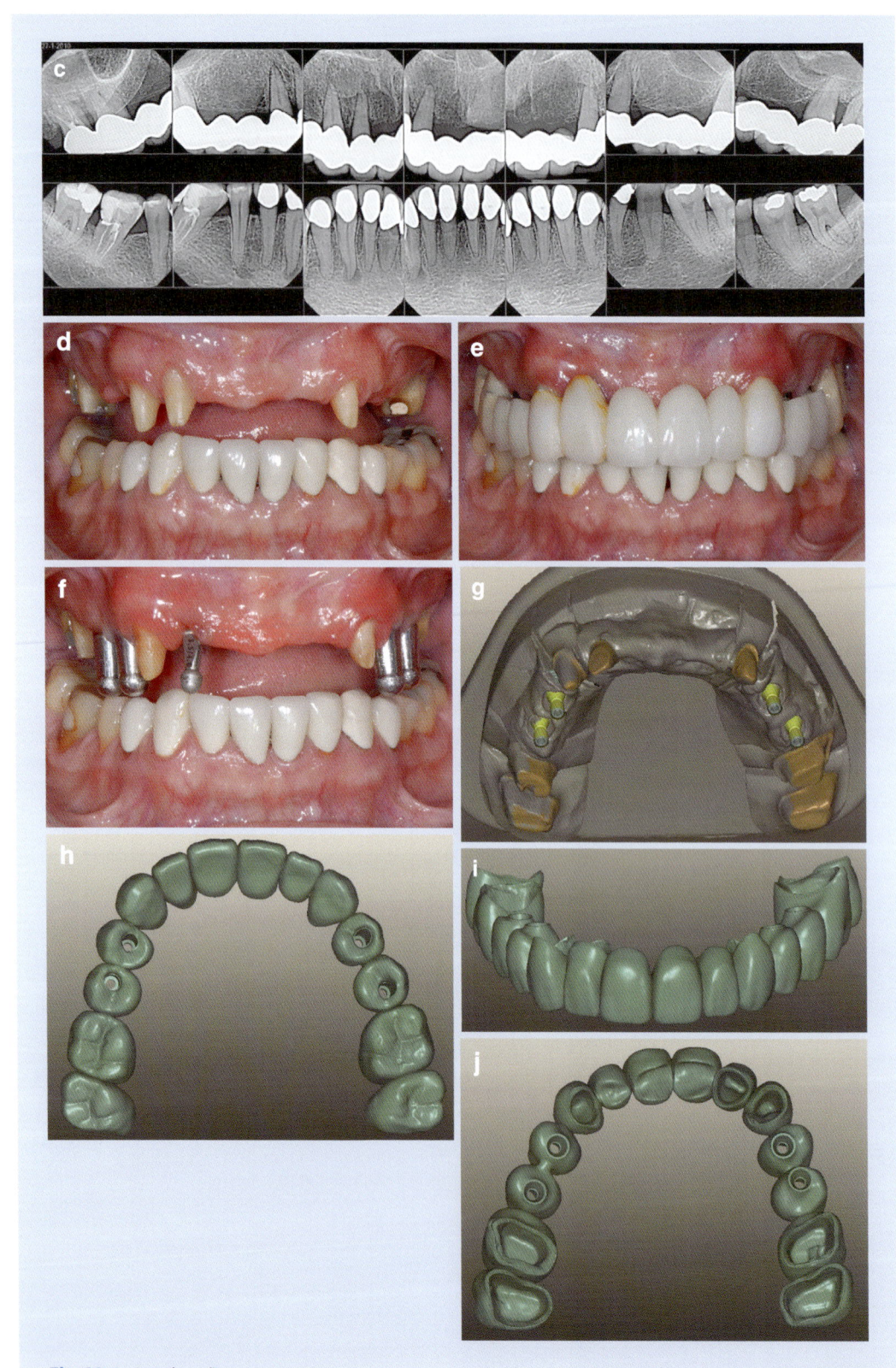

Fig. 22.6 (continued)

22 Challenging Maxillary Anterior Implant-Supported Restorations

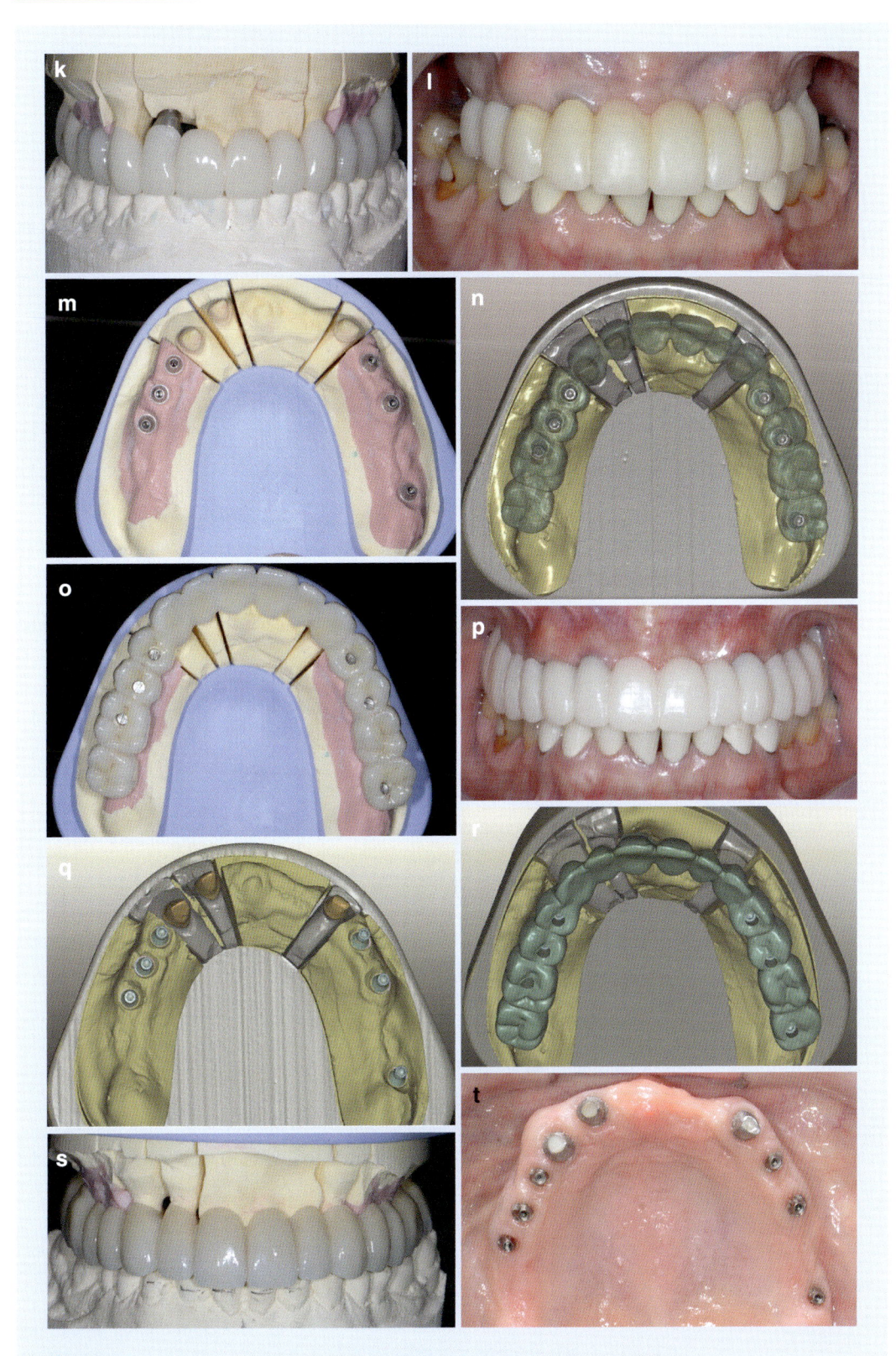

Fig. 22.6 (continued)

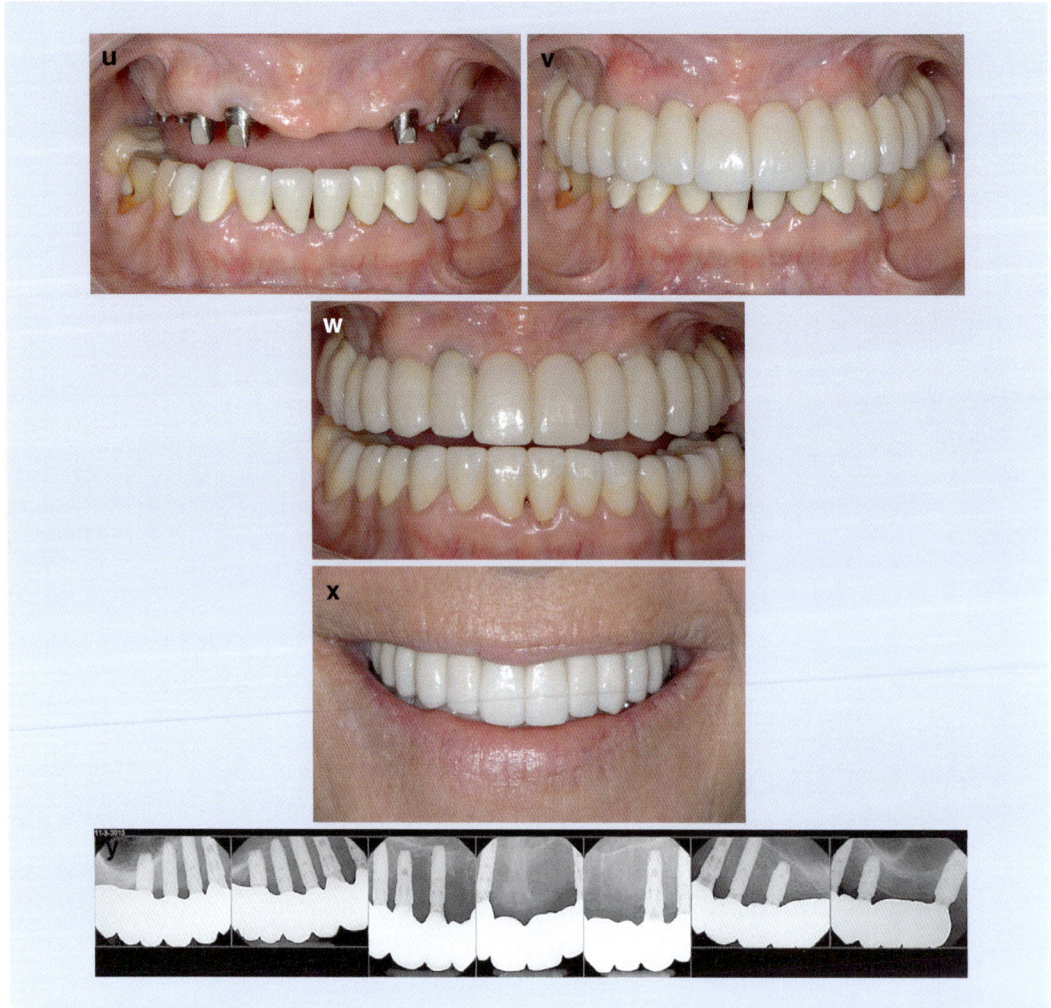

Fig. 22.6 (continued)

Case 22.6: Full-Arch, Monolithic and Pink Gingivae

A female patient aged 69 presented with the following clinical considerations: a maxillary removable partial denture supported by seven teeth with advanced periodontal bone loss (Fig. 22.6) and clinically sound mandibular teeth present from lower right second molar to lower left first molar. The patient's expectation was to replace the maxillary partial denture and failing maxillary remaining teeth with a fixed implant-supported reconstruction.

In consideration of the above conditions, the remaining maxillary teeth were extracted and eight implants were placed in the following positions: right first molar, first and second bicuspids and canine and left first and second bicuspids, canine and lateral incisor. The patient was restored with a maxillary provisional full denture during the healing phase of the implants. After integration of the eight implants, a PMMA prototype-provisional was placed to confirm the functional and aesthetic parameters of the proposed definitive restoration. Following this procedure, a monolithic zirconia maxillary reconstruction was completed from the right first molar to the left first molar (12 teeth). Pink feldspathic porcelain was used to compensate for soft and hard tissue loss (Fig. 22.7).

22 Challenging Maxillary Anterior Implant-Supported Restorations

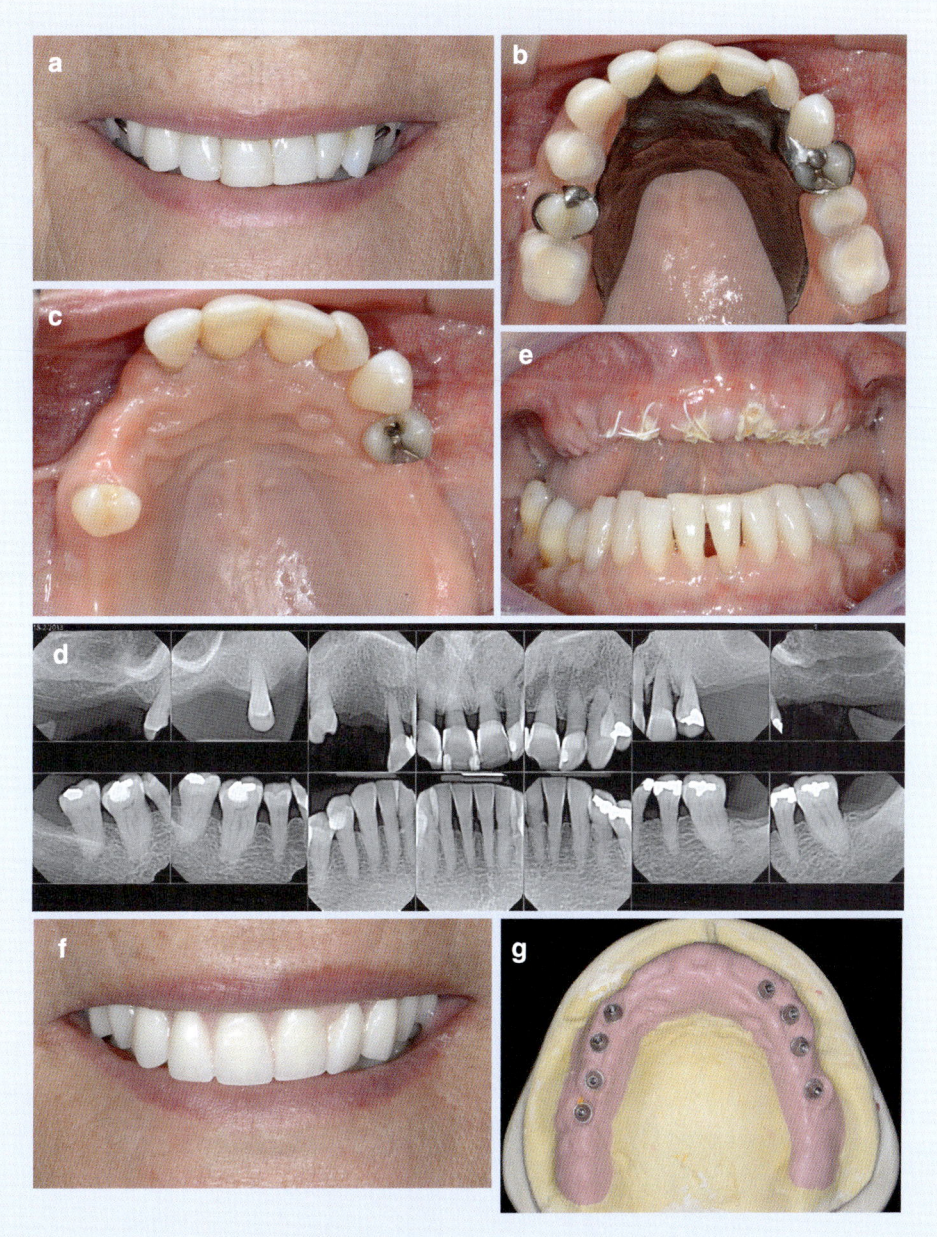

Fig. 22.7 Case 22.6: Full-arch, monolithic and pink gingivae. (**a**) Pretreatment full smile. (**b**) Pretreatment intraoral occlusal view with maxillary removable partial denture. (**c**) Pretreatment intraoral occlusal view without the maxillary removable partial denture. (**d**) Pretreatment radiographs. (**e**) Intraoral view 1-week post-implant placement. (**f**) Full smile with provisional complete upper denture. (**g**) Laboratory view of master cast with eight implant abutments. (**h**) Digital view of master cast with PMMA prototype-provisional design. (**i**) Laboratory view of the master cast with the PMMA prototype-provisional. (**j–l**) Digital view of STL files for the definitive zirconia restoration. (**m**) Laboratory view of the zirconia restoration with pink feldspathic gingivae. (**n**) Laboratory occlusal view of the zirconia restoration. (**o**) Laboratory view of the intaglio surface of the zirconia restoration. (**p**) Intraoral occlusal view of soft tissue and implant abutments. (**q**) Intraoral occlusal view of the zirconia restoration and screw channels sealed with composite and PTFE tape. (**r**) Intraoral facial view of soft tissue and implant abutments. Note mandibular teeth previously bleached. (**s**) Intraoral facial view of the monolithic zirconia restoration with pink feldspathic gingivae. (**t**) Posttreatment radiographs. (**u**) Posttreatment *right lateral* view of full smile. (**v**) Posttreatment facial view of full smile. (**w**) Posttreatment *left lateral* view of full smile

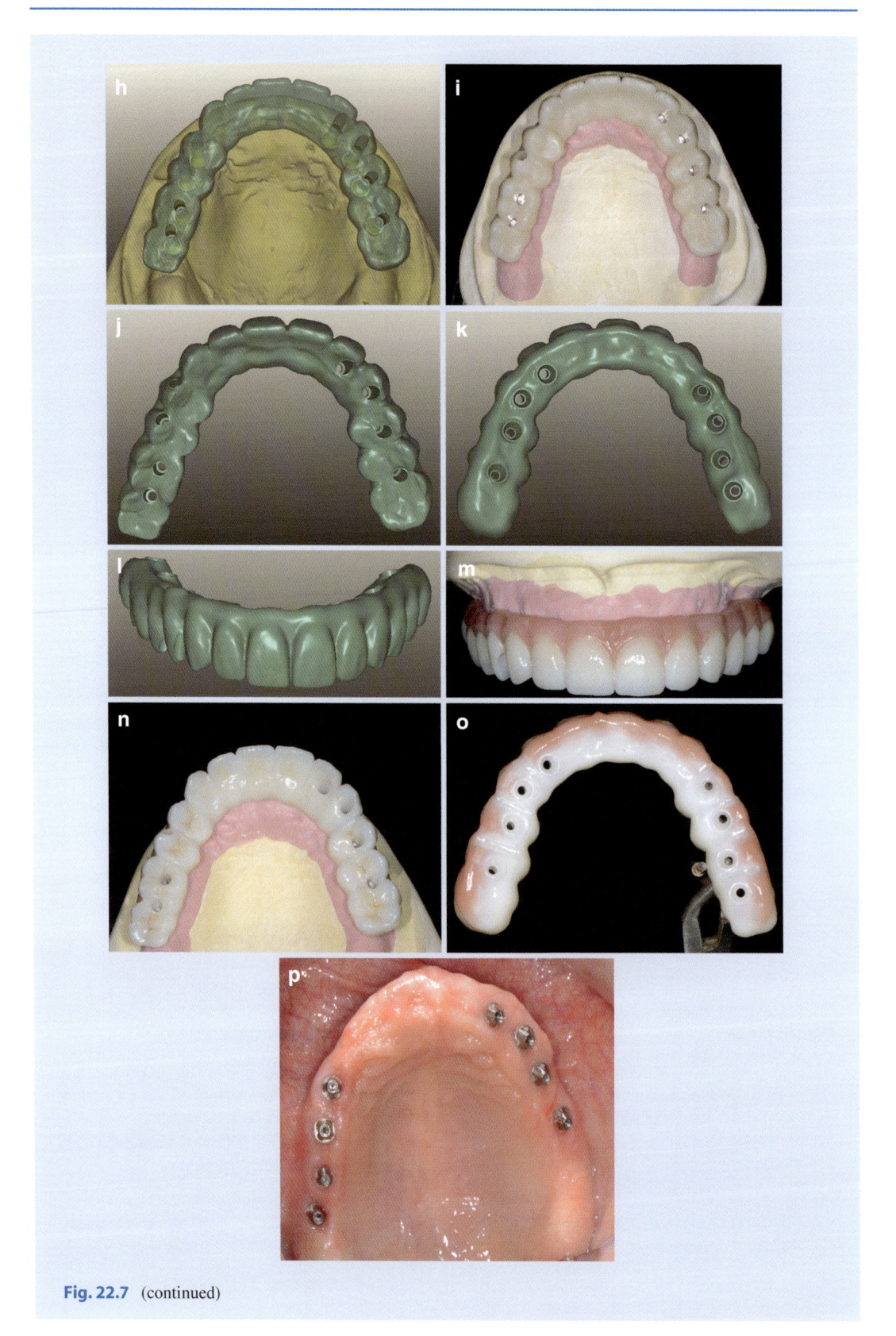

Fig. 22.7 (continued)

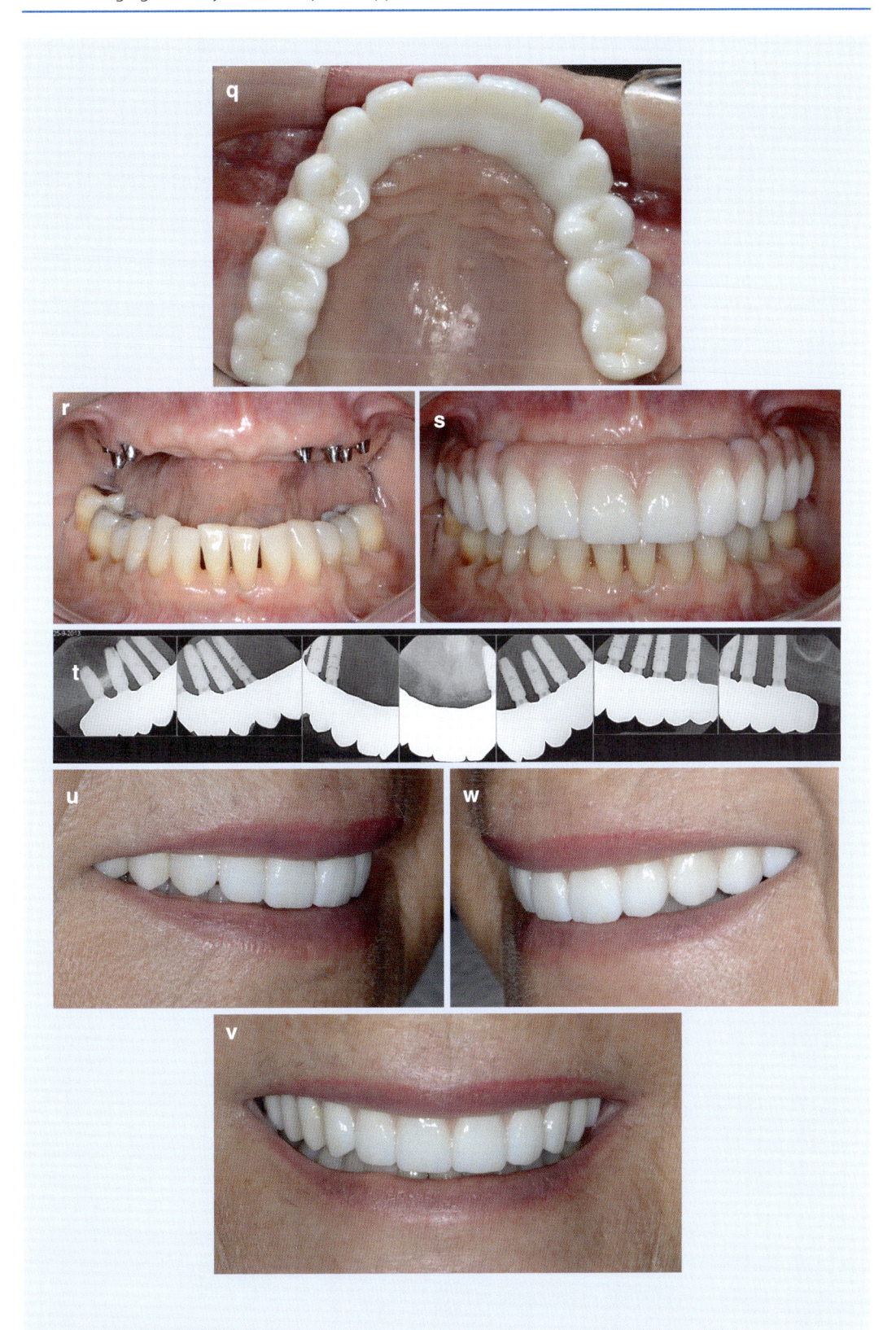

22 Challenging Maxillary Anterior Implant-Supported Restorations

Fig. 22.7 (continued)

Acknowledgements The author would like to thank Hiam Keren, MDT, for the laboratory support in the production of the restorations and Danae Sandoval for the technical assistance in the preparation of this manuscript. The author reported no conflicts of interest.

References

Al-Amleh B, Lyons K, Swain M (2010) Clinical trials in zirconia: a systematic review. J Oral Rehabil 37:641–652

Alghazzawi TF, Lemons J, Liu PR, Essig ME, Bartolucci AA, Janowski GM (2012) Influence of low-temperature environmental exposure on the mechanical properties and structural stability of dental zirconia. J Prosthodont 21:363–369

Alqahtani F. Full-mouth rehabilitation of severely worn dentition due to soda swishing: A clinical report. J Prosthodont 2013;23:50–57.

Barewal R, Stanford C, Weesner T (2012) A randomized controlled clinical trial comparing the effects of three loading protocols on dental implant stability. Int J Oral Maxillofac Implants 27:945–956

Cassetta M, Stefanelli L, Giansanti M, Di Mambro A, Calasso S (2013) Accuracy of a computer-aided implant surgical technique. Int J Periodont Rest Dent 33(3):316–325

Chevalier J, Gremillard L (2009) The tetragonal-monoclinic transformation in zirconia: lessons learned and future trends. J Am Ceram Soc 92:1901–1920

Cho S, Schaefer O, Thompson G, Guentsch A (2015) Comparison of accuracy and reproducibility of casts made by digital and conventional methods. J Prosthet Dent 113:310–315

Christensen GJ (2012) Indirect restoration use: a changing paradigm. J Am Dent Assoc 143:398–400

Cohen M (ed) (2008) Interdisciplinary treatment planning: principles, design, implementation, 1st edn. Quintessence, Chicago

Conrad HJ, Seong WJ, Pesun IJ (2007) Current ceramic materials and systems with clinical recommendations: a systematic review. J Prosthet Dent 98:389–404

Dym H (2015) Implant procedures for the general dentist. Dent Clin 53(2):255–528

Flinn BD, deGroot DA, Mancl LA, Raigrodski AJ (2012) Accelerated aging characteristics of three yttria-stabilized tetragonal zirconia polycrystalline dental materials. J Prosthet Dent 108:223–230

Gökçen-Röhlig B, Saruhanoglu A, Cifter ED, Evlioglu G (2010) Applicability of zirconia dental prostheses for metal allergy patients. Int J Prosthodont 23:562–565

Goodacre C, Bernal G, Rungcharassaeng K, Kan J (2003) Clinical complications with implants and implant prostheses. J Prosthet Dent 90(2):121–132

Guess PC, Att W, Strub JR (2012) Zirconia in fixed implant prosthodontics. Clin Implant Dent Relat Res 14:633–645

Güth JF, Almeida E, Silva JS, Beuer FF, Edelhoff D (2012) Enhancing the predictability of complex rehabilitation with a removable CAD/CAM-fabricated long-term provisional prosthesis: a clinical report. J Prosthet Dent 107:1–6

Harris D, Horner K, Gröndahl K, Jacobs R, Helmrot E, Benic G, Bornstein M, Dawood A, Quirynen MEAO (2012) Guidelines for the use of diagnostic imaging in implant dentistry 2011. A consensus workshop organized by the European Association for Osseointegration at the Medical University of Warsaw. Clin Oral Implants Res 23:1243–1253

Hisbergues M, Vendeville S, Vendeville P (2009) Zirconia: established facts and perspectives for a biomaterial in dental implantology. J Biomed Mater Res B Appl Biomater 88:519–529

Janyavula S, Lawson N, Cakir D, Beck P, Ramp LC, Burgess JO (2013) The wear of polished and glazed zirconia against enamel. J Prosthet Dent 109:22–29

Jokstad A, Braegger U, Brunski JB, Carr AB, Naert I, Wennerberg A (2004) Quality of dental implants. Int J Prosthodont 17(6):607–641

Jung YS, Lee JW, Choi YJ, Ahn JS, Shin SW, Huh JB (2010) A study on the in-vitro wear of the natural tooth structure by opposing zirconia or dental porcelain. J Adv Prosthodont 2:111–115

Kapos T, Evans C (2014) CAD/CAM technology for implant abutments, crowns, and superstructures. Int J Oral Maxillofac Implants 29(suppl 1):117–136

Karl M, Graef F, Wichmann M, Krafft T (2012) Passivity of fit of CAD/CAM and copy-milled frameworks, veneered frameworks, and anatomically contoured, zirconia ceramic, implant-supported fixed prostheses. J Prosthet Dent 107:232–238

Kelly JR, Denry I (2008) Stabilized zirconia as a structural ceramic: an overview. Dent Mater 24:289–298

Keren H, Caro S. Das beste material. Dent Lab. 2009

Klasser GD, Greene CS, Lavigne GJ (2010) Oral appliances and the management of sleep bruxism in adults: a century of clinical applications and search for mechanisms. Int J Prosthodont 23:453–462

Ko N, Mine A, Egusa H, Shimazu T, Ko R, Nakano T, Yatani H (2014) Allergic reaction to titanium-made fixed dental restorations: a clinical report. J Prosthodont:1–3

Lang N, Berglundh T, Heitz-Mayfield L, Pjetursson B, Salvi G, Sanz M (2004) Consensus statements and recommended clinical procedures regarding implant survival and complications. Int J Oral Maxillofac Implants 19:150–154

Larsson C, Wennerberg A (2014) The clinical success of zirconia-based crowns: a systematic review. Int J Prosthodont 27:33–43

Moráguez OD, Belser UC (2010) The use of polytetrafluoroethylene tape for the management of screw access channels in implant-supported prostheses. J Prosthet Dent 103:189–191

Moscovitch MS (2015a) Monolithic zirconia fixed prostheses. In: Beumer J, Faulkner R, Shah C, Moy P (eds) Fundamentals of implant dentistry, volume 1: prosthodontic principles. Quintessence Books, Hanover Park, pp 94–101

Moscovitch MS (2015b) A complex implant-supported reconstruction with monolithic-minimally veneered zirconia: a clinical report. Compendium 36(7):496–502

Moscovitch MS (2015c) Consecutive case series of monolithic and minimally veneered zirconia restorations on teeth and implants: up to 68 months. Int J Periodont Rest Dent 35(3):315–323

Moscovitch MS, Saba S (1996) The use of a provisional restoration in implant dentistry: a clinical report. Int J Oral Maxillofac Implants 11:395–399

Ozkurt Z, Kazazoğlu E (2010) Clinical success of zirconia in dental applications. J Prosthodont 19(1):64–68

Park JH, Park S, Lee K, Yun KD, Lim HP (2014) Antagonist wear of three CAD/CAM anatomic contour zirconia ceramics. J Prosthet Dent 111:20–29

Pjetursson B, Thoma D, Jung R, Zwahlen M, Zembic A (2012) A systematic review of the survival and complication rates of implant-supported fixed dental prostheses (FDPs) after a mean observation period of at least 5 years. Clin Oral Implants Res 23(6):22–38

Raigrodski AJ, Hillstead MB, Meng GK, Chung KH (2012) Survival and complications of zirconia-based fixed dental prostheses: a systematic review. J Prosthet Dent 107:170–177

Reyes A, Turkyilmaz I, Prihoda TJ (2015) Accuracy of surgical guides made from conventional and a combination of digital scanning and rapid prototyping techniques. J Prosthet Dent 113(4):295–303

Rojas-Vizcaya F (2011) Full zirconia fixed detachable implant-retained restorations manufactured from monolithic zirconia: clinical report after two years in service. J Prosthodont 20:570–576

Sagirkaya E, Arikan S, Sadik B, Kara C, Karasoy D, Cehreli M (2012) A randomized, prospective, open-ended clinical trial of zirconia fixed partial dentures on teeth and implants: interim results. Int J Prosthodont 25:221–231

Schmitter M, Boemicke W, Stober T (2014) Bruxism in prospective studies of veneered zirconia restorations: a systematic review. Int J Prosthodont 27:127–133

Thalji GN, Cooper LF (2014) Implant-supported fixed dental rehabilitation with monolithic zirconia: a clinical case report. J Esthet Restor Dent 26:88–96

Walton TR (2014) Making sense of complication reporting associated with fixed dental prostheses. Int J Prosthodont 27:114–118

Wismeijer D, Brägger U, Evans C, Kapos T, Kelly JR, Millen C, Wittneben JG, Zembic A, Taylor TD (2014) Consensus statements and recommended clinical procedures regarding restorative materials and techniques for implant dentistry. Int J Oral Maxillofac Implants 29:137–140

Wood M, Vermilyea S (2004) A review of selected dental literature on evidence-based treatment planning for dental implants: report of the committee on research in fixed prosthodontics of the academy of fixed prosthodontics. J Prosthet Dent 92(5):447–462

Part IV

Complications and Their Management

Peri-implantitis: Causation and Treatment

Michael L. Schmerman and Salvador Nares

Abstract

The continued increase in the placement of dental implants, while modifying the course of and improving treatment, has spawned a set of problems endemic to the therapy. This chapter explores peri-implantitis including its prevalence and histologic features. Identification of the etiology and microbiology of the entity are traced. Periodontitis has been found to play an important role in susceptibility. The differences between ailing and failing implants are defined. Finally, the history, evolution, and methods of treatment of these problems by various researchers and clinicians are explored. These citations include techniques discussed by Meffert, Lang, and Froum. The complexity of peri-implantitis, as expected, will require much in further study. Of paramount clinical importance is the maintenance phase of implant restoration. By vigilant monitoring, both early detection and interventions can enhance outcomes.

M.L. Schmerman, DDS
Department of Periodontics,
College of Dentistry, University of Illinois at Chicago, 458 Dent MC 859, 801 South Paulina, Chicago, IL 60612, USA

Illinois Masonic Hospital,
Chicago, IL, USA
e-mail: drkool@uic.edu

S. Nares (✉)
Department of Periodontics,
College of Dentistry, University of Illinois at Chicago, 458 Dent MC 859, 801 South Paulina, Chicago, IL 60612, USA
e-mail: snares@uic.edu

While dental implants have in many ways, fundamentally transformed how dentistry approaches replacement of missing teeth, they are not immune to biological complications stemming from microbiological, iatrogenic, and patient factors. Of these, peri-implantitis, defined by the Seventh European Workshop on Periodontology as a condition presenting with peri-implant bone loss and bleeding upon probing with or without suppuration (Lang and Berglundh 2011), can be one of the more difficult complications to effectively manage. Peri-implantitis is most often triggered by plaque biofilm; although iatrogenic elements can serve as etiological factors. This is in contrast to peri-mucositis, which much like gingivitis consists of inflammation limited to changes to mucosal contour and color and bleeding on probing but without involvement of supporting bone. In general, peri-mucositis can be effectively managed using non-surgical approaches including removal of the plaque biofilm, institution of effective oral hygiene measures and professional recalls. However, management of peri-implantitis is more complex, typically involves surgical intervention, and can be unpredictable. As such, an awareness and new discipline is evolving that requires cooperation between the clinician and patient to prevent disease and maintain health.

It is important to note that not all peri-implant bone resorption is caused by peri-implantitis. Early peri-implant bone loss can be a manifestation of physiologic bone remodeling as tissue-implant homeostasis is achieved after implant placement and abutment installation as can occur in two-piece implants (Adell et al. 1981) or as a result of gingival conditioning in the aesthetic zone to create the illusion of an interdental papilla (Gallucci et al. 2011). Bone remodeling can also be a consequence of deep placement of an implant (Hämmerle et al. 1996) or result from the placement of adjacent implants too close to each other (Tarnow et al. 2000). As such it has been recommended that long-term monitoring of dental implants, including radiography, should take place after restoration of the implant and at 1 year instead of immediately after placement of the fixture (Alani et al. 2014). Here we summarize current knowledge and recent advances in our understanding of the pathophysiology of peri-implantitis and review contemporary treatment modalities in use.

23.1 The Prevalence of Peri-implantitis

In the United States, it was recently estimated that 1.3–2 million implants are placed annually, and this number is expected to grow at a rate of 15% (Achermann 2012). Therefore, it is reasonable to assume that the prevalence of peri-implantitis will also increase. Unfortunately, the true prevalence of peri-implantitis has been difficult to accurately estimate, due to variations in the threshold for bone loss or bone levels that clinicians use to define peri-implantitis. This, along with the finding that most studies reported in the literature utilize convenience sampling of limited size (Derks and Tomasi 2015). Nevertheless, recent data (2010–2015) indicates that the prevalence of peri-mucositis ranges from 31% to 63% of patients and 22–38% of implants, while the prevalence of peri-implantitis ranges from 12% to 47% of patients and 5–37% of implants (Table 23.1).

23.2 Histological Features of Peri-implant Tissues and in Peri-implantitis Lesions

While plaque biofilm is the main etiological factor in development and progression of peri-implant disease, it is important to note that fundamental anatomic differences exist between peri-implant and periodontal tissues that likely contribute to the aggressive nature of the disease. In dental implants, the biologic width is established by week 6–8 around transmucosal implants (Sculean et al. 2014) although gingival fibers generally do not attach to titanium and instead can be observed parallel to the long axis or circumferentially around the dental implant (Judgar et al. 2014). In contrast, gingival fibers attach to cementum on teeth and radiate outward into the gingival tissues in a perpendicular or oblique direction. This configuration is believed to impede epithelial migration and help prevent microbial invasion into the underlying connective tissues (Stern 1981). As such, these anatomical differences negate the ability to form a true biological seal of the underlying tissues from plaque biofilm and may also help explain why the tip of the periodontal probe often times penetrates beyond the epithelial attachment into the underlying connective tissues (Mombelli et al. 1997). Immunologically, studies indicate that peri-implant tissues respond more aggressively to similar levels of plaque as demonstrated by a larger and greater apical extension of the inflammatory infiltrate (Carcuac and Berglundh 2014; Berglundh et al. 2011), higher levels of inflammatory cytokines, (Emecen-Huja et al. 2013)

Table 23.1 Recent literature documenting incidence of peri-implantitis

Study	Study design	Time (years)	Number of patients	Number of implants	Prevalence of peri-mucositis: % of patients	Prevalence of peri-mucositis: % of implants	Prevalence of peri-implantitis: % of patients	Prevalence of peri-implantitis: % of implants
Atieh et al. (2013)	Meta-analysis	5–10+	1,497	6,283	63	31	19	10[a]
Cecchinato et al. (2014)	Cross-sectional	10	133	407	NR	NR	12	5
Derks and Tomasi (2015)	Meta-analysis	1–10+	NR	NR	43	NR	22	NR
Dvorak et al. (2011)	Cross-sectional	1–10+	203	967	NR	NR	24	13
Koldsland et al. (2010)	Cross-sectional	Mean: 9 years	108	351	39	27	47	37
Marrone et al. (2013)	Cross-sectional	5–10+	103	266	31	38	37	23
Mir-Mari et al. (2012)	Cross-sectional	1–10+	245	964	39	22	16	9
Mombelli et al. (2012)	Systematic review	5–10	2,720	9,236	NR	NR	20	10

NR not reported
[a] Smokers had a 36.3% frequency of peri-implantitis

and osteoclasts (Berglundh et al. 2011) as compared to periodontitis. Thus, the anatomy and pathophysiology of peri-implantitis is distinct from that of periodontitis (Table 23.2), (Tsao and Wang 2003).

23.3 Etiology and Risk Factor

The prime etiological factor for peri-implantitis is the plaque biofilm (Fig. 23.1) although patient factors such as systemic health (diabetes mellitus, osteoporosis, corticoid therapy, radiation, chemotherapy), behavioral factors (smoking, poor compliance), and iatrogenic factors (cement, occlusion) contribute varying degrees of risk to the onset and progression of peri-implantitis. Components of the biofilm trigger an inflammatory response leading to resorption of bone and subsequent exposure of the implant surface. As discussed above, differences in the anatomy and physiology of tissues approximating dental implants are less likely to contain the infection yet respond more aggressively to the microbial challenge. Compounding the problems are the recent advances in surface technologies and thread design. While these advances have improved the predictability of implant therapy, rougher implant surface and aggressive thread pitches are likely to foster a biofilm that is more robust and challenging to remove (Teughels et al. 2006; Berglundh et al. 2007; Lin et al. 2013).

Table 23.2 Differences between implants and natural teeth

	Natural teeth	Dental implants
Attachment	Cementum, PDL, bone	Osseointegration, functional ankylosis
Junctional epithelium	Basil lamina and hemi-desmosomal	Basil lamina and hemi-desmosomal
Gingival fibers	Perpendicular	Parallel or circumferential
Connective tissue		
Collagen volume	More (85%)	Less (65%)
Fibroblasts number	Less (1–3%)	More (5–10%)
Vascularity	More	Less
Biologic width	JE + CT	JE + SD + CT

Adapted from Alani et al. (2014)
JE junctional epithelium, *CT* connective tissue, *SD* sulcus depth

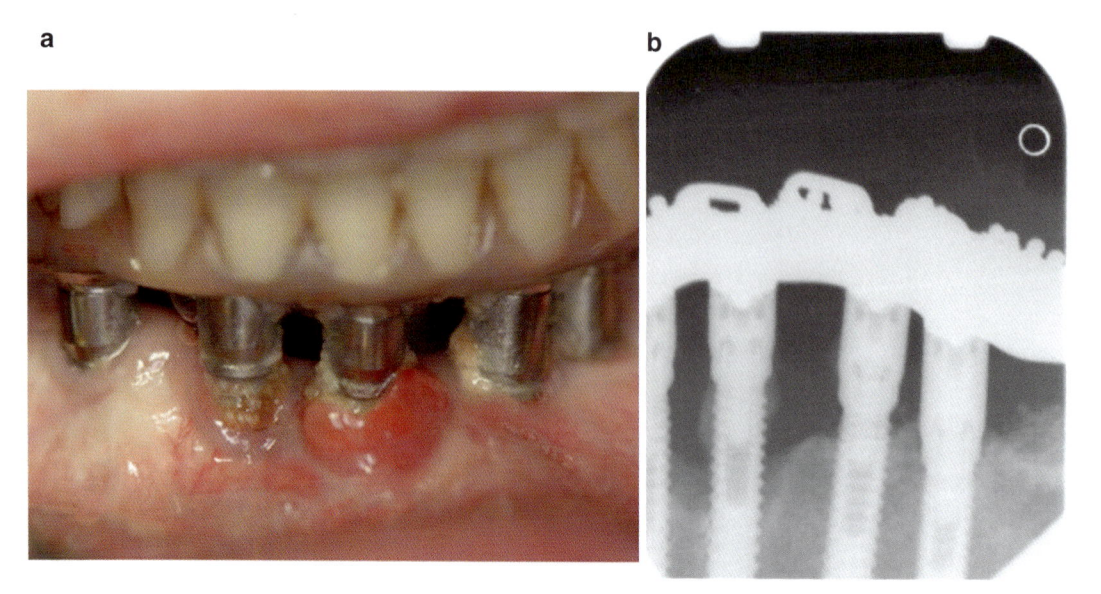

Fig. 23.1 A 57-year-old female referred for treatment of peri-implantitis. (**a**) Note significant quantities of plaque, calculus, and inflammation. (**b**) Periapical image demonstrating significant subgingival calculus and vertical bone loss

Further, implants placed at a failed implant site have been reported to have a diminished probability of survival (Machtei et al. 2008), while thinner gingival biotypes have an increased tendency to loose marginal bone than thick biotypes (Linkevicius et al. 2009).

23.4 Microbiological Features of Peri-implantitis

In the late 1980s, Mombelli and colleagues investigated the microbiological characteristics of successful versus "failing" root form implants (Mombelli et al. 1987). By culture and microscopy, they demonstrated elevated numbers of colony-forming units and numbers of gram-negative anaerobic rods and motile and fusiform microbes in diseased implants as compared to healthy implants which were populated with more facultative coccoids. Importantly, this study also showed that poor oral hygiene and iatrogenic factors such as uncleansable suprastructures contributed to the formation of a pathogenic biofilm resembling that associated with periodontitis (Charalampakis and Belibasakis 2015). Today, advances in molecular technologies have yielded a deeper understanding of the complexity of the microbiome associated with peri-implant disease. Peri-implantitis, much like periodontitis, is an endogenous, opportunistic, polymicrobial infection yet recent evidence suggests both convergence and divergence of the microbial composition. For example, while the plaque biofilm is derived from adjacent teeth and includes non-pathologic and pathologic microbial species, ecological pressures appear to shift an otherwise nonpathogenic flora to one that contributes to the pathogenicity of peri-implantitis (Charalampakis and Belibasakis 2015). The bacterial species such as *S. aureus*, *Peptostreptococcaceae sp.*, and *Desulfomicrobium orale* are not normally associated with periodontitis and are found in greater proportions in peri-implantitis lesions (Maruyama et al. 2014; Heitz-Mayfield and Lang 2010). High concentrations of saccharolytic anaerobes such as *Slackia exigua*, *Filifactor alocis*, *E. saphenum*, *E. nodatum*, and *E. brachy* have been identified indicating that other microbes besides periodontal pathogens appear to be etiologic factors (Tamura et al. 2013). Indeed, recent metagenomic analysis highlights the finding that the peri-implant flora is substantially more diverse than previously believed and includes many uncultivated microbial species (Koyanagi et al. 2013). Recently, Murayama et al. (2014) reported significant differences in the core microbiomes between periodontitis and peri-implantitis lesions. While periodontal pathogens have been identified in peri-implantitis, these appear to be found in significantly fewer number compared to periodontitis (Koyanagi et al. 2013). Thus, it has been proposed that the microenvironment created by dental implants is unique and drives microbial adaptation and selection (Robitaille et al. 2015).

23.5 Periodontitis and Predisposition to Peri-implantitis

A significant body of evidence indicates that smoking and a history of periodontitis are associated with a higher prevalence of peri-implantitis and marginal bone loss (Lang and Berglundh 2011; Mombelli et al. 2012; Casado et al. 2013; Chrcanovic et al. 2015; Saaby et al. 2014). It is estimated that patients with a history of periodontitis are at approximately a fourfold greater risk (odds ratio, 4.7; 95% confidence intervals: 1.0–22) for peri-implantitis (reviewed in Robitaille et al. 2015).

For all patients, but particularly those with a history of periodontitis, it is imperative that meticulous oral hygiene and regular maintenance intervals be instituted. Residual periodontal pockets will likely harbor periodontal pathogens which may place implants at a greater risk of developing peri-implantitis. While a history of periodontitis coincides with a greater risk of developing peri-implantitis, a systematic review by Zangrando and colleagues (2015) indicated implant therapy can be successful in this population. These patients were effectively treated for periodontal disease and were compliant with regular periodontal maintenance intervals. It does not appear that the same can be said for smokers.

23.6 The Ailing vs. Failing vs. Failed Implant

An ailing implant may be defined as those problems limited to the mucosa surrounding the implant without involvement of the supporting bone (Esposito et al. 1999; Kutlu et al. 2016). The inclusion of biologic complications is a corollary to that description. These are all descriptive terms borrowed from the periodontal literature and include increases in probing depth, bleeding on gentle provocation, gingival (mucosal) recession, and possible exudate. Much as is the case in chronic gingival disease, probing depths beyond a certain depth in combination with the unique anatomy present in peri-implant tissues afford an environment that is conducive to selection of bacterial biotypes, thus triggering an increased risk for peri-implantitis.

By definition, a failing implant may include bone loss around an implant without mobility. An exception to this environment can be found in failing implants caused by traumatic occlusion which may have a predominantly streptococcal environment, which is frequently seen in periodontal health. Another site of the failing implant is that of retrograde peri-implantitis (Kutlu et al. 2016). This less common event occurs in about 1 in 400 peri-implantitis cases (Kutlu et al. 2016; Tözüm et al. 2006). This was described by McCallister, et al. (1992) and defined by Reiser and Nevins (1995) as bone loss limited to the apical segment of an otherwise osseointegrated implant.

23.7 Conventional Treatment Methodologies

Much thought, effort and description have gone into treatment of the ailing and failing implant. Early depictions by Meffert (1992) discussed the treatment of the hydroxyapatite coated implant in failure with the use of citric acid for detoxification as being effective. Similarly, the use of tetracycline was the preferred method for those implants with a metallic outer surface. Various autograft, allograft, and xenograft materials have been used to attempt bone regeneration. A protective membrane of either resorbable or nonresorbable material was used to aid in clot stabilization and graft containment. The ultimate goal was to retain the implant and restore it to a functionally noninfected state.

Lang (2000) described prevention, diagnosis, and treatment. Reference is made to the origins of peri-mucositis involving infection in the sulcus initially and the resultant intrabony defects formed as a part of the pathogenic process. He further described the need for *Cumulative Interceptive Supportive Therapy* (CIST, Fig. 23.2, Table 23.3). This protocol is based on diagnostic findings and involves escalation of intervention as the pathologic findings become more significant. Mechanical debridement (CIST-A) is used in cases with mild inflammation and no suppuration. Antiseptic treatment (STP-B) may be added if probing depths become uncleansable (4–5 mm in depth). Chlorhexidine gluconate may be used as a gel or rinse for 3–4 weeks in an attempt to re-achieve a healthy sulcular environment. Supportive protocol C (antibiotic therapy) is indicated when pocket depths reach 6 mm or more. Suppuration may or may not be present. Radiography usually indicates bone loss with an increase in the number of implant threads exposed above the crestal bone/implant interface. Antibiotics are prescribed in conjunction with the regimens in STP-A and STP-B. There is a local and systemic attempt intended to reduce pathogens (anaerobic) in the submucosa. Suggested antibiotics include metronidazole or ornidazole (Mombelli and Lang 1992). The use of locally applied antibiotics (tetracycline fibers or Arestin) has also been mentioned as an alternative to systemic antibiotic therapy. Restoration (regenerative) or respective therapy (STP-D) is advised only if the infection is controlled. Regenerative techniques should be based on the biologic principals of guided tissue regeneration.

A recent systematic review (Muthukuru et al. 2012) revealed that "local delivery of antibiotics, submucosal air polishing or EV: YAG laser treatment results in greater reduction in bleeding compared with debridement and antimicrobial irrigation (chlorhexidine)." Further evidence

23 Peri-implantitis: Causation and Treatment

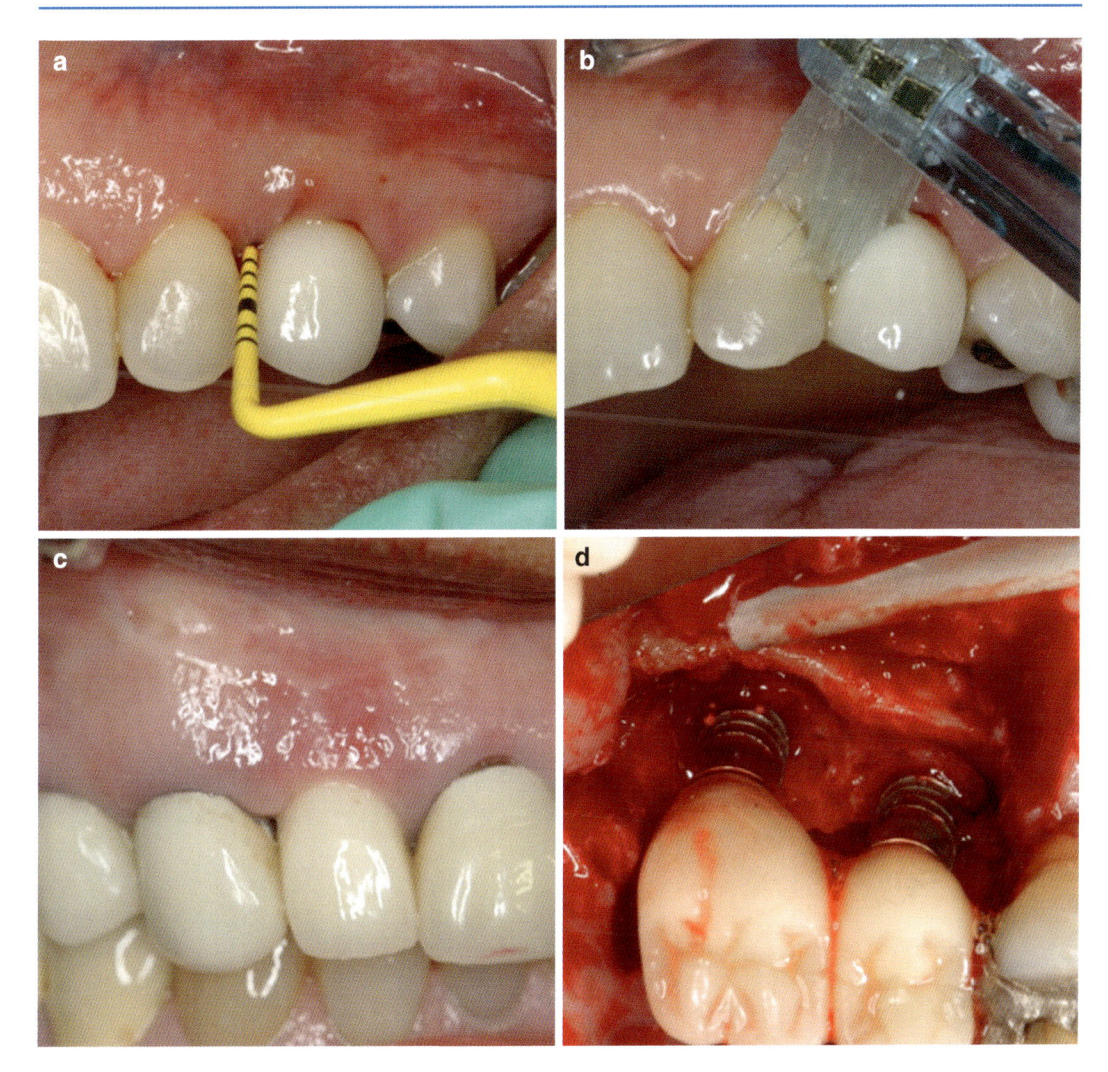

Fig. 23.2 Lang protocol for treatment of peri-implantitis (Teughels et al. 2006). (**a**) Mechanical debridement indicated for CIST-A with PD ≤4 mm, (**b**) mechanical debridement plus antimicrobial therapy indicated for CIST A+B with PD 4-5 mm, (**c**) CIST A+B+C+ antibiotic with PD≥6 mm, and (**d**) CIST A+B+C+D with PD≥6 mm requiring surgical intervention. (**a**, **b** Courtesy of Dr. Ankur Patel)

Table 23.3 Lang protocol for treatment of peri-implantitis Cumulative Interceptive Supportive Therapy (CIST)

Severity pocket depths	Characteristic signs and symptoms	Treatment
≤4 mm	Plaque, calculus, BOP, no suppuration (−)	*MD (CIST − A)
4–5 mm	Possible suppuration (±)	*MD (CIST − A + B) antimicrobial rinse (chlorhexidine-14 days)
≥6	Possible suppuration (±), bone loss present	*MD (CIST − A + B + C)/systemic and/or local antibiotics
≥6	Peri-implant infection controlled	Resective or regenerative (CIST − A, B, C + D)

Adapted from Tarnow et al. (2000)
MD mechanical debridement

Table 23.4 Peri-implantitis classifications

Stages	Characteristics	Amount of bone loss
Early	PD>4 mm, BOP/Supp on 2 or more aspects of implant	BL <25% of IL[a]
Moderate	PD>6 mm, BOP/Supp on 2 or more aspects of implant	BL 25–50% of IL[a]
Severe	PD>8 mm, BOP/Supp on 2 or more aspects of implant	BL >50% of IL[a]

Adapted from Valero (2013)
PD pocket depth, *BOP* bleeding on probing, *Supp* suppuration, *IL* implant length
[a]Compared to time of loading

(Valero 2013) showed that mechanical removal of biofilm should be done through surgical flap and chemical decontamination.

In 2012, Froum and Rosen (2012) published an updated classification on peri-implantitis in which categories were divided into early, moderate and advanced loss around implants. Contemporary information presented in case reports divides treatment into several categories (Eskow and Smith 2010). Those cases were presented in the context of whether the failing implant was deemed retainable and various remedies described versus those in which the failed implant was removed and replaced. Essential initial treatment included direct visualization, debridement, and control of inflammation. Definitive therapy including regeneration and/or resection is designed to create an environment which is conducive in controlling the inflammatory process (Table 23.4).

Apical peri-implantitis is similar in radiographic appearance to apical periodontitis [T. Tozum, personal communication]. Several case reports have offered treatment for the lesion. Common to them are the need for surgical access to the affected area. After debridement, apical resection is presented as one solution. Another mode of treatment includes regenerative allograft material placed at the apex of the implant with a protective collagen membrane cover.

In dealing with peri-implantitis, research indicates decontamination of the implant fixture surface is paramount. Patient compliance with effective plaque control measures and periodic professional maintenance, although consistently difficult to achieve, is critical in long-term success. The clinician has numerous modalities of intervention which basically follow a sequence of mechanical debridement, decontamination/detoxification and regeneration and or resection. Mechanical debridement has proven difficult because of the obstacles in access to instrumentation of surface characteristics of implants. Ultrasonics are recommended for gross debridement followed by hand instrumentation using either plastic or titanium scalers. Rotary titanium brushes are also an alternative. Decontamination has consisted of the use of antibiotics, antimicrobials, and citric acid or ethylenediaminetetraacetic (EDTA). The body of literature discusses bone regeneration that has utilized autografts, allografts, xenografts, and containment membranes. The ultimate goal of all these protocols is to reestablish a healthy environment for the implant to survive and function although no particular method has shown predictable success. The improvements in the field of dental implantology have spawned a whole new area of attendant problems. We are only at the threshold of understanding and treating them.

Conclusions

Peri-implantitis is a complex, polymicrobial, inflammatory condition that is prevalent in approximately 12–47% of patients and 5–37% of implants. It is likely that the increasing demand for dental implants will result in a proportionally higher number of patients seeking treatment for peri-implantitis. While restored dental implants look and function like natural teeth, it is important that both clinicians and patients be aware that periodontitis and peri-implantitis represent distinct entities. This requires an understanding of the histological and microbial differences. As such, treatment modalities used in the treatment of periodontal disease are not as predictive for the treatment of peri-implant disease. It is important that carefully designed maintenance programs be instituted so that early detection and intervention limit the onset and progression of peri-implantitis.

References

Achermann G (2012) How will dentistry look in 2020? Paper presented at the Capital Markets Day, Straumann, Inc., Amsterdam, 16 May 2012

Adell R, Lekholm U, Rockler B, Brånemark PI (1981) A 15-year study of osseointegrated implants in the treatment of the edentulous jaw. Int J Oral Surg 10(6):387–416

Alani A, Kelleher M, Bishop K (2014) Peri-implantitis. Part 1: scope of the problem. Br Dent J 217(6):281–287

Atieh MA, Alsabeeha NH, Faggion CM Jr, Duncan WJ (2013) The frequency of peri-implant diseases: a systematic review and meta-analysis. J Periodontol 84(11):1586–98

Berglundh T, Gotfredsen K, Zitzmann NU, Lang NP, Lindhe J (2007) Spontaneous progression of ligature induced peri-implantitis at implants with different surface roughness: an experimental study in dogs. Clin Oral Implants Res 18(5):655–661

Berglundh T, Zitzmann NU, Donati M (2011) Are peri-implantitis lesions different from periodontitis lesions? J Clin Periodontol 38(S11):188–202

Carcuac O, Berglundh T (2014) Composition of human peri-implantitis and periodontitis lesions. J Dent Res 93(11):1083–1088

Casado PL, Pereira MC, Duarte ME, Granjeiro JM (2013) History of chronic periodontitis is a high risk indicator for peri-implant disease. Braz Dent J 24(2):136–141

Cecchinato D, Parpaiola A, Lindhe J (2014) Mucosal inflammation and incidence of crestal bone loss among implant patients: a 10-year study. Clin Oral Implants Res 25:791–796

Charalampakis G, Belibasakis GN (2015) Microbiome of peri-implant infections: lessons from conventional, molecular and metagenomic analyses. Virulence 6(3):183–187

Chrcanovic BR, Albrektsson T, Wennerberg A (2015) Smoking and dental implants: a systematic review and meta-analysis. J Dent 43(5):487–498

Derks J, Tomasi C (2015) Peri-implant health and disease. A systematic review of current epidemiology. J Clin Periodontol 42(S16):S158–S171

Dvorak G, Arnhart C, Heuberer S, Huber CD, Watzek G, Gruber R (2011) Peri-implantitis and late implant failures in postmenopausal women: a cross-sectional study. J Clin Periodontol 38(10):950–955

Emecen-Huja P, Eubank TD, Shapiro V, Yildiz V, Tatakis DN, Leblebicioglu B (2013) Peri-implant versus periodontal wound healing. J Clin Periodontol 40(8):816–824

Eskow RN, Smith VS (2010) Implant complications related to maintenance therapy. In: Froum S (ed) Dental implant complications: etiology, prevention and treatment, 1st edn. Wiley, Hoboken, pp 422–424

Esposito M, Hirsh J, Lekholm U, Thomson P (1999) Differential diagnosis and treatment strategies for biologic complications and failing oral implants: a review of the literature. Int J Oral Maxillofac Implants 14(4):473–490

Froum SJ, Rosen PS (2012) A proposed classification for peri-implantitis. Int J Periodontics Restor Dent 32(5):533–540

Gallucci GO, Grütter L, Chuang SK, Belser UC (2011) Dimensional changes of peri-implant soft tissue over 2 years with single-implant crowns in the anterior maxilla. J Clin Periodontol 38(3):293–299

Hämmerle CH, Brägger U, Bürgin W, Lang NP (1996) The effect of subcrestal placement of the polished surface of ITI implants on marginal soft and hard tissues. Clin Oral Implants Res 7(2):111–119

Heitz-Mayfield LJ, Lang NP (2010) Comparative biology of chronic and aggressive periodontitis vs. peri-implantitis. Periodontol 2000;53:167–181

Judgar R, Giro G, Zenobio E, Coelho PG, Feres M, Rodrigues JA, Mangano C, Iezzi G, Piattelli A, Shibli JA (2014) Biological width around one- and two-piece implants retrieved from human jaws. Biomed Res Int. doi:10.1155/2014/850120

Koldsland OC, Scheie AA, Aass, AM (2010) Prevalence of peri-implantitis related to severity of the disease with different degrees of bone loss. J Periodontol 81:231–238

Koyanagi T, Sakamoto M, Takeuchi Y, Maruyama N, Ohkuma M, Izumi Y (2013) Comprehensive microbiological findings in peri-implantitis and periodontitis. J Clin Periodontol 40(3):218–226

Kutlu B, Genc T, Tozum T (2016) Treatment of refractory apical peri-implantitis: a case report. J Oral Implantol 42(1):104–109

Lang N (2000) Biologic complications with dental implants: their prevention, diagnosis and treatment. Clin Oral Implants Res 11(S1):146–155

Lang NP, Berglundh T (2011) Periimplant diseases: where are we now? Consensus of the Seventh European Workshop on Periodontology. Working Group 4 of Seventh European Workshop on Periodontology. J Clin Periodontol 38(S11):178–181

Lin HY, Liu Y, Wismeijer D, Crielaard W, Deng DM (2013) Effects of oral implant surface roughness on bacterial biofilm formation and treatment efficacy. Int J Oral Maxillofac Implants 28(5):1226–1231

Linkevicius T, Apse P, Grybauskas S, Puisys A (2009) The influence of soft tissue thickness on crestal bone changes around implants: a 1-year prospective controlled clinical trial. Int J Oral Maxillofac Implants 24(4):712–719

Machtei EE, Mahler D, Oettinger-Barak O, Zuabi O, Horwitz J (2008) Dental implants placed in previously failed sites: survival rate and factors affecting the outcome. Clin Oral Implants Res 19(3):259–264

Marrone A, Lasserre J, Bercy P, Brecx MC (2013) Prevalence and risk factors for periimplant disease in Belgian adults. Clinl Oral Implants Res 24: 934–940

Maruyama N, Maruyama F, Takeuchi Y, Aikawa C, Izumi Y, Nakagawa I (2014) Intraindividual variation in core microbiota in peri-implantitis and periodontitis. Sci Report. doi:10.1038/srep06602

McCallister BS, Masters D, Meffert RM (1992) Treatment of implants demonstrating periapical radiolucencies. Pract Periodontics Aesthet Dent 4(9):37–41

Meffert R (1992) How to treat ailing and failing implants. Implant Dent 1(1):25–33

Mir-Mari J, Mir-Orfila P, Figueiredo R, Valmaseda-Castellón E, Gay-Escoda C (2012) Prevalence of peri-implant diseases: a cross-sectional study based on a private practice environment. J Clin Periodontol 39: 490–494

Mombelli A, Lang H (1992) Anti-microbial treatment of implant infections. Clin Oral Implants Res 3(4):162–168

Mombelli A, van Oosten MA, Schurch E Jr, Land NP (1987) The microbiota associated with successful or failing osseointegrated titanium implants. Oral Microbiol Immunol 2(4):145–151

Mombelli A, Mühle T, Brägger U, Lang NP, Bürgin WB (1997) Comparison of periodontal and peri-implant probing by depth-force pattern analysis. Clin Oral Implants Res 8(6):448–454

Mombelli A, Müller N, Cionca N (2012) The epidemiology of peri-implantitis. Clin Oral Implants Res 23(S6):67–76

Muthukuru M, Zainvi A, Esplugues EO, Flemmig TF (2012) Non-surgical therapy for management of peri-implantitis: a systematic review. Clin Oral Implants Res 23(S6):77–83

Reiser GM, Nevins M (1995) The Implant periapical lesion: etiology prevention and treatment. Comp Cont Educ Dent 16(8):768 770, 772 passim

Robitaille N, Reed DN, Walters JD, Kumar PS (2015) Periodontal and peri-implant diseases: identical or fraternal infections. Mol Oral Microbiol 31(4):285–301

Saaby M, Karring E, Schou S, Isidor F (2014) Factors influencing severity of peri-implantitis. Clin Oral Implants Res 27(1):7–12

Sculean A, Gruber R, Bosshardt DD (2014) Soft tissue wound healing around teeth and dental implants. J Clin Periodontol 41(S15):S6–S22

Stern IB (1981) Current concepts of the dentogingival junction: the epithelial and connective tissue attachments to the tooth. J Periodontol 52(9):465–476

Tamura N, Ochi M, Miyakawa H, Nakazawa F (2013) Analysis of bacterial flora associated with peri-implantitis using obligate anaerobic culture technique and 16S rDNA gene sequence. Int J Oral Maxillofac Implants 28(6):1521–1529

Tarnow DP, Cho SC, Wallace SS (2000) The effect of inter-implant distance on the height of inter-implant bone crest. J Periodontol 71(4):546–549

Teughels W, Van Assche N, Sliepen I, Quirynen M (2006) Effect of material characteristics and/or surface topography on biofilm development. Clin Oral Implants Res 17(S2):68–81

Tözüm TF, Sençimen M, Ortakoğlu K, Ozdemir A, Aydin OC, Keleş M (2006) Diagnosis and treatment of a large periapical implant lesion associated with adjacent natural tooth: a case report. Oral Surg Oral Med Oral Pathol Oral Radiol Endod 101(6): e132–e138

Tsao YP, Wang HL (2003) Periodontal considerations in implant therapy. Int Chin J Dent 3:13–30

Valero (2013) Decontamination of dental implants. Med Oral Path 18(6):e869–e876

Zangrando MS, Damante CA, Sant'Ana AC, Rubo de Rezende ML, Greghi SL, Chambrone L (2015) Long-term evaluation of periodontal parameters and implant outcomes in periodontally compromised patients: a systematic review. J Periodontol 86(2):201–221

Laser-Assisted Treatment of Peri-implantitis

24

Edward A. Marcus

Abstract

Dental lasers are becoming a useful adjunct in the treatment of ailing and failing implants with their ability to remove diseased tissue, decontaminate implant surfaces, and stimulate growth factors, fibroblast attachment, and collagen deposition. When compared to conventional treatment outcomes, reported clinical improvements resulting from laser-assisted treatment of peri-implantitis include reductions in probing depth, bleeding, suppuration, and implant mobility, with evidence of bone formation and reosseointegration. Future research is expected to optimize clinical efficacy and predictability of laser treatment in the long term.

Since their initial intraoral use in the 1970s, lasers have emerged as an instrument of choice for many oral surgical procedures, including the treatment of periodontal disease, whether they are used alone or in conjunction with other treatment modalities (Shafir et al. 1977; Strong et al. 1979; Pick et al. 1985; White et al. 1991; Epstein 1992; Gold and Vilardi 1994; Watanabe et al. 1996; Schwarz et al. 2003; Flax and Radz 2004; Moritz et al. 1998; Borrajo et al. 2004; Kamma et al. 2009). Lasers are also being shown to be a useful adjunct in the treatment of peri-implantitis, as numerous published reports have helped to define the parameters and conditions for use to achieve safety and efficacy (Schwarz et al. 2003, 2005, 2006a, b, 2013; Flax and Radz 2004; Moritz et al. 1998; Borrajo et al. 2004; Kamma et al. 2009; Romanos et al. 2000, 2009; Dörtbudak et al. 2001; Persson et al. 2004; Giannini et al. 2006; Romanos 2006; Takasaki et al. 2007; Lee et al. 2008, 2011; Giannelli et al. 2009; Stübinger et al. 2010; Kim et al. 2010; 2011; Shin et al. 2011; Yamamoto and Tanabe 2013; Marotti et al. 2013; Shin et al. 2013; Nevins et al. 2014).

E.A. Marcus, DDS
University of Pennsylvania
School of Dental Medicine and Temple University
Maurice H Kornberg School of Dentistry,
Philadelphia, PA USA
e-mail: eam1018@aol.com

Private Practice, 712 Floral Vale Blvd.,
Yardley, PA 19067, USA

24.1 Laser Characteristics and Mechanisms of Action

The applicability of lasers for periodontal treatment is dictated by a combination of factors, including their specific light wavelength (e.g.,

660–10,600 nm), interaction with/absorption by specific components within the soft tissue (e.g., water, hemoglobin, melanin), laser light emission mode (e.g., pulsed or continuous wave) and duration of exposure, power level and density, vascularity of tissue, and presence of external cooling (e.g., water spray) (Pang et al. 2010).

In soft tissue procedures, a dental surgical laser's light – whether visible or invisible – produces a thermal reaction when absorbed by the tissue, which is largely composed of water. Ablation (i.e., cutting or vaporization) occurs when the soft tissue approaches 100 °C, the point of water vaporization (Knappe et al. 2004). Other thermal points above 50 °C inactivate nonsporulating bacteria (Russell 2003), while at temperatures above 60 °C, proteins begin to denature and coagulation occurs (Knappe et al. 2004).

Laser capabilities and mechanisms of relevance to their use in treating peri-implantitis include removal of diseased tissue and, as demonstrated in animal and in vitro studies, stimulation of fibroblast attachment, growth factors, and collagen deposition to support healing, bone formation, and osseointegration (Khadra et al. 2005; Yu et al. 1997; Guzzardella et al. 2003; Boldrini et al. 2013; Naka and Yokose 2012; Omasa et al. 2012; De Vasconcellos et al. 2014; Massotti et al. 2015).

A number of in vitro investigations have also examined the capabilities of lasers to reduce the bacterial population. Harris and Yessik (2004) assessed the relative bactericidal effectiveness of an 810-nm pulsed diode laser and a 1064-nm pulsed Nd:YAG laser. The researchers lased the pigmented *Porphyromonas gingivalis* grown on blood agar plates to quantify the efficacy of ablation (tissue removal). Results indicated the Nd:YAG laser was able to ablate the bacteria without visible effect on the blood agar, whereas the diode laser destroyed both the pathogen and the gel. Clinically, the investigators concluded that the pulsed Nd:YAG laser may selectively destroy pigmented pathogens and leave the surrounding tissue intact; the diode laser may not demonstrate this selectivity due to its greater absorption by hemoglobin and/or much longer pulse duration.

Encouraging laboratory investigations of the antimicrobial effects of various laser wavelengths on contaminated titanium implants or disks demonstrate the ability of diode, Nd:YAG, Er:YAG, and CO_2 lasers to reduce the bacterial numbers (Hauser-Gerspach et al. 2010; Gonçalves et al. 2010; Kreisler et al. 2002; Kato et al. 1998). Future clinical studies will determine the extent to which these in vitro findings may apply to the treatment of peri-implantitis in human patients.

24.2 Case Studies

Various lasers have been used clinically or in laboratory experiments in conjunction with other therapies for the treatment of peri-implantitis, as demonstrated in a representative selection of published reports.

24.2.1 Photodynamic Therapy with Low-Level Diode Lasers

A laser-based technique, photodynamic therapy (PDT), has been investigated for its therapeutic potential. PDT refers to the interaction of certain wavelengths of light with a photosensitizing agent that is bound to target cells. In the presence of oxygen, the interaction produces cytotoxic free radicals that selectively destroy the targeted cells.

Bassetti and colleagues (2004) compared adjunctive local drug delivery (minocycline microspheres) to adjunctive PDT in assessing the clinical outcomes in patients presenting with peri-implantitis. For the PDT, they used a low-level 660-nm diode laser at 100 mW in conjunction with a photosensitive dye, phenothiazine chloride, applied submucosally to peri-implant pockets. Both treatment modalities were used subsequent to mechanical debridement with titanium curettes and a glycine-based power air polishing system. At 12 months posttreatment, they observed no statistically significant differences between groups with respect to clinical, microbiological, and host-derived parameters. They concluded that nonsurgical mechanical debridement with adjunctive PDT was equally effective in reducing mucosal inflammation as with adjunctive local drug delivery.

Deppe et al. (2013) performed a 6-month clinical pilot study of the efficacy of nonsurgical antimicrobial photodynamic therapy in moderate and severe peri-implant defects. Involved were 16 patients with a total of 18 untreated ailing implants; 10 implants demonstrated moderate (less than 5 mm) bone loss and 8 showed severe (5–8 mm) defects. All implants received antimicrobial PDT without surgical intervention. After a 3-min residence duration within the peri-implant pocket, the photosensitizer phenothiazine chloride was activated with a 660-nm diode laser at 100 mW for 10s at each of six sites per implant for a total exposure of 1 min. Peri-implant health was evaluated at baseline and at 2 weeks, 3 months, and 6 months after therapy. Their findings indicated that the nonsurgical PDT treatment could stop bone resorption in moderate peri-implant defects but not in severe defects. They recommended surgical treatment of severe peri-implantitis defects, especially in esthetically important sites.

The Bombeccari group (2013) used an 810-nm diode laser at 1 W with the photosensitizer toluidine blue O in their randomized comparative case-control study of 20 patients and 20 controls to compare the efficacy of antimicrobial PDT with surgical therapy in patients with peri-implantitis. Conventional open-flap surgery was performed on both sets of patients, with scaling of implant surfaces and debridement of granulation tissue. Then, the photosensitizer was applied to patients in the PDT group, and they received five separate 20s irradiation exposures along the surfaces of the peri-implant defect, for a total exposure of 100. Microbiologic testing of all patients was done before and after treatment and at 12 and 24 weeks. Results revealed no significant difference in total counts of bacteria between the PDT and conventionally treated patients at 24 weeks. However, the PDT group showed a significant decrease in bleeding on probing and inflammatory exudation.

24.2.2 Diode Lasers

Roncati and colleagues (2013) report a case study of a 45-year-old male presenting with pain and swelling at a mandibular implant site. Clinical evaluation revealed a 7-mm pocket and bleeding on probing with suppuration and gingival inflammatory edema at the implant site. Radiographic evidence showed bone loss of five fixture threads. An 810-nm diode laser was used to treat the site, followed by hand instrumentation with a curette and piezoelectric ultrasonic device and application of chlorhexidine gel. Maintenance debridement visits were scheduled at 3-month intervals. Compared to initial clinical data, the patient showed a decreased probing pocket depth and a negative bleeding-on-probing index. After 5 years of follow-up visits, radiographic evidence showed rebound of the bone level. The authors concluded that conventional nonsurgical periodontal therapy with the adjunctive use of an 810-nm diode laser may be a feasible alternative approach for the management of peri-implantitis.

In their treatment of peri-implant infection in the posterior maxilla of a 55-year-old female, Kutkut and fellows (2011) used an 810-nm diode laser to decontaminate the implant surfaces. The patient presented with a fistula related to implants at sites #11 and 12, and severe bone loss was detected around implants at sites #11, 12, and 14. A full-thickness flap was reflected to access the peri-implant defect, and granulation tissue was removed with hand instruments. The exposed implant surfaces were irradiated with the laser, followed by a 2-min application of tetracycline paste. An allograft of particulate bone substitute was placed in the defected areas, and the graft was covered with a resorbable collagen membrane. At 4 months, signs and symptoms of infection were eliminated, soft and hard tissues regained their natural appearance, and primary implant stability was confirmed. The authors indicated that open debridement, in combination with surface decontamination and the use of a diode laser, can achieve substantial reosseointegration with new bone regeneration of the defects.

In 2014 Papadopoulos and colleagues (2015) reported the results of a randomized clinical trial that compared the effectiveness of open-flap debridement alone with additional use of a 980-nm diode laser for the treatment of peri-implantitis. Nineteen patients were randomly assigned to two groups. In both the control and laser groups, full-thickness flaps were raised, granulation tissue was removed, and mechanical instrumentation of the implant surface was performed. The laser group then received 0.8 W of pulsed laser irradiation with simultaneous sterile saline irrigation to disinfect the exposed implant surface. Pocket depth, clinical attachment level, bleeding on probing, and plaque index were evaluated at baseline and at 3 and 6 months after treatment. Results revealed that the two treatment methods appeared to be equally effective in reducing pocket depth, bleeding on probing, and plaque index. Clinical attachment level improved significantly in the laser group after 3 months only. The investigators concluded that the additional use of a diode laser did not seem to have an added beneficiary effect in the treatment of peri-implantitis.

24.2.3 Erbium Lasers

In 2008 Azzeh (2008) reported on the use of a 2,780-nm Er,Cr:YSGG laser to treat peri-implantitis. A 28-year-old male presented with 2-mm gingival recession and 7-mm probing depth around an implant in the area of the upper left central incisor. An Er,Cr:YSGG laser was used at different power, water, and air settings to open a flap, remove the granulation tissues, perforate the bone, and clean the implant surface. A bone graft and bioabsorbable membrane were used for bone regeneration. At 3, 6, and 12 months postoperatively, no complications were reported; clinical observations revealed probing depths of 3–5 mm, less than 1 mm of recession, no bleeding or implant mobility, and good bone formation. At 18 months probing depth was 2 mm, recession was less than 1 mm, and no bleeding, mobility, or discharge was evident. Azzeh concluded that the laser enabled regenerative osseous surgery around the implant with no complications and with a high level of patient and clinician satisfaction.

The Al-Falaki group (2014) conducted a retrospective analysis of 28 implants with peri-implantitis in 11 patients treated with an Er,Cr:YSGG laser. Implants with probing depths of at least 4 mm and radiographic evidence of bone loss were included. The laser and titanium curette were used to degranulate the pocket epithelium and bony walls, and then the laser was used to irradiate the tissue outside the pocket to disrupt the epithelium around the implant by a distance of at least 5 mm from the gingival margin. Probing depths and bleeding on probing were assessed at baseline and after 2 and 6 months. Reductions in mean pocket depths at baseline (6.64 ± 1.48 mm), after 2 months (3.29 ± 1.02 mm), and after 6 months (2.97 ± 0.7 mm) were statistically significant. Reductions in bleeding from baseline to both 2 and 6 months were also significant. The authors recommended that well-designed randomized controlled trials of the use of Er,Cr:YSGG laser in the nonsurgical management of peri-implantitis be conducted to validate their clinical findings.

Badran and cohorts (2011) reported in 2011 on the clinical management of severe peri-implantitis with adjunctive use of a 2,940-nm Er:YAG laser. Clinical examination of a 70-year-old female showed inflamed mucosa, 5–9 mm pockets, bleeding on probing, and suppuration on the distal surface. The first stage of treatment included ultrasonic scaling and Er:YAG laser debridement with sterile water irrigation. The second stage of treatment included elevation of a full-thickness access flap, ultrasonic and laser debridement of the implant surface, elimination of granulation tissue from the bony defect with bone curettes, and placement of synthetic bone substitute. At 6 months radiographic examination revealed bone formation around the implant. The researchers concluded that nonsurgical treatment with ultrasonic scaling and laser debridement failed to establish acceptable healing, despite reductions in probing depth and bleeding. A surgical approach (including access flap, laser debridement and decontamination of the exposed implant surface, and placement of bone substitute) provided radiographic evidence of newly formed bone.

In 2011 Renvert et al. (2011) reported the results of a randomized clinical trial for the treatment of severe peri-implantitis using an Er:YAG laser or an air-abrasive device for implant debridement. The laser group included 21 subjects with a total of 55 implants; the air-abrasive group had 21 subjects with 45 implants. At 6-week and 3- and 6-month posttreatment examinations, there were no statistically significant differences in the gingival index, plaque scores, or bleeding on probing scores. Both treatment methods resulted in a reduction of probing depth and the frequency of suppuration and bleeding. Their results showed that overall clinical improvement was limited: approximately 50% of the subjects in both groups showed improved clinical conditions.

24.2.4 Nd:YAG Lasers

Nicholson and a group of private practitioners (2014) collaborated on a human clinical study in which a pulsed 1,064-nm Nd:YAG laser was used to treat patients presenting with peri-implantitis and peri-mucositis. Follow-up data collection occurred between 8 and 36 months after laser treatment. Radiographic analysis of 16 cases included in the study revealed an increase in crestal bone mass around the implant and, when reported, reductions in probing depth. In their 2014 published account, all clinicians reported control of infection, reversal of bone loss, and rescue of the incumbent implant. Data also indicated that healing (bone deposition) is not linear; large defects heal rapidly at first, but the healing process gradually slows as the defect disappears. Complete recovery took 1–3 years depending on the size of the lesion. The authors reported a definite trend for larger lesions to heal faster (Figs. 24.1 and 24.2, 24.3, 24.4, 24.5, 24.6 and 24.7).

24.2.5 Carbon Dioxide Lasers

Deppe et al. (2007) assessed the efficacy of a 10,600-nm CO_2 laser-assisted peri-implantitis therapy compared to conventional methodology. The investigation included 32 patients with 73 failing implants. In the laser group, 22 implants were treated with soft tissue resection following laser decontamination, and in 17 implants, bone augmentation was performed with the concomitant use of β-tricalcium phosphate. For the control group, soft tissue resection after conventional decontamination was performed in 19 implants and augmentation in 15 implants. Results were evaluated 4 months after surgery and then at final follow-up (mean duration of 37 months, 5 months minimum, 59 months maximum). Results showed that treatment of peri-implantitis may be accelerated with the use of a CO_2 laser concomitant with

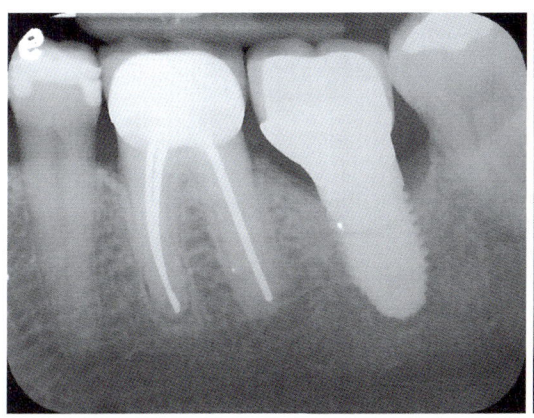

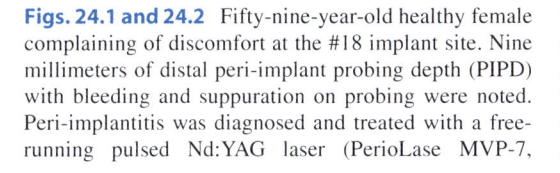

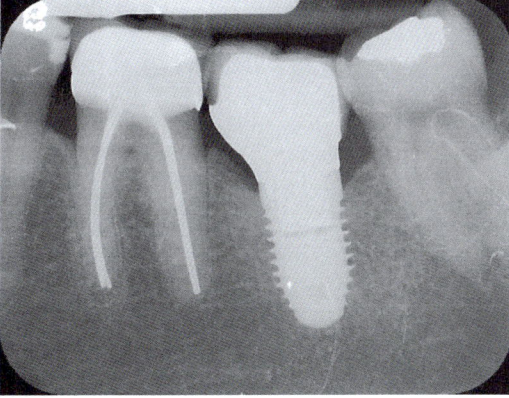

Figs. 24.1 and 24.2 Fifty-nine-year-old healthy female complaining of discomfort at the #18 implant site. Nine millimeters of distal peri-implant probing depth (PIPD) with bleeding and suppuration on probing were noted. Peri-implantitis was diagnosed and treated with a free-running pulsed Nd:YAG laser (PerioLase MVP-7, Millennium Dental Technologies, Cerritos, Calif., USA) and the LAPIP protocol (8-1-2012). Follow-up radiograph (6-3-2013) shows excellent healing, and clinically the site now measures 4 mm PIPD with no bleeding or suppuration. Patient JB (Courtesy, Dr. Edward A. Marcus)

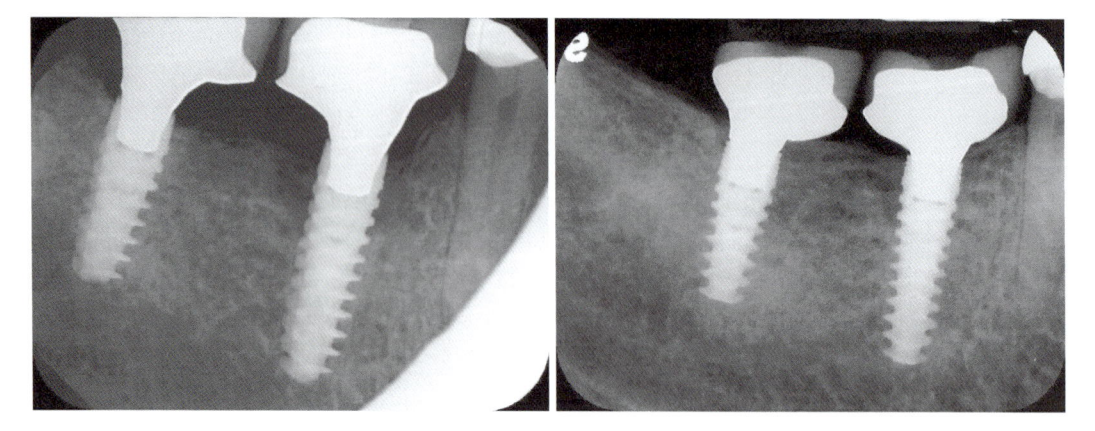

Fig. 24.3 and 24.4 Sixty-two-year-old healthy male referred by his general dentist who noted bone loss on the #30 implant. Clinical examination showed 7–8 mm of PIPD circumferentially with bleeding and suppuration on probing. Peri-implantitis was diagnosed and treated with a free-running pulsed Nd:YAG laser (PerioLase MVP-7, Millennium Dental Technologies, Cerritos, Calif., USA) and the LAPIP protocol (3-9-2013). Follow-up radiograph (7-2-2014) shows excellent healing, and clinically the site now measures 3–4 mm with no bleeding or suppuration. Patient BS (Courtesy, Dr. Karen E. Marcus)

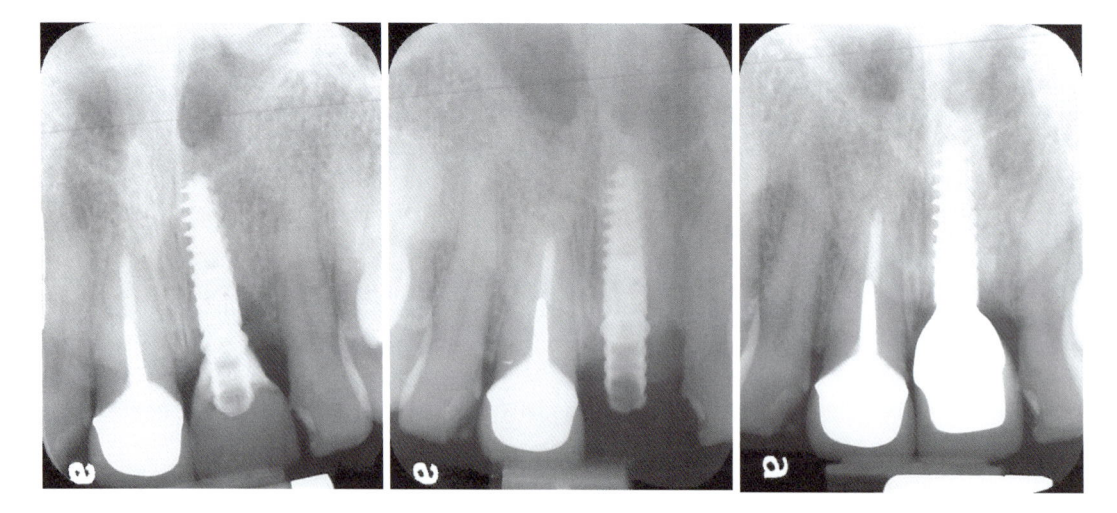

Figs. 24.5, 24.6 and 24.7 Fifty-one-year-old healthy female with a single provisionalized implant at the #9 site which developed peri-implantitis during integration healing. Eight millimeters of distal pocketing with bleeding and suppuration were noted. The site was treated with a new provisional restoration and the free-running pulsed Nd:YAG laser (PerioLase MVP-7, Millennium Dental Technologies, Cerritos, Calif., USA) using the LAPIP protocol (4-5-2012). Follow-up radiograph (2-6-2013) shows excellent healing, and clinically the site now measures 4 mm with no bleeding or suppuration. A posttreatment 3-year follow-up radiograph shows a stable result. Patient JD (Courtesy, Dr. Edward A. Marcus)

soft tissue resection. However, no difference was seen between laser and conventional decontamination with respect to long-term results in augmented defects.

Romanos and Nentwig (2008) evaluated the ability of a 10,600-nm carbon dioxide laser to decontaminate failing implants in 15 patients. A full-thickness mucoperiosteal flap was elevated to access peri-implant bony defects. Titanium curettes were used to remove granulomatous tissue. Then a CO_2 laser was used to irradiate the exposed implant surfaces and promote blood coagulation in the bony defect. Augmentation with autogenous bone grafting material or xenogenic bone grafting material was used, and bone grafts were covered with a collagen membrane.

After 27 months, almost complete bone fill in the peri-implant defect was accomplished. Their results suggest that decontamination of implant surfaces with a CO_2 laser in combination with augmentation techniques can effectively treat peri-implantitis.

24.3 Precautions

Of particular interest when lasers are used around implants (such as for second-stage recovery or treatment of peri-implantitis) is an awareness of the potential for altering the surface characteristics of the implant itself or for overheating the implant, which could lead to undesirable thermal damage to adjacent tissues and ultimately to implant failure.

Several in vitro examinations elucidate the concerns. For example, scanning electron microscopic evaluation of titanium surfaces exposed to an 810-nm diode laser showed scattered markings of a circular nature approximately 50 μ in diameter (Kilinc et al. 2012). Melting, loss of porosity, and other surface alterations were observed on plasma-sprayed and hydroxyapatite-coated titanium dental implants exposed to Nd:YAG laser irradiation (Block et al. 1992). Zirconia implants irradiated by a CO_2 laser at various power settings revealed material cracking and melting, and an Er:YAG laser penetrated through the specimen disks (Stübinger et al. 2008).

Other in vitro studies have investigated surface temperature increases in implants exposed to various levels of 810-nm and 980-nm diode, 1,064-nm Nd:YAG, 2,940-nm Er:YAG, and 10,600-nm CO_2 lasers. All tested wavelengths resulted in temperature increases of varying degrees, depending on the power level and exposure duration used (Leja et al. 2013; Kreisler et al. 2003; Geminiani et al. 2011, 2012; Wilcox et al. 2001; Wooten et al. 1999).

Numerous steps can be taken to mitigate such concerns: Carefully adhering to proper clinical technique, following the manufacturer's recommendations for use, choosing laser parameters judiciously, limiting direct laser exposure to the implant itself, allowing sufficient time for the implant to cool, and using water spray to cool the surgical site (Mouhyi et al. 1999; Monzavi et al. 2014) are some of the methods that can be employed clinically to minimize the potential for inadvertent damage.

Conclusion

Lasers have been used successfully for more than 35 years for various oral and periodontal surgical procedures. When used with appropriate parameters and proper clinical technique, lasers are now demonstrating their utility as adjunctive instruments for the treatment of peri-implantitis.

Based on the findings of numerous in vitro and animal studies in implantology, various laser types have been evaluated for their effectiveness in treating peri-implantitis in human patients. Outcomes assessed included probing depth, bleeding, suppuration, control of infection, bone formation and deposition, reestablishment of reosseointegration, and implant mobility. Overall, results show varying degrees of clinical improvement.

The role of lasers in treating peri-implantitis continues to be a fertile area for future research to optimize clinical efficacy and predictability in the long term.

References

Al-Falaki R, Cronshaw M, Hughes FJ (2014) Treatment outcome following use of the erbium, chromium:yttrium, scandium, gallium, garnet laser in the non-surgical management of peri-implantitis: a case series. Br Dent J 217(8):453–457

Azzeh MM (2008) Er,Cr:YSGG laser-assisted surgical treatment of peri-implantitis with 1-year reentry and 18-month follow-up. J Periodontol 79(10):2000–2005

Badran Z, Bories C, Struillou X et al (2011) Er:YAG laser in the clinical management of severe peri-implantitis: a case report. J Oral Implantol 27(Spec No):212–217

Bassetti M, Schär D, Wicki B et al (2004) Anti-infective therapy of peri-implantitis with adjunctive local drug delivery or photodynamic therapy: 12-month outcomes of a randomized controlled clinical trial. Clin Oral Implants Res 25(3):279–287

Block CM, Mayo JA, Evans GH (1992) Effects of the Nd:YAG dental laser on plasma-sprayed and hydroxyapatite-coated titanium dental implants: surface alteration and attempted sterilization. Int J Oral Maxillofac Implants 7(4):441–449

Boldrini C, de Almeida JM, Fernandes LA et al (2013) Biomechanical effect of one session of low-level laser on the bone-titanium implant interface. Lasers Med Sci 28(1):349–352

Bombeccari GP, Guzzi G, Gualini F et al (2013) Photodynamic therapy to treat periimplantitis. Implant Dent 22(6):631–638

Borrajo JLL, Varela LG, Castro GL et al (2004) Diode laser (980 nm) as adjunct to scaling and root planing. Photomed Laser Surg 22(6):509–512

De Vasconcellos LMR, Barbara MAM, Deco CP et al (2014) Healing of normal and osteopenic bone with titanium implant and low-level laser therapy (GaAlAs): a histomorphometric study in rats. Lasers Med Sci 29(2):575–580

Deppe H, Horch H-H, Neff A (2007) Conventional versus CO_2 laser-assisted treatment of peri-implant defects with the concomitant use of pure-phase β-tricalcium phosphate: a 5-year clinical report. Int J Oral Maxillofac Implants 22(1):79–86

Deppe H, Mücke T, Wagenpfeil S et al (2013) Nonsurgical antimicrobial photodynamic therapy in moderate vs severe peri-implant defects: a clinical pilot study. Quintessence Int 44(8):609–618

Dörtbudak O, Haas R, Bernhart T et al (2001) Lethal photosensitization for decontamination of implant surfaces in the treatment of peri-implantitis. Clin Oral Implants Res 12(2):104–108

Epstein SR (1992) Curettage revisited: laser therapy. Pract Periodontics Aesthet Dent 4(2):27–32

Flax HD, Radz GM (2004) Closed-flap laser-assisted esthetic dentistry using Er:YSGG technology. Compend Contin Educ Dent 25(8):622 626, 628–630, 632, 634

Geminiani A, Caton JG, Romanos GE (2011) Temperature increase during CO_2 and Er:YAG irradiation on implant surfaces. Implant Dent 20(5):379–382

Geminiani A, Caton JG, Romanos GE (2012) Temperature change during non-contact diode laser irradiation of implant surfaces. Lasers Med Sci 27(2):339–342

Giannelli M, Bani D, Tani A et al (2009) In vitro evaluation of the effects of low-intensity Nd:YAG laser irradiation on the inflammatory reaction elicited by bacterial lipopolysaccharide adherent to titanium dental implants. J Periodontol 80(6):977–984

Giannini R, Vassalli M, Chellini F et al (2006) Neodymium:yttrium aluminum garnet laser irradiation with low pulse energy: a potential tool for the treatment of peri-implant disease. Clin Oral Implants Res 17(6):638–643

Gold SI, Vilardi MA (1994) Pulsed laser beam effects on gingiva. J Clin Periodontol 21(6):391–396

Gonçalves F, Zanetti AL, Zanetti RV et al (2010) Effectiveness of 980-nm diode and 1064-nm extra-long-pulse neodymium-doped aluminum garnet lasers in implant disinfection. Photomed Laser Surg 28(2):273–280

Guzzardella GA, Torricelli P, Nicoli-Aldini N et al (2003) Osseointegration of endosseous ceramic implants after postoperative low-power laser stimulation: an in vivo comparative study. Clin Oral Implants Res 14(2):226–232

Harris DM, Yessik M (2004) Therapeutic ratio quantifies laser antisepsis: ablation of Porphyromonas gingivalis with dental lasers. Lasers Surg Med 35(3):206–213

Hauser-Gerspach I, Stübinger S, Meyer J (2010) Bactericidal effects of different laser systems on bacteria adhered to dental implant surfaces: an in vitro study comparing zirconia with titanium. Clin Oral Implants Res 21(3):277–283

Kamma JJ, Vasdekis VGS, Romanos GE (2009) The effect of diode laser (980 nm) treatment on aggressive periodontitis: evaluation of microbial and clinical parameters. Photomed Laser Surg 27(1):11–19

Kato T, Kusakari H, Hoshino E (1998) Bactericidal efficacy of carbon dioxide laser against bacteria-contaminated titanium implant and subsequent cellular adhesion to irradiated area. Lasers Surg Med 23(5):299–309

Khadra M, Kasem N, Lyngstadaas SP et al (2005) Laser therapy accelerates initial attachment and subsequent behavior of human oral fibroblasts cultured on titanium implant material. A scanning electron microscopic and histomorphometric analysis. Clin Oral Implants Res 16(2):168–175

Kilinc E, Rothrock J, Migliorati E et al (2012) Potential surface alteration effects of laser-assisted periodontal surgery on existing dental restorations. Quintessence Int 43(5):387–395

Kim S-W, Kwon Y-H, Chung J-H et al (2010) The effect of Er:YAG laser irradiation on the surface microstructure and roughness of hydroxyapatite-coated implant. J Periodontal Implant Sci 40(6):276–282

Kim J-H, Herr Y, Chung J-H et al (2011) The effect of erbium-doped:yttrium, aluminium and garnet laser irradiation on the surface microstructure and roughness of double-acid-etched implants. J Periodontal Implant Sci 41(5):234–241

Knappe V, Frank F, Rohde E (2004) Principles of lasers and biophotonic effects. Photomed Laser Surg 22(5):411–417

Kreisler M, Kohnen W, Marinello C et al (2002) Bactericidal effect of the Er:YAG laser on dental implant surfaces: an in vitro study. J Periodontol 73(11):1292–1298

Kreisler M, Al Haj H, d'Hoedt B (2003) Temperature changes induced by 809-nm GaAlAs laser at the implant-bone interface during simulated surface decontamination. Clin Oral Implants Res 14(1):91–96

Kutkut A, Andreana S, Al-Sabbagh M (2011) Treatment of periimplant infection in the posterior maxilla, with 810-nm diode laser decontamination of the implant surfaces: a case report. J Laser Dent 19(3):270–275

Lee J-H, Heo S-J, Koak J-Y et al (2008) Cellular responses on anodized titanium discs after laser irradiation. Lasers Surg Med 40(10):738–742

Lee J-H, Kwon Y-H, Herr Y et al (2011) Effect of erbium-doped: yttrium, aluminium and garnet laser irradiation on the surface microstructure and roughness of sandblasted, large grit, acid-etched implants. J Periodontal Implant Sci 41(3):135–142

Leja C, Geminiani A, Caton J et al (2013) Thermodynamic effects of laser irradiation of implants placed in bone: an in vitro study. Lasers Med Sci 28(6):1435–1440

Marotti J, Tortamano P, Cai S et al (2013) Decontamination of dental implant surfaces by means of photodynamic therapy. Lasers Med Sci 28(1):303–309 Erratum in: (2013) Lasers Med Sci 28(3):1047

Massotti FP, Gomes FV, Mayer L et al (2015) Histomorphometric assessment of the influence of low-level laser therapy on peri-implant tissue healing in the rabbit mandible. Photomed Laser Surg 33(3):123–128

Monzavi A, Shahabi S, Fekrazad R et al (2014) Implant surface temperature changes during Er:YAG laser irradiation with different cooling systems. J Dent (Tehran) 11(2):210–215

Moritz A, Schoop U, Goharkhay K et al (1998) Treatment of periodontal pockets with a diode laser. Lasers Surg Med 22(5):302–311

Mouhyi J, Sennerby L, Nammour S et al (1999) Temperature increases during surface decontamination of titanium implants using CO_2 laser. Clin Oral Implants Res 10(1):54–61

Naka T, Yokose S (2012) Application of laser-induced bone therapy by carbon dioxide laser irradiation in implant therapy. Int J Dent 409496:1–8

Nevins M, Nevins ML, Yamamoto A et al (2014) Use of Er:YAG laser to decontaminate infected dental implant surface in preparation for reestablishment of bone-to-implant contact. Int J Periodontics Restor Dent 34(4):461–466

Nicholson D, Blodgett K, Braga C et al (2014) Pulsed Nd:YAG laser treatment for failing implants due to peri-implantitis. In: Rechmann P, Fried D (eds) Lasers in dentistry XX, San Francisco, Calif., February 2, 2014, vol 8929. Society of Photo-Optical Instrumentation Engineers, Bellingham, pp 89290H-1–89290H-14

Omasa S, Motoyoshi M, Arai Y et al (2012) Low-level laser therapy enhances the stability of orthodontic mini-implants via bone formation related to BMP-2 expression in a rat model. Photomed Laser Surg 30(5):255–261

Pang P, Andreana S, Aoki A et al (2010) Laser energy in oral soft tissue applications. J Laser Dent 18(3):123–131

Papadopoulos CA, Vouros I, Menexes G et al (2015) The utilization of a diode laser in the surgical treatment of peri-implantitis. A randomized clinical trial. Clin Oral Investig. doi:10.1007/s00784-014-1397-9

Persson LF, Mouhyi J, Berglundh T et al (2004) Carbon dioxide laser and hydrogen peroxide conditioning in the treatment of periimplantitis: an experimental study in the dog. Clin Implant Dent Relat Res 6(4):230–238

Pick RM, Pecaro BC, Silberman CJ (1985) The laser gingivectomy. The use of the CO_2 laser for the removal of phenytoin hyperplasia. J Periodontol 56(8):492–496

Renvert S, Lindahl C, Roos Jansåker A-M et al (2011) Treatment of peri-implantitis using an Er:YAG laser or an air-abrasive device: a randomized clinical trial. J Clin Periodontol 38(1):65–73

Romanos G (2006) 980-nm diode laser-assisted treatment of peri-implantitis. J Acad Laser Dent 14(1):13–15

Romanos GE, Nentwig GH (2008) Regenerative therapy of deep peri-implant infrabony defects after CO_2 laser implant surface decontamination. Int J Periodontics Restor Dent 28(3):245–255

Romanos GE, Everts H, Nentwig GH (2000) Effects of diode and Nd:YAG laser irradiation on titanium discs: a scanning electron microscope examination. J Periodontol 71(5):810–815

Romanos G, Ko H-H, Froum S et al (2009) The use of CO_2 laser in the treatment of peri-implantitis. Photomed Laser Surg 27(3):381–386

Roncati M, Lucchese A, Carinci F (2013) Non-surgical treatment of peri-implantitis with the adjunctive use of an 810-nm diode laser. J Indian Soc Periodontol 17(6):812–815

Russell AD (2003) Lethal effects of heat on bacterial physiology and structure. Sci Prog 86(Pt 1–2):115–137

Schwarz F, Berakdar M, Georg T et al (2003) Clinical evaluation of an Er:YAG laser combined with scaling and root planing for non-surgical periodontal treatment. A controlled, prospective clinical study. J Clin Periodontol 30(1):26–34

Schwarz F, Sculean A, Rothamel D et al (2005) Clinical evaluation of an Er:YAG laser for nonsurgical treatment of peri-implantitis: a pilot study. Clin Oral Implants Res 16(1):44–52

Schwarz F, Nuesry E, Bieling K et al (2006a) Influence of an erbium, chromium-doped yttrium, scandium, gallium, and garnet (Er,Cr:YSGG) laser on the reestablishment of the biocompatibility of contaminated titanium implant surfaces. J Periodontol 77(11):1820–1827

Schwarz F, Bieling K, Nuesry E et al (2006b) Clinical and histological healing pattern of peri-implantitis lesions following non-surgical treatment with an Er:YAG laser. Lasers Surg Med 38(7):663–671

Schwarz F, Hegewald A, John G et al (2013) Four-year follow-up of combined surgical therapy of advanced peri-implantitis evaluating two methods of surface decontamination. J Clin Periodontol 40(10):962–967

Shafir R, Slutzki S, Bornstein LA (1977) Excision of buccal hemangioma by carbon dioxide laser beam. Oral Surg Oral Med Oral Pathol 4(3):347–350

Shin S-I, Min H-K, Park B-H et al (2011) The effect of Er:YAG laser irradiation on the scanning electron microscopic structure and surface roughness of various implant surfaces: an in vitro study. Lasers Med Sci 26(6):767–776

Shin S-I, Lee E-K, Kim J-H et al (2013) The effect of Er:YAG laser irradiation on hydroxyapatite-coated implants and fluoride-modified TiO_2-blasted implant surfaces: a microstructural analysis. Lasers Med Sci 28(3):823–831

Strong MS, Vaughan CE, Healy GB et al (1979) Transoral management of localized carcinoma of the oral cavity using the CO_2 laser. Laryngoscope 89(6 Pt 1):897–905

Stübinger S, Homann F, Etter C et al (2008) Effect of Er:YAG, CO_2 and diode laser irradiation on surface properties of zirconia endosseous dental implants. Lasers Surg Med 40(3):223–228

Stübinger S, Etter C, Miskiewicz M et al (2010) Surface alterations of polished and sandblasted and acid-etched titanium implants after Er:YAG, carbon dioxide, and diode laser irradiation. Int J Oral Maxillofac Implants 25(1):104–111

Takasaki AA, Aoki A, Mizutani K et al (2007) Er:YAG laser therapy for peri-implant infection: a histological study. Lasers Med Sci 22(3):143–157

Watanabe H, Ishikawa I, Suzuki M et al (1996) Clinical assessments of the erbium:YAG laser for soft tissue surgery and scaling. J Clin Laser Med Surg 14(2):67–75

White JM, Goodis HE, Rose CL (1991) Use of the pulsed Nd:YAG laser for intraoral soft tissue surgery. Lasers Surg Med 11(5):455–461

Wilcox CW, Wilwerding TM, Watson P et al (2001) Use of electrosurgery and lasers in the presence of dental implants. Int J Oral Maxillofac Implants 16(4):578–582

Wooten CA, Sullivan SM, Surpure S (1999) Heat generation by superpulsed CO_2 lasers on plasma-sprayed titanium implants: an in vitro study. Oral Surg Oral Med Oral Pathol Oral Radiol Endod 88(5):544–548

Yamamoto A, Tanabe T (2013) Treatment of peri-implantitis around TiUnite-surface implants using Er:YAG laser microexplosions. Int J Periodontics Restor Dent 33(1):21–29

Yu W, Naim JO, Lanzaframe RJ (1997) Effects of photostimulation on wound healing in diabetic mice. Lasers Surg Med 20(1):56–63

Prosthetic Solutions to Biological Deficiencies: Pink and White Aesthetics

25

Pinhas Adar

Abstract

The digital information age has made knowledge plentiful. With just a "click" of a mouse, our patients can take an active role in their own dental health. How wonderful it would be if knowledge were the only requirement needed. Proper processing of newly learned knowledge is needed to form an action plan or the knowledge helps with nothing. Keeping up with the latest products in the dental field is a full-time job in and of itself. These different options change the demands of our patients, making our job of knowing, with a certain accuracy, all of the products as well as the options and possible implications of the dental care that we choose for that particular patient.

Since the mere action of telling a patient what is needed in their particular case is not just "selling" a product, but we are actually asking them to invest in our expertise in the procedure. So we owe it to our patients to know which product is the best for their particular case but also how that product works, what is the preparation design needed for that product and what are the limitations of it. Knowing all of this is necessary to know what is needed to get the best possible result and make for a happy patient and doctor and technician. A treatment plan is anything said prior to doing the treatment. Once the treatment has been completed, everything which is then said, is an excuse. If a dental professional offers a patient a treatment option and does not know how the product will react in that patient's particular scenario, a disservice is done to all involved.

25.1 Introduction

Digital technology definitely is a time-saver and a source of profit. But technology is also constantly changing and quite expensive. So to be successful in investing in technology pieces, several things need to be considered. What makes

P. Adar, MDT, CDT
Adar Dental Network, Oral Design Center, Atlanta, Atlanta, GA, USA
e-mail: pinhasadar@adar.net

this particular piece of technology unique, what are the learning curves and will the patients like it? Will the manufacturer be around when needed; are they reliable and what is the return on investment in that piece of technology?

The patient should feel and know that technology is only a small part and only an enhancement of the care provider's personal service and should never feel that it dictates their patient care. Communication is one of the key ingredients to achieving this and allowing the patient to feel that they will get what they want the first time.

An "illusion of reality" is what we all are striving for. Thanks to all of the new materials on the market, it is no longer an impossible task to achieve. Proper ceramic selection as well as the skills of the ceramist is the foundation to this. The key to aesthetics in restorative dentistry, regardless of the particular restoration being provided, be it a veneer, crown, pontic or implant, is the soft tissue profile. The topography of the gingival interface is essential to create an illusion of reality (Adar 2014). However, this critical piece of the puzzle is often compromised by trauma or disease making optimal restorative dentistry not an easy task to perform.

25.2 Diagnosis and Treatment Planning

There are several modalities of treatment that can be offered to repair these essential "pink" regions (Fig. 25.1a). Surgical techniques along with orthodontic procedures can manipulate both the hard and soft tissue making for a more optimal site, possibly even including the papilla in the right circumstances (Schweiger and Sorenson 2011) (Fig. 25.1b). All of these scenarios demanding optimal aesthetics make good team members a necessity, including the restorative dentist, a surgeon, orthodontist, skilled laboratory technician and willing patient (Fig. 25.1c). The skill of each of the team members is equally important.

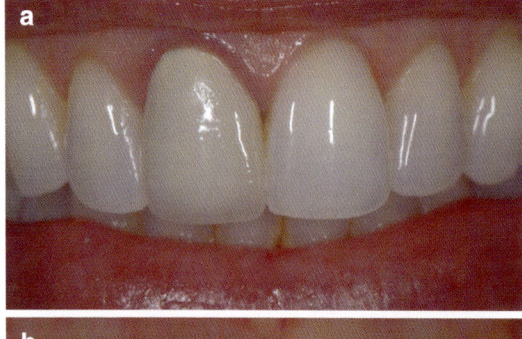

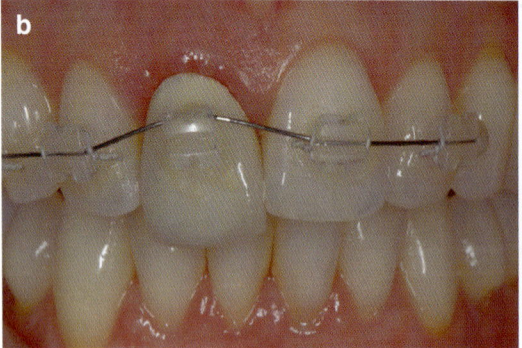

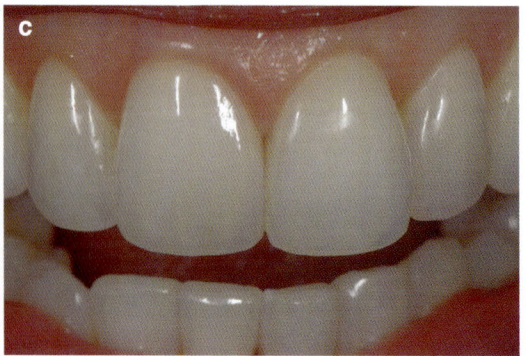

Fig. 25.1 (a) Asymmetry tissue. (b) Using orthodontics to enhance soft tissue. (c) Post-op of new ceramic crown on #8

For instance, the surgeon uses his incredible skills to manipulate the tissue for papilla reconstruction, and then the technician or the restorative dentist makes a temporary that cuts off the blood supply to the newly developed papilla – not a good scenario yet one that happens quite often. Predictable dental aesthetics does *not* happen by chance. It requires an essential relationship between the patient, the clinicians involved and the ceramist (Adar 2014). All parties involved need a definitive vision of the desired end result that satisfies the elements of smile design and appropriate laboratory technology. All must know exactly what to use, when to use it and why to use it to have a successful outcome.

The tissue is always the issue! We need to recognize that there are typically three different types of tissue scenarios. The most challenging type of tissue to deal with is *thin tissue*. This tissue tends to recede more than other tissue types and will show anything that is subgingival on the restoration causing "bleed through" of colour through the tissue. In the scenario shown in Fig. 25.2a, the proper choice would be an all-ceramic restoration built out to create a root eminence with no bleed through.

In comparison to this, the easiest tissue to work on for any type of restoration is *thick tissue*. Thick tissue has no bleed through or translucency (Fig. 25.2b). This figure illustrates the ability of thick tissue to block out the metal substructure subgingivally.

The third type is *no tissue* shown in Fig. 25.2c. Pink ceramic is an option and if done correctly is most likely to be hygienic as well as kind to the remaining soft tissue. However, in this case, the challenge lies within the ability of the ceramist to create both pink and white ceramics with three-dimensional effects so that it looks natural. Another challenge with this is that the ceramic shrinks during baking, so it is difficult to adapt to the soft tissue. Some advocate uses pink composite to restore defects such as that shown in Fig. 25.2c. One of the benefits of using composite

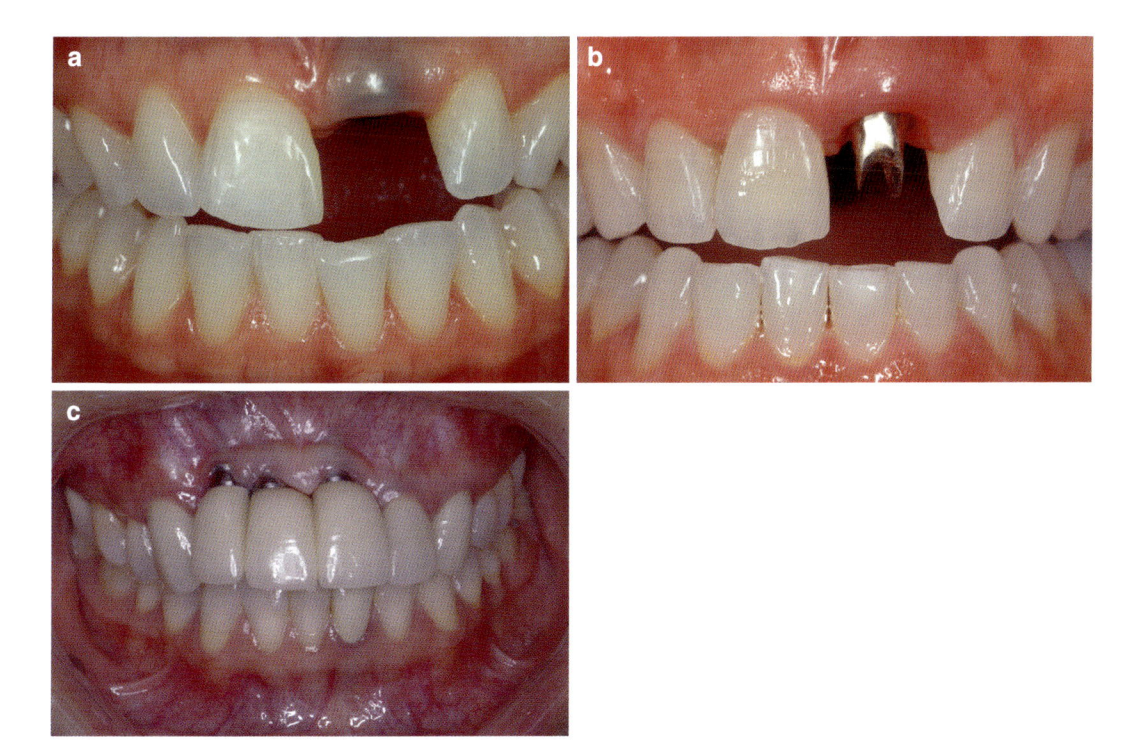

Fig. 25.2 (**a**) Thin tissue showing bleed through of the implant. (**b**) Thick tissue blocking out the implant colour underneath. (**c**) Defective tissue

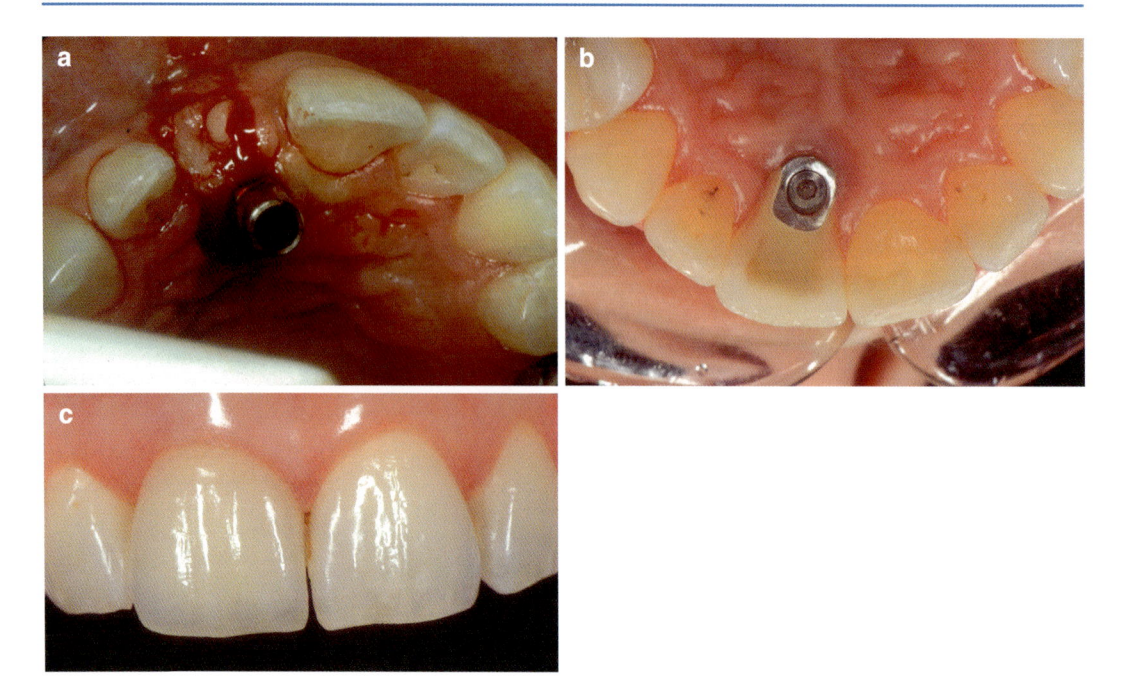

Fig. 25.3 (**a**) Implant fixture placed too far lingually. (**b**) Screw on the lingual; buccal portion of the crown was created similar to an ovate pontic. (**c**) Integration of the soft tissue and the symmetry of the papilla with the adjacent dentition

vs. ceramic is its plasticity. Composite can be moulded to anything intraorally and then light cured. The composite solution can be used only when the restoration is screw retained and therefore retrievable for maintenance purposes. The cons are that composite wears out, loses its lustre, stains and collects odours. Maintenance must be routinely performed on composite materials. The best way to deal with these types of tissue defects is with surgery, if possible.

The lingual positioning of implant #8 shown in Fig. 25.3a makes restoring to mimic nature a challenge. However with the correct team members, this challenge can be overcome. A flap procedure was done to create a root eminence and then a restoration was created, by the ceramist, as a half pontic on the buccal. (Figure 25.3 shows the screw on the lingual, and it can be seen how the buccal portion of the crown was created similar to an ovate pontic. Long-term success can be achieved by integrating multiple disciplines (Ahmed 2002). Figure 25.3 shows the integration of the soft tissue and the symmetry of the papilla with the adjacent dentition along with the ceramic crown blending in with the adjacent teeth.

The existing condition shown in Fig. 25.4a illustrates how thin tissue allows bleed through of the implant. The patient and her parents expressed their dislike of the greyness of the tissue as well as greyness of the screw-retained restoration and positioning of the lateral due to the screw access hole being at the incisal edge.

A flap procedure was done to augment and plump out the root eminence and to thicken the gingival soft tissue. The restoration was then converted to a customized UCLA-type abutment with the metal cast and then customized with ceramic going subgingival to eliminate the greyness in the tissue. The abutment was then prepped (Fig. 25.4b) and an all-ceramic crown was fabricated and cemented in place (Fig. 25.4c).

The patient shown in Fig. 25.5a presented missing tooth #8. A bone augmentation was done and implant was placed. After healing, a screw-retained restoration was placed. Because the surgeon was able to place the implant ideally and slightly lingual, we were able to preserve the subgingival contour with the abutment that was then shaped as a mini pontic (Fig. 25.5b). Figure 25.5c

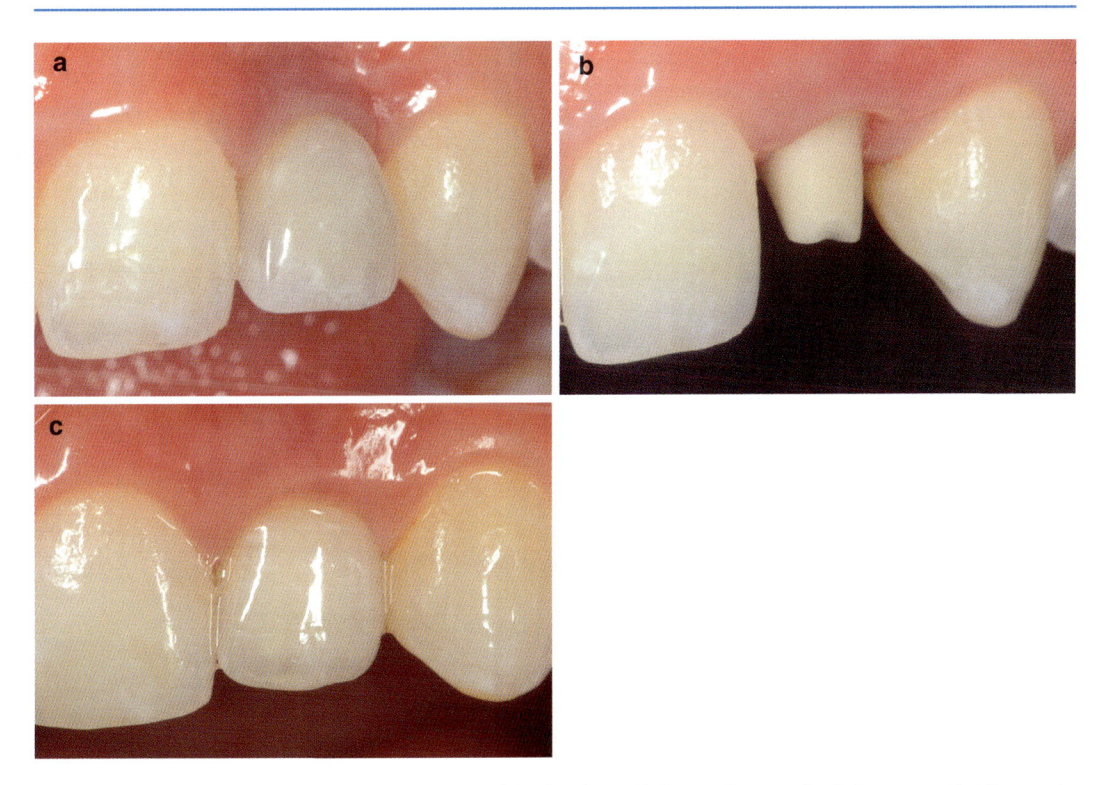

25 Prosthetic Solutions to Biological Deficiencies: Pink and White Aesthetics

Fig. 25.4 (**a**) Thin tissue allowing bleed through of the implant. (**b**) Prepped customized abutment. (**c**) All-ceramic crown cemented into place

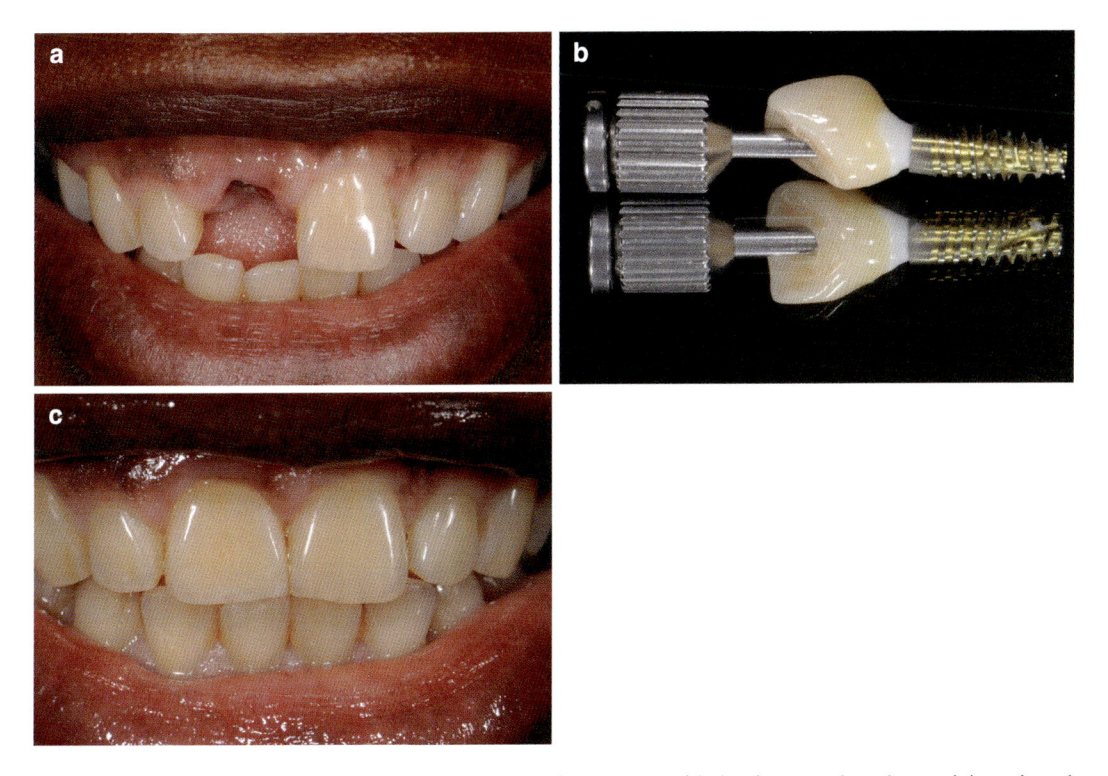

Fig. 25.5 (**a**) Missing tooth #8. (**b**) Preserving the subgingival contour with the abutment shaped as a mini pontic and e.max. (**c**) Healing and integration of the soft tissue

shows the healing and integration of the soft tissue, as well as the symmetry, support of the root eminence as well as the papilla on both the mesial and distal as well as the illusion of reality of the final IPS e.max restoration with the adjacent teeth.

25.3 Defining Patient Expectations

Entering into the market of implant dentistry using CAD/CAM technology can have enormous potential for dentistry. It not only increases business resources, but it offers exposure to new types of patients and other opportunities as well as to some, possibly, unexpected risks dealing with these new materials.

Implant with CAD/CAM dentistry still follows the basic rules of any restorative type of dentistry (Adar 2014).

25.3.1 Types of Materials

25.3.1.1 Lithium Disilicate and Zirconia

Zirconia materials are a metal-free practical alternative for traditional ceramic and in certain clinical situations can be ideal for light transmission. Longevity of restorations using zirconia frameworks has been supported by the University of Zurich (Haemmerle) as well as the University of Goettingen (Huels) (Adar 2014). Fixed partial monolithic zirconia denture frameworks can span up to 14 units on natural teeth as well as edentulous implant restorations. The Zirkonzahn 5× CAD software allows one to design virtually or as a copy mill design from a wax up or a denture set-up (Fig. 25.6a).

When comparing IPS e.max, composed of 70% needle-like crystals held in a glassy matrix to traditional all-ceramic materials, the IPS e.max affords optional strength with durability and

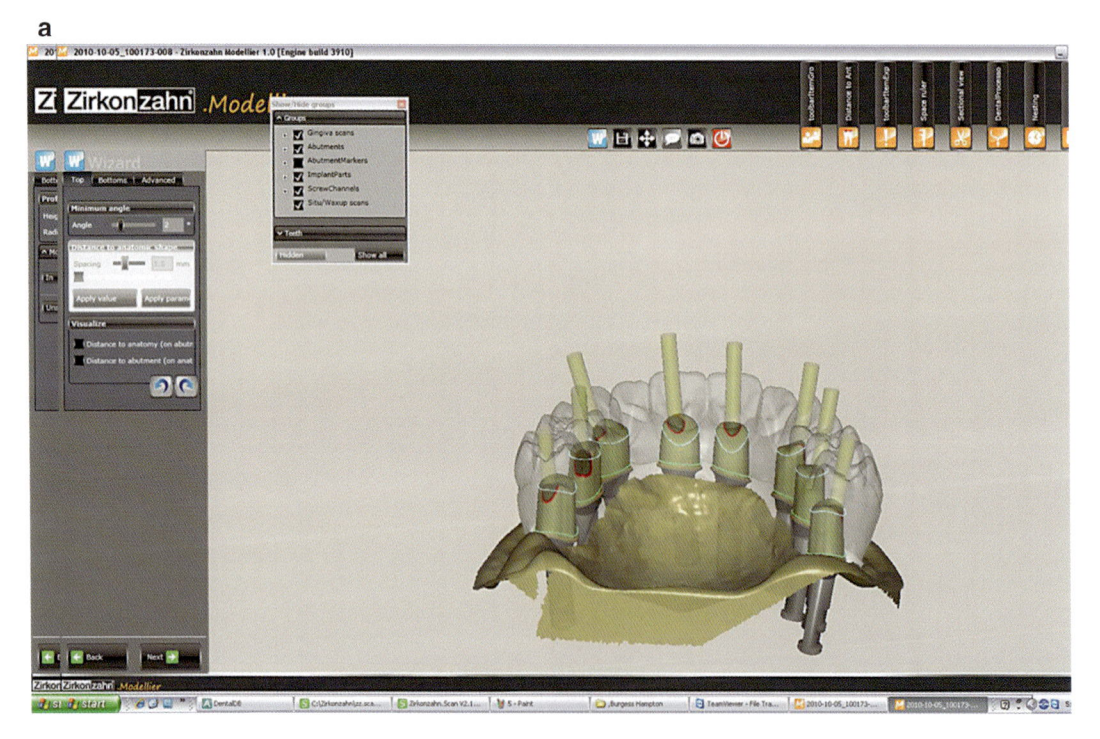

Fig. 25.6 (a) Zirkonzahn 5× CAD design software for screw-retained hybrid restorations. (b) Full-arch zirconia, minimally layered bridge that cracked due to not following protocol. (c) Flanges are contraindicated. (d) What flange designs do to the soft tissue and potential implant failure due to bacterial accumulation, inflammation of soft tissue and debris that accumulates due to lack of cleaning. (e) New design of full-arch zirconia, without flanges

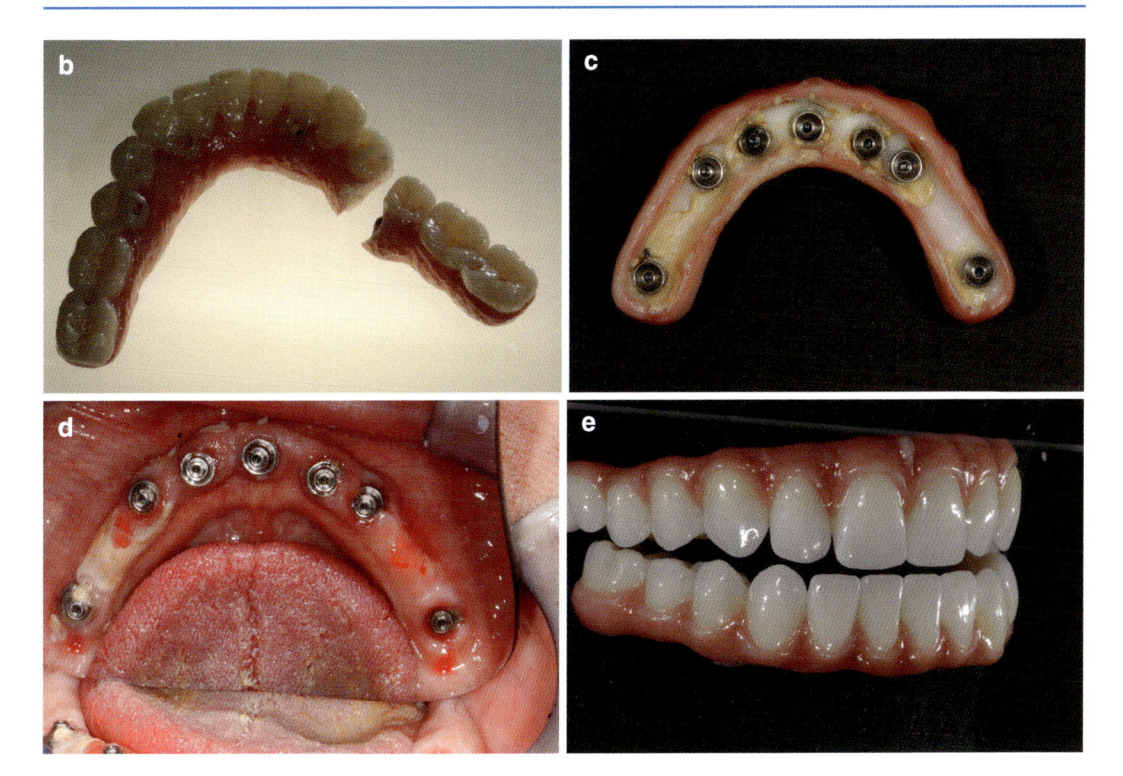

Fig. 25.6 (continued)

aesthetics. E.max has a flexural strength of 360–400 MPa (Culp and McLaren 2010) and is up to three times more durable than other glass ceramic systems. IPS e.max has true-to-nature shades all while having a low refractive index that provided optimal optical properties such as translucency and light transmission. IPS e.max restorations can also be further characterized by using a cutback and layering with porcelain or staining and glazing it. Also for seating of these restorations either an adhesive bonding method or conventional cementation can be used. Dual curing adhesives can be used to create a bond between the prepped tooth and the IPS e.max restorations.

Currently zirconia is the strongest all-ceramic material available, higher in strength than the IPS e.max material – but not quite as lifelike as e.max either. The higher-strength CAD/CAM materials appear chalky and not very aesthetic. However, not all zirconia materials are created equal. The Prettau Zirconia material is more translucent and can produce full contour single crowns as well as implant-supported, screw-retained restorations.

Many CAD/CAM systems are capable of milling full arches in full monolithic zirconia. The crucial, and the human element of this, is the design. An executable plan is needed that will allow proper function for the patient one that does not violate any of the rules of zirconia. Figure 25.6b is a full-arch zirconia, minimally layered bridge that cracked at delivery due to the lack of the proper process that must be followed through the entire fabrication of the zirconia bridge. Every step is important, and abusing the principles, including the necessary slow cooling after baking in the furnace, can lead to disaster.

A correct design is imperative. Some companies are fabricating screw-retained hybrid restoration with either plastic or all zirconia and designing flanges on the soft tissue as shown in Fig. 25.6c. Flanges are contraindicated for hygiene and health purposes and will keep the implant and tissue unhealthy (Adar 2014). This also has the potential of implant failure due to bacterial accumulation, inflammation of soft tissue and debris that accumulates due to lack of cleaning (Fig. 25.6d).

The new design, without flanges, is shown in Fig. 25.6e. The patient is put first in a PMMA as a temporary to allow for tissue adaptation. The patient now has the ability to floss and use adjunctive tools to clean the soft tissue area and the implant junctions allowing for long-term success. This picture also illustrates the aesthetics of the new product, even with using full monolithic with *no* ceramic layering, except for the pink tissue area. We can update these unhealthy hybrids with a skilled technician and get a reasonably aesthetic outcome using the strongest restoration with no chipping or staining.

25.4 Qualifying Differentiators

Poor aesthetics and design concepts are promoted everywhere, all while blaming CAD/CAM technology for it. "Good enough" does not make sense in CAD/CAM dentistry either. We must hold ourselves to the same exacting aesthetic levels as we do with any other type of restorations.

The patient shown in Fig. 25.7a was excited about converting her denture into a full zirconia monolithic Prettau bridge. However, the lab that produced this restoration, lacked the design communication and the interpretation process and also had a lack of artistic ability with this new material. They delivered a smile that was worse than the denture that she previously had.

Besides the unaesthetic look of the new restoration, the patient was also unhappy with the fact that she could not speak as before; certain sounds including the "ch" sound was impossible for her to make. She stated that she felt embarrassed when talking even in simple interactions.

The pink is unnatural with no dimension, texture or finish (Fig. 25.7b). The integration of the papilla into the anatomy of the tooth is non-existent. In Fig. 25.7c the roughness caused to her tissue can be observed, as well as a ridge lap that violates the rules of hygiene and is potential cause for failure of her implant fixtures.

The first step in helping this patient (Fig. 25.7d) was to design the first PMMA restoration virtually through a wax up to establish all the likes and dislikes of the patient's desires (Gratton and Aquilo 2004). The PMMA is a monolithic plastic material that is milled and will be screw retained, and the soft tissue will be developed using anaxdent composite to create a three-dimensional look. The dentist can sit chairside to manipulate the composite and will be able to see the adaptation of the tissue to the new restoration ensuring that it is cleanable.

In Fig. 25.7e observe the natural look of the PMMA used as a temporary for the patient to "test drive", function with it, critique the aesthetics and allow tissue integration. Figure 25.7f shows how the bone and tissue were manipulated by the periodontist and general practitioner to form shapes similar to that of an ovate pontic to allow access for the patient to clean.

After several months of "test driving" the PMMA and upon patient approval, the PMMA was then put on the master model without the soft tissue, and new gingival material was injected to create the new scenario that currently exists in the mouth. Once all the info is transferred, either a duplicate of the temporary or the temporary itself is placed on the model and scanned into the computer with the Zirkonzahn scanner and is designed as a copy mill in the exact shape and adaptation and occlusion of the PMMA that was tested in the mouth as a temporary. It is then milled in full zirconia.

Figure 25.7g presents the full zirconia after sintering in the oven over night, and notice that a cutback was done on the *non-functional areas only*, to create depth and translucency as well as an illusion of reality.

Figure 25.7h shows the last of multiple bakes after adjusting and adding effects on both the pink region and the teeth to create a natural three-dimensional look.

The final product is shown in Fig. 25.7i, after glazing, polishing and cementing the titanium metal cylinders in the restoration to maintain as a screw-retained restoration.

Figure 25.7j illustrates the comparison of the two bridges that were both made using the same technology, with the same zirconia product, but with a different approach and design interpretation and with cohesive teamwork as well as a skilled laboratory technician. All of this is essential for the

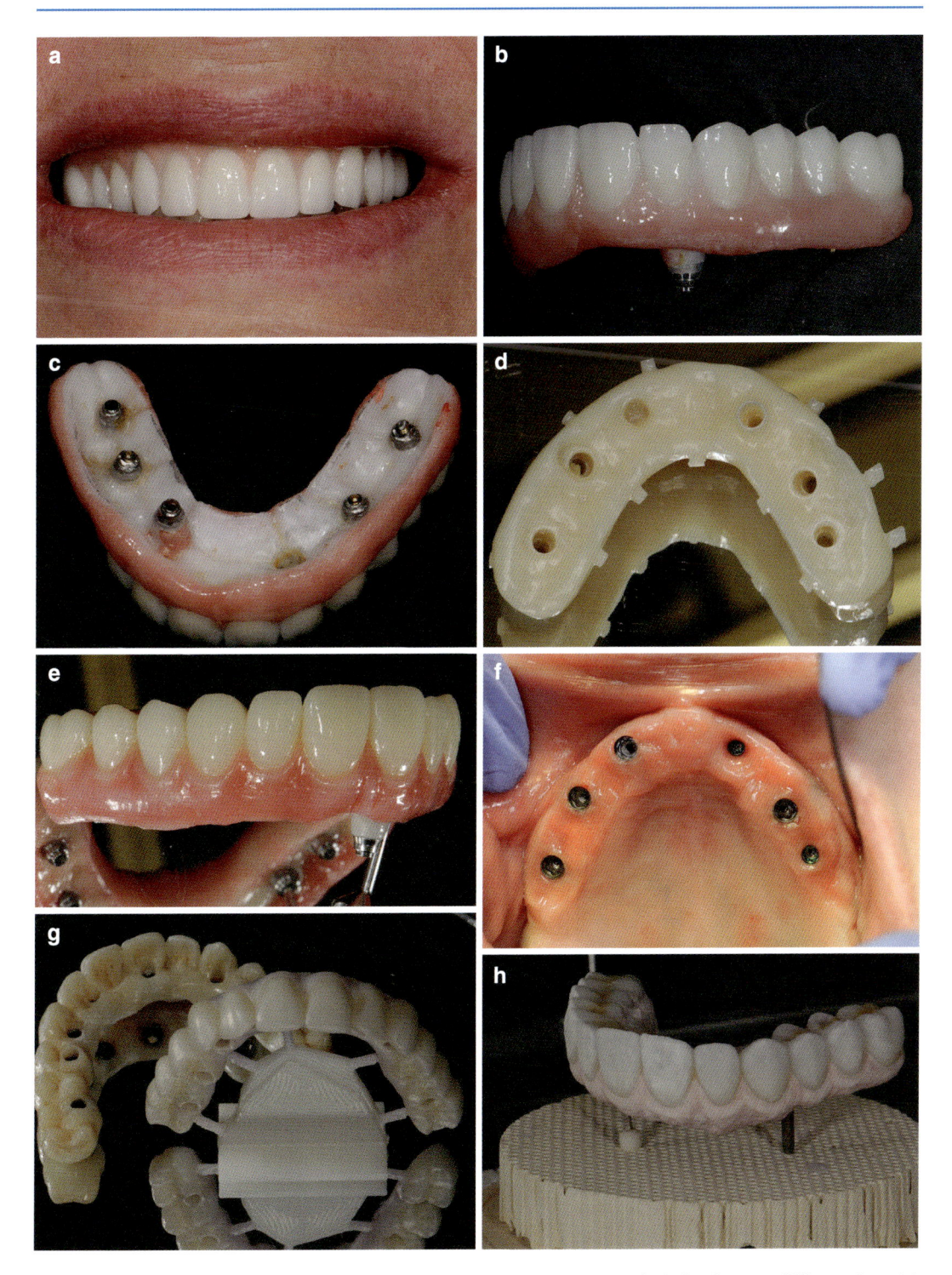

25 Prosthetic Solutions to Biological Deficiencies: Pink and White Aesthetics   435

Fig. 25.7 (**a**) Patient converted her denture into a full zirconia monolithic Prettau bridge and did not like the function or the aesthetics and design. (**b**) Unnaturalness of the pink with no dimension, texture or finish. (**c**) Roughness caused to her tissue as well as a ridge lap design. (**d**) PMMA restoration as a temporary guide blueprint. (**e**) Natural look of the PMMA with *pink*. (**f**) Bone and tissue manipulation creating shapes similar to ovate pontic design for accessibility to clean. (**g**) Full zirconia after sintering in the oven overnight. (**h**) The last of multiple bakes to create a three-dimensional look. (**i**) Final zirconia screw-retained restoration. (**j**) Comparison of the two bridges made with same technology, same material and different laboratories. (**k**) Floss can be easily threaded. (**l**) Patient's smile with final zirconia-retained bridge

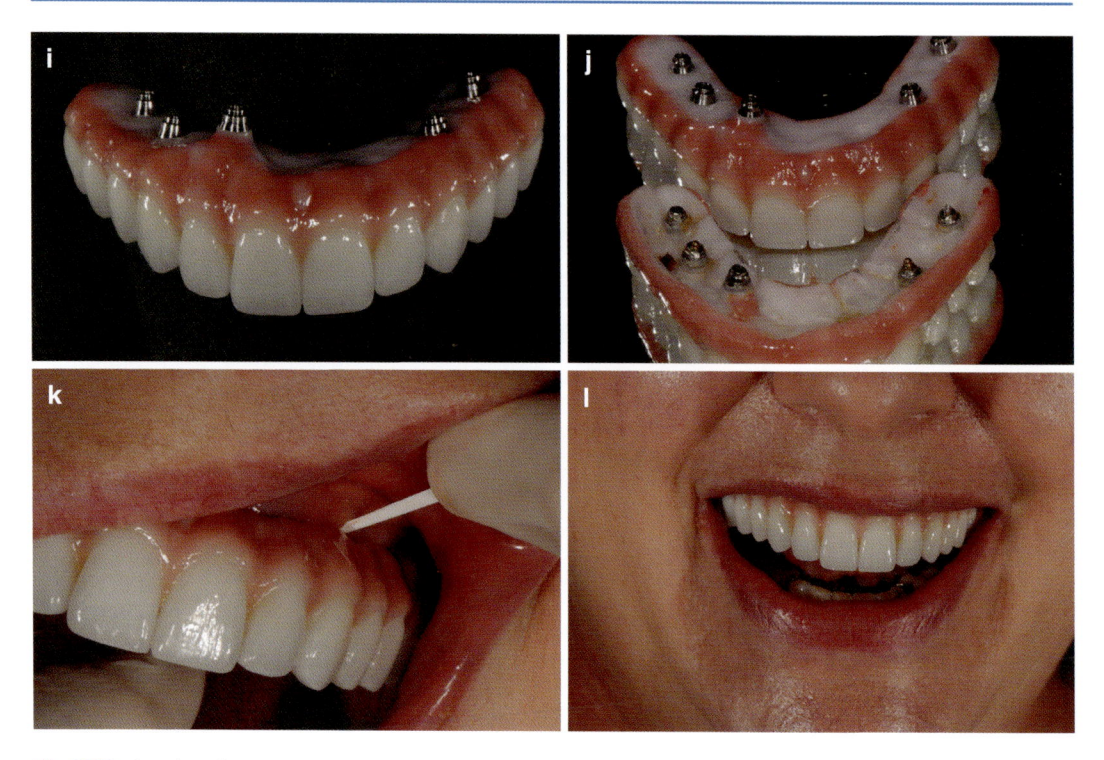

Fig. 25.7 (continued)

success of the final restoration and reaching or exceeding patient expectations.

Floss can easily be threaded between the tissue and Prettau restoration, so the patient has the ability to clean the area to maintain proper hygiene (Fig. 25.7k).

The patient now has a the natural, more youthful and attractive smile (Fig. 25.7l) that makes her feel more confident and comfortable as well as the ability to enunciate her words properly while interacting in her life.

Due to its strength these restorations can be used for single unit up to 14-unit bridges using either full contour monolithic or with minimal cutback on non-functional areas only for ceramic layering to enhance aesthetics. The final restoration shown here is fabricated using the CAD/CAM technology. This is both a computer-aided design (CAD) and milling from a zirconia disc. Once it is milled, the zirconia in the green stage is soft making the necessary "human touch" of shaping, enhancing and colouring an easy task. The bridge is then sintered for 8–13 h at a high temperature and then custom stained and layered by a skilled laboratory technician with pink ceramic on an implant-supported screw-retained bridge to create the illusion of soft tissue. Many cases may be cut back to enhance aesthetics on non-functional areas only.

With CAD/CAM, the human touch and human concepts are the most important aspects. Aesthetic signature lines providing aesthetics, consistency and efficiency at an affordable value are available and are possible. The right human touch can change the rule of thumb for monolithic crowns and bridges.

When large implant bridges are being fabricated, it is extremely important to follow a proven protocol step by step. If one step is overlooked or done incorrectly, the case will need to be redone and that is very frustrating as well as costly. Something like an inaccurate impression can cause the implant bridge to break, or fabricating the bridge without a verification jig is also contraindicated, because, as strong as zirconia is, it is still very brittle. This seems counterintuitive.

When using Prettau, be sure to obtain a certificate of authenticity that comes with each disc – one must ensure that it is present, and if not, a counterfeit material is being passed off as the Prettau product.

We all need to be, not just on a team, but on the RIGHT team; not just using different disciplines, but using the right team members for those different specialties who work together cohesively. The same vision and an ability to interpret and understand each other with different processes, including technology, will enhance our ability to create a better experience for our patients so that we can deliver superior results with the utilization of technology but not with technology replacing the human touch.

Conclusion

If technology and information were the solution for everyone, then everyone would be skinny, rich and happy. Information is not the panacea – humans still need to use the tools correctly just as with any other tool. Thinking properly in the diagnosis stage as what to do, what not to do and with which product and teaming up with others who have skill, passion and the ability to execute and exceed patients' expectations.

Cases 25.1, 25.2, 25.3 and 25.4 Figures 25.1a, 25.2, 25.3 and 25.4c (Dentistry by Dr. David Garber, private practice, Atlanta, GA)

Case 25.5 Figure 25.5a–c (Dentistry by Dr Marilyn Gaylor, private practice, Atlanta, GA)

Case 25.6 Figure 25.6a–e (Dentistry by Dr. Aldo Leopardi, private practice, Greenwood Village, CO)

Case 25.7 Figures 25.7a–l (Dentistry by Dr. Cheryl Pearson, private practice, Lexington, KY)

References

Adar P (2005) Lab talk. Communication: the ultimate in synergy. Insid Dent 1:82–83
Adar P (2014) Incorporating the human touch in restorative outcomes. Insid Dent Technol 4:52–56
Ahmad I (2002) Synaesthetic restorations: a psychological perspective for surpassing aesthetic dentistry. Pract Proced Aesthet Dent 14(8):643–649
Beuer F, Schweiger J, Edelhoff D, Sorensen JA (2011) Reconstruction of esthetics with a digital approach. Int J Periodontics Restor Dent 31(2):185–193
Culp L, McLaren EA (2010) Lithium disilicate: the restorative material of multiple options. Compend Contin Educ Dent 31(9):716–720 722, 724–5
Gratton DG, Aquilino SA (2004) Interim restorations. Dent Clin N Am 48(2):vii 487–97

Further Reading

Adar P (1997) Avoiding patient disappointment with trial veneer utilization. J Esthet Dent 9(6):277–284
Feeley RT (1995) Cosmetics and the esthetic patient and laboratory communication. Oral Health 85(8):9–12 14
Haddad HJ, Jakstat HA, Arnetzl G et al (2009) Does gender and experience influence shade matching quality? J Dent 37(Suppl 1):e40–e44 Epub 2009 May 22
Hatai Y (2008 Winter) Reproducing nature: understanding the composition of natural dentition. Eur J Esthet Dent 3(4):372–380
Herrguth M, Wichmann M, Reich S (2005) The aesthetics of all-ceramic veneered and monolithic CAD/CAM crowns. J Oral Rehabil 32(10):747–752
Ishikawa-Nagai S, Yoshida A, Sakai M, Kristiansen J, DaSilva JD (2009) Clinical evaluation of perceptibility of color differences between natural teeth and all-ceramic crowns. J Dent 37(Suppl 1):e57–e63 Epub 2009 Apr 18
Joiner A (2004) Tooth colour: a review of the literature. J Dent 32(Suppl 1):3–12
Kahng LS (2006) Patient-dentist-technician communication within the dental team: using a colored treatment plan wax-up. J Esthet Restor Dent 18(4):185–196
Luo XP, Zhang L (2010) Effect of veneering techniques on color and translucency of Y-TZP. J Prosthodont 19(6):465–470 Epub 2010 Jun 8
Mayekar SM (2001) Shades of a color. Illusion or reality? Dent Clin N Am 45(1):155–172 vii
Raptis NV, Michalakis KX, Hirayama H (2006) Optical behavior of current ceramic systems. Int J Periodontics Restor Dent 26(1):31–41
Reynolds JA, Roberts M (2010) Lithium-disilicate pressed veneers for diastema closure. Inside Dent 6(5):46–52
Santos GC Jr, Boksman LL, Santos MJ (2013) CAD/CAM technology and esthetic dentistry: a case report. Compend Contin Educ Dent 34(10):764 766,768
Tortopidis D, Hatzikyriakos A, Lokoti M, Menees G, Tsiggos N (2007) Evaluation of the relationship between subjects' perception and professional assessment of esthetic treatment needs. J Esthet Restor Dent 19(3):154–162
Volpato CA, Monteiro S Jr, de Andrada MC, Fredel MC, Petter CO (2009) Optical influence of the type of illuminant, substrates and thickness of ceramic materials. Dent Mater 25(1):87–93 Epub 2008 Jul 7

Appendix: Implant Checklist

Compiled by Satheesh Elangovan, Chris Barwacz, Gustavo Avila-Ortiz, Georgia K. Johnson, and Clark M. Stanford

Pre-Surgical Visit

1. Systemic Evaluation
- ☐ General physical and systemic health assessment (medications, gait, posture, pregnancy status, renal, hepatic, respiratory, etc…)
- ☐ Routine cardio-vascular assessment (blood pressure, pulse, etc…)
- ☐ Coagulation assessment (International Normalized Ratio, bleeding time, etc…)
- ☐ Risk factor assessment - smoking, diabetic status, family History (genetics), etc…
- ☐ Assessing the need for antibiotic prophylaxis (joint replacement, cardiac conditions, etc…)

2. Clinical Evaluation
- ☐ *Extra-oral evaluation*
- ✓ TMJ, lymph node, facial symmetry, tumors etc.

- ☐ *Intra-oral evaluation*
- ✓ Mouth opening measurement
- ✓ Oral cancer screening
- ✓ Oral hygiene status: plaque index / gingival index
- ✓ Periodontal examination (probing depth, attachment level, bleeding on probing, furcation involvement, mobility, gingival recession)
- ✓ Specific implant site evaluation
    - o Ridge dimensions assessment (bucco-lingual width , mesio-distal space and apico-coronal height)
    - o Amount of keratinized mucosa (thickness/width)
    - o Frenal or muscle pull assessment
    - o Vestibular depth measurement
    - o Inter-occlusal space
    - o Arch length, arch shape, tooth proportions relative to edentulous site
    - o Occlusal analysis / para-functional habits evaluation
    - o Ectopic migration / supra-eruption of adjacent / opposing dentition
    - o Incisal/occlusal plane, lip line in repose and full smile
    - o Clinical crown form (square, square-tapering, ovoid) of adjacent dentition

3. Additional Care Planning Steps
- ☐ Mounted diagnostic casts and diagnostic wax-up(s) of implant site(s)
- ☐ Radiographic/surgical guide(s) fabrication and intraoral assessment
- ☐ Imaging assessment (peri-apical, bitewings, panoramic radiographs and computed tomography)
- ☐ Clinical photographs (extra / intra-oral)

4. Surgeon-Restoring Dentist Discussion
- ☐ Strategizing treatment options/alternatives
- ☐ Review of ideal placement based on desired prosthetic outcome
- ☐ Timing/sequencing of treatment based on other restorative needs

5. Patient – Surgeon/Restoring Dentist Discussions
- ☐ Communicate care plan with patient
- ✓ Discussing the findings
- ✓ Developing a care plan, sequencing and timing of steps
- ✓ Planning and execution of disease control phase
- ✓ Planning and execution of corrective phase (restorations, orthodontic, etc…)

- ☐ Pre-operative instructions and treatment information
- ✓ For the surgical procedure
- ✓ For conscious sedation (if applicable)

- ☐ Prescribing medications (if needed)
- ✓ Antibiotic prophylaxis
- ✓ Corticosteroids
- ✓ Oral sedatives

Surgical Visit

1. Pre-operative Check
- ☐ Baseline vital signs assessment
- ☐ Baseline systemic health re-evaluation (diabetic and coagulation status, etc...)
- ☐ Checking if all emergency drugs /cart are readily available
- ☐ Checking the implant kit and surgical instruments for completeness
- ☐ Checking the fit of surgical guide

2. Communicating Informed Consent
[for implant surgery and ancillary procedures or conscious sedation (if necessary)]
- ☐ Discussion of biologic/esthetic prognosis and timing of procedures
- ☐ Discussion of risks/benefits of the procedures

3. Pain and Anxiety Control
- ☐ Proper selection and usage of conscious sedation (if planned)
- ☐ Proper selection and usage of local anesthetics

4. Implant Installation
(As per manufacturer's instructions)
- ☐ Drilling sequence - Verify that peri-implant bone dimensions are adequate according to clinical, radiographic and restorative plan:
  - ✓ Facial and lingual/palatal wall: For example 1.5 to 2 mm
  - ✓ Inter-proximally between implant and tooth: For example 1.5 to 2 mm
  - ✓ Inter-proximally between implants: For example 3 to 4 mm
  - ✓ Minimum distance of approximately 2 mm between implant body and adjacent structures (neurovascular bundles, periodontal ligament, etc...)

5. Making Decisions Before Suturing
- ☐ One stage or two stage procedure: Based on the primary stability of the implant and the need for additional augmentation
- ☐ Additional augmentation
  - ✓ Soft tissue only (connective tissue graft or allograft)
  - ✓ Hard tissue only (autogenous, allografts or xenografts with or without membrane)
  - ✓ Combined soft and hard tissue augmentation

6. Immediate Provisionalization (IP) - If Desired
- ☐ Confirmation of adequate insertion torque and primary stability of the implant fixture at the time of surgery. Confirm occlusion can accommodate IP.
- ☐ Clinical judgment to evaluate indications for either immediate *functional* or *non-functional* loading with a provisional restoration.
- ☐ Establish indications for screw or cement-retained provisional restoration.

7. Final Check Before Discharging the Patient
- ☐ Checking if hemostasis is achieved
- ☐ Checking the vital signs
- ☐ Checking if patient has adequately recovered (if applicable)
- ☐ Post-operative instructions

* The intention of this checklist is to provide general guidelines while planning for implant surgery. It is the clinician's responsibility to make appropriate changes to the checklist as required by the case.

Index

A

Absorbable collagen sponge (ACS), 252
Abutment
  biological considerations on materials, 302–304
  cement retention, 359–361
  ceramic, 315–316
  complications of materials, 363
  custom
    base surfaces treatment, 359
    clinical advantages, 358
    coloration, 358
    form and function of, 357
    merits, 359
    subgingival contour, 358
    supragingival contour, 357
    surface texture, 359
  design, 296
  final, 306–307
  flat interproximal design, 35
  healing (see Healing)
  implant superstructure and, 353
  materials of, 355
  metal, 315–316
  plasma treatment, 359
  pre-made, 357
  screw retention, 361–363
  selection, 355–357
  superstructure characteristics, 359–361
Acellular dermal grafts (ADG), 242–244
Acrylic provisional restoration, 340, 342, 345, 348
ACS. *See* Absorbable collagen sponge (ACS)
ADG. *See* Acellular dermal grafts (ADG)
Aesthetic contour graft, 210–218
"Aesthetic mock-up" process, 262–264
Aesthetic zone, 58
  anterior, 337, 340, 342, 344, 354, 358
  digital impression, 369–373, 376
  implant-abutment crown, 313
  implant position
    apical-coronal, 270–275
    buccal-lingual, 268–270
    improper angulation, 272–275
    mesial-distal, 268
  implant superstructure and abutment, 353
  incision/flap design in, 275–276
  treatment planning, 262–264
  zirconia, 354
Ailing implant, 412
Allograft, 225, 236, 242
  advantages, 22
  autograft *vs.*, 201
  central incisor extraction, 25–27
  gingival contour, 25, 27–28
  labial bone loss, 23–25
  postoperative methods, 23
  soft tissue grafts, 23
  sterile procedures, 22
  thin gingiva, 23–25
Alveolar dimensions
  aesthetic concerns, 184–185
  anatomic limitations, 172
  dental heroics, 172
  dentists and hygienists, 171
  goals, 172
  growth factors/enhancers, 181–182
    calcium sulfate, 182
    L-PRF, 183–184
    rhPDGF-BB, 182
  historical record, 171
  ideal therapy, 172
  after implant restoration, 173
  socket filling materials
    amnion/chorion barrier membrane, 176, 178
    bioexclusive barriers, 179–181
    biphasic calcium sulfate, 176, 177
    bovine bone-grafted sockets, 175
    demineralized freeze-dried bone allograft, 176, 177
    facial fenestration, 176
    grafting of extraction sockets, 175
    guided tissue regeneration, 179
    human study, 179
    ideal location and orientation, 176, 178
    platelet rich fibrin, 175
    site collapse, 173
    vital bone, 175, 176, 178

Alveolar dimensions (*cont.*)
  surgical approach
    astute dentists, 173
    atraumatic extraction, 174
    bone loss, 173
    flap elevation, 173–174
    immediately after extraction, 173
    non-vital maxillary central incisor, 174
    resorption, 173
Alveolar ridge atrophy
  after tooth loss, 58
  classification, 59
  implant placement, 59
Alveolar ridge preservation procedures, 8
Alveolus
  clinical assessment, 104
  general assessments
    anatomic landmarks, 104–105
    esthetics, 106
    occlusion/prosthesis considerations, 105–106
    pathologies, 106–108
  hard tissue assessments
    clinical evaluation, 110–111
    dynamic process, 110
    edentulous ridge deformities classifications, 111–113
    ridge dimension, 111
  soft tissue assessments
    biologic width, 110
    charting, 107, 109
    KM, 109–110
    periodontal/peri-implant health, 108
    tissue biotype, 108, 109
Amalgam tattoos, 235, 240, 241
American Academy of Oral and Maxillofacial Radiology (AAOMR), 57–58
Angulation of implant, 272–275
Anterior alveolar ridge
  accessory foramina, 71–72
  anterior loop, 71
  classification, 60–61
  foramina, 73
  horizontal morphology, 61
  incisive canal, 69–71
  lingual aspect, 72
  lingual canal, 72–73
  mandible, 67
  mandibular canal, 67–68
  maxillary anterior implant region, 61
  maxillary sinuses, 66–67
  mental foramen, 68–69
  nasal cavity/floor, 65–66
  nasopalatine canal, 61–64
  paranasal sinuses, 66
Anterior edentulous sites, 58
Anterior mandible, 192
Anterior maxillary aesthetic zone
  bilateral concave appearance, 80
  different shapes, 81

3-D planning concepts
  abutment margin, 94, 96
  CAD-CAM, 93, 94
  CBCT, 83
  ceramo-metal restorations, 93, 95
  clipping, 87
  desired trajectory, of transfer coping, 93, 94
  digital workflow, 88
  emulation of root eminence, 93, 96
  final restoration, 93, 96
  fixture level impression transfer copings, 92, 93
  full-flap design, 89, 90
  healing collars, 91
  implant placement, 87, 89
  implant position, 84, 86–89
  interactive treatment planning software, 84, 85
  laboratory phase, 93
  left central incisor, 82–83
  lip-lift technique, 82–84
  maxillary and mandibular casts, 93, 94
  noninvasive verification method, 94, 97
  optical scan, 88
  polyether impression material, 93
  postoperative radiograph, 93, 97
  post-trauma, 82
  preexisting bridge, 88, 89
  restorative planning, 91, 92
  right lateral incisor, 82–83
  segmentation, 86, 87
  selective transparency, 86, 94, 98
  soft tissue cast, 93, 94
  soft tissue sulcus, 92
  software tools, 88, 89
  sufficient bone volume, 84–86
  teeth and roots, 86, 87
  tension-free closure, 91
  tooth-borne template, 90
  transitional restorations, 92
  treatment planning software, 91, 92
restorative dilemma, 81
retracted view, 80
root morphology, 81
segmentation, 81
surgical and restorative treatment, 80
three-dimensional imaging, 80
tooth extraction, 79
two-dimensional imaging, 80
Aperture, 155–157
Apical-coronal implant position, 270–272
Artifacts, 75
Atraumatic extraction, 174
Atrophy, alveolar ridge
  after tooth loss, 58
  classification, 59
  implant placement, 59
Auro Galva Crown (AGC)-electroformed gold crown, 362
Autograft, 236
  vs. allograft, 201

B

Basilar process, 61
Beam-harden artifacts, 75
Biological width
    establishment of, 337–338
    micro-gap junction, 354
    peri-implant, 293, 338
Block allografts. *See also* Hard tissues
    autogenous, 194–197
    flap design, 193
    keys, 193
BMPs. *See* Bone morphogenetic proteins (BMPs)
Bone adaptation, 34
Bone augmentation, 209
    barrier membranes, 209
    defect configuration, 204
    dental implant, 234, 253, 421, 430
    mucogingival junction, 192
Bone formation, 253, 254, 418, 420
Bone graft, 248, 251, 253, 254, 274, 296
    autogenous/xenogenic, 422
    connective tissue placed over, 274
    dental implant, 234
    materials, 253
        autogenous, 206
        biomaterials, 205
        freeze-dried bone allografts, 206–209
        ideal, 205
        xenograft, 206, 209
    procedure, 254, 290
    vertical and horizontal, 295
Bone healing pathway
    hybrid
        description, 49
        healing mode shift, 50
        surgical drilling dimension, 50
        time point, 51
    interfacial remodeling
        higher insertion torque, 45
        human retrieved sample, 47
        vs. intramembranous-like, 49
        mechanical stability, 45
        microcracking and compression necrosis, 45
        optical micrographs, 45–46
        substantial region, 46
    intramembranous-like, 47–49
    parameters, 44–45
    software, 52–53
    surgical drilling technique, 52
Bone morphogenetic proteins (BMPs), 252–253
Bone regeneration, 185
Buccal-lingual implant position, 268–270
Buccal plate, 265–267, 289, 291–293

C

Canalis sinuosus, 66
Carbon dioxide (CO_2) lasers, 421–423
CBCT. *See* Cone beam computed tomography (CBCT)
Cementoenamel junction (CEJ), 104
Cement-retained restorations
    final crown reconstruction, 312–314
    implant position, 268, 269, 272, 274
Cement retention, 359–360
Ceramic abutments, 315–316
Chin graft, 198–200
Chlorhexidine gluconate, 412
CIST. *See* Cumulative Interceptive Supportive Therapy (CIST)
Collar design, implant, 294
Computer-aided design/computer-assisted manufacturing (CAD/CAM), 354, 432
    advantages and disadvantages, 379
    ceramic crowns, 379–380
    CEREC® 1 system, 373
    digital scanner, 373–375
    immediate implant provisional placement, 380
    implant abutments, 373–377
    interdisciplinary treatment planning, 124
    LAVA COS system, 373
    lithium disilicate, 330, 380, 432–434
    material selection for, 377–380
    milling machine, 376
    NobelProcera Software, 375
    qualifying differentiators, 434–437
    standard transformation language (STL), 370, 373, 375
    surgical guide, 372–373
    3D design software, 376
    TRIOS, 373, 374
    use of, 377
    zirconia, 432–434
Concha bullosa, 65
Cone beam computed tomography (CBCT), 20, 235, 254
    beam-harden artifacts, 75
    and digital impression, 369–373
    hard tissues development, 189, 190
    immediate implant placement, 344, 345
    implant site evaluation, 264–267
    implant sites, quantification of bone, 73–74
    partial volume average artifacts, 75
    postoperative, 93, 97
    potential for, 57
    preoperative, 94, 97
    with radiographic guide, 265, 266, 277–278
    soft tissue contour and, 306
    utilization, 58
    ZAC protocol, 347
Conical cone connection, 339–340, 350
Connective tissue (CT)
    facial defect, 123
    graft, 23
    harvest, 123
    loss, 6
    SECT graft, 238–242
Core-binding factor α (Cbfa1), 38
Cover screw, delayed implant loading, 308–310

Cumulative Interceptive Supportive
    Therapy (CIST), 412, 413
Cupping effect, 337
Custom abutment
    base surfaces treatment, 359
    clinical advantages, 358–359
    coloration, 358
    form and function of, 357
    merits, 359
    subgingival contour, 358
    supragingival contour, 357–358
    surface texture, 359

D
DAM. *See* Digital asset management (DAM)
Delayed implant loading
    cover screw, 308–310
    healing abutment, 307–308
Delayed implant placement, 310–311
Demineralized freeze-dried bone
    allograft (DFDBA), 176, 177
Dental digital photography
    anterior dentition, 153–154
    aperture, 155–157
    auto-controls, 151
    basics, 155
    exposure, 155, 156
    flash, 159
    focus area modes, 159–160
    goals, 151
    high-quality images, 152–153
    implant restoration, 154–155
    ISO, 158, 159
    light meter, 158–159
    shutter speed, 155
    white balance, 161
        advantages, 162
        bit depth, 162
        catalog backup, 166
        color space and management, 163–164
        DAM, 164
        develop module, 166
        digital workflow, 165–166
        dilemma, 164–165
        disadvantages, 162
        exposure modes, 161–162
        image formats, 162
        intra oral camera setting, 163
        lightroom, 165
        output, 166, 167
        RAW, 162
Dental implants, 3, 247
    abutment design, 296
    biological reality
        alveolar ridge preservation procedures, 8
        buccal soft tissue, 6–7
        clinical capabilities, 10–12
        clinical presentation, 6–7

diagnostic imaging, 9–10
gingival display, 6
gingival health and architecture, 6
occlusion, 9
peri-implant mucosa, 8
ridge augmentation procedures, 8
tissue/bone sound, 8
tooth display, 6
biologic width, 408
bone augmentation, 235, 253, 421, 430
bone grafting, 234
checklist, 439–440
clinicians, 103
complications, 103–104
comprehensive esthetic diagnosis, 4–6
esthetic therapy
    diagnostic waxing, 13
    interproximal tissue loss, 14
    progressive elimination, 15
    protocols, 13
    risk factors, 12–13
    soft tissue architecture, 14
    surgical planning software, 13–14
gingival biotype, 234
immediate non-occlusal loading, 340, 344
long-term monitoring, 408
and natural teeth, 354, 410
patient esthetic expectations, 4
restoration (*see* Restoration, dental implant)
site development, 11, 13
therapy, 261–262
titanium abutment, 268, 269
use of, 117
zirconia abutment, 268, 269
Dental management software, 164
Dental photography, 151
Dental radiation dose, 74–75
Digital asset management (DAM), 164
Digital dental photography. *See* Dental digital photography
Digital impression, 369–373, 376
Digital radiographic technology, 58
Digital scanning, 373–375
Digital technology, 427–428
Diode lasers, 419–420
Double concavity concept, 308, 315
DSLR cameras, 159
Dual-curing resin cement, 316, 317

E
E.max ceramics, 297, 431–433
Erbium lasers, 420–421

F
Failing implant, 412
Flap design
    aesthetic zone, 136, 275–276
    buccal attached gingiva, 141, 143, 144

elements, 136
horizontal defects management, 218, 219
immediate implant placement
   delayed, 138–139
   one-stage, 138
   two-stage, 136–138
papilla reconstruction, 139, 141–143
second-stage implant surgery, 139, 140
Flap procedure, 430
Floss, 434–436
Foramina, 73
Free gingival graft, 236–238
Freeze-dried bone allografts (FDBA), 206–209
Full-thickness flap, 275, 277, 419

G

GBR. *See* Guided bone regeneration (GBR)
Gingiva
   aesthetics, 233
   biotype
      dental implants, 234
      identification, 234–235
      significance of, 234
      thin to thick, 235–236
   clinical assessment, 104
   general assessments
      anatomic landmarks, 104–105
      esthetics, 106
      occlusion/prosthesis considerations, 105–106
      pathologies, 106–108
   grafting
      indications for, 235
      sources, 236
      techniques, 236–238
   hard tissue assessments
      clinical evaluation, 110–111
      dynamic process, 110
      edentulous ridge deformities classifications, 111–113
      ridge dimension, 111
   margin, 272, 343, 350, 357, 420
   soft tissue assessments
      biologic width, 110
      charting, 107, 109
      KM, 109–110
      periodontal/peri-implant health, 108
      tissue biotype, 108, 109
Greater palatine foramen (GPF), 104
Greater palatine neurovascular bundle (GPB), 104
Growth factors, 181–182, 249
   calcium sulfate, 182
   L-PRF, 183–184
   PDGF, 252–253
   rhPDGF-BB, 182
Guided bone regeneration (GBR), 244, 252, 254, 308
   achieving predictable success, 203
   barrier membrane, 209
   bone graft materials
      autogenous, 206
      biomaterials, 205
      freeze-dried bone allografts, 206–209
      ideal, 205
      xenograft, 206, 209
   defect configuration, 204–205
   horizontal defects management
      aesthetic contour graft, 210, 212–218
      alveolar ridge dimensions, 209–210
      flap design, 218, 219
      implant position, 220
      open-book flap procedure, 219–220
      particulate bone, 210
      ridge augmentation, 210–212
   implantology, 203
   vertical alveolar ridge defects
      allograft, 225
      anterior maxilla, 222–224
      autogenous bone graft, 221
      particulate grafting, 221
      patients with, 220
      single missing tooth span, 225, 227–229
      surgical procedures, 230
Guided tissue regeneration (GTR), 244, 252

H

Hard tissues
   development
      autograft *vs.* allograft, 201
      block allografts, 194–197
      block concepts, 200
      buccal bone augmentation, 191
      CBCT, 189, 190
      chin graft, 198–200
      clinicians, 191
      complications, 200–201
      decision tree for donor site, 192–194
      diagnosis, 191–192
      ramus graft, 197–198
      scan appliance, 189, 190
      surgical guide, 189, 191
   gingiva and alveolus, assessments
      clinical evaluation, 110–111
      dynamic process, 110
      edentulous ridge deformities classifications, 111–113
      ridge dimension, 111
Healing
   abutment
      decision for, 305
      delayed implant loading, 307–309
      modified, 333, 334
      placement of, 309
      removal of, 325
   inflammatory phase, 147, 149
   principles, 146, 147
   proliferative phase, 149
   remodeling phase, 149

Horizontal defects, 205
   aesthetic contour graft, 210, 212–218
   alveolar ridge dimensions, 209–212
   flap design, 218, 219
   implant position, 220
   open-book flap procedure, 218–220
   particulate bone, 210
   ridge augmentation, 210–212
Horizontal mattress suturing, 146
Hounsfield units (HU), 74
Hybrid healing pathway
   description, 49
   healing mode shift, 49–50
   surgical drilling dimension, 50
   time point, 51
Hybrid implant screw-retained restoration, 432–433
Hypoplasia, 67

I

IAJ. *See* Implant-abutment junction (IAJ)
Immediate implant loading
   final abutment, 306–307
   provisional abutment, 305
Immediate implant placement, 290, 291, 310–311
   provisional crown, 380
Immediate loading/restoration, 290
Immediate non-occlusal loading, 340, 344
Immediate provisionalization protocol, 342–344
Implant-abutment connection, 339
Implant-abutment junction (IAJ), 280, 281
Implant connection, 295
Implant crowns
   CAD/CAM, 373–376
      final reconstruction, 311–317
         cement-retained implant restorations, 312–314
         digital workflow, 317
         metal/ceramic abutments, 315–316
         platform switching, 314–315
         screw-retained implant restorations, 312–314
Implant loading
   delayed, 305
      cover screw, 308–310
      healing abutment, 307–308
   immediate
      final abutment, 306
      provisional abutment, 305
Implant placement, 58, 59, 69
   immediate *vs.* delayed, 310–311
Implant position, 294
   apical-coronal, 270–272
   buccal-lingual, 268–270
   first stage surgery, 302
   improper angulation, 272–275
   labial and mesiodistal view, 303
   mesial-distal, 268
Implant provisionalization. *See* Provisionalization
Implant selection, 279
   diameter, 280
   length, 280

platform-switched fixtures, 281–282
prosthetic option, 282
traditional platform-matched fixtures, 280–281
Implant site preparation, tissue engineering
   bone morphogenetic proteins, 252–253
   platelet-derived growth factor, 252–253
   platelet-rich fibrin, 248–252
   platelet-rich plasma, 248–252
   stem cells, 253–256
Implant superstructure
   abutment, 353
   characteristics, 359–363
Implant-supported restorations, 341
   aesthetic success of, 233
   provisional, 340–342, 346
Incision
   in aesthetic zone, 275–276
   interdisciplinary treatment planning, 121, 122
   types and techniques, 276–277
Incisive canal, maxillary, 61–64
Inferior alveolar nerve (IAN), 67, 105
Inflammatory phase, 147, 149
Interdisciplinary treatment planning
   advanced dental therapy, 118
   black triangles, 127, 129
   bone harvest, 125, 126
   bone sound, 121
   CAD/CAM, 124, 126, 128, 130, 133
   calipers transferring, 121
   CBCT, 119, 120, 125–127
   cementation, 126, 129
   collagen plug, 129, 132
   computer-generated surgical guide, 126, 127
   connective tissue graft, 122, 123
   contralateral tooth, 124
   dental implant, 117, 122, 123
   diagnostic phase, 118
   diagnostic setup, 125, 126
   diagnostic wax up, 120, 121, 129, 131
   edentulous arches, 124
   eruption of tissues, 129, 130
   Essix retainer provisional place, 129, 132
   facial tissue defect, 119–120
   flap, 121
   gingival margin, 129, 131
   healing surgery, 126, 128
   implant restoration, 119
   incision, 121, 122
   internal bevel gingivectomy, 121
   intra-surgical stent, 125, 126
   maxillary incisors extraction, 129, 131
   orthodontic extrusion, 129, 130
   orthodontic therapy, 119
   orthodontist, 127, 129
   osseous crest, 121, 122
   osseous structures, 129, 130
   osteoplasty, 122
   osteotomy, 126, 127, 129–132
   panoramic radiograph, 127, 130
   patient evaluation, 119

patient's smile, 130, 133
periodontal disease, 127
PFM
    implant bridge, 130, 133
    restoration, 126, 128
provisional design, 122, 123
provisional restoration, 130, 132
ridge preservation procedure, with xenograft, 129, 132
rigid fixation, 126
screw-retained composite resin, 130, 132
screw-retained implant, 122, 123
single-tooth implant-retain, 118
surgical site, primary closure, 126
surgical template, 122, 126, 128
therapeutic concepts, 118
traumatically lost right central incisor, 118
vacuum-formed surgical template, 129, 131
Interfacial remodeling healing pathway
    higher insertion torque, 45
    human retrieved sample, 47
    vs. intramembranous-like, 49
    mechanical stability, 45
    microcracking and compression necrosis, 45
    optical micrographs, 45–46
    substantial region, 46
Intermediate abutment placement, 307, 314, 316
Internal and external grafting (IEG), 290
Intramembranous-like healing pathway, 47–49
IPS e.max restorations, 432–433
ISO, 158

K
Keratinized mucosa (KM), 109–110

L
Laser-assisted treatment, peri-implantitis, 417–418
    carbon dioxide lasers, 421–423
    diode lasers, 419–420
    erbium lasers, 420–421
    Nd:YAG lasers, 421
    PDT with low-level diode lasers, 418–419
    precautions, 423
    in vitro investigations, 418
Leukocyte-and platelet-rich fibrin (L-PRF), 183–184
Lightroom, 165
Lingual cortical plate morphology, 59–60
Lip-lift technique, 82–83
Lithium disilicate, 330, 380, 432–434
L-PRF. *See* Leukocyte-and platelet-rich fibrin (L-PRF)

M
Macrogeometry, 52
Macro-retentive features, 32–34
MAC technique. *See* Minimal abutment change (MAC) technique
Mandibular canal, 67–68
Mandibular incisive canal, 69–71

Mandibular lingual canals, 72–73
Maxillary sinuses, 66–67
Mental foramen, 68–69, 105
Mesial-distal implant position, 268
Metal abutments, 315–316
Microgap, 338–339
Minimal abutment change (MAC) technique, 344–347
Minimally invasive (MI) methods, 289–290
Minimally veneered zirconia, 385, 386, 388–393
Mini pontic, 430, 431
Mock-up, treatment planning, 262–264, 329, 370, 371
Monolithic zirconia, 386, 398, 432–435
Morse taper, 339–340
"M"-shaped flap, 143, 144
Multipotential stromal cells (MSCs), 253

N
Nanotopography, 53
Nasal cavity/floor, 65–66
Nasal meatus, 65
Nd:YAG lasers, 421
Nemcovsky rotated flap, 141
NobelProcera Software, 375

O
Occlusion, 9, 105–106
One abutment-one time concept, 306, 307, 312, 315, 319, 347, 380
Open-book flap procedure, 219–220
Osseointegration, 290, 305, 307–309, 320, 418
    bone healing pathway
        hybrid, 49–50
            interfacial remodeling, 45–47, 49
            intramembranous-like, 47–49
        parameters, 44–45
        software, 52–53
        surgical drilling technique, 52
    clinical end point, 31–32
    description, 43–44
    high success rates, 32
    implantable devices, 44
    macro-surface, 32–34
    micro-retentive features, 38–39
    micro-surface, 32, 34
    oral implants, 31
    peri-implant mucosal health, 34–37
    surface modification, potential role of, 37–38
    wound healing, 37
Osteotomy, 126, 127, 129–132

P
Palacci and Nowzari technique, 141, 143
Papilla reconstruction, 139, 141–143
Papillary loss, 107
Papilla-sparing incisions, 277
Paranasal sinuses, 66
Partial volume average artifacts, 75

Patient expectations, 432–424
PDGF. *See* Platelet-derived growth factor (PDGF)
Peri-implant
    ADG, 242–244
    biologic width, 110
    gingival biotype
        dental implants, 234
        identification, 234–235
        significance of, 234
        thin to thick, 235–236
    gingival grafting
        indications for, 235
        sources, 236
        techniques, 236–238
    SECT graft, 238–242
    tissues
        collar design, 294
        final abutment design, 296
        histological features of, 408, 410
        histology, 289–293
        implant connection, 295
        maintaining health and volume of, 297
        platform switching, 294–295
        provisional abutment/crown, 296
        surgical technique, 295–296
Peri-implantitis, 297, 357, 407–408
    ailing *vs.* failing *vs.* failed implant, 412
    apical, 414
    CIST, 412, 413
    classifications, 414
    conventional treatment methodologies, 412–415
    etiology, 410–411
    histological features of, 408, 410
    laser-assisted treatment, 417–418
        carbon dioxide lasers, 421–423
        diode lasers, 419–420
        erbium lasers, 420–421
        Nd:YAG lasers, 421
        PDT with low-level diode lasers, 418–419
        precautions, 423
        in vitro investigations, 418
    microbiological features, 411
    periodontitis and predisposition to, 411
    prevalence, 408, 409
    risk factor, 410–411
    treatment, 410
Peri-implant probing depth (PIPD), 420–422
Periodontal disease, cellular allograft, 254
Periodontitis, 411
Photodynamic therapy (PDT), 418–419
Photosensitizer, 419
Pink aesthetic score (PES), 288
Pink ceramic, 429
Platelet-derived growth factor (PDGF), 252–253
Platelet-rich fibrin (PRF), 248, 249
    clinical applications, 251–252
    extraction sockets with, 252
    preparation, 249–252
    proposed applications, 248
    in vitro characteristics, 249–251

Platelet-rich plasma (PRP), 248–249
    clinical applications, 251–252
    and mononuclear cells, 253
    in vitro characteristics, 249–251
Platform-matched implant, 280–281, 338
Platform switching
    final crown reconstruction, 314–315
    fixtures, 281–282
    peri-implant tissues, 294–295
    provisionalization, 338
    randomized control trial, 314
Polymethyl methacrylate (PMMA) restoration, 384, 387, 434–435
Polytetrafluoroethylene (PTFE), 209
Posterior mandible, 193
Pouch roll technique/modified roll flap technique, 141, 143, 144
Prefabricated abutment, 306, 314–316, 357
Premaxilla, 192
Prettau Zirconia, 433, 434
PRF. *See* Platelet-rich fibrin (PRF)
Proliferative phase, healing, 149
Provisional abutments/crown, 296, 341, 342, 345–346
    immediate loading, 305
    placement, 309
Provisionalization, 337–338
    abutment, 341
    bone remodelling effect, 337–338
    early/conventional technique, 341–342
    immediate protocol, 342–344
    implant-abutment connection, 339
    MAC protocol, 344–347
    microgap, 338–339
    platform switch concept, 338
    PMMA/bis-acryl material, 341
    restoration, 339–340, 343, 345
    ZAC protocol, 347–351
PRP. *See* Platelet-rich plasma (PRP)

R
Ramus graft, 197–198
Recombinant human bone morphogenetic proteins (rhBMPs), 252–253
Recombinant human platelet-derived growth factor (rhPDGF), 252–253
Recombinant human platelet-derived growth factor BB (rhPDGF-BB), 182, 253
Remodeling phase, healing, 149
Restoration, dental implant, 428
    in aesthetic zone, 301
    biocompatibility of, 355
    conventional provisional protocol, 341–342
    immediate provisionalization protocol, 342–344
    MAC protocol, 344–347
    materials of, 362
    provisional, 339–340, 343, 345
    ZAC protocol, 347–351
    zirconia, 384, 386–390
        full arch, anterior facial veneers, 395–398

Index 449

full-arch, monolithic and pink gingivae, 398–401
multi-tooth, facial veneered and pink gingivae, 391–393
multi-tooth, facial veneered and pink papillae, 388
multi-tooth, facial veneers, 393–394
single tooth, facial veneers, 388
rhBMPs. *See* Recombinant human bone morphogenetic proteins (rhBMPs)
rhPDGF. *See* Recombinant human platelet-derived growth factor (rhPDGF)
rhPDGF-BB. *See* Recombinant human platelet-derived growth factor BB (rhPDGF-BB)
Ridge augmentation, 8, 210
Ridge deformities, 111–113
Ridge dimension, 111
RUNX-2, 38

S

Sandwich technique, 292
Scanning electron microscopy (SEM)
    fractured zirconia abutment, 363
    turned surface implant, 33
Screw-retained restorations, 430, 433
    final crown reconstruction, 311–314
    hybrid implant, 432–433
    implant position, 268, 269, 271, 272, 274
Screw retention, 361–363
SECT graft. *See* Subepithelial connective tissue (SECT) graft
Sequence of therapy
    bovine/equine sintered xenograft, 22
    clinical problem
        data collection, 19–21
        goals, 19
        labial bone loss, 21
        normal to thin bone, 21
        surgical methods, 21–22
    grafting material characteristics, 22
    mineralized bone allograft
        advantages, 22
        central incisor extraction, 25–27
        gingival contour, 25, 27–28
        labial bone loss, 23–25
        postoperative methods, 23
        soft tissue grafts, 23
        sterile procedures, 22
        thin gingiva, 23–25
Shutter speed, 155
SIMPLANT immediate smile concept, 380
Single implant rehabilitation, digital workflow, 317
Single-tooth defects, 204
Single tooth implant (STI), 344
Soft tissue, 136
    alveolus, assessments
        biologic width, 110
        charting, 107, 109
        KM, 109–110
        periodontal/peri-implant health, 108
        tissue biotype, 108, 109

biotype, 293
cast, 93, 94
with free gingival graft, 237
grafts, 235, 270, 291
    autogenous, 242
    bone and, 295
quality, 233
sulcus, 92,
Split-Finger technique, 141, 143
Standard transformation language (STL), 370, 373, 375
Stem cells
    implant site preparation, 252–256
    ridge augmentation with, 254–256
STL. *See* Standard transformation language (STL)
Subepithelial connective tissue (SECT) graft, 238–242
Subgingival contour, 358
Supragingival contour, 357
Surface topography design, 52
Surgical drilling technique, 52
Surgical guides
    CAD/CAM, 372, 373
    for implant therapy, 277–279
Suture
    implant dentistry, 143
    tension-free closure, 143
    variables, 143–145
        knots, 146
        material, 145–146
        needle, 146
        techniques, 146–149
        thread diameter, 145

T

3D digital radiology, 74
3-D planning concepts
    abutment margin, 94, 96
    CAD-CAM, 93, 94
    CBCT, 83
    ceramo-metal restorations, 93, 95
    clipping, 87
    desired trajectory, of transfer copings, 93, 94
    digital workflow, 88
    emulation of root eminence, 93, 96
    final restoration, 93, 96
    fixture level impression transfer copings, 92, 93
    full-flap design, 89, 90
    healing collars, 91
    implant placement, 87, 89
    implant position, 84, 86–89
    implants, 91, 92
    interactive treatment planning software, 84, 85
    laboratory phase, 93
    left central incisor, 82–83
    lip-lift technique, 82–84
    maxillary and mandibular casts, 93, 94
    noninvasive verification method, 94, 97
    optical scan, 88
    polyether impression material, 93
    postoperative radiograph, 93, 97

3-D planning concepts (*cont.*)
  post-trauma, 82
  preexisting bridge, 88, 89
  restorative planning, 91, 92
  right lateral incisor, 82–83
  segmentation, 86, 87
  selective transparency, 86, 94, 98
  soft tissue cast, 93, 94
  soft tissue sulcus, 92
  software tools, 88, 89
  sufficient bone volume, 84–86
  teeth and roots, 86, 87
  tension-free closure, 91
  tooth-borne template, 90
  transitional restorations, 92
  treatment planning software, 91, 92
Through-the-lens (TTL) flash, 159
Tissue biotype, 108, 109
Tissue engineering, 247–248
  bone morphogenetic proteins, 252–253
  platelet-derived growth factor, 252–253
  platelet-rich fibrin, 248–252
  platelet-rich plasma, 248–252
  stem cells, 253–256
Titanium, 43
Titanium abutment, 268, 269, 355, 363
  advantages and disadvantages, 379
  CAD/CAM, 377, 378
  gold hue, 379
  milling residue of, 359
  surface treatments for, 359
  use of, 377
Tooth extraction, 174, 288–289
Topical bovine thrombin (TBT), 248–249
Tunneling technique, 290

V

Vascularized interpositional periosteal connective tissue (VIP-CT) graft, 242
Vertical alveolar ridge defects
  allograft, 225
  anterior maxilla, 222–224
  autogenous bone graft, 221
  particulate grafting, 221
  patients with, 220
  single missing tooth span, 225, 227–229
  surgical procedures, 230
Vertical interdental bone loss, 292–293
VIP-CT graft. *See* Vascularized interpositional periosteal connective tissue (VIP-CT) graft
Vital structures, identification, 68

W

Wall defects, 204
Wax-up
  dental implants, esthetic therapy, 13
  treatment planning, 120, 121, 262–264, 329, 370, 371, 384, 386
White aesthetic score (WES), 288
White balance (WB), 161
  advantages, 162
  bit depth, 162
  catalog backup, 166
  color space and management, 163–164
  DAM, 164
  develop module, 166
  digital workflow, 165–166
  dilemma, 164–165
  disadvantages, 162
  exposure modes, 161–162
  image formats, 162
  intra oral camera setting, 163
  lightroom, 165
  output, 166, 167
  RAW, 162
White ceramics, 429
Wound healing, 37

X

Xenograft, 206, 209

Z

Zero Abutment Change (ZAC) protocol, 347–350
Zirconia
  abutment, 268, 269, 353, 355, 360
    advantages and disadvantages, 379
    in anterior aesthetic zone, 354
    CAD/CAM, 377–379
    coloration, 358, 379
    in green stage, 436
    milling residue, 359
    positive and negative characteristics of, 356
    restorations, 384, 385
    SEM images of fractured, 363
    white, 379
    with zircobond crowns, 360, 361
  clinical considerations, 384–385
  dental, 385–386
  lithium disilicate and, 432–434
  monolithic, 386, 398, 432–435
  qualifying differentiators, 434–437
  restorative workflow, 384, 386–391
    full arch, anterior facial veneers, 395–398
    full-arch, monolithic and pink gingivae, 398–401
    multi-tooth, facial veneered and pink gingivae, 388–389
    multi-tooth, facial veneered and pink papillae, 390–391
    multi-tooth, facial veneers, 391–393
    single tooth, facial veneers, 388
  technology, 385–391